WEBSTER'S
MEDICAL
SECRETARIES
HANDBOOK

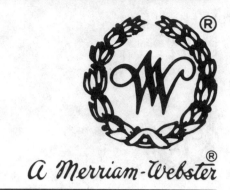

A Merriam-Webster ®

WEBSTER'S MEDICAL SECRETARIES HANDBOOK

JOHN RHODES HAVERTY, MD, FAAP • Consulting Editor

Merriam-Webster Inc., Publishers
Springfield, Massachusetts 01102

A GENUINE MERRIAM-WEBSTER

The name *Webster* alone is no guarantee of excellence. It is used by a number of publishers and may serve mainly to mislead an unwary buyer.

A *Merriam-Webster*® is the registered trademark you should look for when you consider the purchase of dictionaries and other fine reference books. It carries the reputation of a company that has been publishing since 1831 and is your assurance of quality and authority.

Library of Congress Cataloging in Publication Data
Main entry under title:

Webster's Medical secretaries handbook.

    Previously published as: Webster's Medical
office handbook. c1979.
    Bibliography: p.
    Includes index.
    1. Medical secretaries—Handbooks, manuals, etc.
2. Medical offices—Management—Handbooks, manuals,
etc. I. Haverty, John Rhodes, 1926–
II. Title: Medical secretaries handbook.   [DNLM:
1. Medical secretaries—Handbooks. W 80 W382]
R728.8.W43   651'.961   81-9521
ISBN 0-87779-135-X   AACR2

Printed and bound in the United States of America

6789RRD919089

Design/Carolyn McHenry
Illustrations/Charlotte A. Bridgeman; Julie A. Collier
Index/Eva Weber

CONTRIBUTORS

ANNE H. SOUKHANOV
General Editor
Merriam-Webster Incorporated

SUSAN E. ABBE, RN, MS
Instructor, Ona M. Wilcox School of Nursing
Middlesex Memorial Hospital (CT)

LORENE EULER BERMAN, CMA-AC
Administrative Assistant
Los Angeles County Medical Association

AILEEN J. BLACK, RRA
Director, Medical Records Department
Medical University Hospital
Medical University of South Carolina

KEITH D. BLAYNEY, PhD
Dean, School of Public and Allied Health
University of Alabama in Birmingham

HELEN G. BURZYNSKI, RN, MA
Chairman, Allied Health Sciences
Springfield (MA) Technical Community
College

RITA M. FINNEGAN, RRA, MA
Director, Curriculum in Medical Record
Administration
University of Illinois
at the Medical Center

J. F. FOLLMANN, JR.
Vice President (Retired)
Health Insurance Association of America

CHARLES WILLARD FORD, PhD
Associate Dean (Acting)
School of Health Related Professions
State University of New York at Buffalo

JOHN RHODES HAVERTY, MD, FAAP
Dean, College of Allied Health Sciences
Georgia State University

JOSEPH M. HEALEY, JD
Assistant Professor (Law)
University of Connecticut Medical School

MELVIN MORGENSTEIN, EdD
Professor of Accounting and Business
Administration
Nassau (NY) Community College

SUSAN A. ORLOWSKI, RN, BSN,
CMA-C
Coordinator, Medical Assisting
Edmonds (WA) Community College

DONALD D. SCRIVEN, PhD
Professor, Information Systems
Northern Illinois University

JOLENE D. SCRIVEN, EdD
Assistant Professor, Business Education
and Administrative Systems
Northern Illinois University

TABLE OF CONTENTS

MEDICAL OFFICE FINANCIAL MANAGEMENT

WRITTEN COMMUNICATION IN THE MEDICAL OFFICE

ACKNOWLEDGMENTS

The individuals and groups listed alphabetically below gave valuable assistance during the development and production of this book, and to them we express our gratitude:

Joseph I. Bernstein, MD, FAPA
Springfield, MA

Alfred H. Carter, MD
Springfield, MA

Mildred S. Cash, RRA
Director, Medical Record Administration Program
Medical University of South Carolina

Yolande Croteau, MA
Assistant Professor/Business Administration
Springfield (MA) Technical Community College

Susan S. Croy
Editor
The Professional Medical Assistant

Polly A. Fitz, RD, MA
Dean, School of Allied Health Professions
University of Connecticut

John J. Godfrey, MBA
Associate Professor
Business Administration
Springfield (MA) Technical Community College

Hampshire Obstetrical & Gynecological Associates, Inc.
Northampton, MA

Ernst R. Jaffé, MD
Professor of Medicine
Head, Division of Hematology
Albert Einstein College of Medicine of Yeshiva University

John C. Robinson, MD
Chief Medical Director
The Travelers Insurance Company

Robert M. Rodgers, JD
Assistant Professor
Springfield (MA) Technical Community College

Judith Weilerstein, RRA, MPH
Director, Medical Record Administration Program
Northeastern University

PREFACE

The book that you are reading is a product of Merriam-Webster Inc., publisher of the Merriam-Webster® dictionaries and reference books. As such, *Webster's Medical Secretaries Handbook* is also the result of Merriam's collaboration with 15 specialists in the fields of medicine, law, nursing, medical record administration, health insurance, business administration, data processing, and of course medical assisting. The combined experience and technical expertise of these specialists have produced the 18 chapters in the book.

Direction and scope *Webster's Medical Secretaries Handbook* is directed to medical secretaries and medical assistants/administrative who are employed or expect to be employed in single- or multi-physician practices. For this reason, the book concerns itself mainly with the administrative procedures, tasks, and responsibilities that these persons are expected to carry out. All major nonclinical functions are given here in a detailed manner that could not have been achieved had clinical tasks also been delineated. Some of the very important topics of interest to practicing medical assistants and secretaries are these: appointment scheduling, telephone techniques, staff and patient interaction, supply and task organization, medical record administration, accounting/billing/collection procedures, and routines for insurance claims processing. Assistants and secretaries employed by dentists will want to examine the appointments illustrations in Chapter 8 and especially the illustrated guidelines for the completion of attending dentists' statements in Chapter 10.

Medical secretaries, medical transcriptionists, and typists employed by the larger health care and allied health organizations such as clinics, hospitals, foundations, medical schools, HMOs, insurance-company medical claims departments, medical publishers, research organizations, and medical/pharmaceutical product manufacturers will also find the book very useful. These readers will be particularly interested in the material devoted to medical English, manuscript format, correspondence typing, dictation/transcription systems and techniques, and office copying equipment.

In addition, the book is directed to those readers enrolled in programs for medical secretaries and assistants and to those considering reentry into the profession. Chapter 1 introduces the reader to the educational and skill requirements and the career opportunities now prevalent in medical assisting. Chapter 2 takes the reader through every major step in the preemployment process. The proper ways of presenting oneself to a prospective employer by telephone, by letter, by résumé, and in person are explained. Sample interviews are given, accompanied by guidelines for the applicant. *Webster's Medical Secretaries Handbook* is a useful reference source not only for students but also for instructors who are preparing curricula, course outlines, and lectures in medical assisting.

It is equally important to mention the material in this book that is of interest to physicians themselves: the material in Chapter 2 regarding the writing and placement of employment ads and the proper ways to conduct interviews with applicants; the discussions of medical law, medical ethics, and bioethics in Chapters 3 and 4; the data on professional liability insurance in Chapter 10; the guidelines in Chapter 14 for improving one's dictation techniques; the section of Chapter 16 devoted to medical journal article manuscripts; another section of the same chapter where the correct ways of setting up the physician's curriculum vitae, list of publications, and invited presentations are given; and the detailed discussion of medical English in Chapter 17.

Textual organization Each chapter is introduced by its own table of contents listing in numerical order all of its major sections. In turn, the subsections of the chapters are introduced by highly visible boldface subheadings that alert the reader to the particular topics under discussion. When specific data are sought, one need only consult the detailed Index which will guide one quickly to the desired information. Furthermore, the text is copiously illustrated with drawings, diagrams, charts, tables, facsimiles, and lists that offer abundant information in a concise, readable form.

Special features   This book is committed to a realistic, detailed presentation of the administrative functions performed in the physician's office. It takes into account all of the realities that face its readers from day to day: scheduling problems, unexpected disruptions in appointment bookings, problematic patients, time-consuming insurance paperwork, collection problems, problems of physical storage space in medical record management, supply inventory and organization problems, and transcription problems—to name only a few. The book provides tested, workable problem-solving tips and procedures tailored to the single-physician practice and to the group practice as well. A prime example of its realistic guidance is the discussion in Chapter 6 of special problems with patients who are overly emotional or difficult. The chapter does not gloss over this touchy subject; instead, it gives specific, practical, and understandable advice as to the management of such patients. The section was written in consultation with two practicing psychiatrists.

Chapter 10, "Insurance," merits special attention. Coauthored by a health insurance executive and an experienced medical assistant, this ten-part chapter first surveys private and government health insurance plans and then provides concrete guidance for expediting insurance claims. It also offers simple yet complete answers to the questions about insurance that are most often asked by patients.

Accurate and coherent written communication continues to be vitally important to physicians due to the wealth of research being carried on, the vast numbers of patients being treated, and the acute competition among physicians and researchers to publish their findings. For this reason, over 100 pages have been devoted to medical writing, grammar, and the development and styling of medical journal article manuscripts. Chapter 17 contains, for example, charts listing many rules for the use of capitalization, italics, numerals, and punctuation in medical and scientific communications. Each rule is exemplified by at least one verbal illustration. Many of the illustrations are short quotations from a broad spectrum of American medical journals. These quotations are part of the Merriam-Webster file of over 12 million printed citations showing word usage. Similarly, the illustrations of manuscript format in Chapter 16 are examples of published medical journal manuscripts. The suggestions regarding the setup of manuscripts are based on interviews with a dozen medical journal editors.

A physician's practice can run smoothly only insofar as the staff members accept and carry out all assigned tasks competently and with minimal supervision. *Webster's Medical Secretaries Handbook* has been written to help you accomplish this goal.

Editorial credits   *Webster's Medical Secretaries Handbook,* like other Merriam-Webster® publications, represents a collective effort. It would therefore be ungracious and unfair not to recognize those Merriam staff members who have contributed greatly to the value of the book. Dr. Mairé Weir Kay and Dr. Frederick C. Mish, Joint Editorial Directors, gave valuable guidance throughout the project. Claire O. Cody, Secretary to the President, and Helene A. Gingold, Editorial Department Secretary, prepared the typewritten facsimiles. The manuscript was typed by Frances W. Muldrew and Barbara Quimby under the direction of Gloria J. Afflitto and Evelyn G. Summers (retired).

1

CHAPTER ONE

CAREER-PATH DEVELOPMENT

CONTENTS

1.1

MODERN HEALTH CARE: New Opportunities for the Medical Assistant/Administrative

INTRODUCTION

If you would ask which health occupation is most critically lacking in qualified personnel, the unequivocal answer would be Medical Assisting, and particularly the segment of it that offers the Medical Assistant/Administrative a broad spectrum of positions. Whether you are a student, a currently employed assistant, or a person considering reentry into the field, you are indeed fortunate because the opportunities for growth and development in the American health care system are unlimited. If you are educationally and professionally qualified, you should be able to find a wide variety of positions with ease. This situation shows no signs of reversal in the near future.

A number of factors have contributed to the increased employment opportunities for medical assistants. A key factor is this: The number of graduates from American medical schools has more than doubled in the last 10 years, thus doubling the number of practicing physicians requiring office staffs. In addition, the vastly increased public concern about quality health care has made more administrative inroads on physicians' time. American doctors are now confronted with a tremendous amount of paperwork emanating from various organizations (such as fiscal intermediaries and government regulatory agencies). In fact, the volume of this paperwork has recently quadrupled. As a logical result, most doctors must now rely more and more on their medical assistants to perform administrative tasks under a minimum of supervision. These two important developments affecting the knowledge and skills required in today's medical office practice underlie the renewed public recognition of the true importance of the medical assisting profession. It is with these and other such facts in mind that this chapter and indeed the entire book have been written.

EMPLOYMENT OPPORTUNITIES

Well over four million persons are employed in health service and related fields with the number of jobs growing rapidly. Administrators of health facilities, physicians, and other employers are constantly looking for workers because of the growing demand for health care and because of heavy labor turnover. Health service is one of the largest industries in the United States. Career opportunities are excellent.

In making a decision about where to seek employment, the medical assistant should decide initially whether he or she wishes to work directly for a physician or for a group of physicians; or whether other medical organizations such as hospitals, pharmaceutical companies, or insurance-company medical claims departments are preferable. The following material has been developed within these general classifications.

PHYSICIANS' OFFICE PRACTICES

Single practitioners Employees of a single practitioner are expected to perform many different duties. Generally, there are at least two employees in most offices, with their duties divided into administrative and clinical. However, a medical assistant responsible for administrative duties is often expected to perform some clinical tasks (such as taking temperatures and blood pressures, and giving injections).

Group practices The term *group practice* refers to an association of two or more physicians. These practices may be single specialty or multispecialty. In contrast to employment opportunities with single practitioners, the medical assisting positions in group practices are often more clearly defined. For example, a group practice may have on its staff a receptionist, a bookkeeper, a medical secretary, a nurse, and one or more laboratory and X-ray technicians. A very large office may also have a business manager.

A group practice encompassing a single specialty is generally formed so that two or more physicians in one specialty can share office expenses and an on-call schedule. Since only one specialty is involved, the employees are familiar with the basic tasks to be performed for each physician. Multispecialty group practices permit the concentration of several medical specialties within one locality. Since a medical assistant employed in a multispecialty practice is usually assigned to one specialist physician, each assistant in turn has specialized duties and the easy interchange of duties and responsibilities of the single-specialty group practice is seldom possible.

PHYSICIAN SPECIALTIES AND MEDICAL ASSISTING DUTIES

The following outline shows the 22 medical specialties recognized by the American Medical Association. Subspecialties as noted in the *Directory of Medical Specialties* are given where applicable.

Allergy and Immunology

Anesthesiology

Colon and Rectal Surgery

Dermatology

Family Practice

Internal Medicine
  Cardiovascular Disease
  Endocrinology and Metabolism
  Gastroenterology and Medical Oncology
  Hematology
  Infectious Disease and Nephrology
  Pulmonary Disease and Rheumatology

Neurological Surgery

Nuclear Medicine

Obstetrics and Gynecology

Ophthalmology

Orthopaedic Surgery

Otolaryngology

Pathology
  Dermatopathology

Pediatrics
  Pediatric Allergy
  Pediatric Cardiology
  Pediatric Hematology-Oncology
  Neonatal-Perinatal Medicine
  Nephrology

Physical Medicine and Rehabilitation
Plastic Surgery
Preventive Medicine
   Aerospace Medicine
   Occupational Medicine
   General Preventive Medicine
   Public Health

Psychiatry and Neurology
Radiology
Surgery
Thoracic Surgery
Urology

It is important to say at the outset that many of the subspecialties shown above are often *practiced* as separate medical specialties. Examples of these are Gastroenterology and Cardiovascular Disease (Cardiology). The reason for this is the extensiveness of the subspecialties themselves. Another important point is that surgery per se can be thought of not so much as a specialty but rather as a particular *function* of medical practice. Most doctors can and do perform some kinds of surgery (for example, some busy family practitioners may perform numerous tonsillectomies and appendectomies) as part of their overall practice of medicine. On the other hand, many physicians' practices consist of nothing but surgery. And some surgeons' practices are limited to specific *kinds* of surgery, such as heart surgery, thoracic surgery, plastic surgery, orthopaedic surgery, neurological surgery, abdominal surgery, colon and rectal surgery, urinary surgery, and pelvic surgery. These highly specialized types of surgery may or may not be classified as "official" specialties or subspecialties.

The following paragraphs outline specific administrative duties expected of medical assistants employed by physician-specialists in some of the above disciplines and subdisciplines. The duties given within the highlighted fields are examples only, and as such merely represent a small segment of appropriate responsibilities which can and do vary from physician to physician, and from specialty to specialty. In the upcoming discussion, the specialties and/or subspecialties are treated not in alphabetical order as shown in the detailed outline above. Rather, they are listed one after another in related groupings (as Allergy, Dermatology, and Endocrinology) or they are grouped together under one main heading (as the various types of surgery under the one sidehead **Surgery**). The criteria for grouping these specialties in this way are the administrative responsibilities of the medical assistants working therein. Since the problem of space in a book of this size precludes in-depth discussion of all medical specialties and subspecialties, only the ones requiring particularly unusual or highly developed administrative skills on the part of the assistants have been discussed at any length. Some specialties (as Anesthesiology and Pathology) whose practitioners rarely have individual offices outside a hospital or other institutional setting have not been discussed at all.

Allergy and Immunology   Allergy is concerned with the study, diagnosis, and treatment of human allergies. Immunology is concerned with the phenomena and causes of immunity. Together, these two fields comprise one of the major specialties. If working for an allergist, the assistant has to help the physician obtain complete, detailed patient histories that will assist the doctor in making diagnoses and in prescribing treatments for the particular allergic conditions of the patients. Thus, the assistant must be an excellent transcriptionist and typist, and must also be at ease with patients who are often nervous, generally upset, or ill. The assistant also needs to handle numerous referrals a good part of the time, since most of the physician's patients are referred to him or her by other doctors. Because some tests in this specialty require varying lengths of time and often require that the patients being tested remain in the office for observation afterwards, the assistant must understand the nature and the time requirements of the tests so as to be able to schedule appointments efficiently.

Dermatology   Dermatology is a branch of medicine dealing with the skin, its structure, functions, and diseases. An assistant working for a dermatologist performs much the same tasks as outlined above in Allergy and Immunology. Being a good transcriptionist is especially important in the accurate transcribing and typewriting of the medical histories so essential to specialists in this field. In addition, the assistant has to be a very careful record administrator: this specialty is a high-risk one. Consequently, meticulous and immaculate records must be kept in case litigation occurs. Finally, the assistant must be a person who is not easily upset by the more unpleasant symptoms of some skin disorders. And most importantly, the assistant in this field must not make an already embarrassed patient feel unduly worse because of his or her condition. Tact, diplomacy, and human kindness are essential for staff members in Dermatology.

Endocrinology   Endocrinology is the science dealing mainly with the endocrine (or ductless) glands of the human body. Endocrinology is not a board-certified specialty; it, together with Metabolism, is considered a subspecialty of Internal Medicine. However, it is often practiced as a separate discipline just as Gastroenterology is, for example. Endocrinologists, like dermatologists and allergists, often have patients with especially sensitive and also intimate problems. As such, these physicians require medical assistants whose abilities and attributes must include accuracy in record-keeping, diplomacy, a high degree of trustworthiness, and perhaps even some training in psychology and human relations. For these reasons, the discipline is given special coverage here.

   Some of the patient problems treated by endocrinologists include: obesity, sterility, diseases of the thyroid and adrenal glands, diabetes, and certain menopausal conditions. Since many tests often must be administered, the assistant has to be able to schedule appointment blocks accordingly. Furthermore, since many different kinds of injections and other medications are used in patient treatment, the assistant has to be an excellent supply logistician: medications can never be allowed to run out or to exceed their shelf lives. Just as assistants working in Allergy and Immunology and in Dermatology have to remain unaffected by the sight of patients suffering from diseases having unpleasant symptoms and effects, so must the assistant in Endocrinology be levelheaded and calm. In this type of practice, confidentiality cannot be overstressed. The assistant has to be trusted not to release any information about any patient without the physcian's *written* permission.

Psychiatry and Neurology   Psychiatry is a branch of medicine whose practitioners study, diagnose, treat, and attempt to prevent mental, emotional, and behavioral disorders. Neurology is a branch of medicine that includes the study, diagnosis, and treatment of disorders of the human nervous system. Thus, a psychiatrist is concerned primarily with functional disorders, while a neurologist is concerned primarily with organic disorders. However, assistants working for either of these two specialists have to exercise the same care and restraint in dealings with the physician's patients. Of course, confidentiality and the ability to guard patient information is paramount, as pointed out in the preceding paragraphs. Scheduling patients so that they will not see each other is still another important task (in fact, a great many psychiatrists' offices have separate entrances and exits for this reason). Keeping a vigilant eye on physical office security with respect to the location and storage of patient records and controlled medications is also a requisite. Being able to transcribe and typewrite sometimes lengthy case histories, reports, clinical résumés, and referral correspondence is yet another administrative function. An ability to remain calm and supportive in the face of upset patients sometimes exhibiting bizarre symptoms is also very important. To this end, a course or two in psychology and human relations would be advantageous. Being able to screen telephone calls from disturbed patients is yet another task that the effective assistant must be able to handle without having to put every call through to the doctor or without having to consult the doctor about every call. A genuine liking for people and a feeling of empathy for their problems is essential.

Since most of the patients a neurologist sees suffer from disorders adversely affecting their motor control, the assistant also must be prepared to help the patients into and out of the office, into and out of the examining rooms, and before and after their examinations and treatments. Additionally, the assistant must be able to recognize the symptoms of epileptic seizures, and must be able to give aid to the victims of these seizures, if necessary.

Obstetrics and Gynecology Obstetricians specialize in the care of pregnant women, while gynecologists specialize in the study, diagnosis, and treatment of diseases of women. Most physicians in the field practice both disciplines. Medical assistants in OB/GYN practices—and especially the assistants employed by the large group practices—must be superb managers and organizers. Schedules can be set up only to be obliterated at a moment's notice by births requiring the physician(s) to be at hospitals rather than in their offices during regular hours. Appointments have to be grouped according to the various needs of the patients, too. For instance, it is especially important for the assistant to understand the reasons for all patient visits so that the expectant mothers can be seen on particular days, the patients with gynecological problems can be seen at other times, and the patients simply coming in for physical examinations can be seen at still other times. A good disposition and an easy, cheerful, but highly professional manner is also essential in reducing potential embarrassment among patients before and during examinations. Medical assistants in OB/GYN practices may be asked to explain gynecological procedures to patients; to be present during physician examinations (although a clinical assistant or a nurse is usually the one to do this); and to instruct maternity patients regarding diets, medication, weight control, planning for the delivery process, and subsequent events such as nursing. The assistant also has to arrange for upcoming patient hospitalization and has to transmit patient records to hospitals prior to deliveries or operations. In addition, a good deal of the assistant's time may be spent in typewriting case histories, postpartum reports, and referral correspondence.

Pediatrics Pediatrics is a branch of medicine concerned with the development, care, and diseases of children. The patient population in a pediatrician's office ranges from the infant to the school-age child. In order to be an effective assistant in a pediatrician's office, the individual must be able to: (1) deal calmly with and relate well to infants, toddlers, preschoolers, school-age children, *and* their parents (2) schedule appointments sensibly so that children of approximately the same age groups will be in the office at the same time if at all possible (3) organize (and separate, if necessary) the waiting patients so that the contagious ones won't contaminate the well ones (4) fit emergency patients into packed schedules without too much disruption (5) reschedule appointments more often than is the case in other offices due to unexpected situations (6) work calmly in an often noisy environment, and (7) be able to converse calmly on the telephone to the often distraught parents of ill children (this also includes being able to screen calls well and to take a multitude of messages accurately). And most of all, a genuine liking for children is essential.

Surgery Surgery involves structural alterations of part of the body for health or cosmetic reasons by means of manual or operative techniques. As already mentioned in the introductory paragraphs to this section, the types of surgery practiced today are varied and highly specialized. Although the assistant's duties vary according to the kind and size of the office and according to the nature of the practice, it can be generalized that the assistant to a surgeon spends much time scheduling operations and procedures in the office and at hospitals. Hospital scheduling and admitting procedures must be familiar to the assistant. The assistant must know the surgeon's preference as to operating rooms, staff, and scheduled operating hours. Assistants working in specialist surgical offices must also exercise special skills as required. For example, in a plastic surgeon's office, the assistant may have to explain procedures to patients about to undergo treatments. Assistants working for orthopaedic surgeons must be willing and able to help physically disabled patients enter, move around in, and exit the office. Such patients have to be assisted before and after treatments and examinations. Since many orthopaedists see infants and children, the assistant has to be able to get along with these patients, too.

Surgical patients have to be scheduled according to the physician's preferences, which usually means that presurgical patients are seen at certain times, postsurgical patients are seen for dressing changes and follow-ups at other times, and so on. Excellent appointment organization is thus essential.

Assistants employed by surgeons also have to have excellent dictation, transcription, and typewriting rates, for they have to transcribe and typewrite lengthy case histories, clinical résumés, and pre- and postoperative reports.

Cardiovascular Disease (Cardiology) Cardiology has to do with the study of the heart and its actions and the diagnosis and treatment of its diseases. While Cardiovascular Disease is a subspecialty of Internal Medicine or of Pediatrics, it is often practiced as a specialty. Cardiologists specialize in the diagnosis of medical and surgical heart disease, and also in the medical treatment of all conditions related to the cardiovascular system. The assistant employed by a cardiologist deals mostly with referrals from other doctors. Thus, the assistant has to be an effective liaison between the referring physician and the specialist. One particularly important aspect of the assistant's position with a cardiologist is the fact that cardiac patients are often quite nervous about their conditions. As a result, they can be irritable or highly upset. They also may wish to discuss their symptoms at length with whoever is close at hand. Therefore, the assistant must exercise extreme tact and gentleness in dealing with these patients.

Ophthalmology Ophthalmology is a specialist branch of medicine concerned with the structure, functions, and diseases of the eye. Since the physician uses highly complex diagnostic equipment in such a practice, one of the assistant's prime responsibilities is to be sure that all of the devices are in good working order at all times. The assistant also has to be able to interact well with totally or partially blind patients.

Otolaryngology Otolaryngology is a branch of medicine specializing in the study, diagnosis, and treatment of diseases of the ear, nose, and throat. Since most of the patient population is referred, the assistant has to converse with referring physicians and has to typewrite communications from the specialist to the referring physicians. The assistant also may be responsible for the cleaning and maintenance of equipment and the sterilization of quite a few instruments, if required to do so by the employer. The ability to communicate with deaf or with partially deaf patients is also a useful skill in this profession.

Radiology Radiology is a specialty that concerns itself with the study, diagnosis, and the treatment of disease through the use of radioactive substances (as X rays and radium). The assistant working for a radiologist also is faced with a patient load comprised mostly of referrals. The assistant must be an excellent stenographer, transcriptionist, and typist whose medical vocabulary is quite sound, for the number and length of medical reports and opinions in this specialty are great.

Family Practice   The family practitioner's patient population is generally large and varied as to age and medical problems. Hence, the doctor's responsibilities are broad-based. Because of the numerous medical problems of the patients, the assistant working for a family practitioner must be an excellent organizer both of office routines and of appointments. The assistant must be able to improvise and reorganize schedules when required to do so because of unexpected absences on the part of the doctor. The assistant also has to be an expert at public relations. Since the family practice receives numerous telephone calls, the assistant has to know how to screen, transfer, and/or answer the calls appropriately. The insurance paperwork in such a practice is usually very heavy; thus, the assistant must be an efficient and knowledgeable insurance clerk as well. And finally, the bookkeeping, billing, and collection tasks are unusually time-consuming, especially in large practices.

Internal Medicine   Internal Medicine is concerned with the diagnosis and treatment of usually complex nonsurgical diseases. While internists are in essence consultants or "consulting diagnosticians," most of them also maintain substantial general practices. Therefore, the duties of an assistant working for an internist are just as varied if not more so than those of an assistant working for a family practitioner: the assistant handles referrals, makes appointments for many different kinds of patients with various medical problems, schedules diagnostic tests, processes heavy loads of insurance paperwork, fields numerous telephone calls, transcribes and types rapidly and accurately, and functions as an efficient bookkeeper.

Summary   As you can see from the foregoing material, the practice of medicine can be both broadly based and narrowly restricted, depending on the specialty. The Medical Assistant/Administrative's task orientation depends directly on the nature of the particular physician's practice: thus, an assistant working in Internal Medicine or Family Practice has a broad spectrum of administrative responsibilities as opposed to one employed in a practice restricted to one specialty or to a single subspecialty.

INSTITUTIONAL EMPLOYMENT OPPORTUNITIES FOR MEDICAL ASSISTANTS

Clinics   A clinic is an outpatient facility for the diagnosis and treatment of diseases. Clinics can be part of federal, state, or local government organizations; or they can be part of nonprofit or proprietary organizations. Medical assistants employed at clinics perform any of the general administrative or clinical tasks done in physicians' offices. In addition, medical assistants working in clinics can supervise other employees if their job descriptions call for it.

Hospitals   A hospital is a facility for the diagnosis and treatment of inpatients. A hospital can be owned by the federal government or by a state or local government, or it can be owned by a nonprofit or a proprietary organization. Medical assistants working in hospitals may function as transcriptionists, medical record specialists, laboratory technicians, X-ray technicians, secretaries, or administrative supervisors.

Medical schools   A medical school is a facility for the training of physicians. Medical assistants employed by medical schools generally are involved in the administrative details of the school's operation; however, depending on the interests of the physicians for whom they work, they also may be involved in some clinical research.

Foundations These institutions are generally associated with research activities. They may be funded through private and/or public donations. Medical assistants employed by foundations can perform either secretarial or supervisory functions.

Nursing homes Nursing homes are facilities other than hospitals and boarding homes that provide maintenance and personal or nursing care for people who are unable to care for themselves and who have health problems requiring long-term care. Nursing homes are classified as *skilled, intermediate care,* and *extended care.* Medical assistants employed by nursing homes perform varied tasks similar to those described under *hospitals.*

Department of Health, Education and Welfare (HEW) This is a federal government department encompassing many federally sponsored health programs. Opportunities exist in HEW for medical assistants in all administrative aspects of health care, health policy development and implementation, and medical writing.

The Social Security Administration The Social Security Administration is the administrative arm of HEW managing the federal Social Security program. One example of the program is Medicare. Employment opportunities are available on the national level and on the local level for the administration of these programs.

Pharmaceutical and chemical companies These companies are responsible for the development and distribution of drugs and chemicals within the health field. Medical assistants employed by them can perform secretarial duties, can assist in research programs, and can perform laboratory functions.

Drug/surgical/hospital supply houses These are the local companies from which physicians, clinics, and hospitals obtain their supplies. Employment opportunities therein include positions for secretaries, inventory clerks, buyers, and bookkeepers.

Biomedical engineering and research firms Companies in this field develop the equipment needed to perform research concerning animal and human biology. It is a new field offering varied employment opportunities from secretarial positions to technical positions.

Insurance-company medical claims departments Special branches of insurance companies review medical claims made by policyholders. Most private insurance companies have medical claims departments; however, the largest health insurance company in the United States is Blue Cross, Blue Shield. Employment opportunities in such organizations include secretarial, medical record auditing, and supervisory positions.

Medical publishers Many privately owned companies publish health-related materials. Positions available include secretarial, writing, manuscript review, and proofreading jobs.

1.2

JOB DESCRIPTIONS

Medical assisting is an emerging career. It is a broad-based occupation including duties carried on by receptionists, secretaries, clinical attendants, and, at times laboratory personnel. Medical assisting is now the second largest health profession in the United States—second only to nursing. The American Association of Medical Assistants, Inc. (AAMA), estimates that between 300,000 and 400,000 medical assistants work under the direction of physicians in various medical facilities across the United States. The job requirements of the medical assistant vary according to the employment setting. Sometimes, an assistant in a small office carries the total responsibility for all clinical and clerical support services to the physician; at other times, several medical assistants in a large office are each assigned specific areas of responsibility. In all cases, however, the assistant is supervised by a physician and performs tasks as required by the physician and in accordance with state laws.

When performing clinical duties, medical assistants are often called on to sterilize instruments and check diagnostic equipment for good working order. They may prepare patients for examination or treatment, take temperatures, measure height and weight, perform routine urinalyses or simple blood tests, or collect blood samples. They also may assist physicians during patient examinations, treatments, minor surgery, and emergencies. Giving information to patients about the preparations necessary for tests, X rays, and laboratory examinations is also an important aspect of the job.

Medical assistants perform a wide range of clerical duties which help to keep the office running smoothly. They answer telephones; greet patients and other callers; handle mail; record, correct, review, and file patient data and medical histories; and arrange for hospital admissions and laboratory services. Checking and ordering office and medical supplies and dealing with agents of pharmaceutical firms and other medical suppliers may be part of a day's work along with office record-keeping. In addition, the assistant may take, transcribe, and type dictation, as well as type correspondence and reports.

Accuracy, dependability, a courteous pleasant manner, patience, and a respect for the confidential nature of medical information are necessary traits for these workers, since they have a great deal of daily public contact (see also section 1.4). Considerable time is usually spent working at a desk, but clinical duties require the medical assistant to stand, kneel, and do moderate lifting when working with patients. The average work week is about 35 hours in length, but the hours may be irregular, depending on the individual physician's schedule and the patient load.

Medical assistants specializing in pediatrics work in the area of child-health care under the supervision of pediatricians. Some medical assistants may choose to specialize in the field of ophthalmology. These assistants are trained to gather patient histories related to eye problems following a prescribed format, and they learn how to perform certain eye-function measurement testing under the supervision of ophthalmologists. As shown in section 1.1, still other medical assistants may work for physicians in other specialty areas and may receive additional on-the-job training.

DUTIES OF A MEDICAL ASSISTANT

An AAMA study of the duties of the medical assistant in the average medical office confirms that the medical assistant is one of the most versatile members of the allied health care team. The duties typically performed by medical assistants are listed below:

1. Effectively schedule appointments in person and by telephone.
2. Pull patients' files for the day's appointments.
3. Receive the patients.
4. Take and record a patient's statistical data and medical history at the request of the physician.
5. Prepare and drape patients for examinations.
6. Take blood pressures and temperatures and weigh the patients.

7. At the doctor's request and under his or her supervision:
   a. collect blood samples;
   b. take EKGs;
   c. perform diagnostic tests.
8. Assist the physician with patient examinations, treatment, and minor surgery.
9. Give certain medications and injections under the doctor's supervision.
10. Explain the nature of a particular examination, certain diagnostic tests and/or treatment to the patient at the doctor's request.
11. Know how to handle patients when the physician is away from the office.
12. Assist in the collection of specimens (such as Pap smears or throat cultures).
13. Set up patients' files, enter notes or make corrections on records, and review them for completeness and accuracy.
14. Review, separate, and purge medical record files as instructed.
15. Obtain the patients' signatures on forms granting the physician permission to release records, to operate, or to perform diagnostic procedures.
16. Arrange hospital admissions and/or laboratory and X-ray procedures as requested by the physician, and advise the patients accordingly.
17. Schedule surgery.
18. Prepare medical records from information provided by the physician.
19. Perform simple routine laboratory procedures (such as urinalysis or simple blood tests), and collect and prepare specimens for transportation to a laboratory.
20. Record and maintain laboratory, X-ray, and EKG data on patients' records.
21. Instruct the patients regarding the proper preparation for tests that have been ordered by the physician.
22. Prepare and replenish supplies in the doctor's bag so that it is in constant readiness.
23. Sterilize the instruments and maintain the diagnostic equipment in good working order.
24. Throw away contaminated and used disposable items.
25. Receive and organize the handling of medication samples.
26. Order office, laboratory, and medical supplies and maintain an inventory of all three.
27. Handle emergencies properly:
   a. know how to reach the physician;
   b. seek help from a qualified nurse or another physician when necessary;
   c. be able to describe to the doctor or the nurse the nature of a patient's illness or injury;
   d. put the patient in a safe and comfortable examining position when necessary;
   e. apply first aid if necessary;
   f. call a poison control center if this is indicated;
   g. arrange for use of hospital emergency room treatment if required;
   h. explain the doctor's unavailability to the rest of the patients in the reception room if required.
28. Perform the following telephone tasks:
   a. check with the answering service regularly and record all messages;
   b. make appointments;
   c. make calls for the physician;
   d. receive calls from patients, laboratories, other physicians, solicitors, and the doctor's family;
   e. answer a patient's questions concerning his or her illness and questions regarding the doctor's fees and hours;
   f. take laboratory reports.
29. Deal with pharmaceutical representatives, equipment manufacturers, other physicians, the doctor's family, and other visitors.
30. Be able to handle children accompanying patients.
31. Supervise maintenance people (cleaners and others) and see that the office is kept in a neat, attractive, and sanitary condition at all times.

32. Supervise other office staff members if the job description calls for it.
33. Handle correspondence:
    a. incoming mail
        (1) open, sort, and screen the mail in accord with the doctor's wishes;
        (2) flag important mail;
        (3) summarize articles and other materials as requested.
    b. outgoing mail
        (1) answer the doctor's routine mail if instructed to do so;
        (2) take medical dictation;
        (3) transcribe shorthand or machine dictation;
        (4) typewrite all correspondence, including medical reports to other physicians, insurance reports, and other kinds of reports.
34. File all correspondence and medical records, including X rays and EKGs.
35. Operate business machines and assume responsibility for their maintenance.
36. Perform the daily posting of charges and collections.
37. Prepare monthly statements.
38. Handle credit arrangements with patients.
39. Assist with follow-up collections.
40. Handle payments by cash and/or check and make out receipts.
41. Keep financial records (e.g., a daily record of charges and payments, records of accounts receivable, a trial balance, and monthly profit and loss sheets).
42. Prepare payroll and any necessary government forms (such as withholding, FICA, unemployment, and state disability forms).
43. Pay professional bills.
44. Assume all banking duties (such as making regular deposits and reconciling bank statements).
45. Prepare tax return information for the doctor's accountant.
46. Discuss and explain the doctor's fees to patients.
47. Accept, endorse, and record checks received for payment on account.
48. Establish and control the petty cash fund.
49. Discuss and explain insurance coverage to the patients.
50. Complete these insurance forms:
    a. indemnity insurance forms for a patient to submit a claim;
    b. forms for filing assigned insurance claims;
    c. Medicare payment request forms;
    d. Medicaid claim forms;
    e. Workers Compensation forms;
    f. Blue Shield payment request forms.
51. Review, and if necessary, appeal insurance disallowances to achieve satisfactory resolution.
52. Gather data to complete statutory reports for government agencies.
53. Arrange meetings, conferences and/or travel accommodations if asked to do so.
54. Attend meetings and participate in community activities related to the doctor's practice.

1.3

EDUCATION AND REQUIRED SKILLS

There are a number of ways to become a Medical Assistant/Administrative or a Medical Assistant/Clinical. A 1977 survey of members of the AAMA indicates that most medical assistants (52.8%) acquire their training on the job rather than by way of formal degree or certificate programs. This may change in the future as more and more people seek formal education and training, especially in the two-year college Medical Assisting and Business Practices programs. However, with three or more years of experience and a high school diploma or a high school equivalency certificate, practicing medical assistants can take the AAMA certification examination at a number of locations throughout the United States.

Another way to become a medical assistant is to go to school. Many junior and community colleges offer an Associate of Arts degree in Medical Assisting at the successful completion of two years of study. One-year courses also are available in vocational, technical, or privately owned schools which award certificates upon the successful completion of studies.

The basic content of both types of courses must include the following classroom and clinical areas of study: (1) anatomy and physiology (2) medical terminology (3) medical law and ethics (4) psychology (5) communications (6) administrative practices such as office procedures, correspondence, and typing (7) medical dictation and transcription (8) bookkeeping and insurance (9) clinical procedures including sterilization and examination room techniques, laboratory procedures, principles of pharmacology and drug administration, and diagnostic machine orientation, and (10) externship. Candidates for medical assisting programs must submit to the schools evidence of their good health including the results of a tuberculin-screening test or a chest X ray.

At the present time, no legal licensing, mandatory certification, or continuing education requirements apply to medical assistants. However, certification and/or registration is offered by two organizations upon the successful completion of examinations given to those who qualify. American Medical Technologists offer the RMA (Registered Medical Assistant) credential as well as opportunities for continuing education. The AAMA offers certification (Certified Medical Assistant) and, effective in 1980, a revalidation program for CMAs, as well as continuing education for all medical assistants. Persons who successfully pass the AAMA certification examination are entitled to use the CMA designation after their names. In addition to general certification, candidates may earn specialty certification in administrative (CMA-A) and clinical (CMA-C) categories. Those who hold both administrative and clinical certification may use the designation CMA-AC after their names. In addition, the AAMA has made available two types of special certification to persons who have completed training or have acquired knowledge in pediatrics and ophthalmology. Although certification has been offered to Pediatric Medical Assistants (CMA-P), this examination has been discontinued for the time being. Mechanisms for certifying other specialty medical assistants, as well as in pediatrics, are under study.

The credentials listed below are accompanied by the types of courses and training required of the candidate prior to taking the qualifying examination:

Certified Medical Assistant (CMA)
1. Anatomy and Physiology
2. Medical Terminology
3. Medical Law and Ethics
4. Psychology
5. Written and Oral Communication
6. Bookkeeping and Insurance
7. Administrative and Clinical Procedures

Certified Medical Assistant-Administrative (CMA-A)
1. Administrative Procedures
2. Written and Oral Communications
3. Insurance
4. Bookkeeping

Certified Medical Assistant-Clinical (CMA-C)
1. Anatomy and Physiology
2. Clinical Procedures
3. Laboratory Orientation

Ophthalmic Medical Assistant
1. Ocular Anatomy and Physiology
2. Practical Microbiology
3. Ocular Motility
4. Introduction to Diseases of the Eye

All medical assisting educational programs require an externship or practicum.

The skills required to be an effective medical secretary or Medical Assistant/ Administrative are constantly changing in the medical field due to innovations in health technology. Improvements in patient care technology include the development of new drugs, automated clinical laboratory equipment, improved surgical techniques including outpatient surgery, and the broad use of computers in diagnosing disease and in medical record-keeping.

Advances in information handling also stem from computerization. For example, computers are widely used for patient billing and accounting and for word processing. Computers can be used to improve the information flow so that physicians can get the data necessary for the rapid and accurate writing of orders. Thus the Medical Assistant/Administrative who has basic knowledge of computer applications is an even more valuable member of the health care team.

The adoption of disposable items (such as hypodermic needles and surgical gloves and knives) and the use of improved equipment (such as automated laboratory equipment and automatic typewriters) have resulted in improvements in hospital and physician services. The ultimate effect of this rapid technological expansion on the Medical Assistant/Administrative will be to require of the assistant a lifelong education process to assure that the necessary knowledge and technical skills are continuously maintained.

1.4

PERSONAL ASSETS INVENTORY FOR THE MEDICAL ASSISTANT/ADMINISTRATIVE

The importance of working well with the physician, other staff members, and patients cannot be overemphasized. In fact, an entire chapter in this book is devoted to the assistant's interactions with colleagues, visitors to the office, and employers (see Chapter 6, "Effective Interaction with Patients and Staff"). However, it is appropriate to give at the outset a list of some of the most important positive traits that a truly valuable and successful medical assistant should possess. As you read the following paragraphs, consider honestly the degree to which you possess each of these traits. Listed order is insignificant since all are important. As you think about each one, resolve to increase your strengths and decrease your weaknesses. This is *your* responsibility to the physician, to every person who enters the office, and to yourself.

Polite It's easy to be polite to nice people but it takes the skill of a professional to be gracious to one who is somewhat offensive. Politeness is remembering to praise in public and to reprimand or criticize constructively in private. Politeness can be construed as patronization if your voice inflection is not right. *Tact* and politeness go hand in hand.

Pleasant Using a genuine smile even if you do not feel much like smiling is important. Everyone has personal problems that can be unpleasant, but you should not bring those problems to the office. In short, do not entwine your professional and your personal life. Your ready smile when asked to do something difficult will be appreciated tremendously. A cheerful greeting in the morning to your physician and to your co-workers whom you meet is expected. Even if you do not get an answer, continue the practice. And a cordial "good night" as you leave is proper.

Friendly Be equally friendly to everyone in the office; do not have favorites and do not join cliques. Although you may have an especially good friend in your office, do not share confidential information with that person.

Fair   While you should take credit for your own work, you also should give credit to others for their ideas and their help with your work. In addition, you should mention to your physician the helpfulness of your co-workers and pass along to them any compliments or words of appreciation the physician shares with you about them.

Thoughtful   Opinions that others have are important. It's wise to remember that in any argument or discussion between you and another, there may be your side, his or her side, and "the right side." Thoughtfulness is closely linked with courtesy.

Cooperative   You and the physician or physicians must work together easily. The physician-employer is the most important person in your professional life. He or she is also a human being with traits and behavior that are not always perfect. When the doctor lets off steam and you are around to bear the brunt of the remarks, do not take the words personally and vow inwardly to get even or, worse, hold a grudge. Cooperation extends to working with others to get a job done even though some of the tasks you are asked to do are not "your job." It is always right to offer to help a fellow employee who is overloaded with work when you have time to assist unless you have been given specific instructions not to do so. When your employer asks you to perform a task that you consider to be of a personal nature or to run a personal errand, you should cooperate willingly because you realize that by taking care of these time-consuming details, you free up the doctor's time to practice better medicine.

Humble   Humility means being able to accept justified criticism well and to look at it objectively for what it is meant to be: a signal to you to help you increase your value to the physician and the practice. Humility also includes the ability to accept praise and compliments gracefully and with a genuine "thank you" as the response.

Tolerant and considerate   People differ in mental ability, interests, goals, personality and character, appearance, physical and mental health, and behavior. Consideration of these differences will make your office a more livable place for everyone. Patience, pity, sympathy, empathy, and kindness are traits of the tolerant and considerate person.

Loyal, discreet, and ethical   Dedication to the doctor and the practice is absolutely necessary. If you cannot be loyal to either, you should seriously consider finding another position. Confidential matters *must* remain so—not a hint may you give that you have privileged information that you cannot share. A loyal employee never criticizes the employer's policies to other persons. If you are loyal, you also are *proud* of your position, and you take pride in your employer. At all times you must re-member that as an agent of the physician, you and your actions reflect directly on the physician and the practice.

Sensitive   Sensitivity to those around you will develop on the job. You must be constantly aware, alert, and observant. You learn by trial and error and by experience what pleases and what displeases the doctor, when he or she wants to be interrupted and when he would rather be alone, when the doctor's actions speak louder than words, where the doctor prefers that you sit for dictation or consultation, and where and in what form the doctor likes finished work to be presented for review. You thus begin to anticipate the physician's requirements before you are directed to do something. You are sensitive to the likes and dislikes of your co-workers in the same manner. And you are sensitive to your own foibles, knowing that the tendency exists to look at the self through rose-colored glasses while severely criticizing others who have the same traits.

Courageous   You are not afraid to accept responsibility and you reach out for addi-tional duties that you know you can be responsible for. You give your opinions or ideas when you have sufficient background and experience to have formed a reliable opinion that can be backed up with facts and figures if necessary.

Honest   In your dealings with everyone, never lie. Honesty also extends to not appropriating office supplies for your personal use. As a *trustworthy* assistant, you admit your mistakes and neither make excuses for them nor shift the blame for them to others. You also can be depended on never to feed the office grapevine.

Self-controlled and calm   Self-control is a mark of maturity but not every mature individual is self-controlled! Self-discipline, the engaging of one's brain before putting one's mouth in motion, thinking of the consequences of one's words or acts before saying or doing them, keeping one's temper in check at all times, *never* resorting to tears in the office—these are the attributes of self-control. Calmness in dealing with problematic patients, emergencies, and overloaded schedules is essential in medical assisting. If you lose your cool, you can be fairly sure that those around you will too.

Flexible and adaptable   The ability to accept change *willingly* is of inestimable value. Changes in work surroundings, procedures, equipment, and staff structure may come quickly. A flexible and adaptable assistant accepts changes in a positive way and then does everything possible to see that the new arrangement works.

Diplomatic and observant of etiquette   If first names are customarily used in your office, you must remember to use courtesy titles and last names when visitors are present. Keep personal phone calls and personal visitors to a minimum. You should be careful neither to interrupt others' conversations nor to finish their sentences for them. You should not whistle, hum, chew gum, or mumble and talk to yourself at your desk. Do not smoke at your desk or elsewhere in the office unless the physician gives you permission to do so.

Well-groomed   The really professional medical assistant knows that in no other field is grooming so important as it is in medicine. Therefore, your appearance can be nothing short of immaculate at all times.

Punctual   Observe your office hours scrupulously. If you have permission to begin work at a later hour some day or take an extra-long lunch break or leave early, be sure to let others in your area know the reason. Morale deteriorates speedily when workers see their co-workers supposedly getting special privileges that they don't get. Punctuality also means getting work done when you've promised it; if this is not possible, you notify the physician sufficiently far in advance that his or her plans can be adjusted.

Physically strong and healthy   Overtime and rushed schedules can be commonplace in some medical offices; hence, the assistants working there must be strong enough to work efficiently and accurately under pressure for longer than normal hours. In any case, you cannot neglect your own health at any time; if you do, you will adversely affect your job performance, not to mention your own physical self.

Willing to train another to take your place   If you are inwardly secure in your job, you will see that someone else knows what you do and how you do it. This means training a co-worker or subordinate to take over when you must be absent, or when the opportunity for advancement comes to you. This foresightedness is advantageous to you because your work will not pile up while you are gone, and it is advantageous to the doctor.

Enthusiastic   Although you may score well on the other traits mentioned above, if you are not enthusiastic about what you do, about where you work, and about the possibilities for the future, you are like a cake without frosting—something superb is missing!

Responsible   Responsibility is *personal.* You are personally responsible for accomplishing the tasks assigned to you by the physician promptly and accurately. A valuable assistant is able to fulfill all responsibilities with a minimum of supervision from the doctor—especially in administrative matters. Concomitant with this responsibility is accountability. You are *always* accountable for everything that you have done.

1.5

UPWARD MOBILITY

Numerous opportunities via continuing education courses and/or self-programmed instruction can add impetus to your career and can help you to maintain its momentum. Members and certain non-members of the AAMA can participate in a wide variety of continuing education programs. A revalidation program for all Certified Medical Assistants is in effect as of 1980. This is a program requiring proof of continuing education through earned CEU credits. Also available for the career-minded medical assistant is the AAMA's *Guided Study Course in Anatomy, Terminology and Physiology* which is a workbook with tapes usable at home.

Allied health educators and employers are becoming increasingly aware of the need for generalist health care technicians. The proliferation of separate specialty areas in allied health during the last two decades has resulted in more than 200 separate careers in the field. While these careers do offer the opportunity for upward mobility in medical assisting, nevertheless, many of them are so specialized that the smaller employers have found it difficult to use these workers on a full-time basis. In an attempt to rectify the situation, some universities have developed training programs for multiple competency clinical technicians, or MCCTs.

These new allied health professionals receive more advanced training in radiological technology and basic laboratory functions than Certified Medical Assistants receive. The advanced training is based on a real and urgent need for competent technicians—a need that has been expressed by physicians in small, rural locations. The limited pool of trained allied health professionals available to smaller facilities requires that a generalist approach be taken to staff these facilities. The medical assistant who is interested in upward mobility may wish to consider additional training as a generalist technician.

The medical assistant who does develop an interest in more in-depth training in a specific area can choose from a wide variety of allied health careers. A few examples include: (1) clinical dietetics (2) cytotechnology (3) dental assisting (4) health data processing (5) histology (6) medical record administration (7) medical technology (8) nuclear medicine (9) occupational therapy (10) radiologic technology, and (11) respiratory therapy. The individual can also consider studying to become a Physician's Assistant.

In addition to any one of the above allied health careers, the medical assistant may seek training in nursing either as a Registered Nurse or as a Licensed Practical Nurse.

The broad general nature of the medical assisting position permits one to have a wide variety of career options and choices for future growth and development. It is fortunate that the American health care system provides these numerous opportunities for the medical assistant who desires a career with real growth opportunities.

2

CHAPTER TWO

JOB APPLICATIONS

CONTENTS

2.1 OBTAINING A POSITION
2.2 INTRODUCING YOURSELF TO A PROSPECTIVE EMPLOYER
2.3 INTERVIEWING AN APPLICANT YOURSELF

2.1

OBTAINING A POSITION

INTRODUCTION

Although there is no such thing as complete job security, we are often told that there is security in knowing how to go about finding a job. The various ways in which you can obtain a medical assisting position will differ according to (1) your educational background and the professional contacts you have made during your studies (2) your past or current on-the-job experience, and (3) the nature of your geographical area (is it a city? a suburb? a small town? a rural locale?). If, for example, you live in a small town or in the country where most of the inhabitants know each other, you will probably depend to a great extent on personal contacts with the local physicians. On the other hand, if you live in a city or in a large suburb, you will undoubtedly rely more often on medical and/or general employment agencies and on advertisements in your search for the right position. Obviously, the competition for jobs is more acute in heavily populated areas than it is in rural areas. However, this feature is offset by the greater variety of medical office positions available in urban areas where there are numerous types of health care facilities.

Starting your search for a job In seeking a position, it is always best to explore and evaluate every possible opportunity. Do not settle for the first offer that comes along unless you are absolutely *sure* that the job is right for you and that you are the right person for the job. Think of moving laterally as well as up the career ladder. Seriously consider starting at an entry level that offers a good opportunity for promotion. If you investigate the field thoroughly, you will see that many previously unthought-of opportunities are available to you. In this way, you will also be able to explore a large number of jobs with salary ranges wider than those of only one or two potential positions. Especially in situations where the competition for employment is stiff, you ought to investigate as many openings as you are qualified to fill, since you will thus increase the odds for landing one really excellent job. Remember: looking for a job in the right way takes time, energy, thoroughness, and organization. Visit places where you would like to work. For example, look at the roster of physicians on the board in the lobby of a medical building to see if, perhaps, you should investigate openings in some of these offices.

Sources of guidance and recommendation   If you are or have been enrolled in a medical assisting program, you can obtain guidance from the school counselors and/or from your instructors regarding potential jobs in your area and in other geographical areas where salary ranges are higher. If you are still a student, you ought to find out from your instructors or counselors when you should start looking for a position prior to graduation. The lead time will vary according to the size and the economic profile of your location.

You can ask your instructors if they would be willing to serve as references. Bear in mind that it is very important *not* to give a person's name as a reference to a prospective employer without first getting permission from that person. If you have been previously employed, you can also ask your former employer(s) to serve as reference(s). In some cases these individuals will write blanket "To whom it may concern" letters of introduction and recommendation that you can take with you in sealed envelopes to prospective employers; in other cases they will write directly to each prospective employer; and in still other cases they will expect the prospective employer to telephone them for a recommendation.

SOURCES OF EMPLOYMENT OPPORTUNITY INFORMATION
County medical societies   Whether you are new to a particular area or whether you have been a long-term inhabitant there, you can and should utilize the employment information provided by your local medical society. You can, first of all, obtain general data on the various health care facilities in the area from the local society. Likewise, you can telephone the executive secretary of the society for a list of any immediate employment openings that have been submitted by local physicians or for an indication of long-range employment trends in your area. The medical society, as a rule, publishes a bulletin which is distributed to its membership by the secretary. A notice of your interest in and availability for employment can be included in this periodical, or it can be announced at the next professional meeting.

When you call the medical society, however, be sure that you have writing materials on hand so that you can *accurately* record all pertinent information about an opening: the physician's full name *spelled and pronounced correctly;* the name of the association, practice, clinic, or other organization if applicable; the address; the telephone number and the hours (if specified) that you are expected to call about the position; and the job description or title. Be sure to find out the exact nature of the practice—e.g., is it a specialty or not? Before you pursue the matter further, you should double-check the spelling of the doctor's name, especially if a letter of application will be your introduction to the doctor. It cannot be overstressed that misspellings make a very negative impression upon potential employers, especially in medicine where accuracy is so important.

Medical and general employment agencies   Still other sources of employment information and assistance are the professional placement agencies—both medical and general. Usually an employment agency places newspaper ads for its clients regarding job openings that they need to fill. The agency interviews and screens the candidates for the jobs and then refers the qualified candidates to the prospective employer. There is a fee for this service: if, for instance, an employment ad says "fee paid," it means that the agency fee will be paid by the agency's client—your prospective employer—if you are selected to fill the position. Otherwise, you will have to pay the fee if you are selected for the job. Therefore, it is wise to investigate what you must pay the agency when it finds you a job.

Medical employment agencies specialize in the placement of medical and allied health personnel in a range of positions. Some agencies specialize in medical secretarial and assisting positions; others, in dental and pharmaceutical positions. When working with an agency, be realistic in assessing your own potential. You may have more skills than you give yourself credit for, and thus you may be able to fill positions offered through many different agencies.

Both medical and general employment agencies are listed in the telephone Yellow Pages of the areas where they are located. If you are canvassing all of the opportunities and sources of information in a particular geographical location, you can make unsolicited inquiries about potential jobs by simply calling or writing to the agencies. If you write, be sure to include your résumé with your letter of inquiry so that the agency can act on it right away or call you later when any suitable openings come up.

Employment agencies, as noted earlier, advertise their listings in newspapers and in some medical periodicals. If you see an advertised job for which you are qualified, call the agency that placed the ad right away. Be sure to have on hand your résumé and references. This material is important because the initial screening will take place over the telephone. You will make a better impression with the account executive if you can supply all needed data quickly, crisply, and completely without delays or paper shuffling. Remember, the agency will want to interview you in person before recommending you or sending you to a prospective employer. You should be on time for the agency interview, and you should follow the guidelines for interview etiquette outlined in section 2.2. Take with you to the agency your résumé, your reference list, and any other requested materials. You will generally need two copies of the résumé and the reference list: one for the agency and another for the agency to send ahead to its client. Also be prepared to ask your high school and/or college to submit transcripts of your grades to the agency, if requested. This is *your* responsibility. (You may have to pay the schools a nominal fee for this service.)

Never forget that undoubtedly you are only one among many applicants being screened by the agency for a position. Therefore, be sure to show real interest in the job. Find out as much as you can about the tasks and responsibilities involved. Ask about the nature of the practice or group. If it is a physician's office, determine whether or not the physician is a specialist. If the practice involves more than one doctor, find out how many associates are in it and whether they are all of the same specialty. Obtain the estimated patient load if possible. Find out the office hours and whether weekend work, night work, or other overtime is required. Ask about the presence of any other staff members (does the doctor employ an office manager, a Nurse-Practitioner, or what?).

And most importantly—ask *exactly* what duties you will be expected to perform. Find out, if you can, whether any specialized secretarial skills (as machine dictation/transcription) or clinical skills (as drawing venous blood, doing microscopic urine tests in the laboratory, or performing electrocardiograph procedures for the physician) are required. Ask whether the physician expects to train you further in specialized procedures during the course of the job. While the employment agency may not be able to give you all of the answers to these questions, you will have found out which questions to ask the employer later on, and you will also have demonstrated genuine interest in the job and a thorough knowledge of your field. After you have explored what the job entails, you can then discuss further with the agency the salary range and the benefits offered by the employer. Inquire whether or not the position is fee paid. If it is not fee paid, find out the amount of the fee vis-à-vis the salary, and determine the expected fee payment arrangements. Fees vary according to the job, the salary, and the economic profile of the community.

The agency account executive may decide to send you out to see the prospective employer right away. Otherwise, he or she may decide to call you later to set up an appointment with the employer. This varies according to how many applicants there are and how you shape up in comparison with the competition. Employment agencies generally request that you call your account executive after every interview so that they can obtain an idea of how you feel about the employer. The agencies also call their clients to follow up on these interviews.

Advertisements placed by physicians In all likelihood, you will answer directly newspaper advertisements placed by single physicians, joint practices and associations, clinics, hospitals, medical schools, and others. These ads may be blind or signed. A blind ad is one that lists and describes the job and sometimes the salary, and then gives a post office box to which you are supposed to send a letter of application, a résumé, and any other required material. A signed ad, on the other hand, gives not only the above information about the job but also the name, address, and possibly the telephone number of the prospective employer. (If you are answering a blind ad, be sure that your name and address are on the envelope, the letter, and the résumé.) If references are asked for, supply them. Be certain that your type-written material is letter-perfect, as this is your initial chance to make a positive impression (see also section 2.2).

When responding to a signed ad requesting that you telephone the office for an appointment, make sure that you call only during the hours specified. Have your background material at hand so that you can respond concisely, coherently, and completely to all questions. In some instances, you will be telephone-interviewed by another medical assistant, by a nurse, by an office manager, or by the physician. In general, you should follow the guidelines given earlier for telephone etiquette with employment agency interviewers. However, your responses and your own questions ought to be tailored to the particular individual conducting the interview. For example, in talking with a physician, you should keep your responses and questions brief but inclusive so as to convey all necessary information but not waste the doctor's valuable time. On the other hand, you can pursue important matters with the doctor such as his or her personal expectations of the successful candidate—matters that you ordinarily would not bring up with a staff member. If the interviewer is an office manager or another assistant, you can discuss details of office routines which you might not go into in depth with the doctor or with a nurse.

Remember: the employer is generally searching for the right person. Skills are relative. Go after the job level you prefer if you can realistically convince yourself that you qualify for it. Pursue the medical assisting position that will make you happy because you enjoy your work.

2.2

INTRODUCING YOURSELF TO A PROSPECTIVE EMPLOYER

Making a good impression on employment agency interviewers is certainly important, but it is only half the battle. You must now be interviewed by your prospective physician-employer or a member of the office staff. It is, of course, paramount that you convey the best possible image of yourself to the physician and/or the office staff. First impressions—whether created on the telephone, in writing, or in person—are *lasting* impressions. Therefore, the following matters will require your attention throughout the introductory stages:

1. Telephone etiquette prior to a personal interview
2. The appearance, content, and format of your application letter, your résumé, and your list of references
3. Your manners and personal appearance during the interview.

TELEPHONING A PROSPECTIVE EMPLOYER'S OFFICE

When inquiring about a job that may be open or when responding to an employment ad by telephone, you must be polite and coherent. After all, one of a medical assistant's prime responsibilities is the easy handling of telephone calls in the practice. Thus, the members of the medical office team will be evaluating your telephone performance from the beginning to the end of the conversation. If an applicant shows that he or she cannot converse with aplomb during an initial interview, it is obvious that the applicant may not be able to deal effectively with all of the many calls that come into or originate from a busy medical office. Take into consideration the fact that patients can be frightened, demanding, and often impatient. This is usually the type of telephone call you will be dealing with if you are hired. It is necessary, therefore, to project a smile in your voice and a relaxed, confident manner of self-assurance.

Be sure to prepare yourself before placing your call. If necessary, jot down any special questions you want to ask and any particular points you wish to make. Also, have your personal data information on hand by the telephone. If you are not placing the call yourself but are waiting for the doctor to call you, keep these materials at hand, anyway. Since you can never know what kinds of questions will be asked, you must be ready for anything.

Sample telephone interviews   While it is impossible to provide answers for all questions and guidelines for all situations, the following two dialogues indicate a few of the more typical questions and their responses. The participants in the first dialogue are a medical assistant who is returning to the job market after a few years as a full-time wife and mother and a currently employed assistant who is screening applicants for a busy pediatric group practice. The applicant is calling in response to a newspaper ad placed by the office manager. (NOTE: A specific salary has been stipulated in the ad, so this matter is not brought up in the initial interview.)

DIALOGUE 1

Office: Good morning. Wing Memorial Pediatric Associates. Miss Dow speaking.

Applicant: Good morning, Miss Dow. My name is Ann Mason. I'm calling about the opening for a Medical Assistant/Administrative position that was advertised in yesterday's *Observer*. Is the position still open?

Office: Yes, it is. Would you mind just telling me a bit about yourself—your past experience, if any, and your educational background?

Applicant: I have an AA degree in Medical Assisting from Jonesville Community College. I graduated in 19__. Then, I worked four years for Dr. Martha Brown, a pediatrician in Longmeadow.

Office: Good. When exactly did you work for Dr. Brown?

Applicant: From 19__ to 19__.

Office: Then you moved here?

Applicant: Yes. I got married, moved here with my husband and had a baby. He's of school age now and I'd like to go back to work. I have made tentative child-care arrangements.

Office: That's a help! Now I'd like to ask if you've done any part-time medical work during that interval.

Applicant: No. But I studied for and passed the national certification examination for the CMA-A rating in May of this year.

Office: Well, you are wise to keep current since the whole field of medicine changes so rapidly.

Applicant: May I ask how many doctors are now in the group practice?

Office: Six. Everyone is quite busy, so the Associates decided to hire one other assistant who will deal strictly with filing and correspondence.

Applicant: Yes, the ad indicated that. How many other assistants work there?

Office: The doctors have another administrative assistant while I handle reception, appointments and the telephone. The other person does the bookkeeping. There are also two clinical assistants.

Applicant: Can you expand a little on the office hours and give me an idea of any expected overtime? I'll need to know this when scheduling my child-care needs.

Office: Certainly. Regular office hours for medical assisting staff are from 8:00 a.m. to 5:00 p.m. weekdays, with staggered lunch breaks of 30 minutes each. Although we officially close at 5:00 p.m., quite often at least one of us has to stay until 5:30 or perhaps 6:00 if the patient load is especially heavy on a particular day. The office is not open on weekends except for emergencies. The doctors and the assistants rotate so that the doctor on duty can see emergency patients from 8:00 a.m. to noon on Saturdays and Sundays.

Applicant: All right. I can make adequate arrangements for the care of my son during overtime and weekend hours when needed.

Office: Good. Mrs. Mason, why don't you put your résumé in the mail right away so that the staff can look it over? They would also like to have a list of at least three references. As soon as the staff evaluates your material and assumming the review is favorable, I will call you to arrange for a personal interview.

Applicant: That's fine. I'll get the material in the mail immediately. By the way, can you give me an idea of what time of day you'll be calling back so that I will be sure to be here?

Office: The patient workload is lowest between 4:00–5:00 p.m.; therefore, I will call sometime this week at that time. May I have your address and telephone number?

Applicant: My address is _____ and my number is _____. Thank you for taking the time to talk to me. It certainly sounds like an interesting position. Good-bye.

Office: Good-bye.

COMMENTS

1. In your concern about the job, do not forget to say hello and good-bye.
2. Identify yourself at once and state your reason for calling.
3. Use the other person's name in the conversation and if for some reason it has not been mentioned, ask "To whom am I speaking, please?"
4. Give straightforward, complete, brief answers to all questions.
5. Ask the questions that *you* have, but keep in mind that there are some questions that only the doctor can answer.
6. Be polite and enthusiastic without becoming emotional.
7. If you have small children at home, *do not* try to call when they are in the room, making noise. Such a practice indicates that you aren't well organized. Make your call when they are outside or are napping.
8. If, for some reason, you discover during the conversation that you really are not qualified for the job or that you do not want to pursue the matter further, say so politely.
9. If the interviewer sounds rushed, ask if you can call at another time, or if the interviewer could call you back at his or her convenience.
10. It is usually pointless to discuss salary matters during an initial telephone conversation.

The following is a sample telephone conversation between an applicant and a physician in a single practice. The physician has decided to call the applicant back after reviewing the résumé and consulting with the references.

DIALOGUE 2

Applicant: Hello. Sarah Davis speaking.

Physician: Dr. Bernstein.

Applicant: Oh, yes, Dr. Bernstein. Thanks so much for calling me back!

Physician: I have read your résumé with interest, Miss Davis. Everything seems to be in order. I have, by the way, heard some very positive comments about you from Dr. Crawford and Dr. Roberts. I would like to make an appointment with you for a personal interview.

Applicant: Fine. When would you like me to be in your office?

Physician: Let's make it on Friday, January 6, at 4:45 p.m. Okay?

Applicant: Fine, Dr. Bernstein. I'll look forward to seeing you on Friday, January 6, at 4:45. And thanks again for calling!

Physician: Not at all. Good-bye.

Applicant: Good-bye.

COMMENTS

1. If you are expecting a call or calls regarding employment, don't just answer the telephone with "Hello." Give your name.
2. Answer all questions politely and thoroughly. However, do not ramble: doctors are too busy to waste time with irrelevant conversations.
3. Save most of your questions for the interview if the physician suggests a personal interview. You can, however, mention that you have some questions that cannot wait. That way, you will show your interest but not at the expense of the doctor's valuable time. Also, jot down your questions for future reference.
4. Verify your appointment date, time of day, and location.
5. Let the physician terminate the conversation by saying good-bye first.

APPLICATION LETTERS, RÉSUMÉS, AND REFERENCE LISTS

The job application letter   A properly formatted and well-written letter of application will greatly assist in preselling you to a prospective employer. This type of letter is a concrete indication of your verbal and technical skills and of your general personality and intelligence.

You should typewrite the letter on plain bond paper. (*Do not* use social stationery or personalized letterhead.) Exotic typefaces should be avoided. Either the Block or the Modified Semi-block styling is appropriate. The letter ought not to exceed one page. Under no circumstances should you prepare and photocopy a form letter to be sent to numerous physicians. Such a procedure will create a most unfavorable first impression on those evaluating your application. The applicant lacking the time and the common courtesy to write a personal letter will most probably not receive careful consideration.

Before typewriting the letter, you should plan your approach in detail. An outline or a draft of the points to be made will assist you. If the letter is solicited (i.e., you are responding to an advertisement), you should mention in the first paragraph the specific position for which you are applying and the date and source of the advertisement. If the letter is unsolicited (i.e., you are applying on your own initiative), you should say as much in the first paragraph and indicate why you are interested in working for the particular practice. Next, you ought to focus on and develop your best assets. A concise statement of your technical skills (such as shorthand and typewriting rates) may be given along with mention of any more specialized skills (as clinical procedures, if you have been so trained). Another sentence or even a

A Letter of Application

```
                                        123 Smith Lane
                                        Jonesville, ST 98765
                                        June 1, 19—


        Ms. Ann Stone
        Director, Personnel
        ABC Insurance
        81 Albany Towers  Suite 12
        Smithville, ST 12345


        Dear Ms. Smith:

            The ABC Insurance employment ad on page 48E of the May 30, 19—
        issue of the Sunday Republican has attracted my immediate interest.
        Because I believe that I am qualified for the executive secretarial
        position in your Medical Claims Department, I am sending you a copy
        of my résumé.

            My shorthand rate is —— wpm; and my typewriting rate —— wpm.
        I am experienced in the use of machine dictation and transcription
        equipment — both cassette and belt.  I am also thoroughly familiar
        with the use of electronic printing and display calculators.

            As you can see from the attached résumé, I am currently employed
        as Medical Office Manager for Dr. Helen P. Thornton who is retiring
        from practice at the end of July.  I believe that the experience
        gained in this position would be quite useful in medical claims work.

            I look forward to a personal interview at your convenience, if
        you decide to follow up on this initial application.  ABC Insurance
        is indeed a fine company — one for which I know I would enjoy
        working.

                                        Sincerely yours,


                                        Carol C. Mannington

                                        Carol C. Mannington
```

Résumé

RÉSUMÉ

Carol Conners Mannington
123 Smith Lane
Jonesville, ST 98765
(300) 567-8910

<u>Employment Experience</u>

October 1974 - present	Helen P. Thornton, MD
	129 Main Street
	Jonesville, ST 98765
	Medical Office Manager
June 1965 - October 1974	BR Pharmaceuticals
	12 Industrial Park Drive
	Smithville, ST 12345
	Secretary to Dr. Kenneth Preston
	Group Leader, R&D
June 1960 - June 1965	Jonesville Municipal Hospital
	Jonesville, ST 98765
	Director, Surgical Secretarial Services
	1963 - 1965
	Secretary, Surgical Services
	1962 - 1963
	Typist, Business Office
	1960 - 1962

<u>Education</u>

1958 - 1960	Mason County Community College	Associate in Arts
	Jonesville, ST 98765	Business Education
1954 - 1958	Jonesville High School	Diploma
	Jonesville, ST 98765	

<u>Special Skills</u>

medical stenography
fluency in German

<u>References</u>

References will be provided on request.

References

REFERENCES

Helen P. Thornton, MD   telephone: (222) 123-4567
129 Main Street
Jonesville, ST 98765

Kenneth Preston, MD, PharmD   telephone: (333) 890-1234
Group Leader
Research & Development
BR Pharmaceuticals
12 Industrial Park Drive
Smithville, ST 12345

Mary A. Samuels, RN, CMA-AC   telephone: (222) 124-4444
Chairperson, Medical Assisting
Mason County Community College
Jonesville, ST 98765

Personal reference

The Reverend Donald D. O'Leary   telephone: (222) 125-9898
The Rectory
St. Mary's Church
North Street
Jonesville, ST 98765

paragraph expanding on some aspect of your education or on your previous employment experience not already developed fully in the résumé can be included in the letter. The tone throughout should be straightforward, yet modest and sincere. Of course, the material should be carefully proofread so that there will not be any grammatical or typographical errors. You should keep a copy of the letter for your records. (See the illustration of a sample job application letter that is found on page 24 of this section.)

The résumé   Your résumé is the complete statement of your professional advancement and accomplishments to date. As such, it is a key factor in achieving your employment objectives. Although books have been written on this subject, there are elements essential to all well-written résumés which can be set down here. These elements are: (1) personal identification: your full name, address, and telephone number (home and/or office) typewritten at the top of the résumé (2) employment experience: each job that you have held listed chronologically from present to past, including the name and address of each doctor, practice, or organization (such as a clinic, a hospital, or a health maintenance organization), applicable employment dates, your job title and a *brief* job description if the responsibilities are not obvious from the title itself, and perhaps a concise summary of your special accomplishments in each position if space permits (3) educational background: a list of the institutions that you have attended or from which you have graduated, starting with the highest level (as college) and concluding with high school (4) special skills: a list of special skills (as machine dictation/transcription or clinical skills) that might prove a valuable asset to a prospective employer should you be hired, and (5) references: the sentence, "References will be provided on request," included at the end of the résumé. NOTE: If you have no previous employment experience, you can supplement your education category with a list of the business and secretarial courses that you have successfully completed, you can mention your typewriting and transcription rates, and you can list any academic or professional honors that you have been awarded. If you have completed any special free-lance secretarial projects (as the typing of manuscripts and theses), you can mention them under the heading "Special Projects" following the educational section.

The following data should *not* be given on the résumé itself: (1) names and addresses of references: references should be typewritten separately and should be provided by you at the interview or in an interview follow-up letter (2) salary: it is best to discuss salary requirements and ranges during the interview itself, since you will not want to undersell yourself ahead of time or possibly price yourself out of a job market that you may be unfamiliar with (3) your reasons, if any, for changing jobs: since wording can often be misunderstood without personal clarification, it is best to discuss this matter with the interviewer and only if you are asked, rather than committing yourself on paper (4) your reasons for present unemployment, if applicable: this topic is also tricky and is therefore best dealt with in person or in a telephone conversation, since adequate explanations often require valuable page space that can be better used to highlight your assets, and (5) a photograph: a photo can work for or against you, depending on the subjectivity of the person evaluating your application; hence, it is best not to risk a premature negative reaction on the part of the employer before you have had a chance to present yourself in person.

Your résumé normally should not exceed one page. To achieve maximum brevity and at the same time attain comprehensiveness, you should plan the material and then write it out in draft form before typewriting it. All facts should be double-checked. Use plain, straightforward English devoid of technical jargon and superlatives. The material ought to be typewritten on plain standard bond paper. Margins should be balanced on all four sides.

Although there are many acceptable résumé formats, the simplest and cleanest treatment is to block all the material flush left. Entries should be single-spaced internally, with double- or triple-spacing between entries, depending on the page space available. Underscoring and capital letters may introduce main and secondary headings. Copies *must* be clean and legible; for this purpose, offset copies or photocopies are suggested. Avoid mimeographed copies and carbons. Your typewriter typeface must be sharp and clean. Avoid exotic typefaces (including italic). See the illustration of a sample résumé.

Professional and personal references   When you typewrite a list of references, follow the general format and style that you have used for your résumé. Do not change paper size or color and do not use a different type style. White bond paper is appropriate. Head the list REFERENCES. Single-space each entry and double- or triple-space between entries. Include the full name, address, and telephone number of each person who has consented to recommend you. Include at least one supervisor and/or doctor from each former place of employment. Include one former instructor if possible. You should not have unexplained gaps that will show up when the résumé and reference list are compared. Personal character references can be listed at the bottom of the sheet, if necessary. Give the physician the reference list when it is asked for but do not staple this list to your résumé. Make sure that you have enough names in the list to satisfy the individual doctor's requirements.

MANNERS AND APPEARANCE DURING INTERVIEWS
Your manners   Since the medical assistant is usually the first and the last member of the office medical team seen by the patients and other visitors, it is essential that the assistant be a credit to the practice. Thus, impeccable manners are requisite. Since an applicant's manners will be carefully observed by an interviewer, the following are some of the most important points to remember:

1. **Punctuality**   Be on time for your interview. If you don't know exactly where the office is located, get directions beforehand. If the office is in a large city where traffic and parking are a problem, ask a staff member for the best driving or public transportation route and find out where you can park. This can be done when your appointment is being made. If you are still unsure of the directions, you can make a dry run in advance to make sure that you know the way. In any event, give yourself plenty of time to get there with minutes to spare. The longer you wait in the office, the more you can observe about the office routines.

2. **Arrival**   When you enter the office, identify yourself to the receptionist or assistant and state your business ("I'm here to see Dr. Yowell at 4:30 about a job"). Be cheerful and polite. If the weather is bad and you need to doff heavy outerwear, find out where to hang it up so that you won't be burdened with coat, scarf, mittens, hat, or the like during the interview.

3. **Waiting to see the doctor**   If you have to wait for a while before seeing the doctor or doctors, sit quietly and observe as much of the routines as possible without appearing nosy. This process may provide you with additional questions to ask later in the interview, and it will also give you a fairly accurate reading on the practice itself.

4. **Introductions**   When introduced to the doctor or doctors as well as to other staff members, smile, repeat their names ("How do you do, Dr. Lee," or "It's nice to meet you, Ms. Smith"), and appear enthusiastic but not gushy. The other extreme to avoid is appearing glum or sick (even if you *feel* that way!).

5. **Posture**   When sitting, do not sprawl. On the other hand, do not sit rigidly like a store mannequin. Try to relax and enjoy the experience.

6. **Smoking**   Many waiting rooms and private offices are now no-smoking areas. It is best not to smoke at all unless the doctor asks if you would like to do so.

7. **Chewing gum**   Taboo!

8. **Termination of the interview** Let the physician end the interview. When he or she stands up, then you may do the same. Shake hands, thank the physician for the time spent with you, say that it has been interesting or enjoyable or whatever seems most appropriate and then say good-bye. Don't forget to say good-bye to the assistant or the receptionist on your way out.

Personal appearance In medicine, personal appearance and hygiene are particularly important. You should dress carefully for your interview. Although it is not necessary for you to wear whites to an interview, it is essential that the clothing you do wear be clean, pressed, and conservative. Exotic attire (such as jumpsuits, dirty jeans, or dashikis) is definitely out of place. If you are a woman, avoid excessive makeup. Hair should be clean, combed, and generally neat. Be especially careful in cleaning your hands and manicuring your fingernails. A sloppy, unkempt appearance is often taken as an indicator of a sloppy worker.

THE INTERVIEW ITSELF: General Pointers

While it is impossible to offer cut-and-dried guidelines to cover every eventuality in interviews, the following paragraphs give general suggestions that, if followed, will make your experience more positive.

Eye contact Look directly at the interviewer when you are speaking. Avoiding someone's eyes, especially when you are answering questions, can be interpreted as evasiveness. On the other hand, don't stare blankly at the interviewer.

Speech mannerisms Try to avoid those annoying verbal tics that many people use to cover up pauses or to give themselves time to think of what to say next. Some of the more irritating mannerisms are the use of "ah" or "uh" at the beginning or end of sentences; the use of "Like . . ." at the beginning of sentences; and the repetition of "you know" or "OK" throughout a conversation.

Interview direction and the asking of questions Don't try to lead the conversation since the doctor undoubtedly will have decided what is to be asked and discussed. Follow the doctor's lead. You can interject your own questions during appropriate lulls in the conversation, or you can save them for the end when the physician will probably ask if you have any questions. However, feel free to ask intelligent questions about such matters as the nature of the practice, the patient load, and the specialty or specialties (if any). Another good question to ask the doctor is his or her particular dislikes regarding routines. Many applicants fail to mention this (or the doctor forgets to discuss it), and then the newly hired assistant inadvertently does things that the doctor dislikes during the first weeks on the job. It is much better to find out what you are expected *not* to do as well as what you are expected to do right in the beginning.

Your job description and on-the-job training Be sure that you get a clear idea of just what you will be doing in the office. Understand the expected hours of work and any required overtime. Find out if the doctor intends to give you any on-the-job training and, if so, what kind. During the interview, you should ascertain all the employee benefits available to you, and any orientation training necessary.

Questions you can't answer Many people are embarrassed when they discover during an interview that they don't know everything an interviewer expects them to know. If you are asked something that you cannot answer, say so honestly. Sometimes interviewers ask questions that they *know* you can't answer, just to see whether they will get an honest reaction.

Weaknesses (if any) in your skills   If the doctor mentions a required skill in which you know you are weak, admit it right away. Be prepared to say that you are willing to improve in that area, whether by programmed self-study, by taking a refresher course, or by learning on the job. In some cases, the doctor will prefer the latter.

Salary, fringe benefits, and insurance   The physician will tell you your base pay and will undoubtedly outline the fringe benefits and insurance provisions. Feel free to bring up any one of these topics if the doctor doesn't. However, it is bad practice to argue with a prospective employer about a salary that you feel is too low. You can ask about the doctor's raise policy (for example what is a standard raise and when are employees considered for them?). You can ask about staff promotions if the office is large enough to accommodate a large staff.

A recent survey by the AAMA reveals the following data on medical assisting salaries: In 1974, eight out of 10 medical assistants received an average weekly salary of $120; but in 1977, eighty-four percent of them received an average weekly salary of $184. Almost 8% of them were earning in 1977–1978 salaries ranging from $12,500 to $25,000 annually in large urban communities. Although it is obvious from these figures that salaries for medical assistants have improved markedly, it still should be kept in mind that an assistant's salary will be governed by: (1) the size of the practice (2) the economic profile of the area in which the physician practices, which in turn affects his or her fee profile (3) the assistant's educational qualifications (4) the assistant's past experience and the recommendations of previous employers, and (5) the nature and the number of the tasks that will be assigned to the assistant.

Open salaries   Sometimes an employment ad that you are responding to will have stipulated that the salary is *open* (i.e., open to negotiation). If you have familiarized yourself beforehand with the usual and customary salary ranges for medical assistants in your area, you ought to be able to discuss the issue intelligently with the physician. In cases like this, it is even more important to highlight your education, experience, and any specialized skills that you feel would place you as close as possible to the top range.

If you can see that the interview is about to end with the doctor's still not having brought up the matter of salary, you might say, "Oh, by the way, Dr. _____ , what do you feel is a reasonable salary based on your expectations and my qualifications?" Or you could say, "What will the starting salary be for this position?" Another way of wording your question could be, "May I ask what the salary will be?" You can also convey your knowledge of the usual and customary salary ranges in the particular geographical area by mentioning those ranges in round numbers. Example: "When I spoke recently with the Medical Society, it was suggested that the going salary for this type of position is currently _____." You should not be pushy or insistent, however. Just state the facts objectively.

Professional liability insurance   Determine during the interview whether or not you will be covered in the physician's professional liability insurance policy. This is very important, for as an agent of the physician, you too can be liable to litigation. (See also Chapters 3 "Medical Law," sections 3.5 and 3.9; and Chapter 10, "Insurance," section 10.10.)

Fringe benefits   Fringe benefits occasionally include discounts on pharmaceutical prescriptions or fee discounts when you require the services of the physician's colleagues. Inquire about the policies regarding holidays, vacations, and sick leave. Find out whether or not occasional personal days are allowed (as for house closings or deaths in the family).

Introductions to other members of the medical team   If you are introduced to and are given time to talk with other staff members, be sure to use this time to your advantage by asking pertinent questions regarding their tasks and routines. In this way, you can get a valid idea of what it would be like to work for and/or with them. You can also find out how efficiently the office is managed.

Office tour   If your prospects look good or if you have been offered the job, try to get a brief tour of the office suite. Becoming generally familiar with the location of various rooms and equipment will ease your first day on the job. Another good idea is to borrow an extra copy of the procedures manual, if there is one, so that you can familiarize yourself with the actual management of the office prior to your first day on the job.

The offer   At the end of the interview, you may be offered a job on the spot or the doctor may tell you that he or she will get back to you in a day or so, after all other applicants have been interviewed. If you would like a day or two to think about the offer, say so. However, you should set up a specific day and hour when you will call the doctor back. Do not delay your return call more than one or two days.

If the doctor indicates that you will be called regarding a possible offer, accept this decision politely. Try to get some idea of when you will be contacted so that you will be at home. You might also mention that you need to complete your own plans rather soon.

If you don't get the job   If the doctor says that you are not quite qualified for the position, thank the doctor for the candid evaluation and be sure to mention that the interview has been a pleasant as well as an informative experience. Say good-bye politely. Don't be needlessly discouraged: appreciate the honest evaluation, work to improve any indicated deficiencies, and keep on looking for the right position.

2.3

INTERVIEWING AN APPLICANT YOURSELF

INTRODUCTION
Once you have obtained the position you really want, it may sometimes become one of your duties to conduct interviews of applicants for other positions on the doctor's staff. The following discussion should help you to handle interviews effectively on the other side of the desk. Many busy physicians prefer to assign the *initial* screening of job applicants to their assistants if they feel that the assistants can competently evaluate their peers in such situations. Therefore, you may have to interview your potential replacement if you are being promoted or if you are planning to leave your current position. You also may have to screen a prospective addition to the office assisting staff.

EQUAL OPPORTUNITY LAWS
Since the content of employment advertisements and the questions asked of applicants in preemployment interviews are greatly affected by federal and state Equal Employment Opportunity laws, you should be generally familiar with the major aspects of this legislation. However, since state laws vary, this section discusses only the federal laws applicable all over the United States.

The main thrust of the federal legislation is that it is illegal to discriminate against any individual in any employment practice on the basis of race, color, sex, religion, national origin, or age (between 40 and 65, specifically). The most comprehensive federal enforcement legislation is Title VII of the Civil Rights Act of 1964. Age discrimination is specifically prohibited by a separate federal statute—the Age Discrimination in Employment Act of 1967. Almost any employer and especially an employer having more than five employees is subject to this legislation. Title VII is administered by the Equal Employment Opportunity Commission (EEOC), whose headquarters is in Washington, DC. The EEOC also has district and regional offices across the country and individual questions regarding the implementation of this legislation can be directed to the EEOC offices in your area.

Regarding hiring the handicapped, federal laws prohibit an employer's refusing to hire any handicapped person so long as the handicap does not prevent appropriate performance of the job requirements. (For example, if the only job requirement were to type material from a dictated source, a blind person could not be refused employment based on his or her handicap.) Further, HEW regulations require that employers must make "reasonable accommodation" for such handicapped persons hired, so long as this accommodation would not impose undue hardships on the operation of the office or clinic. This makes it even more important that the physician-employer spells out clearly the job requirements and competencies needed to perform them, and then hires employees whose selection is based solely on these criteria.

Recruiting and hiring practices   The EEOC has set down specific regulations to be followed by employers during the recruiting and hiring processes. For instance, employment ads may not stipulate employer preference as to race, national origin, sex, or age. Furthermore, some states have their own regulations affecting the preemployment inquiries made of applicants by prospective employers. Any questions asked of an applicant that would directly or even indirectly reveal the applicant's race, color, religious preference, national origin, or age are unlawful in some states.

Therefore, interviewers and prospective employers should remember to ask *only* questions directly relating to the applicant's qualifications (as opposed to extraneous matters) and questions relating specifically to those qualifications relevant to the performance of the particular job under consideration. Examples of questions to be avoided concern:

1. The applicant's birthplace or that of the applicant's spouse, parents, or other close relatives
2. The applicant's citizenship
3. The applicant's religion
4. The place of employment of the applicant's spouse or relatives
5. The maiden name of the applicant if the applicant is a woman
6. The applicant's age and height.

It is now generally prohibited for an employer to require that a photograph of an applicant be submitted prior to employment. (Remember the comments earlier regarding the voluntary submission of photographs by applicants.)

As for inquiries regarding an applicant's criminal record, the EEOC currently does not take the position that such an inquiry is illegal; however, the EEOC does say that there can be no comprehensive prohibition against the employment of individuals with criminal records and that any inquiry into this matter must be shown to be required by the nature of the job. Example: an applicant for a medical assisting position in a physician's office where medications are kept could be asked if he or she had ever been arrested or convicted on a drug charge.

Since the restrictions on preemployment inquiries are so numerous, it is advisable for employers to review their employment application forms and current employment procedures to ensure compliance with the law. It is also wise to become thoroughly familiar with the state laws affecting employment practices.

Postemployment follow-up Postemployment questions regarding an employee's age, sex, race, etc., are perfectly legal. These data are used in the filling out of Equal Employment forms, and in the compilation of data for pension and insurance purposes. However, the questions should *not* be posed until *after* the individual has been formally employed, and the data obtained should be kept in files separate from individual personnel files.

ADVERTISEMENTS: How to Write and Place Them

If the physician is working with a medical or general employment agency, the agency will write and place the advertisements according to the physician's directions. If, on the other hand, the physician asks you to work up a draft for a blind or signed ad, you should first find out where the doctor wishes the ad to appear and then you should read that publication's Information to Advertisers in order to ascertain costs. If you cannot understand this material or if you find it incomplete for your purposes, call the publication's advertising department for further details. In general, though, costs are determined by the number of words, the typesize (i.e., boldface capitals may cost more than capitals and lowercase regular type), and the column size and column placement of the ad (i.e., a two-column box will definitely cost more than an unboxed single-column ad). Tailor the text so as to convey maximum information in a minimum number of words.

Ad copy should be typewritten on plain white bond paper separate from the covering letter accompanying the ad. Use 1½-inch margins with triple line spacing. Typewrite the material exactly as the doctor wishes to see it in print. Explain in the covering letter when and for how long the ad should run (give specific dates). It is better to write this information down than to telephone the ad in because the chance of errors is decreased if the publication editors can see just what the doctor desires.

The physician should check and approve the final copy before mailing and should also approve the costs and other financial details. You and/or the physician should check the ad on its first day in print: some newspapers, for instance, refuse to make free corrections of printer's errors if they have not been notified of the errors on the first day of publication.

The following illustrate the wording of several typical blind and signed ads designed for newspapers:

MEDICAL TYPIST $563
         Dowville area
Process Case Histories - Corresp - Reports - Use Dictaphone - Group OB/GYN practice - Bnfits. Résumés to Box 180, Dowville *Trib.*

MEDICAL ASSISTANT Full-time chairside & receptionist duties to podiatrist. Exp. preferred but will train right person. Résumés to Box 4545, Huntsville *Rocket.*

MEDICAL ASSISTANT/ADMIN $650
Exp. Med. Asst./Admin. Dictaphone, heavy typing, filing. Call Hamilton Orthopaedic Associates, Ltd., Dr. Warren, (456) 789-1010, 9–10 a.m., Mon–Fri.

MEDICAL SECRETARY exp'd only. Résumés to Box C, Martinsville *Leader.*

MEDICAL RECEPTIONIST   Exp'd for busy group practice. Must relate well to young patients. Typing-forms. Résumés to Carter City Pediatric Associates, 444 Lee Highway, Carter City, ST 12345.

MEDICAL SECRETARY exp'd only. Call Dr. Lee, 444-5555, 9–10 a.m., weekdays.

MEDICAL RECEPTIONIST
Wanted recpt. w/Medical exp. Heavy phones, multi-MD practice. Some typing, salary open. Résumés to Box 4A, Johns. *Star.*

SCREENING APPLICANTS FOR THE PHYSICIAN
Telephone evaluations   A good way to weed out unacceptable applicants is to talk to all job candidates by telephone before taking the time to interview them personally. Set up specific call-in hours (as an hour or so before regular office hours or at times when the doctor is not seeing patients). However, if you use this technique, you must expect to sit by the telephone for the entire period. Keep all conversations brief and to the point. Don't be brusque or curt, though. Make sure that when you ask questions, you adhere to the guidelines given in the previous section discussing Equal Opportunity Employment. Just because you are talking on the telephone to an applicant, you do not have the right to ask prying or potentially discriminatory questions. Be sure to write down your interview questions leaving space for comments so that you may relay the desired information to other staff members at a later time. A preprinted form containing necessary and appropriate questions with space for answers and comments after each may be useful. It is also possible to save time by using a tape recorder after you have completed the interviews.

Listen to the person. For example, if you were a patient calling your employer's office, would you like this person's attitude and telephone mannerisms if he or she were the medical assistant or receptionist? Does the person use good grammar? Is the voice clear and well modulated? Is the applicant well enough organized to answer your questions quickly and completely? Does the applicant have the requisite educational background? How much previous medical assisting experience does the individual have and in what medical specialties? Reread the telephone interviews in section 2.2, this time from the standpoint of the interviewer.

Résumé evaluation: good and bad signs   One of the most important ways of judging a person's concern for on-the-job accuracy is to evaluate the written material submitted by the candidate prior to an interview. If misspellings, typographical errors, areas of broken or smudged type, creases and tears, messy formats, poor photocopy reproduction, and other such gaucheries abound in a candidate's application letter and résumé, you can be fairly certain that these factors are symptomatic of the individual's potential job performance. Does the physician want the office correspondence and records to reflect these negative characteristics? The individual who is so lazy as to send a mimeographed or photocopied form letter of application does not deserve serious consideration in a profession where precision and careful attention to the details of professional etiquette are so important. Avoid applicants with such sloppy presentations.

The résumé should have a clean and neat format devoid of errors (see the material in 2.2); in addition, it should not contain any chronological gaps that have not been explained therein or in the covering letter. All dates of employment and names of previous employers should be given.

Watch out for résumés that are longer than one page and that are unnecessarily verbose. Inflated language and the use of incomprehensible jargon are negative signs. Heavy emphasis on extracurricular activities at the expense of hard professional background data are also favorite ways to fill gaps or to gloss over weaknesses in skills and formal education.

CONDUCTING PERSONAL INTERVIEWS
The key to interviewing a number of applicants in a short time is to get yourself together beforehand. Set up specific personal interview hours, just as you would for telephone interviews. Space the appointments to avoid overlaps. No single appointment should exceed 30 minutes at the most. Don't try to see everyone on the same day. Interview the applicants before office hours, when the physician is out of the office, or at whatever other time the physician prefers. Have a typewritten

synopsis of the job description on hand—one copy for the candidate and another for you to refer to. If your office has a procedures manual, keep it at hand for consultation if necessary. If the doctor desires that all applicants fill out an application form, have the form on a clipboard to be given to the person as soon as he or she arrives.

Putting the applicant at ease   Treat the applicant politely and in a relaxed manner. Use the person's name when you say hello, and call the person by name during the interview. Offer coffee or whatever refreshments you may have at hand. See that the person is comfortably seated in a private area before you begin the interview. Outline the nature of the practice, the nature of the job, the salary as stipulated by the doctor, and then give the applicant a copy of the job description to look over. Ask the applicant the necessary questions or the questions that the doctor has directed you to ask. Verify any unclear data, and ask for a list of references. Be sure that you adhere to the Equal Opportunity guidelines given earlier in this section. Try at all times to keep the conversation relaxed: a staccato inquisition will unnerve the most easygoing applicant!

Evaluation   Evaluate the applicant according to the following: (1) punctuality for the interview (2) neatness of personal appearance (3) degree of expressed interest in the job (4) personality: the ability of this person to relate well to the doctor, the other team members, and the patients (5) formal education (6) past medical assisting experience and the nature of that experience relative to your physician's practice (7) any special additional skills held by the applicant (8) a discerned willingness to work beyond the call of duty if necessary (9) honesty in responses (10) the ability to communicate clearly and accurately by telephone, in person, and on paper (11) organizational ability and efficiency (12) enough knowledge of the field so that he or she can ask intelligent questions about the job. Jot down your impressions in shorthand or in short phrases either during the interview or just after the interview has ended. Later, you can typewrite the material briefly on a cover sheet for the individual's file. The doctor can then evaluate it.

Interview termination   After you have concluded the interview, you should tell the individual approximately when the office will get in touch regarding the status of the job. It's up to you to end the conversation by standing up and saying something like "Thanks so much for coming by, Ms. (name). It's been nice to chat with you. Dr. (name) will evaluate your material and then we'll get back to you on (date)." Then mention that you've enjoyed talking to the person, and escort the person to the door. Never commit yourself about hiring someone: THIS IS THE DOCTOR'S RESPONSIBILITY.

INTRODUCING AN APPLICANT TO THE PHYSICIAN
Make sure beforehand that the doctor has on the desk all data relating to the applicant whom you are going to introduce. Bring the applicant to the doctor's private office and say something like "Dr. (name), I'd like to introduce Ms. (first + last name). Ms. (surname) is one of our applicants for the (description) job." After you have seen that the person is comfortably seated and that the physician is ready to proceed, excuse yourself and leave the room.

POST-INTERVIEW FOLLOW-UP
Reference checking   Be sure to give the applicant's reference list to the physician: the physician will usually call or write to these individuals. Make sure that all telephone numbers and addresses are complete beforehand.

Call-back to applicants   If it is office policy to call all interviewed candidates regarding the job, try to set up a definite time to do it. For those people whom the doctor has eliminated from consideration, you can write brief letters (some busy practices have preprinted form letters for this purpose). Or you can call them and say something like "Dr. (name) has asked me to tell you that the job has been filled. We had many well qualified applicants, so it was a real chore to make a final decision. We do, however, intend to keep your résumé on file, in case something else develops. Dr. (name) has asked me to tell you that we thank you for your interest in the position." Be friendly and polite. You can also wish the person luck in future endeavors. Also, you may mention that the reason for telephoning is to notify the person that the position has been filled so that he or she can make other plans.

The doctor may, on the other hand, decide not to call anyone except the successful applicant. If this is the case, you must tactfully explain the policy to all interviewed applicants during the interview. Tell them that if they don't hear from the office by (date), they can assume that the job has been filled. This is the quickest and easiest way of handling the situation.

In your dealings with all applicants, you should remember to treat them as you yourself would expect to be treated, were you applying for the job. This requires politeness, good organization, and forthright honesty on your part.

3

CHAPTER THREE

MEDICAL LAW

CONTENTS

3.1

INTRODUCTION

Legal aspects of medical practice have become increasingly significant for physicians and medical assistants during the past 30 years. Since the end of World War II, there has been a dramatic upsurge in the regulation of health care providers, their employees, and the health care process. It is essential for you to be aware of the problem areas which may lead to potential liability of either the physician or the medical assistant, and the material in this chapter will help meet that need.

Chapter 3 contains basic information about the physician's legal rights and obligations; about medical licensure, registration, and certification; about federal regulations affecting the practice of medicine; and about the medical assistant's legal obligations as an employee of the physician. The material should enable you to help the physician limit or eliminate potential liability in medical practice by encouraging the development of appropriate office policies that satisfy legal requirements. These policies should be developed by the physician and the attorney for the practice. Since the process of lawmaking changes over time, the office policies—once established—should be reviewed and updated by the physician and the attorney.

Understanding the functions of the law   Several things will become clear to you as you read this chapter. First of all, the law is not always what some people think it is. It is not simply a collection of easy, cut-and-dried solutions to all problems. In fact, there are many questions for which no clear legal answers are available. In many ways the law is more a process of finding answers to certain problems than an embodiment of the answers themselves. The process of finding legal answers to difficult questions is complicated by the various mechanisms which are the sources of law: judicial opinions, agency regulations, legislative enactments, and executive orders. Many sources of law need to be examined before conclusions can be drawn about what the law requires. This process is further complicated by the American structure of government which recognizes us both as citizens of the nation and as citizens of the state of our residence. The effect of this "dual citizenship" is that each of us is accountable in important respects both to the federal government and to one of the 50 state governments. Since laws may vary from state to state, one must be very careful not to generalize about the law too freely. Questions frequently arise as to which government—federal or state—has the authority to deal with a certain subject matter. Thus, everyone has to recognize the complexity inherent in determining what the law requires in a specific situation.

Terminology   It should be mentioned at the outset that the terms *medical law, legal medicine, medical jurisprudence,* and *forensic medicine* are frequently used by some writers without due attention to their proper meanings. For the purposes of this chapter, the term *medical law*—the substantive area of law dealing with the legal regulation of medicine and medical practice—is appropriate to describe the focus of the following material.

3.2

LEGAL REGULATION OF THE HEALTH CARE PROCESS

The law has two chief interests in regulating the health care process: (1) the protection of the public health, safety, and welfare, and (2) the protection of the rights of health care providers and their patients. Authority to protect the public health, safety, and welfare is called *police power;* it is an inherent power possessed by each of the 50 states. Each of the states has exercised this power by passing a wide range of health care regulations ranging from physician licensure acts (see section 3.3) to statutes that require the reporting of child abuse (see section 3.7). Since the responsibility for this type of legislation rests with each of the states, there is much variation among them. Authority to protect the rights of health care providers or patients may be exercised either by federal or by state governments depending on the source and nature of the right at issue. The federal constitution or a state constitution, federal legislation or state legislation, and a federal judicial opinion or a state judicial opinion could be the source of such a right.

In its regulation of the health care process, the law functions as a restraint on health care decisions, a source of human values to be respected and protected in the health care process, and an influence on the quality of health care provided. Each of these functions of the law can be important for physicians and medical assistants. Certain values have been historically identified as important in the Anglo-American legal tradition. These values include self-determination and freedom of choice. The discussion of the physician-patient relationship which follows (see section 3.4) demonstrates the influence of these values in medicine. Physicians and other health care providers are subject to limitations contained in state practice acts and licensure laws as to the determination of *who* may do *what* to *whom* in the pursuit of health. These limitations exemplify the restraints that the law imposes on health care decision-making. Another legal mechanism to influence the quality of health care is the malpractice system (see section 3.5).

Some physicians feel that legal regulation of the health care process is a relatively recent phenomenon, but this regulation has existed since the time of the ancient classical civilizations. What is new is the staggering amount of regulation. In light of the quantity of regulation, it becomes increasingly important for the physician and the medical assistant to appreciate the sources and the requirements of the laws that must be adhered to.

3.3

LICENSURE, REGISTRATION, AND CERTIFICATION

INTRODUCTION

The terms *licensure, registration,* and *certification* refer to the key steps in permitting individuals to provide health care in the 50 states. The medical licensure system—the cornerstone of the legal regulation of the American health care process—is the mechanism that determines who satisfies the state licensing criteria and who is eligible to practice medicine. Each of the 50 states has its own statute that defines the practice of medicine and that requires the licensing of candidates by a state administrative agency before they may practice. These statutes are called *medical practice acts.* Obviously, it is important for you to become familiar with the medical practice act in your own state.

LICENSURE

Although the licensing criteria vary from state to state, they generally include graduation from an AMA–AAMC-accredited medical school, the successful completion of graduate medical training (such as internship and/or residency), endorsement of the National Boards, and/or the successful completion of a written (or sometimes oral) individual state-administered examination. The majority of American medical school graduates now qualify to be licensed through their successful completion of the National Boards (prepared by the National Board of Medical Examiners). Parts I and II of the Boards are often taken when the candidates are still in medical school. All states except Louisiana and Florida currently endorse the certificate of the National Boards when they license new physicians. Those medical school graduates who are candidates for licensure but who have not passed the National Boards must pass an individual state board exam (the exam most often used is the Federation Licensing Examination, called *FLEX*). American citizenship is no longer a requisite for licensure since the Supreme Court ruled that lack of U.S. citizenship was an unconstitutional reason for denying an otherwise successful candidate a license.

Licensure reciprocity among the states   When the state medical licensure boards originally made up their individual licensing examinations, each board had to be familiar with the tests used by other states in order to evaluate candidate physicians from these states prior to awarding them licenses without an additional exam. Thus, the states entered into reciprocity agreements among themselves whereby they agreed to endorse the qualifications of the doctors who had successfully passed the examinations of other states.

Physicians not having licenses   Many doctors engaged in research and administration do not hold licenses to practice. Similarly, there are many foreign doctors employed as residents or house staff members in American hospitals who have not yet been awarded full, unrestricted medical licenses. Many of the latter group do hold temporary licenses, however. These doctors work under the supervision of licensed physicians. According to the current edition of *Physician Distribution and Medical Licensure in the United States,* published by the AMA, there are over 38,000 physicians in the United States not holding full and unrestricted licenses.

Continuing education for license renewal   In July 1976 some 16 states had passed laws requiring doctors practicing there to prove that they have completed minimal amounts of continuing education before their licenses can be renewed. Several other states have similar legislation on the drawing boards. In fact, the state medical societies currently predict that before the next decade begins most states in this country will have passed continuing medical education laws. The usual continuing education requirements in the states having such laws is 150 hours of course work or an equivalent credit every three years.

Retention and revocation of licenses   No individual has a legal *right* to practice medicine. The *privilege* to practice may be granted by a state board only if the board is convinced of the candidate's competence. However, once a person has been granted a license to practice medicine, that license may not be revoked without satisfying due process of law. A state board retains the power to revoke a license from a physician—but only for good reason and only after the physician has had the opportunity to present a defense at a hearing. Although the criteria for revoking a license to practice vary from state to state, they generally include conviction of a felony, violation of ethical standards, or repeated gross and wanton negligence.

REGISTRATION
Licensure and *registration* are closely tied in together. Almost all state boards require physicians who are licensed in their states to register with them each year or every two years. A variable fee is required of the registering physician. Registration forms are sent to the physician every year or every two years by the state licensing board. When the physician receives such a form, he or she should fill it out promptly and return it with the required fee. If your physician is licensed to practice in several neighboring states (such as in Maryland, Virginia, and the District of Columbia), be sure that all of the annual registration renewal forms are neither misplaced in the office nor delayed in being mailed. It is also important to remember that not all states send out these forms at the same time of year.

CERTIFICATION
Certification in its most basic sense refers to the mechanism by which an individual health profession or a medical or other specialty identifies those of its members who have achieved a certain level of excellence according to the standards held by the profession or specialty. Certification is awarded by boards in the 22 medical specialties and by boards in eight dental specialties, 12 osteopathic specialties, one podiatric specialty, and seven veterinary specialty organizations. In addition, over 25 other independent and allied health professional organizations perform certification.

After having completed postgraduate training (such as internship and residency) or after having achieved a stated amount of experience or a combination of both, a physician can be recognized as a board-certified specialist upon successful completion of an examination administered by the specialty in which he or she wishes to practice.

Certification, though voluntary on the part of the candidate, is professionally necessary for the following important reasons: (1) most hospitals require a specialist to be board-certified before he or she will be granted staff privileges (2) health care accrediting groups use board certification as a way in which to evaluate the quality of the staff in hospitals and clinical laboratories (3) federal agencies consider certification an important factor in the hiring and promotion of specialist federal physicians (4) certification is one way in which a doctor can be granted a license to practice medicine in some states, and (5) Medicare regulations require board-certified or board-eligible specialists in certain hospital and clinical laboratory staff positions.

In short, certification has become in recent years much more than a recognition of excellence in a specialty discipline: it is now considered representative of an *essential minimal standard of specialist competence* that a candidate must possess before hoping to practice medicine within a specialty.

3.4

THE PHYSICIAN-PATIENT RELATIONSHIP

The law considers the physician-patient relationship to have three essential aspects: the contractual aspect, the consensual aspect, and the quality assurance aspect. Medical assistants should understand and appreciate each of these. Many problems in the physician-patient relationship occur because of a failure by either party or both to recognize the importance of one or more of these aspects.

THE CONTRACTUAL ASPECT
The law considers the physician-patient relationship to be contractual. This means that the relationship is voluntary both for the physician and for the patient. Generally speaking, physicians do not have a legal obligation to accept a person as a new patient; conversely, patients have the right to choose their own physicians. Neither can be coerced into the physician-patient relationship. However, two exceptions to the general rule should be identified. First, if a physician is responsible for providing emergency medical care in the emergency room of a hospital, the physician has been required by recent decisions to provide care for any person seeking emergency care who comes to the emergency room with an identifiable emergency. The reasoning behind this departure from the voluntary nature of the physician-patient relationship is rooted in the hospital's obligation to treat emergency patients since the presence of an emergency room encourages the people seeking emergency care to come to the hospital in the first place. The second departure from the rule is not so much an exception as it is a *waiver* of the physician's right to refuse to accept a person as a new patient. A physician who enters into an agreement to provide medical care to certain people (e.g., by accepting employment at a Veterans Administration Hospital) has the obligation to treat those persons who are eligible to receive this kind of care. Thus, physicians are free to waive their right to refuse to accept a person as a patient by entering into such agreements.

Up to this point, the discussion of the contractual aspect of the physician-patient relationship has dealt with the acceptance of new patients. But if a physician has already accepted a person as a patient, he or she then is obliged to provide appropriate treatment for as long as is necessary or to terminate the relationship in a manner consistent with the safety of the patient. (Termination of the relationship is discussed in section 3.5.)

A second element of the contractual aspect is the right of a physician to receive compensation for the services he or she has provided. Patients should be aware that they are responsible for the cost of the services rendered by physicians. Medical assistants should be aware of potential problems in identifying the party responsible for providing this compensation in cases (such as the treatment of minors) where the identification of the responsible party is not readily apparent. Many problems in the nonpayment of physicians' fees result from poor communication with the patient. (See also Chapter 12, section 12.1 for guidance in communicating fee information to patients.)

A third element of the contractual aspect is the existence of reasonable expectations on the part of each contracting party about the conduct of the other party. Patients have the right to expect that physicians will treat them in a manner consistent with the appropriate professional standard (see section 3.5). On the other hand, physicians have the right to expect that their patients will comply with the proposed treatment regimens and will keep their assigned appointments. This third element—patient compliance or noncompliance—also has been the source of many difficulties between physicians and patients.

THE CONSENSUAL ASPECT

The law also considers the physician-patient relationship to have a consensual aspect. This generally means that before physicians begin treatments, they must obtain the informed, voluntary, and competent consent of their patients. It is important to recognize that the essence of consent is *assent*—the agreement of the patient. Proper consent is not obtained simply by having a patient sign a written form. While written consent forms are important in the consent process (see section 3.5), they nevertheless are not sufficient by themselves. Obtaining the consent of a patient also requires clear <u>verbal</u> communication between the physician and the patient.

The law of consent is established by each of the 50 states for its citizens. Though individual state standards vary, it is nonetheless possible to examine elements of consent as a general policy. (Medical assistants should know what the laws of consent are in their specific states.)

By *competent consent,* the law means that the assent (the agreement to treatment) must be provided by a legally competent person. Generally speaking, an adult of sound mind is capable of providing the necessary consent. The age of adulthood is typically 18, but each medical assistant should determine what this age is in the individual practice setting. By and large, minors (those who have not reached the age of adulthood) do not have the legal authority to consent to treatment for themselves. Thus, the consent of a parent or a legal guardian is necessary in such cases. (However, a number of states do allow minors to consent to treatment in some or all cases.) Adults who have been declared legally incompetent and for whom a court has appointed a guardian cannot themselves give a competent consent. It is generally true that the consent of the legal guardian should be obtained before treatment can be provided to such people. By *voluntary consent,* the law means that the assent of the patient has been given freely and without duress or compulsion. By *informed consent,* the law means that the assent of the patient has been obtained after the physician has made an appropriate disclosure of the diagnosis, the prognosis, the proposed treatment, the risks of the proposed treatment, any alternatives to the proposed treatment, the risks of the alternatives, and the risks of nontreatment. A critical factor in determining what information is sufficient to satisfy this disclosure requirement is the standard required by each state. The traditional standard embraced by a majority of American states requires that the physician disclose what "a reasonable" physician would disclose in the same or in similar situations. This standard thus reflects the acceptable community standard. During recent years, several states have recognized an alternative standard requiring the physician to disclose the information that a "reasonable" patient needs to know in order to make an intelligent decision. It is evident, then, that the focus of this alternative standard has shifted from the medical community to the general community of citizens. The medical assistant should know which is the appropriate standard in his or her state.

Three special situations in the consent process need to be appreciated. First of all, patients who are unconscious are by definition incapable of consenting to treatment. Nonetheless, these individuals generally retain the right to expect that health care will be provided them. Especially in an emergency situation, a physician should not hesitate to give the necessary medical care because of the patient's unconsciousness. In general, the law allows the physician to act on the patient's implied consent and to proceed with treatment.

Emergency situations involving conscious patients who are not legally competent should be handled in a similar fashion. A patient should not be allowed to suffer without treatment in an emergency situation simply because the parent or legal guardian cannot be reached for consent. The existence of an emergency generally will allow a physician to imply the consent of a parent or guardian and to provide the necessary treatment.

THE QUALITY ASSURANCE ASPECT

The law considers the physician-patient relationship to have a quality assurance aspect legally obligating the physician to provide medical care of appropriate quality. The physician is required to provide health care of the same quality as that of a "reasonable" physician in the same or similar circumstances. The most important mechanism for ensuring quality care is the medical malpractice aspect of the law. (See section 3.5.)

PATIENT RIGHTS

Patients undergoing health care do not sacrifice their human rights by virtue of their having become ill or injured. In recent years, the patients' rights movement has had a dramatic influence on the physician-patient relationship. Some patients' rights arise out of the three legal aspects of the physician-patient relationship. Others merely represent an application of the more general rights that citizens in our society possess. But regardless of their source these legally enforceable rights play a key role in protecting the patients' interests.

The most famous statement of patients' rights was set forth by the American Hospital Association in November 1972. It is given below.

STATEMENT ON A PATIENT'S BILL OF RIGHTS
Affirmed by the Board of Trustees
American Hospital Association
November 17, 1972

The American Hospital Association presents a Patient's Bill of Rights with the expectation that observance of these rights will contribute to more effective patient care and greater satisfaction for the patient, his physician, and the hospital organization. Further, the Association presents these rights in the expectation that they will be supported by the hospital on behalf of its patients, as an integral part of the healing process. It is recognized that a personal relationship between the physician and the patient is essential for the provision of proper medical care. The traditional physician-patient relationship takes on a new dimension when care is rendered within an organizational structure. Legal precedent has established that the institution itself also has a responsibility to the patient. It is in recognition of these factors that these rights are affirmed.

1. The patient has the right to considerate and respectful care.
2. The patient has the right to obtain from his physician complete current information

concerning his diagnosis, treatment, and prognosis in terms the patient can be reasonably expected to understand. When it is not medically advisable to give such information to the patient, the information should be made available to an appropriate person in his behalf. He has the right to know by name, the physician responsible for coordinating his care.

3. The patient has the right to receive from his physician information necessary to give informed consent prior to the start of any procedure and/or treatment. Except in emergencies, such information for informed consent, should include but not necessarily be limited to the specific procedure and/or treatment, the medically significant risks involved, and the probable duration of incapacitation. Where medically significant alternatives for care or treatment exist, or when the patient requests information concerning medical alternatives, the patient has the right to such information. The patient also has the right to know the name of the person responsible for the procedures and/or treatment.

4. The patient has the right to refuse treatment to the extent permitted by law, and to be informed of the medical consequences of his action.

5. The patient has the right to every consideration of his privacy concerning his own medical care program. Case discussion, consultation, examination, and treatment are confidential and should be conducted discreetly. Those not directly involved in his care must have the permission of the patient to be present.

6. The patient has the right to expect that all communications and records pertaining to his care should be treated as confidential.

7. The patient has the right to expect that within its capacity a hospital must make reasonable response to the request of a patient for services. The hospital must provide evaluation, service, and/or referral as indicated by the urgency of the case. When medically permissible a patient may be transferred to another facility only after he has received complete information and explanation concerning the needs for and alternatives to such a transfer. The institution to which the patient is to be transferred must first have accepted the patient for transfer.

8. The patient has the right to obtain information as to any relationship of his hospital to other health care and educational institutions insofar as his care is concerned. The patient has the right to obtain information as to the existence of any professional relationships among individuals, by name, who are treating him.

9. The patient has the right to be advised if the hospital proposes to engage in or perform human experimentation affecting his care or treatment. The patient has the right to refuse to participate in such research projects.

10. The patient has the right to expect reasonable continuity of care. He has the right to know in advance what appointment times and physicians are available and where. The patient has the right to expect that the hospital will provide a mechanism whereby he is informed by his physician or a delegate of the physician of the patient's continuing health care requirements following discharge.

11. The patient has the right to examine and receive an explanation of his bill regardless of source of payment.

12. The patient has the right to know what hospital rules and regulations apply to his conduct as a patient.

No catalogue of rights can guarantee for the patient the kind of treatment he has a right to expect. A hospital has many functions to perform, including the prevention and treatment of disease, the education of both health professionals and patients, and the conduct of clinical research. All these activities must be conducted with an overriding concern for the patient, and, above all, the recognition of his dignity as a human being. Success in achieving this recognition assures success in the defense of the rights of the patient.

Reprinted with the permission of the American Hospital Association.

The primary focus of those interested in asserting and protecting patients' rights has been directed to a person's right of self-determination. The doctrine of consent, as earlier described, is designed to allow the patient to exercise this right. However, not all rights claimed by the patient are legally enforceable. In fact, some of them are more accurately called *moral rights*. Even though moral rights may not be enforceable under the law, nonetheless they must be identified and respected as well as those which are legally enforceable.

The existence of patients' rights also raises questions as to the physician's responsibility in a case where the patient refuses to comply with the physician's orders or when the patient fails to appear at scheduled appointments. Since the patient has the right to refuse treatment and to change physicians, cases of noncompliance or broken appointments would appear to be the patient's and not the physician's responsibility. However, this is true only if it is clear that the physician has communicated to the patient the seriousness of the situation and the importance of compliance and/or follow-up.

3.5

PROFESSIONAL LIABILITY OF PHYSICIANS

In daily life, all citizens are expected to act in a reasonable fashion toward each other. Many normal activities—driving a car, maintaining a house, operating machinery, and others—have the potential to inflict harm on others if the activities are not carried out prudently. The Anglo-American legal system has long recognized the many ways in which one person's conduct is capable of causing harm to another. The general legal mechanism designed to prevent the injury of other people is called the *negligence* area of the law of torts. The specific application of the general rules of negligence to a professional relationship with a client is called *malpractice*. Medical malpractice is, therefore, one aspect of the larger concept of negligence. *Black's Law Dictionary* defines *malpractice* in its broadest sense as "any professional misconduct, unreasonable lack of skill or fidelity in professional or fiduciary duties, evil practice, or illegal or immoral conduct." It then goes on to say that with regard to physicians and surgeons, the word generally means "professional misconduct towards a patient which is considered reprehensible either because [it is] immoral in itself or because [it is] contrary to law or [is] expressly forbidden by law." Even more specifically, the term means "bad, wrong, or injudicious treatment of a patient, professionally and in respect to the particular disease or injury, resulting in injury, unnecessary suffering, or death to the patient, and proceeding from ignorance, carelessness, want of proper professional skill, disregard of established rules or principles, neglect, or a malicious or criminal intent."

The elements that have to be demonstrated in order to prove that a physician or other health care provider has been guilty of malpractice are the same as those that have to be proved in any case of negligence. The five elements include:

1. **Duty**   The defendant physician owed a duty of reasonable care to the plaintiff patient;
2. **Breach of Duty**   The conduct of the defendant physician was such that it breached the duty owed to the plaintiff patient;
3. **Causation I**   The conduct of the defendant physician was the direct cause (cause in fact) of the harm suffered by the plaintiff patient;
4. **Causation II**   The conduct of the defendant physician was the proximate cause [the last negligent act contributory to an injury without which the injury would not have resulted] of the harm suffered by the plaintiff patient;
5. **Damages**   The plaintiff patient suffered actual harm.

All five elements must be present in a case in order for malpractice to be established.

It is obvious that malpractice is a major concern of physicians. Consequently, medical assistants should be aware of opportunities to avoid problems that might lead to malpractice liability. First of all, it is important that the patient's medical record be accurate, up-to-date, and legible. The medical record should contain all relevant information about the patient. In the event that a question arises about the care that has been provided the patient, the medical record will become the key resource in resolving differences. In this regard, it cannot be overemphasized that the medical assistant should ensure that all materials are properly filed. Furthermore, there is no substitution for good communication in the physician-patient relationship; good communication can prevent misunderstandings which can lead to more serious medicolegal problems. The medical assistant should facilitate the communication process by treating all patients with courtesy and by helping them find appropriate answers to their questions. A third key way to avoid malpractice problems is by use of appropriate written forms. As part of their office policies, physicians should develop, in consultation with their attorneys, written forms dealing with incidents that should be recorded and made part of the patients' medical records. Examples of such forms include:

1. consent forms
2. parental consent forms for minor children
3. consent forms for the performance of autopsies
4. permission forms for a patient to allow the physician to disclose confidential information
5. form letters announcing to a patient that the physician is withdrawing from the case
6. form letters to patients who habitually miss appointments or who fail to comply with the physician's instructions.

These forms should be written in a way enabling the doctor to adjust them to meet the needs of each specific case. The forms are not illustrated here because their wording depends on the laws of the various states. Form letters are not illustrated for the same reason. However, it is important to mention that local and state medical societies, specialty societies, and hospitals frequently have developed specific forms that have proved satisfactory for their particular locales. The physician and the medical assistant should look into the possibility of using these materials if they are available. Another solution is for the doctor and the doctor's attorney to develop the wording of the forms and the form letters. Regardless of how the material is drawn up, it should be checked and updated once a year. It is the assistant's responsibility to see that the material is properly typed, proofread, and signed. All such forms should be mailed promptly, and photocopies of them should be kept in the physician's files.

Medical assistants should be familiar with some of the terminology used in malpractice cases. For instance, the term *statute of limitations* refers to the time period within which a malpractice suit must be filed by the patient. This period varies from state to state. A suit filed after the period has expired cannot be prosecuted. Physicians accused of malpractice may allege in response that they were not responsible for the injuries to the patient because the patient was also negligent (*contributory negligence*) or that the patient accepted the risk of harm (*assumption of the risk*). Medical assistants should at least know whether these defenses are available in their respective states.

Virtually all of the states have *good samaritan statutes* designed to encourage physicians to provide emergency medical care to persons injured in automobile accidents. These statutes afford the physician protection against certain types of liability. Medical assistants should know whether there is a good samaritan statute in their states and if so, what type of immunity the statute provides.

The physician should always remember that while a patient may terminate a physician-patient relationship at any time, the physician is nevertheless obliged to terminate the relationship in a way consistent with the best interests of the patient's health. This usually requires that a transition period be allowed so that the patient may obtain a new physician. Failure to provide for such a transition period could render a physician liable for abandonment.

3.6

REGULATION OF NARCOTICS AND OTHER MEDICATIONS

Practicing physicians may prescribe, dispense, or administer drugs or narcotics in the treatment of their patients. However, the prescribing, dispensing, or administering of drugs or narcotics must be made in compliance with federal and state laws regulating such practices. It is important for medical assistants to understand the basic elements of this regulation and to assist their physicians in satisfying the legal obligations required of them. Several goals are sought in the laws influencing this segment of medical practice. They are:

1. the safeguarding of the interests of consumers using dangerous products;
2. the prevention of fraud by keeping impure, mislabeled, or adulterated drugs out of the marketplace;
3. the promotion of the public health, safety, and welfare;
4. the prevention of drug addiction or dependency when possible.

To achieve these goals, the United States Congress and the individual state legislatures have passed laws regulating the manufacture, possession, sale, prescription, administration, and dispensing of a range of medicines. A comprehensive system of regulation has therefore emerged. Medical assistants should know and understand the laws regulating drugs and narcotics in their specific states.

The cornerstone of the federal regulation of drug use is The Federal Food, Drug and Cosmetic Act (21 *U.S.C.* 321). This statute follows in the tradition of its predecessor, The Food and Drug Act of 1906.

The general purpose of The Federal Food, Drug and Cosmetic Act is to control the movement in interstate commerce of impure and adulterated food and drugs. For the purpose of the Act, the term *drug* means:

Those articles recognized in the official *United States Pharmacopeia,* official *Homeopathic Pharmacopeia of the United States,* or official *National Formulary,* or any supplement to them; articles, other than food, intended to affect the structure or any function of the body of man or other animals;

and articles intended for use as a component of any articles specified in the above clauses.

The Statute forbids, among other things: (1) the introduction or delivery for introduction into interstate commerce of any drug that is adulterated or misbranded (2) the adulteration or misbranding of any drug in interstate commerce (3) the receipt in interstate commerce of any drug that is adulterated or misbranded, and (4) the failure to maintain the required records or to permit inspection of these records by authorized agents.

Of particular importance to the medical assistant are the required reports and records that must be established and maintained in the doctor's office. The report and record requirements may be modified or eliminated by subsequent changes in either the statute or the regulations. The Federal Food, Drug and Cosmetic Act requires the establishment, maintenance, and reporting to the Secretary of Health, Education and Welfare of data (including analytical reports by investigators) obtained during the investigational use of a new drug. Such reports are used to evaluate the safety and effectiveness of the new drug. Medical assistants should aid their physicians in complying with these requirements.

The cornerstone of federal regulation of narcotic use is The Comprehensive Drug Abuse Prevention and Control Act (21 *U.S.C.* 801), which superseded or repealed earlier statutory provisions such as The Jones-Miller Act and The Harrison Narcotic Act. The principal goal of this Act is to regulate the manufacture, distribution, dispensing, or possession of controlled substances. The Statute authorizes the attorney general to promulgate and enforce rules and regulations concerning the registration and control of the manufacture, distribution, and dispensing of controlled substances. The Statute sets forth five schedules of controlled substances. Each of the five schedules is discussed below.

SCHEDULE I.
(A) The drug or other substance has a high potential for abuse.
(B) The drug or other substance has no currently accepted medical use in treatment in the United States.
(C) There is a lack of accepted safety for use of the drug or other substance under medical supervision.

Schedule I includes (unless specifically excepted by the attorney general or unless listed in another schedule) any of the following opiates including their isomers, esters, ethers, salts, and salts of isomers, esters, and ethers, whenever the existence of such isomers, esters, ethers, and salts is possible within the specific chemical designation:

1. Acetylmethadol	15. Diethylthiambutene	29. Morpheridine
2. Allylprodine	16. Dimenoxadol	30. Noracymethadol
3. Alphacetylmathadol	17. Dimepheptanol	31. Norlevorphanol
4. Alphameprodine	18. Dimethylthiambutene	32. Normethadone
5. Alphamethadol	19. Dioxaphetyl butyrate	33. Norpipanone
6. Benzethidine	20. Dipipanone	34. Phenadoxone
7. Betacetylmethadol	21. Ethylmethylthiambutene	35. Phenampromide
8. Betameprodine	22. Etonitazene	36. Phenomorphan
9. Betamethadol	23. Etoxeridine	37. Phenoperidine
10. Betaprodine	24. Furethidine	38. Piritramide
11. Clonitazene	25. Hydroxypethidine	39. Proheptazine
12. Dextromoramide	26. Ketobemidone	40. Properidine
13. Dextrorphan	27. Levomoramide	41. Racemoramide
14. Diampromide	28. Levophenacylmorphan	42. Trimeperidine.

Schedule I also includes (unless excepted by the attorney general or unless listed in another schedule) any of the following opium derivatives, their salts, isomers, and salts of isomers whenever the existence of such salts, isomers, and salts of isomers is possible within the specific chemical designation:

1. Acetorphine	12. Methyldesorphine
2. Acetyldihydrocodeine	13. Methylhydromorphine
3. Benzylmorphine	14. Morphine methylbromide
4. Codeine methylbromide	15. Morphine methylsulfonate
5. Codeine-N-Oxide	16. Morphine-N-Oxide
6. Cyprenorphine	17. Myrophine
7. Desomorphine	18. Nicocodeine
8. Dihydromorphine	19. Nicomorphine
9. Etorphine	20. Normorphine
10. Heroin	21. Pholcodine
11. Hydromorphinol	22. Thebacon.

Also included in Schedule I (unless specifically excepted by the attorney general or unless listed in another schedule) is any material, compound, mixture, or preparation containing any quantity of the following hallucinogenic substances or any of their salts, isomers, and salts of isomers whenever the existence of such salts, isomers, and salts of isomers is possible within the specific chemical designation:

1. 3,4-methylenedioxy amphetamine
2. 5-methoxy-3,4-methylenedioxy amphetamine
3. 3,4,5-trimethoxy amphetamine
4. Bufotenine
5. Diethyltryptamine
6. Dimethyltryptamine
7. 4-methyl-2,5-dimethoxyamphetamine
8. Ibogaine
9. Lysergic acid diethylamide (LSD)
10. Marihuana
11. Mescaline
12. Peyote
13. N-ethyl-3-piperidyl benzilate
14. N-methyl-3-piperidyl benzilate
15. Psilocybin
16. Psilocyn
17. Tetrahydrocannabinols.

SCHEDULE II.

(A) The drug or other substance has a high potential for abuse.
(B) The drug or other substance has a currently accepted medical use in treatment in the United States or a currently accepted medical use with severe restrictions.
(C) Abuse of the drug or other substances may lead to severe psychological or physical dependence.

Schedule II includes (unless specifically excepted by the attorney general or unless listed in another schedule) any of the following substances, whether produced directly or indirectly by extraction from substances of vegetable origin, or independently by means of chemical synthesis, or by a combination of extraction and chemical synthesis:

(A) Opium and opiate, and any salt, compound, derivative, or preparation of opium or opiate.
(B) Any salt, compound, derivative, or preparation thereof which is chemically equivalent or identical with any of the substances referred to in clause (A), except that these substances shall not include the isoquinoline alkaloids of opium.
(C) Opium poppy and poppy straw.
(D) Coca leaves and any salt, compound, derivative, or preparation of coca leaves, and any salt, compound, derivative, or preparation thereof which is chemically equivalent or identical with any of these substances, except that the substances shall not include decocainized coca leaves or extraction of coca leaves, which extractions do not contain cocaine or ecgonine.

Schedule II also includes (unless specifically excepted by the attorney general or unless listed in another schedule) any of the following opiates, including their isomers, esters, ethers, salts, and salts of isomers, esters and ethers, whenever the existence of such isomers, esters, ethers, and salts is possible within the specific chemical designation:

1. Alphaprodine
2. Anileridine
3. Bezitramide
4. Dihydrocodeine

5. Diphenoxylate
6. Fentanyl
7. Isomethadone
8. Levomethorphan
9. Levorphanol
10. Metazocine
11. Methadone
12. Methadone-Intermediate, 4-cyano-2-dimethylamino-4,4-diphenyl butane
13. Moramide-Intermediate, 2-methyl-3-morpholino-1,1-diphenylpropane-carboxylic acid
14. Pethidine
15. Pethidine-Intermediate-A,4-cyano-1-methyl-4-phenylpiperidine
16. Pethidine-Intermediate-B,ethyl-4-phenylpiperidine-4-carboxylate
17. Pethidine-Intermediate-C,1-methyl-4-phenylpiperidine-4-carboxylic acid
18. Phenazocine
19. Piminodine
20. Racemethorphan
21. Racemorphan.

Schedule II also includes (unless specifically excepted by the attorney general or unless listed in another schedule) any injectable liquid containing any quantity of methamphetamine, including its salts, isomers, and salts of isomers.

SCHEDULE III.

(A) The drug or other substance has a potential for abuse less than the drugs or other substances in Schedules I and II.
(B) The drug or other substance has a currently accepted medical use in treatment in the United States.
(C) Abuse of the drug or other substance may lead to moderate or low physical dependence or high psychological dependence.

Schedule III includes (unless specifically excepted by the attorney general or unless listed in another schedule) any material, compound, mixture, or preparation containing any quantity of the following substances having a stimulant effect on the central nervous system:

1. Amphetamine, its salts, optical isomers, and salts of its optical isomers
2. Phenmetrazine and its salts
3. Any substance (except an injectable liquid) which contains any quantity of methamphetamine, including its salts, isomers, and salts of isomers
4. Methylphenidate.

Schedule III also includes (unless specifically excepted by the attorney general or unless listed in another schedule) any material, compound, mixture, or preparation containing any quantity of the following substances having a depressant effect on the central nervous system:

1. Any substance which contains any quantity of a derivative of barbituric acid, or any salt of a derivative of barbituric acid
2. Chorhexadol
3. Glutethimide
4. Lysergic acid
5. Lysergic acid amide
6. Methyprylon
7. Phencyclidine
8. Sulfondiethylmethane
9. Sulfonethylmethane
10. Sulfonmethane.

Schedule III also includes Nalorphine (and unless specifically excepted by the attorney general or unless listed in another schedule) any material, compound, mixture, or preparation containing limited quantities of any of the following narcotic drugs, or any salts thereof:

1. Not more than 1.8 grams of codeine per 100 milliliters or not more than 90 milligrams per dosage unit, with an equal or greater quantity of an isoquinoline alkaloid of opium;
2. Not more than 1.8 grams of codeine per 100 milliliters or not more than 90 milligrams per dosage unit, with one or more active, nonnarcotic ingredients in recognized therapeutic amounts;
3. Not more than 300 milligrams of dihydrocodeinone per 100 milliliters or not more than 15 milligrams per dosage unit, with a fourfold or greater quantity of an isoquinoline alkaloid of opium;
4. Not more than 300 milligrams of dihydrocodeinone per 100 milliliters or not more than 15 milligrams per dosage unit, with one or more active, nonnarcotic ingredients in recognized therapeutic amounts;
5. Not more than 1.8 grams of dihydrocodeine per 100 milliliters or not more than 90 milligrams per dosage unit, with one or more active, nonnarcotic ingredients in recognized therapeutic amounts;
6. Not more than 300 milligrams of ethylmorphine per 100 milliliters or not more than 15 milligrams per dosage unit, with one or more active, nonnarcotic ingredients in recognized therapeutic amounts;
7. Not more than 500 milligrams of opium per 100 milliliters or per 100 grams, or not more than 25 milligrams per dosage unit, with one or more active, nonnarcotic ingredients in recognized therapeutic amounts;
8. Not more than 50 milligrams of morphine per 100 milliliters or per 100 grams with one or more active, nonnarcotic ingredients in recognized amounts.

SCHEDULE IV.

(A) The drug or other substance has a low potential for abuse relative to the drugs or other substances in Schedule III.
(B) The drug or other substance has a currently accepted medical use in treatment in the United States.
(C) Abuse of the drug or other substance may lead to limited physical dependence or psychological dependence relative to the drugs or other substances in Schedule III.

Schedule IV includes:

1. Barbital
2. Chloral betaine
3. Chloral hydrate
4. Ethchlorvynol
5. Ethinamate
6. Methohexital
7. Meprobamate
8. Methylphenobarbital
9. Paraldehyde
10. Petrichloral
11. Phenobarbital

SCHEDULE V.

(A) The drug or other substance has a low potential for abuse relative to the drugs or other substances in Schedule IV.
(B) The drug or other substance has a currently accepted medical use in treatment in the United States.
(C) Abuse of the drug or other substance may lead to limited physical dependence or psychological dependence relative to the drugs or other substances in Schedule IV.

Schedule V includes any compound, mixture, or preparation containing any of the following limited quantities of narcotic drugs, which shall include one or more non-narcotic active medicinal ingredients in sufficient proportion to confer on the compound, mixture, or preparation valuable medicinal qualities other than those possessed by the narcotic drug alone:

1. Not more than 200 milligrams of codeine per 100 milliliters or per 100 grams;
2. Not more than 100 milligrams of dihydrocodeine per 100 milliliters or per 100 grams;
3. Not more than 100 milligrams of ethylmorphine per 100 milliliters or per 100 grams;
4. Not more than 2.5 milligrams of diphenoxylate and not less than 25 micrograms of atropine sulfate per dosage unit;
5. Not more than 100 milligrams of opium per 100 milliliters or per 100 grams.

The Statute also requires the registration of any manufacturer, distributor, dispenser, or clinical investigator of controlled substances with the attorney general. Medical assistants should ensure that their physicians are properly registered. Failure to be properly registered could lead a physician to significant criminal and civil liability.

Failure to comply with the regulations promulgated under either The Federal Food, Drug and Cosmetic Act or The Comprehensive Drug Abuse Prevention and Control Act may lead to the physician's loss of the right to prescribe and dispense medicine. Narcotics officers have the right to visit the physician's office and, upon presentation of valid identification, to review the physician's records and his or her office policy. Medical assistants should play a major role in helping their physicians avoid potential liability by carefully keeping appropriate records, by guarding the prescription pads and preventing their misuse by nonphysicians, by locking storage cabinets and other places where medications are kept to prevent stealing, and by placing drug samples in an appropriately secure location. The assistant can also help the physician avoid potential liability by ensuring that drugs whose shelf lives have been exceeded are properly removed and destroyed.

The medical assistant also should be aware that an individual state may supplement the federal legislation with its own laws. It is therefore critical for the assistant to learn what laws in the specific state need to be followed with respect to medication.

3.7

REPORTS REQUIRED BY LAW

In addition to the specific responsibilities which they have to their patients, physicians also have responsibilities to society in general. Often these responsibilities are formulated in mandatory reporting statutes. Mandatory reporting statutes obligate doctors to file a report with a designated local or state official each time a specific problem is encountered. Required reports include those for births, deaths, fetal deaths, gunshot wounds, the occurrence of certain contagious diseases (as venereal diseases), and incidents of child abuse. Reporting requirements vary from state to state. Medical assistants should make every effort to identify the cases in which such reports should be filed, the agencies to which the reports should be forwarded, the forms required, and the specific information that must be included in the reports. Medical assistants should help their physicians in speedily complying with these requirements. (Failure to comply with them could result in the imposition of a fine.) One way to assist the physician in the forwarding of these reports to the appropriate agencies is to have on hand an adequate supply of the various kinds of report forms used by state and federal organizations. The assistant also should proofread the completed reports and should ensure that they have been signed by the doctor prior to transmittal. Office copies of all such documents should be made and kept.

3.8

THE PHYSICIAN IN THE COURTROOM

In an era of widespread reliance on the courts to resolve conflicts, it is increasingly likely that the physician will become personally involved in litigation as a defendant, as a plaintiff, or as an expert witness. Medical assistants should appreciate the differences in these roles and should provide their physicians support if the doctors have to participate in court actions.

Physicians are considered defendants in the legal system when they have been sued by another party. For instance, a physician accused of malpractice is the defendant in that case. Physicians are considered plaintiffs in the legal system when they sue another party. As an example, a physician who sues a patient for non-payment of bills is a plaintiff in that case. Physicians are considered expert witnesses when they are called on to testify to such matters as the appropriate standard of care in a given case or to the extent and nature of injuries in an accident case. Either a plaintiff or a defendant has the right to use an expert witness to establish this standard. For example, if J.D. (plaintiff) sues Dr. X (defendant) for malpractice and calls on Dr. Y to establish what a "reasonable" physician of the community would do in the same or similar circumstances, Dr. Y would be functioning as an expert witness in this particular case.

A physician who is a defendant in a legal case needs to prepare a line of defense carefully. The most important information available to the physician in a medical lawsuit will be derived from the medical record. The physician will often be asked to describe what was done in a specific case, based solely on what is contained in the record. The litigation may occur some years after the treatment was performed. It is therefore critical that medical records be kept accurately, that they be filed appropriately, and that they be available to the physician who is a defendant.

A physician who is a plaintiff also needs to have sufficient information to present the case effectively. Medical records may play a key role in this situation as well, especially when a question arises as to what services the physician has provided. Again, the importance of proper medical record administration cannot be overemphasized.

The physician who is an expert witness is expected to discuss the case in terms of what actually happened and what should have happened. This assignment requires broad knowledge of the current state of practice in the community. In all three examples, the medical assistant should take steps to aid the physician in preparing for court activity. The physician will inform the assistant of the tasks that must be performed in each situation.

3.9

LEGAL RESPONSIBILITIES OF THE MEDICAL ASSISTANT/ADMINISTRATIVE

The medical assistant is not a *licensed* health care provider even though the assistant may hold certification from a professional medical assisting organization; hence, in the eyes of the law the physician-employer is the individual ultimately responsible for all acts carried out by the assistant as his or her employee. This responsibility is delineated under the doctrine of *respondent superior* whereby an employer is considered liable for the negligent actions of the employee. If the assistant is aware of the potential medicolegal problems which could create liability for the doctor and for the assistant, these problems can be avoided. Of prime importance is the assistant's legal obligation to respect the rights of the physician's patients. Failure to do so can result in the assistant's liability as an individual or as an employee of the physician, or it can result in joint liability with the physician.

Familiarity with the state's medical practice act is also essential, as stated earlier in this chapter. For example, some procedures and seemingly routine assignments may be carried out in some states only by licensed health providers (such as registered nurses, physicians, and physicians' assistants). For a medical assistant to perform such acts even if directed to do so could constitute the illegal practice of medicine, interference in a medical case, or both.

Aside from becoming familiar with the medical practice act of the state where the assistant is employed, the assistant has other obligations. One of them is to carry out all reasonable and lawful orders of the physician. Another is to avoid at all times the performance of any act that may prove dangerous to a patient. A third is never to overstep the task boundaries established by the physician for the assistant. A fourth obligation is to know one's level of competence and not to exceed it.

The physician ought to give the assistant a written outline of the tasks the assistant is expected to perform and a list of those tasks the assistant is not to perform. Such lists are especially important to medical assistants whose job descriptions include clinical responsibilities. In this regard, the clinical task list should be annotated by the physician to indicate the procedures that must be accomplished under his or her direct personal supervision and the procedures that may be carried out unsupervised but only under his or her direct orders. The nature of the lists and the ways in which the tasks are to be carried out depend on the medical practice act of the state where the office is located and on the professional judgment and personal wishes of the physician.

LIABILITY OF THE MEDICAL ASSISTANT

It is very important for the medical assistant to understand that supporting or aiding another individual in the commission of an illegal act—albeit unwittingly or unintentionally—can make the assistant liable as an accessory or even a conspirator. For instance, an individual who, being absent at the time that a crime is committed, still assists, encourages, or induces another person to commit the act is deemed an *accessory before the fact.* A person who stands by without interfering or attempting to prevent a criminal offense is deemed an *accessory during the fact.* Likewise, an individual who knows fully that an unlawful act has been committed but nevertheless chooses to conceal that information or decides to protect the offender is considered an *accessory after the fact.* A *conspirator* is an individual who joins with one or more other persons to jointly commit an unlawful act or an act which, though innocent in itself, becomes unlawful when carried out by the concerted action of the individuals.

These definitions bear clear implications to the medical assistant: any assistant who helps—knowingly or unknowingly—a physician in the committing of an unlawful act can be held liable for prosecution as an accessory or as a conspirator, depending of course on the nature of the act. While the assistant is indeed expected to be loyal to the physician and to carry out all reasonable and lawful orders issued by the physician, the assistant nevertheless must not support, aid, encourage, or protect the physician-employer or any member of the office staff in the performance of an unlawful act even if instructed to do so. Furthermore, the assistant should resist any requests by the physician or by a patient which involve carrying out acts beyond the scope of the assistant's competence and responsibility. Medical assistants also should avoid delegating responsibility to any other employee if that responsibility is beyond the competence and ability of the employee.

LEGAL PRECAUTIONS FOR THE MEDICAL ASSISTANT: Specific Examples

Careless chatter   Be very careful what you say and to whom you say it—both on duty and off duty. Although this is an ethical matter (see Chapter 4), it is also a legal matter that can have grave consequences. Your position requiring constant interaction with patients, physicians, and other office callers as well as your knowledge of confidential data can make you vulnerable to charges of slander or libel if you are not extremely careful in your oral and written communications.

Black's Law Dictionary defines slander as "the speaking of base and defamatory words tending to prejudice another in his reputation, office, trade, business, or means of livelihood." The same dictionary defines libel as "a method of defamation expressed by print, writing, pictures, or signs . . . . malicious falsehood expressed by writing, painting, or by signs and pictures, which tends to bring any person into disrepute, contempt, or ridicule." Obviously, all of your written and spoken communication must be above legal reproach. The following examples illustrate the dangers of untrue statements and loose talk. Take, for instance, Ms. X who is bitter about her past employment with Dr. Y, for whom she no longer works. To get even, Ms. X spreads the false story that Dr. Y dispensed narcotics to known addicts in the neighborhood. By doing this, Ms. X has left herself open to possible litigation. In fact, any false statement denigrating the professional ability or conduct of the physician can constitute grounds for litigation.

In the same way, loose talk on the part of a well-meaning, loyal, but unthinking medical assistant can embroil the physician in a lawsuit. Consider the case of Ms. A who commented to one of Dr. B's new patients thusly, "I can't see why Dr. Z didn't put you on [drug name] and then have you hospitalized. Oh, well, at least you've come to Dr. B. She'll have you back on your feet very soon." Ms. A's remarks are doubly dangerous: (1) the patient could interpret the comments to mean that Dr. Z has been negligent—and if the patient is already dissatisfied with the care received from Dr. Z, the patient may be in the mood to litigate the matter, and (2) the patient could construe the last remark as a guarantee that Dr. B will "cure" the illness when in fact the assistant is in no position to evaluate the case or to guarantee the patient anything.

Careless, offhand remarks on the telephone or in person in a busy office situation can also cause untold damage. For example, if a patient comes in with pains and you ask him or her whether any medication has been taken, you should never comment positively or negatively on the medication that the patient may indicate has been taken. Saying "That's good," or "That's bad for you" is taboo. Only the doctor can make such judgments and remarks. Simply note the medication on the record and inform the doctor before the examination proceeds. In busy offices, patients will frequently call in for telephone consultations about their conditions or parents will seek advice about the conditions of their sick children. No matter how much you may be tempted to offer advice, DO NOT PRESUME TO DIAGNOSE THE COMPLAINT OR TO PRESCRIBE MEDICATION. This could be taken as an attempt on your part to practice medicine.

In summary, the medical assistant should never try to evaluate a case, a condition, or the competence and decisions of any health care provider. Never offer a medical recommendation: an inaccurate or inappropriate word or comment may fail to take into account the complexity of the case or it may suggest that the assistant possesses sufficient expertise to play a role in the patient's care. Such actions can jeopardize the patient's care and can result in injury to the patient. A malpractice suit or an allegation of the illegal practice of medicine can also result.

NOTE: Chapter 6 offers ways by which you can avoid or terminate conversations with patients about other physicians when the patients insist on drawing you into such discussions.

Office safety   Remember that patients can have accidents in the office and that the physician can be sued as a result. Do the following to ensure maximum office safety:

1. See that the floors are not slippery after they have been washed and/or waxed.
2. Help those patients who require assistance in walking, undressing and dressing, and preparing for examinations. (This includes helping them onto the examining table.)
3. Never leave very ill, infirm, infant, or very young patients unattended in examining rooms or toilet areas.
4. Ensure that all equipment is in clean, safe operating condition.
5. Make sure that the doctor's accident liability insurance policies are kept up-to-date and that the premiums are paid on time.

Prescription pads and medications   Although the point is repeated over and over in this book, the repetition is justified: DO NOT LEAVE PRESCRIPTION PADS AND MEDICATIONS (INCLUDING SAMPLES) IN EXAMINING ROOMS WHERE PATIENTS CAN HAVE FREE ACCESS TO THEM. This rule is ignored by many individuals. With the current emphasis on drug law enforcement (see section 3.6) and the stiff penalties one can pay for noncompliance with the letter of the law, it is frightening to observe the carelessness of some staff members and physicians with regard to the security of these kinds of items.

Diplomacy with potentially litigious patients   Be especially conciliatory and diplomatic with overly emotional patients whom you know or suspect are dissatisfied with the treatment ordered by your physician. Your responsibility is to foster and not impair the physician-patient relationship. If a particular situation becomes unmanageable, inform the doctor at once, but in the meantime try to do your part to soothe the upset or angry patient. (See also Chapter 6 for specific suggestions that may be of help to you in dealing with various kinds of problematic patients.)

Record-keeping   Section 3.5 and Chapters 4 and 9 all discuss the importance of keeping accurate, complete medical records. From the legal standpoint alone, the importance of good medical record management cannot be overstressed. A patient's record may be needed at any time as evidence attesting to the nature and the quality of care rendered by the doctor and whether or not the patient followed the treatment program recommended by the doctor.

Third-party inquiries   No data on any patient may be released by the medical assistant to a third party without written permission of the patient and the physician's knowledge and approval. Record confidentiality is a prime legal concern of the medical assistant. (See also Chapter 9.)

Professional liability insurance   Make sure that you are covered in the doctor's professional liability (malpractice) insurance policy. As indicated at the beginning of this section, you could become a party to litigation against your employer, so you do need this sort of coverage.

4

CHAPTER FOUR

MEDICAL ETHICS

CONTENTS

4.1

INTRODUCTION

Any discussion of medical ethics must be introduced by a definition of *ethics* itself. In its most basic sense, the word *ethics* means the discipline dealing with what is good and bad or right and wrong or with moral duty and obligation. More specifically, the word means the principles of conduct governing an individual or a group. These principles of conduct are used especially by groups to regulate or control the actions and activities of the individual members and to establish general standards of conduct which the membership is obligated to meet.

Ethics as applied to medicine   The term *medical ethics* is used in two related, though different, ways. First of all, the term refers to the system of ethical standards of conduct of the medical profession. Specifically, medical ethics refers to the body of rules, regulations, oaths, and codes that have been developed by physicians and that have to do with their conduct in the practice of medicine. But the term *medical ethics* also encompasses *bioethics*—the study of moral issues, questions, and problems arising in the practice of medicine and in biomedical research. The many sophisticated scientific developments in recent years have been accompanied by increased concern both in the scientific community and in lay circles about the moral questions and the social implications particularly of biomedical research. Some of the more important problems have to do with the legality and/or the morality of research and procedures involved in organ transplantation, genetic engineering, and artificial insemination. Other crucial issues are the definitions of *life* and *death*. Obviously, bioethical problems are of great concern to physicians, life and physical scientists, social scientists, and attorneys. The medical assistant should be conversant with these problems.

In this chapter, the term *medical ethics* is used to encompass both of the two specific senses outlined above except in instances when the individual senses of the single term are being considered separately. In the latter case, the terms *professional ethics* and *bioethics* are used to distinguish the two senses from each other.

Ethical obligations of physicians and their medical assistants It is vitally important that physicians and medical assistants identify, respect, and observe both their legal and their ethical obligations and responsibilities to the patients they serve. Unfortunately, this is not a cut-and-dried task that can be easily fulfilled. Just as it is often difficult to know what the law requires in certain situations, so is it often difficult to know what one's ethical obligations are. The reason is that many different perspectives exist with regard to ethical problems, responsibilities, and obligations—both from the viewpoint of the medical community and from that of society in general. Nevertheless, it is important for the individual physician to evaluate his or her ethical duties and to formulate concrete office management policies fulfilling those duties. It follows that the medical assistant should understand the reasons for the physician's policies and should be vigilant in implementing them at all times.

One way that physicians and other health care practitioners can meet their ethical responsibilities is to be aware constantly of their patients' human rights as discussed in Chapter 3, section 3.4 (see the Statement on a Patient's Bill of Rights). Physicians must realize too that society expects them to be not merely objective scientists but also sensitive humanists acting as moral agents and allowing their patients to function as moral agents also.

Content of this chapter This chapter provides the medical assistant with very basic information about the doctor's ethical obligations in the practice of medicine and concomitant guidance as to the assistant's own ethical obligations to the doctor's patients.

4.2

THE ETHICS OF THE MEDICAL PROFESSION

Concern about medical ethics is not a recent phenomenon. From the earliest days of the healing art, there has been serious concern about ethical issues in medicine. The Oath of Hippocrates is an early indication of this concern:

The Oath of Hippocrates

I swear by Apollo, the physician, and Aesculapius and health and all-heal and all the Gods and Goddesses that, according to my ability and judgment, I will keep this oath and stipulation:

TO RECKON him who taught me this art equally dear to me as my parents, to share my substance with him and relieve his necessities if required; to regard his offspring as on the same footing with my own brothers, and to teach them this art if they should wish to learn it, without fee or stipulation, and that by precept, lecture and every other mode of instruction, I will impart a knowledge of the art to my own sons and to those of my teachers, and to disciples bound by a stipulation and oath, according to the law of medicine, but to none others.

I WILL FOLLOW that method of treatment which, according to my ability and judgment, I consider for the benefit of my patients, and abstain from whatever is deleterious and mischievous. I will give no deadly medicine to anyone if asked, nor suggest any such counsel; furthermore, I will not give to a woman an instrument to produce abortion.

WITH PURITY AND WITH HOLINESS I will pass my life and practice my art. I will not cut a person who is suffering from a stone, but will leave this to be done by practitioners of this work. Into whatever houses I enter I will go into them for the benefit of the sick and will abstain from every voluntary act of mischief and corruption; and further from the seduction of females or males, bond or free.

WHATEVER, in connection with my professional practice, or not in connection with it, I may see or hear in the lives of men which ought not to be spoken abroad I will not divulge, as reckoning that all such should be kept secret.

WHILE I CONTINUE to keep this oath unviolated may it be granted to me to enjoy life and the practice of the art, respected by all men at all times but should I trespass and violate this oath, may the reverse be my lot.

Notice that the Oath places primary value on the proper use of medicine to help the sick and not to injure or harm them. In the third paragraph of the Oath, the expression of unwillingness to comply with requests (as for "deadly medicine") represents a declaration by physicians that they must use their professional judgment and not merely be agents of someone else's will. Bear in mind also that from the fifth century B.C., when the Oath was written, confidentiality has been afforded a central role in the physician-patient relationship. The Oath is still taken at many American medical schools.

Under the Oath, the physician's patients have a right to receive health care from the physician according to the best of his or her ability. Patients also have a right to expect that any confidences shared with their physician will be treated as secrets by the physician. Furthermore, doctors have the ethical obligation to avoid injuring their patients.

In 1803, Thomas Percival published his *Code of Medical Ethics,* which became the foundation for the formulations of modern medical professional ethics. Dr. Percival attempted to describe four types of conduct that doctors should adhere to in medical practice: professional conduct in hospitals, professional conduct in private or general practice, professional conduct in relationships with apothecaries, and professional duties in cases involving legal programs.

The principles developed by Percival reflect his sense of what a physician should do in the health care process. But his focus was more on etiquette than on ethics, as compared with modern-day treatment of the subject. The physician's deportment; the physician's bedside manner; the physician's conversations with patients, relatives, or other physicians; the need for punctuality—these are the real subjects that concerned him. (His book provides enormous insight into the practice of medicine in mid-nineteenth century America.)

In 1847, the American Medical Association adopted the first form of its Code of Ethics. This Code has been reissued several times since then, and its latest form has 10 major sections. The Code is given in full below. It is reprinted from pages 4 and 5 of *Judicial Council Opinions and Reports* by permission of the American Medical Association.

Principles of Medical Ethics

PREAMBLE
These principles are intended to aid physicians individually and collectively in maintaining a high level of ethical conduct. They are not laws but standards by which a physician may determine the propriety of his conduct in his relationship with patients, with colleagues, with members of allied professions, and with the public.

SECTION 1
The principal objective of the medical profession is to render service to humanity with full respect for the dignity of man. Physicians should merit the confidence of patients entrusted to their care, rendering to each a full measure of service and devotion.

SECTION 2
Physicians should strive continually to improve medical knowledge and skill, and should make available to their patients and colleagues the benefits of their professional attainments.

SECTION 3
A physician should practice a method of healing founded on a scientific basis; and he should not voluntarily associate professionally with anyone who violates this principle.

SECTION 4
The medical profession should safeguard the public and itself against physicians deficient in moral character or professional competence. Physicians should observe all laws, uphold the dignity and honor of the profession and accept its self-imposed disciplines. They should expose, without hesitation, illegal or unethical conduct of fellow members of the profession.

SECTION 5
A physician may choose whom he will serve. In an emergency, however, he should render service to the best of his ability. Having undertaken the care of a patient, he may not neglect him; and unless he has been discharged he may discontinue his services only after giving adequate notice. He should not solicit patients.

SECTION 6
A physician should not dispose of his services under terms or conditions which tend to interfere with or impair the free and complete exercise of his medical judgment and skill or tend to cause a deterioration of the quality of medical care.

SECTION 7
In the practice of medicine a physician should limit the source of his professional income to medical services actually rendered by him, or under his supervision, to his patients. His fee should be commensurate with the services rendered and the patient's ability to pay. He should neither pay nor receive a commission for referral of patients. Drugs, remedies or appliances may be dispensed or supplied by the physician provided it is in the best interests of the patient.

SECTION 8
A physician should seek consultation upon request; in doubtful or difficult cases; or whenever it appears that the quality of medical service may be enhanced thereby.

SECTION 9
A physician may not reveal the confidences entrusted to him in the course of medical attendance, or the deficiencies he may observe in the character of patients, unless he is required to do so by law or unless it becomes necessary in order to protect the welfare of the individual or of the community.

SECTION 10
The honored ideals of the medical profession imply that the responsibilities of the physician extend not only to the individual, but also to society where these responsibilities deserve his interest and participation in activities which have the purpose of improving both the health and the well-being of the individual and the community.

The American Medical Association has established a Judicial Council which has jurisdiction over all questions of professional medical ethics and the interpretation of the AMA *Constitution, Bylaws,* and *Rules.* Among the procedures available to it in responding to violations of the Principles of Medical Ethics is a disciplinary proceeding to revoke membership. Physicians and medical assistants alike should try to avoid any such problems by respecting and carrying out their ethical obligations.

The medical assistant should be conversant with the material contained in the current volume of *Judicial Council Opinions and Reports* and especially those sections dealing with referrals, office practices, confidentiality, record administration, fees and billing, and civil rights.

4.3

BIOETHICS

Bioethics is the examination of moral issues, questions, and problems arising in the practice of medicine and in biomedical research. It is extremely complex and requires a thorough knowledge of not only medicine and science but also philosophy and theology. Bioethical considerations have to do with controversial research, opinions, and practices with regard to abortion, sterilization, contraception, organ transplantation, and human experimentation. Other bioethical concerns are the definitions of *life, death,* and *dying.* Obviously, bioethical problems are of primary concern to physicians and scientists. However, the medical assistant should be aware of this aspect of medical ethics especially as it affects the conduct of the physician's practice. The assistant must have general knowledge of the physician's position with regard to the areas of controversy already mentioned, because this position will influence the entire physician-patient relationship.

It is also worth saying at the outset that with recent advances in medicine and in biomedical research, bioethics has now become a recognized academic discipline. Several university programs having been established wherein controversial biomedical issues are examined at length and in detail with a view toward their resolution.

From the viewpoint of bioethics, it is assumed that the physician and the patient are ethical agents whose actions have ethical consequences. In this connection, it is worth repeating that physicians have ethical obligations to their patients and that patients have the right to expect that their physicians will behave in an ethical manner toward them. Many ethical obligations emerge from sources similar to those of legal obligations. For example, the need to obtain a patient's consent for treatment and for release of information has an ethical as well as a legal dimension, because the patient's moral right to autonomy is protected by the consent requirement. Similar derivations can be made with regard to ethical rights such as the patient's right to hear the truth from the doctor, to have privacy and confidentiality respected, and to refuse treatment.

Although it is well beyond the scope of this book to treat the subject of bioethics in detail, it is important to mention five critical questions which doctors should consider when studying and attempting to resolve bioethical problems arising in the course of the physician-patient relationship. As a medical assistant, you too should be aware of the questions and should think about their implications for the daily conduct of your own work. The questions—identified by Robert Veatch in his *Case Studies in Medical Ethics* (Cambridge: Harvard University Press, 1977)—are:

1. What makes right acts right?
2. To whom is moral duty owed?
3. What kinds of acts are right?
4. How do rules apply to specific situations?
5. What ought to be done in specific cases?

These questions form the basis for analysis of bioethical problems. They also can be thought of as the general basis on which patients can make moral claims. And they should be considered by all health team members before any action affecting the well-being of the patients is taken.

In conclusion, it is suggested that physicians and their staffs review the bioethical problems specific to their individual practices and that they be prepared to discuss these problems with their patients if and when the need arises. (See also the References section of the Appendix for a list of titles treating the topic of bioethics.)

4.4

MEDICAL ETHICS AND THE MEDICAL ASSISTANT

INTRODUCTION

The medical assistant is not only a legal agent of the physician-employer but also an *ethical* agent of the doctor. As such, the assistant has the responsibility to respect the rights of all patients, just as the physician does. The overriding ethical obligation of the assistant in this respect is therefore to treat all patients at all times with respect and dignity, in spite of any external pressures that might encourage the assistant to behave otherwise.

Although individual ethical considerations involving the assistant's professional behavior are treated throughout this book in their appropriate chapters (as in the chapters dealing with staff and patient interaction, appointments, record administration, insurance, transcription, and medical office financial management), it is felt that the importance of these considerations demands a full discussion of them here. The following paragraphs detail the ethical responsibilities of the assistant. You will see that ethics and law are closely related.

Financial arrangements with patients   The assistant ought to be cognizant of the AMA's position regarding appointment charges and collection agencies. First, with regard to appointment charges, the AMA Judicial Council feels that charging for a missed appointment or for one that the patient has not cancelled 24 hours ahead of time is ethical, providing that the physician has already advised the patient that such charges will be levied in these circumstances. A wall sign to this effect, notices in office newsletters to patients, notations on appointment cards and patient reminder cards, and oral notification of the policy can be used to inform the patients of the doctor's appointment charge policy. If this kind of charge policy is operative in your employer's office, you are responsible for seeing that the patients are aware of it.

With regard to collection agencies, you should realize that it is considered unethical for a physician to sell his or her delinquent patient accounts to a collection agency. If you are given the responsibility for investigating and then recommending a collection agency for the doctor's consideration, keep this fact in mind. Remember also that it is unethical for a physician to enter into any contract with a collection agency whereby the physician loses full control over the delinquent accounts or the collection methods and techniques used by that agency. In choosing an agency, the doctor should understand the collection techniques and methods that will be employed: they must not be "unfair" or "abusive," according to the AMA. Thus, if you are supposed to screen several agencies for the doctor, be sure that you find out the details of the collection process so that you can brief the doctor accurately. His or her later evaluation and decision with regard to the choice of an agency may depend on your report. And most importantly, no account should be assigned to a collection agency until the patient's ability to pay the fee has been fully evaluated by the doctor. If you are asked to provide data for this decision-making process, be sure that the data are accurate and that both sides of the case have been fully presented to the doctor for his or her final decision.

Rebates   A doctor can ethically receive from his or her patients payments only for medical services rendered. It is absolutely unethical for a doctor to accept a rebate of any kind from anyone. Furthermore, a physician cannot ethically accept "gifts" (rebates in another guise) from manufacturers or distributors of pharmaceuticals, remedies, or equipment. This practice is considered unethical because it could be used by the donor to influence the doctor to prescribe a particular product manufactured or distributed by the donor. If, in the absence of the doctor, an agent of any such firm attempts to leave a rebate for the doctor with you and you know what the item is, you should avoid accepting it. Tell the individual to discuss the matter with the doctor in person or by telephone later. Explain also that it is the doctor's policy not to accept such items. Then tell the physician what has happened as soon as possible.

Insurance form completion   As is indicated in Chapter 10, the physician ought to complete the simplified Health Insurance Council forms and similar forms without levying a charge to the patient. The completion of such forms is considered part of the service afforded the patient. However, in accordance with local custom, the doctor may levy a charge for the completion of the more complex forms. The local medical society should be consulted for an opinion before a charge policy is implemented. The assistant should ensure that the patients understand the charge policy (if there is one) and the reasons for it.

Confidentiality   This ethical consideration cannot be overstressed. The medical assistant cannot discuss a patient's case with third parties or reveal any aspect of a patient's record to unauthorized individuals. The medical assistant is responsible for ensuring that no unauthorized person ever removes, reads, copies, or otherwise tampers with any record at any time. Since you often collect and file sensitive medical information, you should ensure always that the information is secure. This can be accomplished by (1) never leaving open files without cover sheets on desks or in unattended rooms (2) locking file cabinets and desk drawers and rooms containing medical records at the end of each working day (3) refraining from answering queries regarding patients from third parties (4) referring all third-party inquiries about patients to the doctor (5) shredding any unusable duplicates of photocopied records or any records being disposed of before they are actually put into waste containers (6) avoiding conversations about patients with fellow employees when within hearing distance of other patients and visitors, and (7) refraining from any discussion of patients' cases in off-duty hours.

In general, medical information may be disclosed only if the patient has signed a waiver of rights (see also Chapter 9, section 9.7, the subsection entitled "Consent to Release Medical Information"). Furthermore, no information should be given out without the doctor's prior knowledge and approval. (Note also that although the records are the physician's property the patient nevertheless has a right to the information contained in his or her record.) The importance of medical record confidentiality applies to computer-stored records and to computerized billing systems as well. Thus, when evaluating a computer file or billing system for the doctor, it is imperative that you make certain that the system has built-in safeguards for data confidentiality. Consult the local medical society for recommendations and standards to be followed in evaluating these kinds of systems.

If an insurance company investigator or nurse requests a patient's history, the doctor's diagnosis or prognosis regarding a patient, or any other such data, consider this as a third-party inquiry and remember that the data may be released only if the patient or a lawful representative of the patient has consented to the disclosure. It is also your duty to double-check all disclosure releases to ascertain that the correct signatures have been properly affixed to them.

When a colleague of your physician treats a patient formerly treated by your employer, the other doctor can ask to see the patient's records. After proper authorization has been obtained from the patient, the records should be made available promptly to the other doctor, but you must tell your employer about the request before releasing the material. Your duty is to ensure that the patient's authorization is complete and correct. You also may have to make the arrangements for the other doctor to examine the record, as directed by your employer. Be sure to read carefully Chapter 9, section 9.7, the subsection entitled "Medical Ethics in Record Management."

Knowing and adhering to your responsibilities   From your initial contact with a patient to your last encounter, you should never engage in any activity outside the scope of your responsibilities and competence. This means that you should refrain from making an evaluation of any patient's case and from dispensing any medication whatsoever. Even innocuous-sounding statements like "I'm sure the doctor will make you well/feel better" are not only unethical but also could constitute interference in a medical case—interference that could be misunderstood as an attempt to practice medicine or to guarantee that the doctor will indeed "cure" a particular patient. Obviously, these kinds of statements could have serious medicolegal repercussions for the doctor and for you. This sort of thing is a good example of the interrelationship of law and ethics.

Furthermore, you must refrain at all times from discussing with patients the advantages and disadvantages as well as the side effects and contraindications of any drug, device, remedy, treatment, procedure, operation, or therapy. This is the doctor's prerogative only.

It is highly unethical for an assistant to discuss other physicians with patients. You may be tempted to comment either in defense of or in opposition to another doctor, especially if you are drawn or pressured into a conversation with a patient who is angry or dissatisfied with the other doctor for some reason. The best advice is to avoid such conversations to begin with; however, if you *do* become drawn into one, simply refrain from commenting on the matter at all and then end the conversation politely yet firmly by saying, "I'm very sorry but I simply cannot comment on that. It is unethical for me to do it, and I'm sure you can understand that."

The necessity for accuracy in your work   This point is reemphasized again and again in the upcoming chapters, and especially in those dealing with written medical communications. However, it bears stressing here that inaccuracies in any aspect of your work can have far-reaching legal implications for your employer, who bears the ultimate responsibility for your actions. Thus, you are ethically obligated to give paramount attention to the achievement and the constant maintenance of accuracy in letters, reports, insurance forms, filing, record-keeping, billing, appointments, and any other task designated by the doctor for you to perform. When corrections are necessary in medical records, you should follow the correction procedures given in Chapter 9. In short, you must behave so as to inspire the doctor's complete trust in your accuracy.

OVERALL CONCERNS

As a medical assistant, you have two overall ethical concerns that you must never lose sight of: your obligations to the patients and your obligations to your physician-employer. It is therefore recommended that you read the current edition of the AMA *Judicial Council Opinions and Reports* with a view toward how its guidelines directed primarily to physicians also can apply to your own professional performance as an agent of the physician.

With regard to your employer, you should always keep in mind the necessity of absolute loyalty to him or her. Regard all conversations with your employer about patients or others as privileged communications. Avoid discussing your employer with others. In short, strive to be worthy of the trust imparted to you by your physician.

A code of ethics for medical assistants   No chapter on medical ethics would be complete without inclusion of the Code of Ethics contained in Chapter 18 of the *Constitution and Bylaws* of the American Association of Medical Assistants, Inc. The following material is reprinted by permission of the AAMA:

Members of this Association dedicated to the conscientious pursuit of their profession, and thus desiring to merit the high regard of the entire medical profession and the respect of the general public which they serve, do pledge themselves to strive always to:

(a) Render service to humanity with full respect for the dignity of person.

(b) Respect confidential information gained through employment unless legally authorized or required by responsible performance of duty to divulge such information.

(c) Uphold the honor and high principles of the profession and accept its disciplines.

(d) Seek to continually improve our knowledge and skills of medical assisting for the benefit of patients and professional colleagues.

(e) Participate in additional service activities which aim toward improving the health and well-being of the community.

Whether or not you actually are a member of the AAMA, you ought to think about the principles outlined above and strive to follow them in your daily tasks, for they are relevant to all medical assistants.

5

CHAPTER FIVE

THE TELEPHONE:
A Public Relations
Instrument

CONTENTS

5.1

THE TELEPHONE AND MEDICAL PUBLIC RELATIONS

Have you ever examined the way you felt after talking to a telephone operator? How did you respond to the attitude that the operator projected over the telephone? Irritation, frustration, or simple unresponsiveness at the operator's end of the line often produces a similar internal reaction at the caller's end. The opposite is also true. Have you ever had your call placed on HOLD, only to have the other person then offer a brief word of apology that immediately calmed your irritation over the delay? Have you ever called a telephone operator for information and found that, with only an incomplete name or little or no address to go on, the operator can become a personal detective who will do everything possible to help solve your problem? As a result, you feel better cared for.

Some people say that they can sense what a person looks like from the way he or she talks on the telephone. Perhaps the documentation for such a generalization is weak, but the underlying point may be useful especially when considered in the context of medical office telephone usage. Do you project in your conversations an image of the kind of person you would actually like to *be*? Do you also think about the person at the other end of the line? It is especially important that you consider the feelings and the reactions of every caller because many of them are ill or upset. The same careful attention that is given to the patients who visit the office should be afforded the patients who telephone the office.

A person in a state of panic, or even acute distress, is not always able to convey accurate information to you. That is one reason why the initial response of a medical assistant—just like that of a telephone operator—can determine the success or failure of an emergency telephone communication. Politeness and caring on your part will make the caller feel better emotionally and will allow him or her to better answer the questions that you, as a medical assistant, must ask to gain essential information.

What you say and how you say it are representative of the doctor and the quality of the care rendered by the practice, as far as callers are concerned. A negative impression created by a medical assistant on the telephone is hard if not impossible to dispel later during office visits. Therefore, the patients must be made to feel that they are not so unimportant as to be rushed, put on HOLD, or abruptly disconnected when they telephone the doctor's office. This point cannot be overstressed, for it is one that patients most often complain about. In short, the telephone is the voice of the practice.

GOOD TELEPHONE USAGE

It is entirely appropriate to introduce this section with an example of an actual conversation that did take place—a conversation exemplifying how an assistant misused the telephone to the detriment of the entire practice:

Assistant: Dr. _____'s office. Miss _____ speaking.
Caller: May I please speak with Dr. _____?
Assistant: Of course not.

Sadly enough, this sort of inexcusable rudeness is not all that uncommon, especially in situations where the assistant is very rushed or distracted. In the case exhibited above, it so happened that the physician's policy was never to accept calls unless the callers identified themselves to the assistant beforehand. Nevertheless, the assistant made no effort to ask politely for the caller's name or to explain the doctor's policy regarding call transfers. When a caller experiences this and other types of rudeness, he or she can be reasonably expected never to call or visit the office again. At the very least, the office can expect to receive a complaint about the assistant's lack of manners.

The following paragraphs containing guidelines to good telephone usage have been written to help you improve your telephone techniques and avoid potential problems with callers.

Answer promptly   Answer on the first ring, if possible. If you are already talking on another line, mention this to the second caller by saying, "Please hold the line for a moment and I'll be right with you." Never say "Hold" or, worse, depress the HOLD button before saying anything.

Use proper identification   Always identify the office and yourself. This saves time. Example: "Dr. Sawyer's office. Ms. Deaven speaking." If you work for five or six physicians, it may be necessary to say, "Doctors' Office" or to name the group practice or the building, but be prepared for the inevitable response from the caller, "Is this Dr. Sawyer's office?"

Do not answer the telephone while talking to someone else in the office   There is nothing more annoying to a caller than to hear loud garbled voices in the background, followed by a shuffling of papers or other extraneous noise, and finally a reluctant if not rushed voice saying, "Yes?".

Try not to speak rapidly when answering the telephone   All too often a caller is faced with an undecipherable spurt like this: "HudsonvilleOB/GYNAssociatesMissDownspeakingMayIhelpyou?" If you are so rushed as to be unable to answer the telephone coherently, what kind of care can the patient expect to get on an office visit?

Obtain the name of the caller As soon as possible before you become involved in a conversation, obtain the name of the caller. Write the name down so that you can use it later in the conversation, so that you can transmit a complete message to the physician if necessary, and so that you can pull the patient's record if there is one. Avoid asking for the name in an abrupt manner. These kinds of questions are absolutely unacceptable:

"Name?"
"Who is this?"
"Who's calling?"
"What's your name?"

The following ways of asking for the caller's name are correct and courteous:

"May I please have your name?"
"Will you please give me your name?"
"May I ask who is calling, please?"
"May I tell Dr. _____ who is calling?"

When the person does give the name, be sure to respond by saying "Thank you."

Project a pleasant telephone personality The telephone company recommends that you hold the telephone so that its mouthpiece is about one inch from your lips. Speak directly into it in a low-pitched, normal tone of voice. Your voice should convey a caring attitude. If you imagine that you are speaking face-to-face, you will avoid affectation. Do not use slang or overly technical medical expressions. For instance, saying "Okay, hon, see ya tomorrow" is apt to insult the patient. By the same token, technical jargon will only confuse the patient. Listening effectively on the telephone is just as important as speaking effectively. Take notes on the conversation, and if necessary, refer to them when replying. You would not want to be embarrassed by having to ask the patient what the complaint is again after he or she has just told you and has described all the symptoms.

Use proper HOLD techniques If you *must* leave the line, tell the caller why and approximately how long it will take. If the delay is likely to take more than a few minutes, offer to call back. Examples: "Please hold the line a minute while I get your ledger card, Mr. Jones" or "I'll have to check our inactive files for that information, Ms. Watson. May I call you back in an hour?" or "Dr. Sawyer is on another line just now, Mrs. Lee. Would you rather wait or call back in half an hour?" When you leave the line, depress the HOLD button. When you return to the line, alert the caller by saying something like "Thank you for waiting, Mr. Jones. I have the information now." If a caller is placed on HOLD while he or she is waiting to speak with the doctor, try to return to the line about every minute with the following statement: "I'm sorry to keep you waiting, but Dr. Sawyer is still busy."

Handle the call yourself Most of the calls to a physician's office can be handled by the medical assistant. The following list provides examples of such calls.

1. **Appointments** More than half of all calls received in a doctor's office are for appointments. The amount of information required will differ in various offices, but the following items are usually considered minimal:

Item	You Say	Why You Say it
Name	"May I please have your name?"	You will need the complete name correctly spelled in order to pull an existing chart or to prepare a new chart.

Availability	"Would you prefer mornings or afternoons, Mr. Brown?"	This information narrows the scheduling options.
Telephone Number	"May I have your telephone number, please?"	This information allows you to contact the patient later.
Reason for Visit	"May I tell Dr. Sawyer why you are coming in?" *or* "What seems to be the trouble?"	You will need this information to decide the urgency of an appointment and to schedule the appropriate amount of time for it.

Additional information such as where the patient lives, who referred the patient, or what insurance the patient has may be obtained during the patient's visit.

2. **Questions about test results**   If test results are within normal limits, the doctor will usually authorize you to inform the patient of this. Example: "Your Pap smear is negative, Ms. Cooke. That means that everything is normal." However, most doctors prefer to discuss unfavorable or questionable test results directly with the patients. In these cases, the physician may call a patient or have you immediately transfer the telephone call when the patient calls the office. Should a patient ask you for test results when the doctor is unavailable, you might say, "The doctor has not seen the mail reports yet. May I call you after two o'clock?"

3. **Favorable progress reports**   Frequently, a doctor will ask the patient to call in a progress report. If the patient is progressing satisfactorily (e.g., the patient feels better, the rash is gone, the medicine is working), take the message and relay it to the doctor. Do not transfer the call. Example: "Dr. Sawyer will be so happy to hear that, Mrs. Downs. I'll tell the doctor right after the next patient leaves."

4. **Requests for home visits**   Most doctors prefer to treat patients in the office or at the hospital because it saves time. For this reason, you should encourage patients to come to the office by saying, "Can you possibly bring in your son, Mr. Eccles? Dr. Sawyer can examine him and treat him much more efficiently in the office."

   If the patient insists that the doctor make a house call and the doctor's policy is to do so, be sure to obtain the following information: the name and age of the patient, the telephone number, the address, a description of the exact problem, and explicit directions to the address. (See also Chapter 8, section 8.6.)

5. **Cancellations**   If a patient cancels an appointment, immediately offer to make another. Occasionally, you may have a patient who consistently cancels or does not show up for appointments. If applicable, you might say, "You have missed several appointments, Ms. Franklin. Dr. Sawyer thinks it's very important to your progress that you be examined (or whatever) regularly. Is there some problem in getting to our office?" Many offices require a notation on the patient's chart if an appointment is canceled or missed. (See also Chapter 8, section 8.3.)

6. **Questions about insurance and bills**   If you are familar with major community policies, you can answer many insurance questions over the telephone. When in doubt, you can ask the patient to mail in the policy (see also Chapter 10, section 10.9, for a list of typical questions and answers about health insurance).

   Questions about bills may be reduced if the patient receives itemized statements. If a patient is upset over the fee charged, you can point out that the fee is fairly typical in the community (assuming that it is).

7. **Incoming laboratory and X-ray reports**   Many hospitals and laboratories telephone results to a doctor prior to mailing a written report. In order to save time, you may wish to obtain copies of the forms so that you can fill them out during the initial telephone transmittal.

8. **Inquiries about patients**   Attorneys, insurance examiners, and friends of a patient may call to request medical information. You *must* explain that you cannot give any information regarding a patient. You can express it this way: "I'm sorry, Mr. Goode, but I must have written consent from the patient before I can release any information."

9. **Miscellaneous calls** Occasionally, you may get a caller who refuses to give a name but demands to speak with the doctor. To screen such a call effectively, you might say this: "I'm sorry, but Dr. Sawyer has requested that I not interrupt him unless I know who is calling. May I suggest that you write him a letter and he will contact you."

You may also receive calls from unfamiliar salespeople and from charities asking for donations. You may want to say, "Please mail your literature to the doctor. I am sure it will be reviewed."

Shoppers may call to inquire about the doctor's fees, procedures, and so on. Questions about procedures may be easily answered, but a discussion of fees over the telephone is a delicate matter. You might say, "It's very difficult to say until the doctor examines you, Ms. Hall, because you may need special tests. However, $30.00 is the usual charge for the first office visit, and $15.00, for subsequent visits."

A patient may ask where the office is located or where to park. Be sure that you are familiar with bus routes and nearby major streets.

Screen calls carefully Few physicians will take *all* incoming calls. That's your job! The appropriate time to transfer a call to the doctor will depend on the doctor's personal preference—often determined by the specialty—and on your own good judgment and experience (see also section 5.2). Many callers will ask to speak with the doctor. Usually, you should respond by saying, "The doctor is with a patient just now (or is at the hospital or at a medical conference, or whatever is the case). May I help you?" Frequently, you *can* help—by making an appointment for the patient, by solving an insurance problem, or by answering a routine question.

Take messages and get them right Obtain printed message forms or use a steno pad to record the details from each telephone call requiring that a written message be taken. The minimum information required is the time and the date, the name of the caller, the caller's telephone number, the message, and the action required.

Follow up the message Has the action required been taken? the patient contacted? the insurance form filled out? You may also find it necessary to make a notation on the patient's chart or attach a message slip to the chart.

Transfer the call to the doctor Most telephone calls to a physician's office can be handled by the medical assistant. However, the following paragraphs illustrate calls that should be transferred immediately to the doctor or that should be handled by the doctor later.

1. **Emergency calls** While most new medical assistants worry about emergency calls, few such calls are actually received. Because an emergency may occur, however, you should always know how to locate your doctor or the doctor on call.

The symptoms that constitute an emergency will be identified by your employer, but the following symptoms definitely should be considered as potentially serious: extreme abdominal pain, excessive bleeding, high fever over several days, prolonged vomiting, and severe chest pain.

If the doctor is in the office, obtain the name of the patient and transfer the call immediately.

If the doctor is *not* in the office, be sure to obtain the name, the location, and the telephone number of the patient, an exact description of what is wrong, and the name of the caller. You may wish to place the caller on HOLD while you use another line to contact the doctor.

2. **Calls from other physicians** Medical etiquette dictates that such calls be transferred to your doctor immediately and without screening. If immediate transfer is impossible, explain why and offer to have your employer call back as soon as possible.

3. **Calls from the doctor's immediate family**   Do not screen calls from the doctor's immediate family, but do transfer them at once (unless you have been directed otherwise).

4. **Calls to report poor progress**   If a patient calls to report adverse side effects from a prescription or a worsening condition, refer the call to the doctor.

5. **Calls to complain about care**   You may try to soothe a patient by listening calmly and nonjudgmatically to the complaint, but in most instances you should refer the call to the doctor.

6. **Calls from concerned relatives**   Calls from close relatives of acutely ill patients should be referred to the doctor. The doctor either can take the incoming call immediately or can promise to return the call at the first opportunity. Legally, you *cannot* give information regarding a patient to *anyone* without the doctor's permission.

7. **Calls to get prescriptions**   Since a medical assistant cannot authorize a prescription or its refill without the doctor's permission, such calls are usually transferred to the doctor. Moreover, federal law states that a prescription for a controlled substance must be issued *directly* to the patient by the doctor. In such a case, you might say to the caller, "I'm sorry, Mrs. Abbott, but that drug cannot be prescribed over the telephone. Can you come into the office this afternoon?"

In summary, remember that when a call must be transferred, you should explain to the caller what you are doing and why. Example: "The bookkeeper has that information, Mr. Lawton. I'll transfer your call to her. Will you hold, please?"

When transferring a call to the physician, it is also useful to ask the patient if the call relates to his or her illness. If it does, you ought to get the chart for the physician. Similarly, if another doctor (or perhaps an insurance company representative) calls, it will be wise to ask whether or not the call is about a patient. If it is, you should get the appropriate chart for the physician.

5.2

INCOMING CALLS

The moment the telephone rings is not necessarily the time to consider conversational responses. However, planning in advance is possible even though the actual conversations are still unknown. This process is particularly important for the neophyte or for the person who has difficulty responding in an unstructured situation. By considering the general categories of possible conversations and the alternative responses, a medical assistant can quickly develop a telephone routine that is both efficient and effective.

CATEGORIES OF CALLS
By person   Is the caller a patient calling about a patient-related problem or is the caller a nonpatient? The latter could be anyone from a drug salesperson to a maintenance person.

By content   Is the caller (whether a patient or a nonpatient) requesting information or providing information? A patient may be supplying a medical insurance number or requesting an appointment. A nonpatient may be supplying a price estimate or requesting the cooperation of the physician in setting up a clinical education program for a student.

By action   Is the caller purposely or unknowingly demanding a decision and/or action on the part of the medical assistant?

Discussion of categories The first two categories can be handled in a relatively straightforward way. The calls can be screened as soon as you have enough information. However, the action category requires screening of a higher order. An action response requires special judgment on the part of the medical assistant.

Before deciding on an appropriate action, the medical assistant must systematically make the following decisions:

1. Is the information that I have gathered so far from the caller enough for me to decide on an action?
2. Is an action required of me immediately or should I delay taking action?
3. Am I knowledgeable enough about the subject to seek the necessary information and decide on an action response or should my response be to seek aid from somone else in the office?

A medical assistant cannot prepare for every contingency that can occur during a telephone conversation, but by systematically thinking through a typical conversation, the medical assistant can very soon develop a pattern that will help to ensure consistency and completeness. The guidelines suggested are, of course, based on a model caller who is both rational and coherent. Most callers will fit into this category. However, for the irrational and/or incoherent caller, the first action of the medical assistant is to calm the caller enough to collect information that will be useful in making some tentative judgments.

It has been suggested that, for the most part, incoming calls predictably fall into a number of major categories. By thinking through a typical response, the medical assistant can be efficient and effective. In the literature of organization and administration, this process of planning ahead for possible alternatives is called *contingency management*. Alternative contingencies are considered and responses to each contingency are planned.

On the other hand, *crisis management* occurs when contingencies are *not* considered and responses are not planned. The office of a physician may periodically face a crisis that begins with an emergency telephone call, but it is the well-organized office that keeps the crisis response to a minimum.

TAKING ACTION

Once the medical assistant has decided that action is required, the assistant must assume responsibility for formalizing the action. The formalization could be as simple as writing an appointment in an appointment book or it could entail transferring the call to the physician or to someone else in the office. These immediate, uncomplicated responses do not normally lead to any serious communication breakdown, because the possibilities are so limited. However, situations requiring later follow-up contain greater possibilities for incomplete communication. Because of time lapses, the medical assistant must avoid depending on memory. The medical assistant should immediately write down all pertinent data provided by the caller along with any observations made during the call. Furthermore, the assistant should gather for the physician any supplemental information on the patient that is available in the office. Having received a morning call while the physician was out of the office, the medical assistant could report a particular matter to the doctor in this way:

Call: Barbara Johnson
Time: 8:30 a.m.
Subject: Son, Jerry 3 years old, had high temperature all
            night, starting at 10 p.m. Temperature
            taken twice— 10:00 p.m., 100 F; 7:00 a.m., 101 F.
Direction: Advised B. Johnson to record hourly temperatures and provide
            alcohol bath if temperature exceeds 102 F. Recommended she

call back if temperature exceeds 103 F. Reported that you
would be back between 2:00 and 4:00 p.m.

Comment: B. Johnson highly upset. Jerry is her first child, and she has had
no previous experience with high temperature.

Attachment: Medical record, Jerry Johnson

This report should be arranged with reports of calls from other patients in the order
of their urgency.

CALL-IN HOURS

One way of reducing the number of nonemergency calls and of handling them
systematically is the establishment of call-in hours. These are times set aside during
the workday in which the doctor is most likely to take immediate action on requests
from patients and nonpatients. Call-in hours can be particularly beneficial in a small
office not having a full-time receptionist. The medical assistant will be better able
to plan the workday if telephone interruptions are kept to a minimum during the
day. Thus, call-in hours contribute to the running of a more efficient office.

ANSWERING SERVICES

Most physicians have answering services to receive and record calls made during
nonworking hours and during vacation times. Because most answering services do
not normally hire personnel with training in the health care field, the medical assistant
is most likely to be responsible for maintaining liaison with the answering service.
For example, in some offices the medical assistant's first responsibility in the morning
is to call the answering service for messages. These messages may often require a
telephone response. The medical assistant can make those initial calls and answer
them just as though they had come directly into the office.

The last thing the medical assistant does before closing the office is to report
its closing to the answering service so that the telephone service to the office can
be continuous. Many offices now have automatic relays that will forward all telephone calls to the answering service if the telephone in the office of the physician
is not answered within a specified number of rings. Other offices have a switch
providing an automatic relay only when the office is closed. Whatever the system,
the medical assistant should understand how it functions and how it relates to the
normal office routine.

TELEPHONE REFERRALS

The word *referral* means the process of directing or redirecting a patient to another
physician or to an institution for appropriate care, including diagnosis and treatment.
Referrals are typically made when a patient's problems seem beyond the scope or
bounds of a physician's practice. Referrals may be made from physician to physician
concerning a patient, or from physician to patient concerning another physician.

Physician-generated referrals   Referrals can be made from one physician to another
by letter (see Chapter 15, section 15.9), by telephone, or by both. As a medical
assistant, you have to be able to deal with these physician referral situations:

1. If you are employed by a family practitioner or an internist, you probably will be directed
    by your physician to transmit referral messages to the offices of other doctors. Although
    your employer might ideally prefer to place all referral calls personally, he or she never-
    theless may ask you to take on this assignment when circumstances make it necessary,
    especially during very busy office hours. In any case, the referral call is usually followed
    up by a letter from the referring physician to the other doctor. Sometimes, the referring
    physician will follow up the initial telephone message with a letter and a personal tele-
    phone call.

2. If you work for a specialist, you must be prepared to receive many telephone referrals from other physicians. You transfer physician referrals immediately to your employer. You take messages when other physicians' medical assistants transmit the referrals for their employers.

When your employer directs you to transmit a referral message to another doctor, give the doctor or the medical assistant the followng data:

1. the name, address, and telephone number of the patient
2. the condition for which the patient is being referred
3. a description of the treatment (if any) that has been given so far.

Include in the message any other data specified by your employer.

When you receive a call placed by a referring doctor, ask the doctor if the call is about a referral that has already been dealt with in the office or if the call has to do with a new patient who has not been seen yet. If the former is the case, pull the patient's chart and give it to your physician. Then transfer the referring physician's call to your employer at once. (It is wise to keep referred patients' charts close to the telephone so that you can pull them quickly.) If the latter is the case, simply put the call through immediately to your physician. If your physician is unavailable, explain this to the other doctor, and ask if you can take a message.

Physician-to-patient referrals   Regardless of the nature of the practice, the office will receive some calls from patients desiring treatment for conditions that fall outside the scope of the practice. For example, a patient with a condition requiring ophthalmic surgery might telephone for an appointment with a general surgeon. If the general surgeon excludes eye surgery from the practice, the assistant would have to refer the patient to the appropriate ophthalmologist who does perform eye surgery. A patient complaining of a painful mole might ask to be seen by a dermatologist whose practice excludes any kind of surgery. Therefore, the assistant should know the name of a general surgeon to whom the patient should be referred. (A list of other doctors to whom patients can be referred should be kept near the telephone. This list should be organized alphabetically by specialty. The doctors' names—alphabetized by surname—should be accompanied by their full addresses and their telephone numbers.) After the patient has been directed to the appropriate physician, the doctor or the assistant calls the other doctor to alert him or her of the recommendation to the patient. Thus, you should have obtained the patient's name, address, and telephone number and a description of the complaint so that you can transmit these data to the other doctor.

The practice also may receive calls from patients requiring treatment when the physician is out of the office for an extended period of time. In the single-physician practice, the assistant should have a list of doctors who have been designated by the physician to take over the regular patients when he or she has to be away from the office for long periods of time (as for vacations, illnesses, emergencies, medical conventions, and so on). This list should be alphabetized, and the physicians' names should be accompanied by their addresses and their telephone numbers.

5.3

OUTGOING CALLS

CALL-BACK HOURS

Just as there may be a most appropriate time during the workday for patients to call in, so may there be an appropriate time for the physician to return calls. Each physician may have a personal preference often limited by hospital rounds or scheduled office hours. Most physicians prefer to leave some time during office hours unscheduled. This time can be used as a safety valve for patient overloads, for correspondence, and for outgoing calls.

CALL-BACK ROUTINES

Each physician should provide the medical assistant with guidelines as to the method of ordering a call-back. For example, most physicians would want patient calls separated from nonpatient calls; they would want those needing immediate attention separated from those that can wait; and they would want all backup information (such as medical records or laboratory reports) on the desk along with the call-back information.

The medical assistant has responsibility for making some calls—from returning calls to setting up conference calls. Just as plans can be made for the handling of each category of incoming call, so can outgoing calls be planned in advance. Return calls ought to be concise, complete as to content, and well organized. The message may be a request for special information, a specific statement, or a response to either of the above. The assistant should develop a fairly routine pattern for each.

Identification comes first; then come all essential details followed by a specific request, a specific declaration, or a response to either of the aforementioned. However, careful planning does not negate the importance of politeness. A brief, direct conversation carried on in a pleasant tone of voice is certainly more thoughtful and useful than a garbled, disjointed message—even if delivered pleasantly.

An appropriately informative way to begin a telephone conversation would be to say, "This is Cynthia Deaven calling for Dr. Sawyer. May I please speak to Mr./Mrs./Miss/Ms._____?" This opening is especially useful when the person on the other end of the line has answered with a simple "Hello." When you have identified yourself and have obtained the proper person, state your message clearly and politely. Do not rush through the message as if the other person is unimportant to you. Avoid staccato questions and responses like "What? I can't hear you" or "Sure. OK. Will do. Bye." Such mannerisms make very poor impressions on patients and others alike. Remember to end all calls politely. The same techniques apply to any telephone call, be it to a telephone operator, to a patient, or to a business person. Identify yourself and state your message clearly and precisely.

TELEPHONE LISTS

One valuable tool in making outgoing calls is a correct and comprehensive list of telephone numbers. The medical assistant automatically has access to the records and the card file for all patients. However, since the physician will often desire to place calls directly, one of the medical assistant's more important tasks is to develop a telephone list for the physician and for other staff members. This list would include the names and numbers of other physicians, of business people, and of any other individuals the physician is likely to wish to call directly. Rotary card files are especially useful for this purpose, since they can be updated easily. The file should be kept in the secretarial work station near the telephone.

5.4

TELEPHONE EQUIPMENT AND SERVICES

The modern medical office testifies that some rather dramatic changes have occurred in a relatively short time. Equipment that did not exist a few years ago is now evident in many offices. Clinical laboratory equipment, radiograph equipment, and respiratory equipment have become common sights in medical offices during the last quarter of the twentieth century. The telephone has been available longer than many other devices, but it too has undergone changes. The old-fashioned switchboard operator has all but disappeared, having been replaced with equipment offering the user far greater flexibility in handling both internal and external messages.

The trend toward more sophisticated telephones has provided individual users with a greater range of choices. For example, in the past office users always had to go through a main switchboard in order to place outside calls. This is no longer the case: now a telephone caller can talk to others in the same office on extensions and can add a third (inside or outside) party to that line for a conference without having to go through a switchboard.

The telephone company is willing to provide full information regarding ways to expand an office's telecommunication equipment. When it is felt that the telephone equipment and/or service is inadequate for the size of the practice, the telephone company's representative should be contacted. A study of the office requirements can be made, and the appropriate systems and equipment recommended.

TELEPHONE EQUIPMENT

Single line telephones   The single line telephone is the basic telephone set that we are all familiar with—it can come in many colors, sizes, and types. It may be a dial or a pushbutton telephone. Its configuration may be desk, wall, Trimline, Candlestick, Cradle, or Ericofon.

Multi-button telephones   The multi-button telephone can feature 6, 10, 20, or 30 buttons. It is typically used by assistants to answer, transfer, or screen calls. Various signals and intercommunications can be installed within these telephone sets.

Hands-free telephones   The hands-free telephone is commonly referred to as a *speakerphone*. Various types of hands-free telephone devices are available: some have individual receivers and transmitters, while others form an integral part of the telephone set. Hands-free devices are ideal when one is having a telephone conversation with three or four people at once. These devices are also helpful to one who is checking data and talking over the telephone at the same time.

Automatic answering device   Telephone answering and receiving devices, such as Electronic Secretary and Code-A-Phone, to name two, answer incoming calls automatically with prerecorded announcements. These automatic systems can tell the caller to leave a message, they can tell the caller where the person being called is or when he or she will be back. Advantages of these devices include the following: (1) the telephone is covered 24 hours a day (2) the expense of an office clerk is saved, and (3) telephone ordering and reporting procedures are speeded up. (See also page 78, "Answering services.")

Automatic dialer   With the use of an automatic dialer, a repertoire of telephone numbers can be stored on magnetic tape or prepunched on plastic cards so that you may poll many locations or continually dial the same number automatically.

Radio paging   Two types of radio paging equipment are available: *tone only* or *tone and voice*. Access is effected by dialing the paging equipment to tone-alert or voice-page pocket radio receivers that are carried by doctors. A common type that is offered by AT&T is called the Bellboy. These pocket radio page receivers are used by physicians and some nurses especially when they are on call.

TELEPHONE SYSTEMS

The wide variety of telephone systems on the market and the great flexibility in features offered today give the customer complete freedom of choice to select the system that suits his or her office best. With stored-program electronic switching and the use of small minicomputers and detailed message accounting techniques, these new telephone systems offer more features and benefits than have ever been available before. The Dimension R of the Bell System and the electronic switches of the interconnect industries such as the Danray CBX 2000, the Northern Telecom Ltd. Pulse, The Rolm CBX, the North Electric NX-1E, and the ITT and Stromberg-Carlson Electronic PABXs, to name a few, give high reliability, are easily maintained, and can provide excellent service. The features of the available telephone systems are numerous and varied. Along with the standard Direct Inward Dialing (DID), Direct Outward Dialing (DOD) and station-to station calling, the following are some of the more exotic features that are offered to customers:

1. Local Automatic Message Accounting (LAMA)—a service providing a magnetic-tape record of all telephone calls except station-to-station calls; information such as the station calling, the number called, the time and length of the call, the trunk used, and the charges may be captured on tape. This is an excellent tool to control toll costs.

2. Automatic Route Selection—the routing of calls over the least expensive trunk (as tie line, WATS, or FX); and the automatic stepping up to the next most expensive route (DDD) if all primary routes are busy.

3. Call Transfer—the ability to transfer to another party inside or outside the telephone system an established incoming or outgoing call without the assistance of an attendant.

4. Add-On Conference—an option that permits the telephone user to add a third party to any established conversation without the assistance of an attendant.

5. Call Forwarding—the capability to have incoming calls rerouted automatically to another telephone number; this feature is activated by dialing a forwarding code and then the number to which the calls are to be forwarded.

6. Camp On Busy—the ability of an operator to camp on an incoming call to your telephone while it is in use; a short burst of tone may be sent to your line to notify you that a call is waiting for your attention.

7. Call Pick-Up—the ability to answer an incoming call directed to another telephone.

8. Abbreviated Dialing—the ability to program one's telephone to accept a set of abbreviated numbers to replace certain telephone numbers; this is a feature that speeds up outside dialing.

9. Automatic Call Back—by dialing a code into the system, the user programs the system to continue to attempt to accept a call on a busy telephone; the first instant that the line is free, the system will automatically put the call through.

OTHER SPECIAL TELEPHONE SYSTEMS

The following paragraphs outline some of the special systems being used today which can be installed in medical offices having specialized requirements.

Centrex equipment   In the Centrex system, each extension has its own number that can be reached directly from outside lines. This system normally would not be used in the office of a single physician, but it might be used in a group practice in which each physician has major responsibility for a large group of patients.

Privacy button   Telephones can be equipped with a privacy button that temporarily cuts off extension telephones and conference calls.

Conference calls   Some telephone systems are capable of setting up conference calls with three to eight outside parties by means of the direct-distance dialing network. The telephone company operator can manually arrange for conference calls in which each call is charged at the operator-handled rate. It should be noted, however, that this rate is expensive.

Zero Express Dialing (ZED)   ZED is commonly used for credit card calls, collect calls, or bill-to-third party calls. Dial 0 followed by the telephone number. The telephone operator will request your credit card number or other instructions and then your call will be connected; the call will be charged as an operator-handled call.

Mobile calls   Telephones can be used to communicate with automobiles, trucks, aircraft, and ships. Calls are connected via land-line telephones through radio circuits.

Answering services   Check the Yellow Pages of your telephone directory where there are various answering service advertisements which will help you in your selection. Many local medical societies provide answering services for their members, and may offer more personal attention than the strictly commercial firms do. Most answering services are available 24 hours a day and can answer the telephone in the doctor's name or in the name of the practice. The types of answering services that are available range from relaying messages to two-way radio dispatching or radio paging. An answering service can be contracted for on a month-to-month basis.

Telephone dictation service   Centralized dictation systems have been installed by many large hospitals today. These systems are usually available from any telephone within a PBX telephone system allowing anyone within the system to dictate. When an access code is dialed, a recorder is seized. By following a prescribed procedure, the document that the user dictates is recorded on tape or on a magnetic disk and is ready for transcription. Playback, correction, stop, and operator assistance features are also available. The advantages of these systems are many: dictation can take place at any time of the day, centralized secretarial help reduces a hospital's clerical staff, and centralized dictating equipment reduces the cost of having such equipment installed and operational in individual offices. (See also Chapter 14 for more details regarding the use of this type of system in the dictation and transcription of medical documents.)

LOCAL CALLS
Just as telephone equipment has become more complex, so too have telephone services. Equipment (or hardware) usually accounts for 30% of the monthly telephone bill. The remaining 70% is for local and long-distance message units. Not much can be done to reduce local message units, but substantial savings can be achieved if the medical assistant is aware of the various services that are available and can use them to the fullest extent. For example, in the past several years, free information telephone calls have been limited. Information calls exceeding the limits are charged on a per call basis.

Usually local calls have been charged at a flat rate for unlimited usage in a local area; however, this method is fast disappearing and is being replaced by message units which allot a certain number of calls for a fixed fee. Most large cities throughout the United States are now using message units.

LONG-DISTANCE CALLS
More substantial savings can be made if the medical assistant is aware of the different rates charged for each type of long-distance service. The United States is presently divided into 14 rate steps based on distances ranging from 1 mile to 3,000 miles. Calls are classified as station-to-station, operator station-to-station, and person-to-

Area Codes—by States

State	Area Code	State	Area Code
Alabama	205	Minnesota	218, 507, 612
Alaska	907	Mississippi	601
Arizona	602	Missouri	314, 417, 816
Arkansas	501	Montana	406
Bahamas	809	Nebraska	308, 402
California	209, 213, 408, 415,	Nevada	702
	707, 714, 805, 916	New Hampshire	603
Canada	204, 306, 403, 416,	New Jersey	201, 609
	418, 506, 514, 519,	New Mexico	505
	604, 613, 705, 709,	New York	212, 315, 516, 518,
	807, 819, 902		607, 716, 914
Colorado	303	North Carolina	704, 919
Connecticut	203	North Dakota	701
Delaware	302	Ohio	216, 419, 513, 614
District of Columbia	202	Oklahoma	405, 918
Florida	305, 813, 904	Oregon	503
Georgia	404, 912	Pennsylvania	215, 412, 711, 814
Hawaii	808	Rhode Island	401
Idaho	208	South Carolina	803
Illinois	217, 309, 312,	South Dakota	605
	618, 815	Tennessee	615, 901
Indiana	219, 317, 812	Texas	214, 512, 713,
Iowa	319, 515, 712		806, 817, 915
Kansas	316, 913	Utah	801
Kentucky	502, 606	Vermont	802
Louisiana	318, 504	Virginia	703, 804
Maine	207	Washington	206, 509
Maryland	301	West Virginia	304
Massachusetts	413, 617	Wisconsin	414, 608, 715
Mexico	903	Wyoming	307
Michigan	313, 517, 616, 906		

person. Rates are based on the time of day when the call is placed from the originating station and on the rate mileage. The Day Rate period is Monday through Friday from 8:00 a.m. to 5:00 p.m.; the Evening Rate (currently a 35% discount from the Day Rate) is charged for Sunday through Friday from 5:00 p.m. to 11:00 p.m. The Night and Weekend Rate (currently a 60% discount of the Day Rate) is charged for every night from 11:00 p.m. to 8:00 a.m. and all day Saturday and all day Sunday except for the hours 5:00 p.m. through 11:00 p.m.

Station-to-station calls (Direct Distance Dialing) This is the fastest and least expensive way to place long-distance telephone calls. The charge is based on a one-minute minimum plus an additional charge for each succeeding minute. You dial 1, the Area Code, and the local telephone number.

Operator station-to-station calls These calls can be categorized into credit card, collect, or bill-to-third-party calls. Based on a three-minute minimum plus an additional charge for each succeeding minute, these calls are much more expensive than station-to-station calls. They usually range from a $.15 to a $1.15 increase for a six-minute telephone call. You dial 0, the Area Code, and the local telephone number. The operator will speak with you before completing the connection.

Person-to-person calls   The charge for these calls is also based on a three-minute minimum plus an additional charge for each succeeding minute. Person-to-person is by far the most expensive way of calling, and its use certainly should be minimized. You dial 0, the Area Code, and the local telephone number. The operator will speak with you before completing the connection.

Area Codes—by Numbers

Area Code	State	Area Code	State	Area Code	State
201	New Jersey	413	Massachusetts	703	Virginia
202	District of Columbia	414	Wisconsin	704	North Carolina
203	Connecticut	415	California	705	Ontario, Canada
204	Manitoba, Canada	416	Ontario, Canada	707	California
205	Alabama	417	Missouri	709	Newfoundland
206	Washington	418	Quebec, Canada	712	Iowa
207	Maine	419	Ohio	713	Texas
208	Idaho	501	Arkansas	714	California
209	California	502	Kentucky	715	Wisconsin
212	New York City	503	Oregon	716	New York
213	California	504	Louisiana	717	Pennsylvania
214	Texas	505	New Mexico	801	Utah
215	Pennsylvania	506	New Brunswick, Ca.	802	Vermont
216	Ohio	507	Minnesota	803	South Carolina
217	Illinois	509	Washington	804	Virginia
218	Minnesota	512	Texas	805	California
219	Indiana	513	Ohio	806	Texas
301	Maryland	514	Quebec, Canada	807	Ontario, Canada
302	Delaware	515	Iowa	808	Hawaii
303	Colorado	516	New York	809	Bahamas, Puerto Rico, Virgin Islands
304	West Virginia	517	Michigan		
305	Florida	518	New York	812	Indiana
306	Saskatchewan, Ca.	519	Ontario, Canada	813	Florida
307	Wyoming	601	Mississippi	814	Pennsylvania
308	Nebraska	602	Arizona	815	Illinois
309	Illinois	603	New Hampshire	816	Missouri
312	Illinois	604	British Columbia, Canada	817	Texas
313	Michigan			819	Quebec, Canada
314	Missouri	605	South Dakota	901	Tennessee
315	New York	606	Kentucky	902	Nova Scotia
316	Kansas	607	New York	903	Mexico
317	Indiana	608	Wisconsin	904	Florida
318	Louisiana	609	New Jersey	906	Michigan
319	Iowa	612	Minnesota	907	Alaska
401	Rhode Island	613	Ontario, Canada	912	Georgia
402	Nebraska	614	Ohio	913	Kansas
403	Alberta, Canada	615	Tennessee	914	New York
404	Georgia	616	Michigan	915	Texas
405	Oklahoma	617	Massachusetts	916	California
406	Montana	618	Illinois	918	Oklahoma
408	California	701	North Dakota	919	North Carolina
412	Pennsylvania	702	Nevada		

NOTE: Your telephone directory contains an Area Code map specifying Area Codes for particular states and locales, including those states (as California) that have more than one Area Code.

Time Zone Map

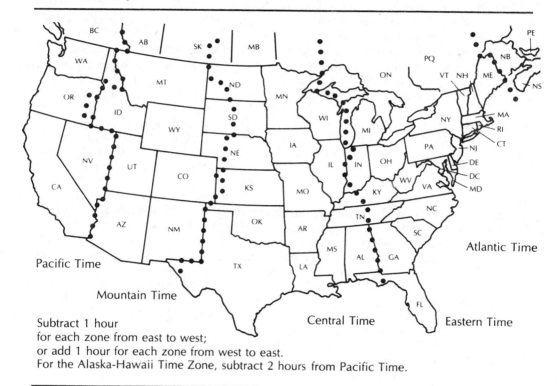

Pacific Time

Mountain Time

Central Time

Eastern Time

Atlantic Time

Subtract 1 hour
for each zone from east to west;
or add 1 hour for each zone from west to east.
For the Alaska-Hawaii Time Zone, subtract 2 hours from Pacific Time.

Wide Area Telephone Service (WATS) WATS is a bulk-use tariff available to large users of telephone service throughout the United States and Canada. The United States is divided into five bands excluding the state in which you are located; Canada is divided into three bands. Presently, each system is independent of the other. Band 1 encompasses all surrounding states and especially bordering states; Band 5 includes the entire United States. Each band is inclusive of the preceding band; that is, Band 4 service includes Bands 4, 3, 2, and 1. Service may be purchased for your own state or for any of the five bands based on a Full Business Day Rate or a Measured Rate. Full Business Day Rates for Bands 1 through 5 are based on a minimum of 240 hours use per month plus overtime. The Measured Rate is for a minimum of ten hours a month plus an overtime rate. Rates vary from state to state depending on the location and distance.

WATS is designated as *inward* or *outward*. Outward WATS will let you place as many calls as you wish, one after another, to a specific band up to the allotted time that you have purchased. Inward WATS permits you to receive as many calls as are needed, one after another, over a specific line. To the number of your inward WATS line is prefixed an 800 Area Code number. With the purchase of inward WATS, the telephone company gives you an additional facility which allows you to receive another call when the primary inward WATS is busy. This call is charged at the overtime rate.

WATS calls are handled over the same telephone switch network as other direct-distance calls. There is no difference in transmission characteristics, since the same telephone network is used. The big difference is that with WATS, a significant reduction in cost can be gained by large-volume telephone users. Most businesses take advantage of the service and use it not only for telephone voice transmission but for data transmission as well. Many state and national medical and allied health associations have WATS lines. It would be useful to ascertain if your physician's organizations have such a service.

Towards the end of 1976, AT&T and Bell of Canada began to offer WATS service covering not only the mainland United States but also Canada, Alaska, and Hawaii. With this new offering, WATS coverage is extended so that Band 6 includes 50% of the Canadian telephones nearest your state. Band 7 includes the remaining 50%.

International dialing   Generally, in order to place a telephone call overseas, you must call the local telephone operator and give the name of the city and country that you wish to call. You will then be connected with the overseas telephone operator who will place the call. The initial charge is for a three-minute minimum, and for each additional minute the charge is approximately one third of the three-minute rate. Rates are determined by the time the call originates and are categorized as *Day* and *Night/Sunday*. The time period may vary for some countries but the Day Rate most often extends from 5:00 a.m. to 5:00 p.m.; the Night Rate, from 5:00 p.m. to 5:00 a.m. Sunday rates apply all day Sunday.

Some areas throughout the United States have access to the International Direct Distance Dialing Service (IDDD). This expands your direct-dialing capability without operator assistance to over 32 countries overseas. IDDD is by far the simplest, fastest, and least expensive way to call abroad. If you have access to an area which has IDDD, you can dial 011 + the country code + the city routing code + the local telephone number and be connected without operator assistance. As an example, a six-minute call to the United Kingdom, dialed directly, would currently cost about $7.20; a call made with operator assistance, about $10.80; and a collect or person-to-person call about $15.00.

5.5

TELEGRAPH SYSTEMS

Periodically a brief, urgent message must be sent from a physician's office. A message like this may be too short to justify a long-distance telephone call. Additionally, the message may require documentation (as in a case of a supply order or an urgent reminder that a patient pay a delinquent bill). Use of a telegram therefore may be in order.

DOMESTIC SYSTEMS AND SERVICES
Western Union provides us with a simple and convenient method of transmitting the written word from one point to another. All one has to do is to telephone one's local Western Union office and dictate the message that is to be transmitted. The cost for this service will be billed to the customer by the local telephone company. Telegrams and cablegrams can also be transmitted from one's office by using the office teletype equipment or FAX machine. If the volume is sizable, one may want a direct line to the Western Union office. Telegrams provide three basic types of service:

Day Letter—usually reaches its destination within two hours. A 15-word minimum charge not including the address and signature is applicable; this service is fast but expensive.

Night Letter—usually delivered to its destination early the following morning on or before the opening of business; the minimum charge is for 100 words, excluding the address and signature. (Keep the three-hour difference in mind when sending a telegram from the East Coast to the West Coast, and vice versa. It may be to your advantage to send a Day Letter in place of a Night Letter.)

Telegraph Money Order—a service which enables money to be transmitted swiftly between Western Union offices at a nominal charge. Most offices have special arrangements with Western Union so that there is no need for a cash advance. Money Orders are transmitted as telegram Day Letters and can reach their destination within a few hours.

Word count is very important in telegrams, because you pay for exactly what you write. The following guidelines may be helpful in the writing of economical messages:

1. The only free words are the address and signature.
2. Dictionary words are counted as one word.
3. Non-dictionary words longer than five letters are counted as two words or more.
4. Abbreviations of less than five letters are counted as one word.
5. Proper names are counted according to the way they are normally written.
6. Punctuation marks are not chargeable, but signs and symbols such as $, &, #, ' (for *feet)* and " (for *inches)* are counted as part of a mixed group used in conjunction with other numbers and letters. Every five characters equals one word.

OTHER TELEGRAPH SERVICES AND SYSTEMS

Telex service   Telex is a service offered by Western Union to give the customer a low-cost worldwide communications system. This service is available in a manual and/or an automatic mode. Most subscribers prefer the automatic unit which can perforate and transmit prepunched tape at a maximum speed of 66 words per minute. Incoming messages as well as hard copy can be received simultaneously on perforated tape. All telex teletypewriters are automatically activated and will automatically respond to a unique preselected identification code. Charges are based on distance and time used. There is no minimum charge. Telex is compatible with the worldwide communication network covering 120 nations throughout the world. Telex equipment can also send messages to TWX equipment by means of a computer interface. In addition, a telex can send multiple address messages and telegrams. Refer to the *Telex Directory* published by Western Union for further details on TWX and a full explanation of current operational procedures.

TWX Service   TWX service is the companion service of telex and is also offered by Western Union. This service also can transmit in a manual or an automatic mode up to a speed of 100 words per minute. Both services can communicate with each other by means of a computer interface. The difference between the two lies in the speed: TWX is faster. There is also a distinct difference in the method of charging: TWX rates are based on a one-minute minimum. This service also can be used in combination with data transmission, since it offers a four-row keyboard very similar to the typewriter keyboard. In contrast, the telex service offers a three-row keyboard limiting the number of characters that the user can transmit. Both teletypewriters can either be leased or purchased.

Mailgram   The Mailgram was developed jointly by Western Union and the U.S. Postal Service to speed written communications. A Mailgram can be prepared at one's teletype terminal, computer terminal or by facsimile machine; or it may be telephoned into one's local Western Union office for transmission. The message is dispatched to the nearest post office and is delivered to the addressee in the first mail the following morning. In addition, a business reply envelope can be incorporated in the Mailgram to ensure a quick response in the shortest time possible. A Mailgram is charged at the standard Western Union rate, plus a special delivery charge.

INTERNATIONAL SYSTEMS

There are two basic ways of transmitting a message overseas, either by cablegram or by International Telex Service. The major international common carriers that can provide this service are as follows:

French Telegraph Cable Company
ITT World Communications, Inc.
RCA Global Communications, Inc.
Western Union International, Inc.

International telegrams (cablegrams)   International telegrams can be sent by way of your local Western Union office to any location in the world. Western Union will file the message with an international carrier of your choice which will then transmit the message overseas. It will then be delivered by the local telegraph company, post office, or government agency of the destination country. The two types of cablegram rates most commonly used are Full Rate Service, which has a seven-word minimum, and Letter Rate, which has a 22-word minimum. Full Rate Service is the most expensive and the message is transmitted immediately. This type of service should be used sparingly. Remember that there is a five- to six-hour time difference between the U.S. and Europe. Don't send a message by Full Rate Service to Europe in the late afternoon or evening. Cablegrams sent by Letter Rate are 50 percent cheaper than the ones sent by Full Rate. These cablegrams usually arrive at the destination after 8:00 a.m. local time the next morning.

Word count is always important, especially if you are sending a Full Rate cable. Rates vary from country to country, of course. *Every word is counted,* including the address and signature as well as the text. Words longer than 10 letters are counted as two words, and each punctuation mark or symbol is counted as one word. Most companies have registered cable addresses; use them. This procedure will certainly reduce word charge. Specify the routing (i.e., name of the international common carrier of your choice) and give delivery instructions (if desired).

International telex   Direct teletype connection can be made to more than 150 countries from any teleprinter that is connected directly to an international carrier. The message can be either directed by keyboard or prepared on punched paper tape and transmitted to your overseas correspondent. You can also have two-way written communication, which provides you with instant confirmation and verification that your message has been received and understood. Rates are about one-fifth those for cablegrams but they vary from country to country. Most European and South American countries are on a one-minute minimum (or approximately 60 words). All others are on a three-minute minimum. Most overseas teletypes are equipped with automatic answer-back features so that no matter what time of day it is, the printer that you call is ready to receive your message.

5.6

USING TELECOMMUNICATIONS SYSTEMS ECONOMICALLY

The office manager in a group practice or the physician in a single practice most often makes policy decisions affecting the kind and cost of the equipment installed. The telephone company can be helpful by providing a communications consultant upon request.

However, the medical assistant can reduce costs in using the equipment. Some helpful hints follow:

1. **Take advantage of the telephone company's discount time periods.** Be sure to remember that calls are charged *at the time* the call is placed. For example, a call placed at 4:59 p.m. is charged as one placed before 5:00 p.m. even if the conversation extends past 5:00 p.m.

2. **Use direct dialing whenever feasible.** Direct dialing rates are considerably lower than operator-assisted rates. Operator-assisted rates are based on a three-minute minimum, compared with a one-minute minimum for direct-dial telephone calls. Operator-assisted rates must be charged *whenever* the operator is on the line; this includes credit card calls, collect calls, and third number calls.

3. **Avoid person-to-person calls.** The cost for person-to-person calls is so high that six station-to-station attempts to reach a person would cost less than one person-to-person call!

4. **Review your toll statement.** Make an attempt to account for all calls listed. In a small office, you should pass the list along to the physician for further scrutiny. In a large office, a telephone log may prove useful.

5. **Report all service disruptions to the telephone company immediately.** This is especially crucial in a medical office, for obvious reasons.

6. **When changes in service are requested, make sure that the work is done to your satisfaction.** Make sure that all equipment is installed exactly as specified. Make sure that service terminations are carried out as required and that the billing coincides with the removal record. The telephone company is known for its expert workmanship, but remember you and your office are the customer and are entitled to satisfaction.

7. **Make sure that credits are applied.** When your service is interrupted or when you have misdialed a toll number, make sure you receive proper credit.

8. **Keep often-used telephone directories on hand.** The trend to charge for Directory Assistance is becoming quite common among telephone companies. It would therefore be wise to keep a supply of telephone directories for major metropolitan areas on hand so that you can look up numbers yourself.

9. **Contact the telephone company if you need a usage study.** Telephone company personnel are always willing and able to perform usage studies and will provide free training for employees in your office.

6

EFFECTIVE INTERACTION WITH PATIENTS AND STAFF

CONTENTS

6.1   STAFF INTERFACE
6.2   MEDICAL OFFICE DIPLOMACY
6.3   HUMAN RELATIONS: Special Problems with Patients

6.1

STAFF INTERFACE

The medical office of today has come a long way from the typical single-physician, single-nurse office of the past. With the current advances in medicine and the advent of various allied health professions, the nature of the medical office staff has been radically changed. For example, a large group practice now may include among its staff members a Registered Nurse-Practitioner, a Physician's Assistant, and several Medical Assistants.

Health care professionals—whether they be nurses or medical assistants—have specific responsibilities based on their academic backgrounds. Consequently, harmony must exist among all office health team members so that they can carry out their assigned tasks efficiently while at the same time creating comfort and a secure atmosphere for the patients. Staff harmony is essential, regardless of the size or the nature of the practice.

The kind of staff necessary for a medical office is determined by: (1) the number of physicians in the practice (2) the patient load, and (3) the particular specialty of the practice. If there is only one physician in the office and you are the only assistant, you then will be responsible for assisting the doctor both administratively and clinically. On the other hand, if you are employed in a joint practice, your duties will depend on your own abilities and your education. If you are a Certified Medical Assistant/Administrative, the clinical duties might be performed by a Certified Medical Assistant/Clinical, a Licensed Practical Nurse, or a Registered Nurse. If you are a Certified Medical Assistant/Clinical, others might perform the more administrative tasks, and you might assist in clinical duties. Since the physician is the one who ultimately decides what you will be doing in the office, it is wise to ask what your duties will be in areas that you are unsure of. Remember: do not overstep your boundaries unless you are specifically told to do so by the physician. Remember also to know your personal limitations and to feel free to ask questions before taking action.

A PROCEDURES MANUAL

Regardless of the size of the staff, a procedures manual is a very important asset to the smoothly run office. While it is helpful to the new employee, it is also a tremendous asset to a person who might be covering for another staff member during illness or vacation. Because it can shorten the orientation period for new employees, a procedures manual can save the physician money. Such a manual also saves time and produces more harmony between the doctor and the patients and among co-workers. However, its most important function is that it spells out the responsibilities of each member of the office team. Thus, the overlapping of responsibilities and the subsequent repetition of procedures are prevented. For example, if no one has been delegated the responsibility for ordering supplies on a regular basis, one staff member may assume that another person has ordered the supplies, when in fact that person had assumed that someone else had ordered them. If the procedures manual has clearly delineated these and other such tasks and has assigned them to specific people, mixups and the costly waste of time can be avoided.

Although it does take time to compile a complete manual, the effort and time expended will result in a more smoothly run office. If your office does not have a manual, you can start one by jotting notes on individual file cards and placing them in an alphabetized and categorized file. With this method, further information can be obtained easily and updated as needed. Later, in spare moments, you can collate the data into a looseleaf binder alphabetized by category.

Unless the procedures manual is updated as procedural changes are made, it will be a useless tool. Updating is necessary: (1) when there are role changes among the staff members (2) when new or additional supplies are ordered (3) when procedures are changed (4) when additional office staff members are hired, and (5) when a new physician joins the practice or a physician leaves the practice. It is wise to take a few minutes now and then to update a section as promptly as the need occurs instead of waiting until the whole book must be updated. (See Chapter 7, section 7.3, for details regarding administrative and/or clinical procedures manuals.)

One person should be assigned the responsibility for ensuring that all employees are aware of any procedural or staff changes. Putting changes on paper does not necessarily make them work if the staff members themselves are not aware that the changes have been made in the first place. One way to increase staff awareness of procedural changes is to have regular meetings before office hours, at lunch, or when the physician is normally out of the office. During the staff meetings, team members can ask questions and can be brought up-to-date.

STAFF COMMUNICATION

One-to-one communication is an integral part of medical office staff interaction. Staff interaction with others occurs in the making of appointments, the greeting of patients, telephone conversations, the greeting of sales representatives, and conversations with the physician's colleagues and family. As stated earlier, a smooth interaction of the staff within itself is absolutely essential to a smoothly run practice. Since patient contentment and security are paramount, it is vitally important that all team members learn to work efficiently and effectively together. You and every other member of the team should have definite responsibilities which you carry out so that you can work together toward two main goals: the best possible patient care and the best possible office routine for the good of the practice. Poor staff relations caused by ineffective or garbled communication can cause tension among staff members which in turn can result in negative patient reactions.

Your attitude and its effect on others   Since some of your training coincides with that of a nurse as well as with that of a Medical Assistant/Clinical, you must fit into the office pattern of work but at the same time you must not be so rigid that a slight change in routine, e.g., an emergency or an illness of a team member, upsets you or causes chaos. All team members must be flexible. Having an alternative plan for such exigencies will prevent any one staff member from becoming unduly burdened.

If tension arises between you and another staff member, it will be much better for you to talk the matter out calmly with the involved person rather than to bear a grudge in silence. Open discussions of personality problems make the persons involved feel better. Also, discussion enables the problems to be resolved early on before they mushroom out of proportion. Of course, no one can be expected to like all of one's colleagues. Nevertheless, a mature person exercises self-discipline in the maintenance of cordial professional relationships. A few of the more basic guidelines to follow are: (1) do not participate in chronic criticism of others (2) avoid office gossip (3) recognize your own shortcomings and try to rectify them (4) be restrained in your speech patterns and in your tone of voice (5) don't try to build a personal empire in the office, regardless of how many important tasks may have been assigned to you, and (6) keep an open mind to useful innovations suggested by other staff members.

As far as the assistant's relationship with the physician is concerned, it goes without saying that the doctor must have implicit confidence in the assistant's ability to carry out assigned tasks with a minimum of supervision. Your behavior, then, must be conducive to that kind of trust. Make a point of finding out the doctor's preferences regarding routines. At the same time, have the doctor tell you what is *not* to be done. Familiarize yourself so well with the doctor's patterns of response to particular questions and situations that you will, in most cases, understand immediately what is to be done without having to ask for a detailed explanation. This is particularly important when a new physician joins a group practice: be sure to learn the doctor's preferences and dislikes at the outset. Make sure that your personal conduct conforms at all times with the wishes of the physician: it is sometimes easy to slip into bad habits (such as tardiness). If you are criticized for making mistakes, accept the criticism politely and resolve to improve. Avoid using the office to conduct your personal business. Do not tie up the telephone at any time with personal calls, do not use the typewriter and the copying equipment for your own material, and do not invite your friends to the office.

6.2

MEDICAL OFFICE DIPLOMACY

First impressions are often lasting ones! Every contact that the medical secretary or the Medical Assistant/Administrative has with patients, medical salespeople, insurance company representatives, and other physicians subtly affects the employer's reputation and practice. Therefore, you are in an excellent position to create a positive office atmosphere since you see the patients and other callers first when they enter the office and last when they leave. A cheerful smile and a professional demeanor will help create confidence in the patients. A happy medium must be reached, though. To this end, a balanced attitude is of utmost importance. A medical assistant or a secretary who is too professional can seem cold or aloof. However, too lax an atmosphere (e.g., gum chewing, gossiping with other staff members, sloppy dress, and undue friendliness with patients) is also bad.

Good public relations skills cannot be developed overnight; rather, it will be a daily effort to cultivate them. You should be aware constantly of what you say, how you react, and how your expressions change—all of which reflect your attitude toward everyone who enters the office. Whenever you speak to a visitor or a patient, that person considers you a representative of the physician's practice.

PUBLIC RELATIONS

Since most patients coming to the office are ill, are in pain, or are simply frightened about their health, the medical assistant can be of great help by calming and reassuring them while they wait to see the physician. Patients' emotional states vary each time they come to the office, and so the same individuals might have to be approached differently on each visit. An alert medical assistant watches for cues from the patients revealing what their feelings are on a particular day and then reacts to them accordingly (see also section 6.3). If you can satisfy the patients' needs, understand their fears, consider their feelings, and look out for their physical well-being, they will respond to you in a more positive way.

Using patients' names   It is nice to get to know patients' names and to learn something about their families: how many children they have, their ages, and the existence of any other live-in relatives. You could also find out about the patients' hobbies, although this is sometimes difficult to do in a large or an extremely busy practice unless the patients or their family members frequently visit the office. To help you remember such information for future office visits, jot down the data in the corner of the patient's ledger card and review it just before the patient is expected. A patient will feel more important if the medical assistant or the secretary says something like "How are the kids today?" when greeting him or her.

Knowing a patient's name and using the name during a conversation adds a personal touch to a purely professional relationship. However, if you're going to use a person's name, be sure that you can pronounce it correctly. If a particular name is difficult to pronounce, it is a good idea to write it phonetically next to its correct spelling on the patient's ledger card so that you will not mispronounce it when you talk with the person.

If you are on the telephone when a patient comes into the office, it is, of course, impossible for you to cut short the conversation so that you can converse with the incoming patient. A simple nod and a smile at the person will indicate that his or her arrival is being acknowledged. After you have concluded your telephone conversation, you can then greet the incoming patient by name.

Personalization instead of depersonalization   With today's scientific advances, with the advent of complex diagnostic equipment, and with the increase in medical specialization, lay criticism of the resulting depersonalization of patients has heightened. This disaffection may be playing a role in some lawsuits against physicians and their staffs. Thus it is doubly important for all staff members to infuse a more personal atmosphere into the office, particularly in a specialist's practice. For instance, a physician-specialist may see a patient only once. Although a single visit to the office is really inadequate to build a substantial relationship of mutual trust, staff members should still approach all such patients with concern and care rather than herding them through the office like cattle.

PATIENTS' FEARS

Patients are often apprehensive, tense, and worried because of fears surrounding office visits. Most patients do not look forward to the visits, so it is important to try to make them feel as comfortable as possible. Remember that they are in an unfamiliar environment surrounded by equipment and smells that they are normally unaccustomed to. Even if a patient is a member of the medical or allied health professions, fear still can erode his or her security. Thus, you should remember that when other health team members come to your employer's office for an appointment, they are coming in *not* as doctors, nurses, or laboratory technicians, but as *patients.* They should be given the same common courtesy afforded any other patient. This includes your giving them thorough explanations and moral support. In fact, do not take any patient for granted, especially if he or she has been coming to the office for some time. These patients too should be shown the same respect and consideration as new patients.

Some common anxieties that patients have include the fear of being hurt, of the diagnosis, of absence from work, of costs, of hospitalization, of surgery, or of death itself. Listen intently and watch carefully to ascertain what the patients are saying and how they are reacting so that you can recognize signs of undue apprehension. However, you also should recognize your limitations. If you feel unable to handle a particular situation, consult a nurse (if one is present) or the physician. If you feel that you can handle the situation, think through your plan of action before proceeding. In all situations, try to put yourself in the patient's place to see how you would react to your own attitudes and statements.

CREATING THE PROPER OFFICE ATMOSPHERE
A medical assistant or secretary must be sincerely interested in people, must enjoy helping them, and must be friendly, courteous, and kind. You will meet many patients whom you will thoroughly enjoy, but you will also meet others who are irritable, unreasonable, and perhaps even rude. Remember that under conditions of stress, people's personalities sometimes change: thus, an ordinarily mild-mannered person may become angry, frightened, or thoroughly uncooperative. Although you yourself may become irritated by such a patient, you *must* remain composed. You cannot take any outburst personally. The patient is probably letting off steam resulting from fears and would probably strike out at anyone conveniently at hand.

PATIENT PREPARATION FOR EXAMINATIONS AND PROCEDURES
The best way to prepare a patient for an examination or a procedure is first to put yourself in the patient's place and treat him or her as you yourself would like to be treated. Choose your words wisely, think before you say anything, and explain the procedure on the layperson's level of understanding. Do not use big words. Medical jargon can frighten patients: most of them know a little about medicine but some of what they know may be misinformation or deficient information. Letting them ask questions after your explanation and having them repeat specific instructions will help to clarify any misunderstandings.

Explaining routines and procedures to patients Do not take for granted that a patient knows the office routine even if he or she has been to see the doctor many times before. If you ask a patient to fill out a form or to prepare for an examination, make certain the patient understands exactly what is to be done and how to do it. Have the patient repeat the instructions as a double-check.

Using preprinted patient information materials Many physicians' offices have on hand preprinted explanations of treatments, instructions for patients, e.g., instructions to be followed prior to X rays or surgery, postoperative orders, special diets, and immunization schedules—to name but a few. Doctors also use product literature provided for patients by pharmaceutical companies. If your physician's office uses such material, be sure first of all that you are familiar with it yourself. When giving this type of material to a patient, go over each instruction or explanation orally to verify that the patient thoroughly understands it.

The importance of not rushing the patient When you are helping to prepare a patient for a session with the doctor, do not give the impression that you are too rushed to do anything more than grab the chart, get the patient in tow, and drop the patient into an empty examination room. If the patient has the impression that you are too hurried to spare even a moment to talk, he or she may then feel that the time to be spent with the doctor will also be rushed. In addition, the patient may forget to ask important questions or mention facts pertinent to the case when the physician does arrive. Therefore, you must try to make every minute spent with the patient a *quality* minute.

Terminating overlong conversations With an overly gregarious patient, you may have to end the conversation politely yet firmly so that you can continue your work and not get behind. You could say, "It's so nice to talk with you, Mrs. (<u>name</u>), and I wish I could keep it up, but you know how it is here, sometimes. I'll just make sure that you're comfortable until the doctor comes in. In the meantime, I must go back to the desk. Don't hesitate to ring the buzzer if you need anything. Dr. (<u>name</u>) will be with you in about (<u>number</u>) minutes."

   If the circumstances are appropriate, you could also say, "It sounds as if you're having difficulty—I'll make a note on your chart so that the doctor will be sure to see that," and then leave the room so that the problem can be charted. If you are polite, calm, and seemingly unhurried, the patients will have a more positive attitude toward their office visits. They must be made to feel that they have had enough time with the staff and the doctor to meet their needs.

Waiting in the examination room If you know that there will be a short wait for patients who are being brought into examination rooms, suggest that they take magazines with them. An alternative is to have a small supply of reading matter in each examination room. If you find that a patient's wait is becoming excessive, check on the patient at regular intervals. On the other hand, if you know at the outset that the wait will be excessive, it is bad policy to take a patient to an examination room. Instead, have the patient stay in the reception room until five minutes before the physician is ready to see him or her. Of course, there are exceptions to this rule, especially when a child becomes noisy in the waiting room or when a patient is ill and would rather wait in the privacy of an examination room. Remember, though, to check on all such patients if they are brought to private areas earlier than usual.

Patients' relatives At times, a patient's relatives can be an asset to the patient's preparation for a procedure; at other times, relatives can be a liability. You will have to use your own judgment in each situation and then tactfully carry through your decision. For example, with pediatric patients, it is often better for toddlers if the parents wait in the reception room. One way of having a parent wait in the reception area is to say, "Johnnie, let's go into the back room," and then to take the child to the room. If another young child is also present, you could also add, "...while Mommy and baby Susie wait here." On the other hand, many pediatricians prefer to have the children's parents in the examination room.

Easing patients' tension before and during procedures and examinations Some procedures and examinations are uncomfortable; others are quite painful. Few patients can anticipate discomfort or pain calmly. Explaining procedures and relating them to accompanying noises, smells, and/or other sensations will help you to allay some fears and will help you to gain cooperation. Many procedures and examinations can be performed with less discomfort to the patient if he or she is relaxed. Therefore, it will be helpful if you have the patient take deep breaths during the procedure so as to aid in relaxing the muscles. An example of a procedure that is often frightening or painful to patients is the insertion of an instrument into a body orifice.

If you will be present during an examination or a procedure, tell the patient so. During the examination or procedure, do not automatically hold the patient's hand for comfort; rather, place your hand *near* his or hers so that the patient can take yours if desired. Not all patients will want to take your hand, but this will give them the opportunity to do so if they wish. Another supportive gesture is to place your hand on the patient's shoulder or arm during a procedure and to stroke it lightly if possible. A reassuring gesture can do wonders for most anxious patients.

If a patient is scheduled for an uncomfortable procedure for the second or third time or more, the level of anxiety will be especially high because the person already knows what to expect. Let the individual know that you too are aware of the impending discomfort and that you sympathize. Encouraging such patients to vent their anxiety (as by crying) is sometimes helpful to them since holding back tears is hard, increases inner tension, and often just intensifies their anxiety. Saying, "It's no crime to let it all out...Just try to relax a bit," beforehand and adding, "I know you're uncomfortable but the doctor is almost through," during the procedure itself are signs that you really care. This is much better than saying curtly, "Don't move."

DEALING WITH VISITORS WHO ARE NOT PATIENTS

Frequently, pharmaceutical and medical equipment representatives and salespeople will arrive with their respective products. These representatives are valuable to the doctor, since they convey information on new products beneficial to patient care. Such products are the concern of all members of the practice. While these representatives should be approached with tact, courtesy, and consideration, they also should be appropriately screened prior to their seeing the physician.

If the callers are new, you might ask for their cards, samples, and/or brochures. Then check with the physician, who will decide whether or not the representatives will be seen. If they do not have something that the physician needs, they nevertheless must be turned away tactfully and courteously, since they may have something of value for the physician in the future. If you are rude, they may never be back. Some physicians prefer to schedule free time each week or every other week to see these representatives. Others like to have a representative wait until a few minutes are free before the next patient is seen. Be sure, in any case, that you know how the physician wishes to handle the situation before it arises. You can help by telling such visitors approximately how long the wait will be or whether they should come back later.

If the physician is a specialist, a list can be compiled of the names of a few selected pharmaceutical and medical supply houses and their representatives. This list will enable you to know whether or not to schedule the visitors for interviews with the doctor. In this way, a representative will not have to wait unnecessarily. You can ask the representative to leave new literature and/or samples and then say that you will contact him or her later. If a representative is coming to confirm a reorder, you can handle the situation yourself if you are routinely in charge of ordering supplies. Otherwise the appropriate staff member should be notified.

If another physician comes to see your physician, quickly usher him or her into an available private room. Notify your physician of the other doctor's arrival so that the visiting doctor can be seen as soon as possible. If it is impossible for your employer to see the visiting doctor, tell the visitor when he or she can be seen, but remember to let your physician make the decision first.

When the physician's family or relatives visit, usher them into an available room and notify the physician. If the physician is busy, you can tell the visiting family that they will have a short (or long) wait. When relatives telephone, connect them with the physician as soon as possible: do not keep them waiting or put them on "Hold" for an inordinately long time.

Occasionally, an insurance company representative will visit the office, requesting additional information on a patient. Be certain that you can identify the representative (as by an identification card) prior to giving him or her *any* information. Check the patient's chart to be sure that the patient has signed a consent form (See also Chapter 3, section 3.5, for a discussion of patient consent forms.) It is illegal to release information without the written permission of the patient. If you are not certain how much information can be released, check with your physician.

Not all insurance representatives are adjustors, salespeople, or general investigators. Many insurance companies have RN-investigators who are assigned by their employers to look into certain health care claims. They typically visit physicians to discuss cases and to examine medical records. It is important for you to know who they are so that you can show them in to see the physician as soon as possible. Nurses should have priority over salespeople, whom you can ask to come back later.

If attorneys arrive requesting information about patients, be sure that you find out whom they represent. Since it is illegal to release information to third parties, a written release must be acquired from the patient or guardian. Many physicians charge attorneys fees for such information; this policy must be explained if applicable.

Government agents (as those from the DEA or the FDA) may visit the office. You should notify the physician immediately so that the agent can be seen by the doctor as soon as possible. Government agents have priority over drug salespeople, insurance company salespeople and other such visitors.

Occasionally, members of the press will come to the office requesting information regarding accident or other cases. Make sure that you see their credentials prior to dispensing any information. Since this is also a third-party inquiry, a release signed by the patient or guardian *must* be obtained. Present the patient's chart to the physician so that some thought can be given to the information before any data are released to the media.

BROACHING FEES

If the physician wishes to stress office payments rather than billing, a system must be devised which will make office payments a natural and routine procedure. An excellent way to do this is to use charge slips. As the physician completes the examination, a charge slip is handed to the patient: included on the slip are the charges for each procedure or service. In this way, the patient can see exactly what has been done during each visit. When the patient leaves the examination room and approaches the exit desk, you take the slip and say, "The charge today is $15.00," or, "Do you have insurance coverage?" Since the patient brings the charge slip to you, you can enter it on the day sheet immediately. Another method of handling office payments is to have a sign in the reception room stating, "We encourage you to pay at each visit to reduce our billing expenses. Thank you." When the patient returns to the desk after seeing the physician, you might say, "Will that be cash or a check today?" Regardless of the method used in your office, you should look up expectantly when the patient approaches the desk. This helps to encourage payment.

SAYING GOOD-BYE

Your last chance to build goodwill is bidding the patient good-bye properly. Patients want to feel that they are important to the staff and that you are interested in them not just as case histories or medical numbers but as human beings. You might end a particular patient's visit by asking if you can call a cab when you know that the patient does not drive. It is nice to say, "We'll be looking forward to seeing you next month, Mrs. Jones," if the patient has just made another appointment.

It is a good idea to have two separate desks in the outside office: an entrance desk and an exit desk. A special layout will be required, including separate doors in and out of the office or a desk situated between two windows with one facing the reception room and the other facing the exit area. After patients have seen the physician, they can stop at the exit desk where other arrangements (as for additional testing) can be made and where the subject of fees can be broached in privacy. Many patients feel uncomfortable when topics such as tests and fees are discussed at a desk opening into a reception room, because other patients can easily overhear the conversations. If the exit desk is in another area, exiting patients are apt to discuss problems or fees more openly. (For additional information on medical suite layouts, see Chapter 7, section 7.1.)

6.3

HUMAN RELATIONS: Special Problems with Patients

INTRODUCTION

The term *human relations* means the study of human problems arising from organizational and interpersonal relationships. In your particular employment situation, human relations involves not only your interactions with your co-workers and your employer's patients but also the understanding and management of your own feelings. As a consequence, you must deal with your personal feelings about illness, pain, and death before you will be able to deal effectively with patients and their problems. This self-understanding is also necessary before you can expect to interact smoothly with other health team members in stressful situations.

In your daily work, you will be handling a variety of patient problems. Some people will be very ill. Others will be extremely anxious or mentally disturbed. Still others will be very young or very elderly. Each patient will have his or her own set of problems. You will also deal with unscheduled emergency patients requiring special treatment. You may also have to handle very angry individuals. In all of these cases it is vitally important that you listen to what the patients say and observe their behavior carefully so that you can inform the physician of any particularly important details prior to examination. You must be able to distinguish medically pertinent information from confidential data having no relevance to the treatment of a patient. At the same time, however, it is important not to break a confidence and lose a patient's respect as a result.

Since medicine is an emotionally charged profession, you must be able to handle your own emotions, or serious problems will be created. Because of the nature of your work, you also will be called on to give support to patients without becoming emotionally involved with them.

You must treat all patients, and especially the very ill ones, with respect and empathy. (Empathy means feeling *with* the patient in an objective way without becoming emotionally involved in the patient's problems.)

This section offers in the following order some practical guidelines for the management of difficult situations with patients:

The Overcrowded Waiting Room   The Non-English-speaking Patient
The Angry Patient   The Emergency Patient
The Infant or Toddler   The Very Ill Patient
The Elderly Patient   The Patient Having a Contagious Disease
The Blind Patient   The Frightened and the Overly Emotional Patient
The Deaf Patient

THE OVERCROWDED WAITING ROOM

One of the chief causes of patients' irritation is a long wait to see the physician. This is especially problematic when the reception area is crowded with patients who have made appointments and who expect to see the doctor on time. Experience shows that most patients are on time or are a little early for their appointments even though they may expect a short wait. It is not uncommon for a patient to wait 20–30 minutes, but since any time longer than that becomes an annoyance, long delays should be avoided.

The medical assistant who makes appointments should be cognizant of the time required for performing procedures so that the appointments can be scheduled accordingly. For example, a first-visit appointment will take twice as long as one for an established patient. No matter how well you schedule the appointments, there will always be something (as a physician's taking longer than expected or being interrupted by an emergency) that will disrupt the patient flow. To remedy this, catch-up time or free time of at least 10 to 15 minutes should be scheduled daily.

When patients come to the office, write down the arrival times next to their names so that you can determine at a glance exactly how long they have been waiting. If the delay is longer than 20–30 minutes, you can express regret for it. For instance, you can tell the patient that the physician has been called away on an emergency, if indeed that is truly the situation. Or you can explain that a very ill patient has arrived and must be seen first, if this is what has really happened. If you know that the wait will be excessive, it is a good policy to inform the patients. Then ask them if they wish to wait or if they would like another appointment. Or you can mention that if they have any other business that they can take care of in a given amount of time, they can do it and then return to the office. Patients find it very annoying to waste time by waiting when they have other things that they could be doing. If you find that the delay will be markedly longer than you originally expected, ask the patient again if he or she wishes to continue waiting, and then apologize again for the inconvenience.

It is also a good policy to learn how to judge time. Never say to patients, "The doctor will be with you in a few minutes." If you really mean a half hour or if the wait will be an hour, say so—or the doctor will be seeing a very angry patient.

THE ANGRY PATIENT

Every office staff at one time or another is confronted with angry patients. The anger may be due to their reactions to pain, fear, or illness itself. Although these situations can be very difficult to handle, remember to approach them calmly. If you raise your voice, the angry individual will simply raise his or her voice even louder. It is best to escort the individual into an empty room and handle the problem there before all of the other patients in the waiting room are disturbed. Letting patients talk out their anger is sometimes a way to help calm them, but if it does not work, notify the physician at once.

Angry patients are in no frame of mind to listen to an explanation of the situation. Letting them air their views without your becoming hooked into the anger is best, although very difficult at times. Recognition of how they are feeling, such as a *yes* followed by a short pause may be all that is needed to help calm them down. For example, "Yes, Mr. Doe, I can understand your viewpoint," or "Yes, Mrs. Smith, I can see that you are upset," or "Yes, Mr. Black, I will check that again" shows them that you are concerned about their problems and are willing to listen. When responding, do not smile since this can give patients a double meaning: "I care, but boy are you wrong!" The worst thing you could do at this time is to try to defend your position, even though you may feel completely justified in doing so. Your defense will probably make the patient even angrier.

During these hypertensive situations, you should be interested primarily in calming the patient rather than in solving the problem per se. It is better to defer full discussion until the patient's emotions have returned to normal, either later that day or on the following day. Before you bring up the problem again, be sure that you have thoroughly investigated the situation and that you understand the problem from the patient's point of view as well as from yours. Since the physician is ultimately responsible for everything that goes on in the office, he or she should be consulted and the situation explained. The physician may wish to deal with the problem by talking with the patient or the physician may give you suggestions on dealing with the problem. No matter what happens—remain calm, poised, and in control of your verbal responses, emotions, and facial expressions.

THE INFANT OR TODDLER

A visit to a physician's office can be a very traumatic experience for young children or infants. Their speech development and their perceptions are limited. Objects such as examination tables, chairs, and instruments look huge to young children. If your physician sees several young children each week, an examination room with child-size furnishings should be set up. This will help to allay some of their fears.

Children's vocabularies are limited, of course. As a result, they are exceptionally sensitive to a person's tone of voice and facial expressions. You must speak slowly and gently to them. If you speak loudly, the children will become frightened. When talking to children, make it a point to get down to their eye level or bring the children up to yours so that you speak to them, not down to them.

If it is important for a child to keep a body part stationary, explain the matter. If the child is in pain, you can explain that it is all right to cry just so long as the affected part is not moved. Explain that moving the injured body part will only increase the pain. Again—don't tower over the child: get down to his or her eye level when you talk so that you won't appear to be so formidable.

It is common practice in many offices to mention to the children that "bravery medals" or other trinkets are given out to the best behaved patients. These rewards often work very well to ensure cooperation. Give infants hugs before and after examinations and procedures if possible. This is especially important because infants and most very young toddlers will not be able to understand why they have been thumped, examined with strange lighted instruments, and stuck with needles. If you do not make sure that you have left the child more or less consoled and calm by way of a sincere hug or a pat, you can be fairly sure that the child will remember it and on subsequent visits will associate you and the office environment with pain. Then, the child will become upset beforehand and will cry.

By the time children are five years old, they start asking *who, what,* and *why.* To deny a child answers to questions especially in a medical office will accomplish nothing more than to magnify the child's fears of the office, the doctor, and the unknown things that may happen there. Some children's fears of people in white are directly related to previous or anticipated frightening incidents in the office. Therefore, you should take the time to answer the child's questions simply and in brief sentences. You must reduce your explanations to the child's level of comprehension. Never lie to the child, but try to answer *only* what is asked. Long irrelevant explanations can only engender more questions and new fears on the child's part. Some children will want to help you with their care (as by undressing all by themselves or by proving that they can climb onto the examining table without your help). If it is safe to do so, let them help. Be sure, however, that you praise them for it.

Some offices have separate rooms for children where they can play and make noise without disturbing the entire waiting room. However, parents are still expected to control their children in these play areas. A polite sign saying as much can be placed at a strategic point in the main reception area if the practice has a heavy load of child patients.

Safe toys should be provided in the waiting room and in the examination rooms for the children to play with while awaiting the doctor. A generous supply of paper, pencils, and crayons as well as a chalkboard can also be kept in the play area or in the main waiting room.

It is extremely unwise to leave any unaccompanied child alone in an examination room because of the instruments and medications that may be stored there. Be sure that this does not happen, even for one or two minutes. The physician and/or staff could be liable for any resulting injury to a child.

THE ELDERLY PATIENT

Since there is a mutual relationship between old age and diseases (and especially degenerative diseases), you may see many elderly persons in the office each day. As with the very young, the aged require a little more time and attention because of changes in their sensory perception. One common mistake made by many health team members is the assumption that once a person reaches an advanced age, he or she automatically becomes deaf. While it is true that an older person's hearing may not be as acute as it was 30 years before, it is not necessarily true that the staff members must shout when talking to the person. Talking slowly and speaking distinctly yet not in a patronizing way while looking directly at an elderly person is much more appropriate. Repetition may be necessary, but the small amount of time it takes to repeat a sentence or two will prevent a longer time being spent in correcting mistakes or misinterpretations. You can tactfully try to have the patients paraphrase important instructions in order to determine whether or not they have really understood what must be done.

Because some elderly patients have difficulty in moving easily, they may require assistance onto examination tables or they may need help in removing their clothing. Most elderly patients are very proud and find it quite difficult to ask for assistance, so if you do offer to help them, do not appear overly insistent or rushed.

THE BLIND PATIENT

Obviously, you will have to give special attention to the physician's totally or partially blind patients. If you know in advance that a particular person is blind, you can plan the appointment so as not to coincide with a heavy patient load, and you can make any other special arrangements deemed necessary.

A few basic guidelines for assisting partially and totally blind patients are given in the list below:

1. Be sure that you approach the blind person immediately upon his or her arrival and identify yourself politely ("Hello. I am Janice Smith, Dr. Lee's assistant. How are you today?").
2. Make the first move to shake hands with an incoming blind patient. This gesture will let the person know where you are, and it will also help you to establish some personal rapport with the patient. It will help orient the patient to his or her surroundings.
3. Speak to the patient in a direct and distinct manner, but do not shout. Never address a blind patient through anyone accompanying him or her, as if the guide were an interpreter of sorts. This is very rude.
4. Tell the patient what you are going to do *before* you do it (e.g., "Mr. Goode, we're going to walk down the hall about 20 paces and then we're going to make a right turn through an open door into the examining room.").
5. When you escort a blind patient, walk moderately slowly, and in a straight line whenever possible. Avoid sudden starts, stops, and changes of direction. Consistency in movement will afford the patient more security.

6. Have the patient take your arm, elbow, or hand while walking or negotiating stairs. Do not pull or push the patient.

7. Alert the patient of upcoming doors (are they open, closed, or swinging?), stairways (up or down?), and corners (right or left?).

8. Walk about a half step ahead of the patient so that it will be easier for him or her to follow you and to sense impending changes in direction even though you will have already alerted the patient of these.

9. When going through doorways, make sure the patient will not be struck by a closing or swinging door and that the patient's fingers will not be caught in a closing door.

10. Keep control of the patient whenever you both are near stairways. Never allow the patient to turn so that his or her back faces a down staircase.

11. When negotiating stairs, tell the patient ahead of time whether the stairs go up or down, whether they are steep, whether they are straight or twisting, and how long they are. Allow the patient to hold to the banister if there is one. Have the patient feel the edge of the first step with his or her foot before you attempt to guide the patient up or down the steps: this will show the patient exactly how far he or she will have to step up or down. Stay one step ahead of the patient and allow the patient to take your arm or elbow.

12. In helping a blind patient into a chair, first put the patient's hand on the back of the chair and then on the seat so that the patient can get an idea of the size of the chair, the direction in which it faces, and the location of its back in relation to the seat. When the patient has been comfortably seated, explain the location of the chair within the office layout so that the patient will feel more secure.

13. Tell the patient whenever you intend to leave, and announce your return. A blind person must never be made to feel abandoned in a strange place.

14. Do not invite a person accompanying the patient as a guide into the examining room unless the blind person gives you express permission to do so.

15. Exercise extreme care when positioning a blind patient on an examining table. Never leave the person unattended after he or she has been situated on the table.

16. Be sure to help the patient in removing and putting on clothes.

17. Help the patient back to the desk after the examination and if there are further instructions, make sure that a written copy of them is given to the patient.

18. Assist the patient to the door, and if travel arrangements need to be made, help out with them.

THE DEAF PATIENT

In dealing with deaf patients, you can simplify matters considerably by using pre-printed questionnaires whose content can be tailored to the particular practice or to the specialty. An example of a very general questionnaire is as follows:

1. What is your medical problem?
2. When did it start?
3. Please give us all symptoms in the space provided:
   a. pain—where and what kind?   f. discharge?
   b. nausea?   g. dizziness?
   c. vomiting?   h. constipation?
   d. bleeding?   i. dehydration?
   e. itching?   j. diarrhea?
4. Please list any other symptoms not given above:
5. How long do the symptoms last?
6. How often do the symptoms occur—regularly? sporadically? constantly? rarely?
7. Is the pain (if any) intense? mild? sharp? dull? throbbing?

Use of this type of material will enable you to communicate with a totally deaf patient without shouting (which is a natural tendency) and without risking misunderstanding through misinterpretation of sign language, gestures, or imperfect speech patterns on the part of the patient.

Remember at all times that some deaf patients experience balance problems. Be sure to watch them carefully so that they do not fall while in the office.

If your physician sees many deaf patients, you might want to use a local interpreter. Contact the local registry for interpreters in your area. A list of these registries can be obtained by writing to Registry Interpreters for the Deaf, 814 Thayer Avenue, Silver Spring, MD 20910.

THE NON-ENGLISH-SPEAKING PATIENT

Occasionally, you may be faced with patients who do not speak English and have not brought interpreters with them. As with elderly patients, you should not shout at them, since this will only tend to raise their anxiety levels and will not help them to understand you any better. Using a type of sign language such as pointing to an object, making an accompanying sound and/or a descriptive gesture will help them to understand better. If you know that patients who speak foreign languages often come to the office, you can use a bilingual book with English sentences and foreign-language translations of them. You can also collect pictures illustrating directions or procedures so that patients who do not understand English can look at them while you make your own explanations. Bilingual questionnaires can be typed with *yes/no* blocks after questions. Blank spaces can be left after longer queries, so that the patients can answer them. Example: the question "Are you allergic to _____, _____, or _____?" or the query "Have you had any of the following diseases: _____, _____, or _____?" are typical items that could appear on a questionnaire in English and in whatever foreign language is spoken predominantly in the area. If the physician sees many non-English speakers, you might consider taking a conversational language course to facilitate communication with these patients. Using a patient's native language will also help you to alleviate his or her anxiety: even learning how to say *hello* and *good-bye* in the person's language will be useful.

THE EMERGENCY PATIENT

You will sometimes be seeing emergency patients in the office. Emergency situations require a somewhat different approach since the patients and their families obviously will not have had time to prepare themselves mentally for the visit. In this situation, their anxiety levels are quite high. If possible, you should bring them at once to available examination rooms. There they can be treated or they can wait for the physician. This procedure will grant them needed privacy and also prevent all the other patients from becoming unduly anxious. Usually a patient's family or a relative will accompany him or her in an emergency situation. Therefore, these people must be dealt with as well. You or another health worker should stay with the patients and their families for moral support. The physician should be notified immediately. The worst thing you can say at this point is, "Don't worry, you are going to be all right." How can you *know* that they will be all right? In the second place, people cannot turn off emotions on command. Patients sense a lack of real concern in these overworked phrases. Your use of bromides like these may only encourage more anxiety. And most importantly, you are legally committing the physician to making them "all right" by such a statement. (See Chapter 3.)

THE VERY ILL PATIENT

Occasionally, very ill patients will come to the office for diagnosis. This can happen before treatment or prior to emergency admittance to a hospital. Since these patients feel physically uncomfortable and tired as well as quite anxious, it is wise to take them as soon as possible to available examination rooms where they can be isolated from other patients, extraneous noise, and other annoyances such as cigarette smoke. Very ill patients might feel more comfortable lying down or sitting in a semi-Fowler's position on the examination table. If a very sick patient must undress for an examination, be sure to give the patient a blanket to cover up with, or allow the patient to wear a coat until the physician comes in for the examination. Notify the physician of the patient's condition so that the person can be seen as soon as possible. Check on very ill patients frequently. Give emotional support with a minimum of words since too much talking will simply tire them even more.

THE PATIENT HAVING A CONTAGIOUS DISEASE

Patients with contagious diseases will often come to the office for treatment. For patients such as these, contagion rooms are invaluable. A contagion room is one that is separate from the general waiting room. It will help to reduce the spread of disease to other patients waiting to see the physician if all patients known to be suffering from contagious diseases are assigned to it. If such a room is available in your office, be sure that the patients assigned to it are checked frequently. Make certain that they too have a supply of magazines and/or toys. In a pediatric contagion room, toys should be disinfected after the patients leave since children have a tendency to put objects into their mouths. Otherwise, the microorganisms from one patient will remain on the surface of the toys for the next child.

THE FRIGHTENED AND THE OVERLY EMOTIONAL PATIENT

As mentioned previously, many patients who are emotional or overemotional in the office are reacting to inner anxiety or fear. Although such emotionalism—whether expressed or repressed—is sometimes unrelated to the patient's health problem, it can equally well be tied in directly with the visit. In this case it can be an adjunct to an existing organic ailment, or it can stem from other anxieties intensified perhaps by the unfamiliar office environment. In a few instances, it can even be the actual cause for the visit to the doctor. At any rate, it is the staff's responsibility to recognize the potential causes of such emotionalism, to not take the patient's behavior personally, and to make the patient feel more secure by showing him or her that the staff cares and is trying to work together for the patient's benefit. You and the other staff members should also remember that fear is contagious: don't allow yourselves to become infected with it. Stay calm so that you can act and react in a coherent, rational manner.

Another important cautionary note: DO NOT GIVE ADVICE. The upset patient has probably heard all possible (and some impossible!) alternatives from well-meaning family and friends but has had far too few listeners. Listening with an objective ear rather than talking is a response less common than it should be and it is one that every patient will appreciate. Many times a patient will feel more comfortable talking with a medical assistant than with the physician and will, therefore, mention to the assistant important facts relevant to the case. In fact, some patients subconsciously withhold important medical information from the doctor but feel free to discuss it with the doctor's office assistant. If this happens to you, listen intently but do not pry. Then be sure to relay to the doctor whatever relevant information you have heard. Sometimes the doctor will ask you later what a particular patient has said and how the patient has behaved with you. If you can help the doctor by remembering as much as possible, you will make a major contribution to the care of the patient. It is vital to keep in mind at all times that good medical teamwork can be sensed by the patients. Good teamwork makes them feel more secure, less anxious, and better cared for.

As mentioned earlier in this chapter, all patients experience a degree of anxiety;

however, it is manifested more obviously in some individuals' behavior than in others'. A typical anxiety/fear manifestation is hypochondriacal complaining about one's medical problems. Although this behavior pattern can be extremely annoying, people exhibiting it have to be treated with empathy yet with professional firmness. Under no circumstances should the complainers be dismissed or ignored just because they are a pain in the neck to the staff. Remember: these patients too should receive the VIP treatment from you. Many times, hypochondriacal patients who are preoccupied with their treatments will ask you about some medication or treatment that the doctor might choose to utilize. Since it is not your responsibility to prescribe, the statement, "I don't know, but the doctor will surely do what is best for you," is the best reply.

Another manifestation of fear or anxiety is anger that may take the form of a tantrum over a bill or over what the patient may consider an excessive wait to see the physician. Even if you do not consider the bill or the wait excessive, the patient—because of his or her irrational state—will not be able to see it any other way . Now is *not* the time to try to explain matters logically to the patient; rather, a simple statement such as, "I can understand why you're upset, and I'm truly sorry for (whatever has irritated the patient)," may help to calm the patient in some instances.

Still another anxiety manifestation is that of excessive stoicism. That a person *appears* to be a Rock of Gibraltar does not necessarily mean that he or she is entirely free of all emotion. In fact, the patient who displays bizarre behavior is in some ways easier to deal with than the stoic, because at least you know right away that something is wrong and you can alert the physician immediately. The fact that the stoic does not exhibit any outward signs of anxiety does *not* give you permission to ignore or to rush the person.

Occasionally you will encounter patients exhibiting overt psychosis. Usually such patients are very scared themselves. It is most unusual for a person of this type to hurt others, yet the myth of the dangerous lunatic still lingers, especially when strange behavior patterns are discernible. If the patient is irritating others in the reception room, it will be best for you to separate that patient from the rest by having him or her wait to see the doctor in an empty examination room. If separated from the other patients, the disturbed person should *never* be left unattended or unobserved. If the patient's relatives or a friend are also in the office, they may stay with the patient. Even then, however, you or another staff member should check on the patient every few minutes.

Because such patients' comprehension and attention spans may be shortened, you may have to repeat your explanations of office procedures. Try to make sure that they understand what is happening, and stay calm when you are talking with them. As mentioned earlier, fear is catching: don't let it get to you, because the other patients will sense it and will in turn become upset. If a situation is beyond your present skill to handle, ask the physician or a nurse to take control.

CONCLUSION

It is appropriate to mention here five of the most important attributes sought in medical team members by physicians interviewed in connection with office staff interactions:

1. maturity
2. empathy
3. flexible efficiency
4. sensitivity
5. calmness

The assistant whose relationships with patients and co-workers reflect these attributes is indeed a valuable asset to the doctor.

7

OFFICE, SUPPLY, AND TASK ORGANIZATION

CONTENTS

7.1

THE OFFICE

Regardless of the medical specialty in which you are employed, your role in the smooth management of the office is vitally important. Good organization—from the arrangement of the physical components of the office complex to the arrangement and management of the equipment and supplies within the office—is essential. Your major responsibilities in achieving this end are to (1) provide a comfortable yet professional office atmosphere (2) arrange the office components in the most efficient manner possible (3) adhere to the principles of sound housekeeping, and (4) accomplish the daily routines effectively, accurately, and on schedule. This chapter is intended to help you with problems of office, supply, and task organization.

OFFICE ATMOSPHERE

There is no longer any need for a medical office to be austere and cold. The white sterile walls and bare rooms of the past are being rapidly replaced by colorful furnishings and decorated walls more conducive to comfort and relaxation for the patients. Wall colors ought to be chosen for their soft, calming effects. It is suggested that the office walls be painted rather than wallpapered because painted walls are easier to clean and are sometimes less disconcerting to the eyes. (Exception: pediatric waiting and examining rooms can be made more attractive to the children if colorful nursery wallpaper is used in decorating them. Washable wallpaper is very handy for this purpose.) The following chart, adapted from Max Lüscher's book *The Lüscher Color Test*, depicts the effects of certain colors on people.

The Effects of Colors on People

Colors	Effects
Blue	has a calming effect; tends to lower blood pressure and to decrease pulse and respiration rates; relaxes the viewer
Green	elicits feelings of firmness, constancy, and control
Red	tends to raise blood pressure and to increase pulse and respiration rates
Yellow	is considered light and cheerful by many; tends to raise blood pressure and to increase pulse and respiration rates (but to a lesser degree than red does)

Brown   sometimes creates physical unease; conveys little security;
             may cause mental unease
Gray   is neutral

Good artificial or natural lighting, or a combination of both, should be devoid of glare and should produce a minimum of shadowing. While overhead lighting is essential in the secretarial work station and in the clinical areas, table and/or floor lamps are sufficient for the reception area. The manner in which the waiting room is lighted can have either a positive or a negative effect on the patients. Consequently, the choices of lighting should aim at achieving a more cheerful environment where possible through a combination of natural lighting and soft artificial lighting.

The arrangement of the office furniture in the waiting area also is important in the creation of a relaxed, informal atmosphere. Small groupings of chairs, with end tables and/or coffee tables interspersed, or a mix of chairs and small sofas will create a warm environment. Although you must provide adequate seating, you should make sure at the same time that you do not create the feeling of overcrowding: avoid lining chairs up in rows or putting furniture too close together. Remember also that small furniture needs to be included if children come to the office.

Draperies should be selected with care. The location of the windows ought to be kept in mind when fabrics are chosen. For instance, when people outside can readily see into the office, heavy fabrics should be used for the draperies to ensure privacy. Heavy fabrics are also useful on windows that take a great deal of strong warm sunlight. A dark green or blue fabric will tone down the intensity and the heat of the sun in cases like this. Conversely, when the room faces north, lightweight fabrics of lighter colors (such as white, cream, or pastels) can be used to allow for more sunlight.

The use of a low-pitched FM radio supplying soft music is yet another way to relieve the monotony of the waiting room atmosphere. Such music is used in many offices. Select the music for its restful qualities and avoid loud music (as rock or even soft rock) that can be distracting to the patients. If your physician sees many older patients, it would be wise to avoid the music altogether.

A few plants can relieve the impersonal quality that ofter pervades reception areas. Nonflowering potted plants are to be preferred. First of all, potted plants are usually a one-time purchase, while fresh flowers need to be bought on a weekly basis. Secondly, the nonflowering potted plants usually require less constant care, while flowering plants must be cut back periodically and their dead blossoms removed. (Exception: if your employer is an allergist, it would be wise not to include plants in the office decoration scheme, since some of the patients may be allergic to them.)

Aquariums and terrariums are also attractive decorative features that can be effectively built into the office decor. However, you must make sure that they are set up so that children cannot reach inside them.

For a full discussion of the intangibles that contribute to a pleasant and professional office atmosphere, see Chapter 6, section 6.2.

COMPONENTS OF THE OFFICE

The most basic physical components of a typical medical suite are as follows:

1. Reception room(s)
2. Secretarial work station(s)
3. Physicians' office(s)
4. Examining room(s)
5. Utility/supply room(s)
6. Laboratory

The following floor plan exemplifies the positioning of these and other office components within the overall layout of the suite. Of course, the number and the size of the rooms depend on the available space within the facility, the number of physicians in the practice, the nature of the practice, and the preferences of the physician. (Additional information and floor plans for medical office suites can be obtained from the AMA.)

Reception room   An individual enters this room first when arriving at the office. It is typically located in the outer area of the office complex, and it is the primary place for patients to wait before seeing the doctor. Some offices have several other reception areas—one for contagiously ill patients and another for children.

Secretarial work station   This is the area in which the office administrative staff performs its work. The area contains desks, file cabinets, chairs, telephones, dictation/transcription equipment, typewriters, and all the other items needed in the performance of secretarial functions. The work station is located next to the reception area in the outer office complex. Although the two rooms are separate, visibility via an inside window must be maintained so that the medical assistant can acknowledge the presence of incoming patients and can talk to the patients when necessary. Many doctors situate the secretarial work station so that there are two windows and two desks—one facing the reception area and the other facing a separate exit area. This arrangement affords more privacy to the outgoing patients when they are discussing bills, payments, and treatments.

Floor Plan of a Medical Office

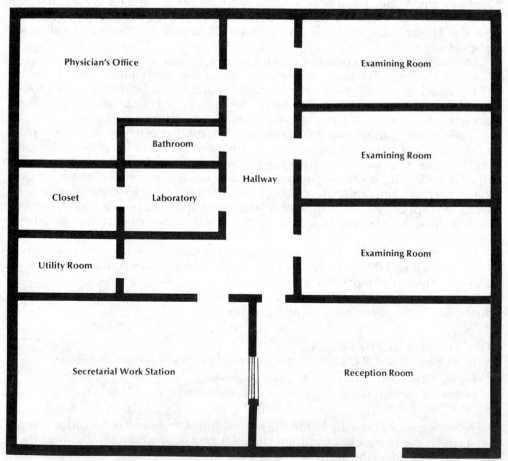

The window to the work station should be kept shut at all times except when the staff members are talking to patients. If the window is shut and the telephone bells are turned down, the patients will not be disturbed by the noise of typewriters and telephones within the work area.

The physician's office   The physician's private office is located in the core of the complex. It provides the doctor with some private space for interviewing patients, counseling and teaching patients, reading and writing professional literature, consulting with other professionals, and managing his or her personal business. The medical library is often located in the doctor's office, too.

Examining room(s)   Examining rooms are designed to be used in the treatment and examination of patients. Individual examining rooms, the size and layout of which vary according to the nature of the practice, are located within the inner core of the office suite. Examining rooms frequently have specific functions within a specialty. For example, in a surgeon's office minor surgery may be performed in one room while dressing changes, suture removal, and follow-up examinations may be accomplished in another room. The functions of each room determine the medical supplies and equipment kept there. However, the minimal furnishings required for an examining room are an examining table, a cabinet, a counter with a sink, two chairs, good lighting, and a writing area.

Utility/supply room   Instruments are cleaned, sterilized, or disposed of in this room. In addition, clinical supplies are stored here. The room should be designed so that clean and sterile supplies do not come into contact with soiled materials and equipment. Cross-contamination is likely to occur if these items are mixed within the same area. The utility/supply room should be readily accessible to the staff, yet removed from proximity to the main patient care areas.

Laboratory   Basic diagnostic tests on urine and blood are performed in this room. In addition, cultures are grown here for the detection of microorganisms. A microscope, a centrifuge, culturing media, an incubator, glassware, Bunsen burners, a refrigerator, and running water are examples of equipment and facilities needed in the laboratory.

PLANNING A NEW OFFICE LAYOUT

Before beginning to help the physician plan for a new office, you ought to read current books or magazines and AMA material on office suite designs and layouts. You can also visit other offices to see how they are laid out. When planning a new office design, make a written inventory of your employer's particular requirements as dicatated by the size and nature of the practice.

In addition to the above, think about the following four points: (1) general space requirements (2) safety considerations (3) comfort for the patients, and (4) room arrangement with respect to ease in accomplishing all daily tasks. Always keep in mind the nature of the practice and the patient population so that you can use the existing space to accommodate the activities and the patients effectively. Also try to plan for the future, because as health care trends change additional space may be needed for the staff to perform all of the services offered by the specialty.

Also consider the principles of microbiology in the placement of rooms in relation to potential cross-contamination. Make sure that all rooms are large enough to facilitate installation of equipment that might be used in them. With today's emphasis on the needs of the handicapped, you also ought to plan for wider doorways and halls and possibly ramps to accommodate wheel chairs.

HOUSEKEEPING TASKS

Microorganisms are always present in the environment. They are found in our bodies, in the air, in food, in water, and on our skin. Since they are often harmful, the medical assistant must understand and practice medical asepsis—the process of reducing the number of microorganisms and the transfer of microorganisms from one person to another. One necessary step is to implement good housekeeping practices. The following are good policies to follow: (1) damp-mop or dust with a bacteriostatic or bactericidal agent (2) avoid using vacuum cleaners unless they are designed so that they do not stir up dust (3) carry all sterile equipment and instruments so that they do not come in contact with your body (4) clean the least soiled areas in the office before the most soiled areas, and (5) place all soiled articles directly into appropriate containers. Additional practices of medical asepsis are proper hand scrubbing and the use of disposable items whenever possible.

Medical offices commonly contract private cleaning firms to perform major cleaning projects on a regular basis. Reliable firms are available in most communities. Before contracting a firm, you should delineate the firm's expected functions and responsibilities and the fee that the office is prepared to pay. The hours of work should also be established. Daily or weekly functions include washing and/or vacuuming the floors, dusting the woodwork, and disposing of wastes. Identify what equipment (e.g., machines and cleaning agents) the firm will provide and what the office will supply. The best hours for cleaning are late in the day when the office is closed.

Two or three times a year the walls and the windows should be washed, the draperies cleaned, and the rugs shampooed. Make arrangements with the cleaning firm for these activities. If the cleaning of the draperies and the rugs does not fall within their responsibilities, make the necessary arrangements for rug and drapery cleaning with an appropriate specialty firm. It is a good idea to plan for this sort of cleaning during vacations and holidays.

Spots, stains, and discolorations are natural in busy offices, but they distract from a pleasant environment and they do not give a good impression of the practice. Take care of them immediately. The following chart, adapted from Kenneth Swezey's book *Formulas, Methods, Tips and Data for Home and Workshop* and Michael Gore's book the *Encyclopedia of Household Hints and Dollar Stretchers*, will assist you in removing common stains.

Directions for the Removal of Common Stains

Cause of Stain	Removal method
Adhesive tape	Remove with a grease solvent or amyl acetate. Rub vigorously with a piece of cheesecloth to avoid rings.
Blood	Soak if possible in cold water; never use hot water. Add a neutral detergent to the water. If necessary and if the fabric can tolerate it, use hydrogen peroxide.
Candy	Sponge the material with plain water. Add a neutral detergent to the water if necessary.
Carbon paper	Sponge the material with a grease solvent.
Chewing gum	Remove as much of the gum as possible with a blunt knife or another instrument. Sponge with a grease solvent or amyl acetate.
Coffee	Soak if possible in warm water with a neutral detergent.
Ink, ball-point	Lubricate the area with Vaseline or white mineral oil. Flush the area with grease solvent. Repeat as often as necessary.
Iodine	Apply sodium thiosulfate to the material. Rinse with cold water.

Pencil, lead	Try a soft eraser first. If necessary, work a heavy detergent solution into the stain. If necessary, use a few drops of ammonia on the stain. Rinse well.
Silver nitrate	Dampen the area with water and add a few drops of tincture of iodine. Soak in cold water if possible. If necessary, use a solution of one tablespoon of sodium thiosulfate in a pint of water. Rinse.

The next chart entitled "Housekeeping Tasks in the Office" is divided into the following segments: Care of the Environment, Care of Equipment, Care of Instruments, and Care of Supplies. This material is intended to assist you in organizing the tasks.

Housekeeping Tasks in the Office

Care of the Environment

Items	Tasks	Special Comments
floors	Damp-mop daily with a bactericidal or bacteriostatic agent. Wax with a nonskid wax.	Highly polished floors are dangerous and can cause injury.
rugs	Shampoo periodically. Vacuum daily.	Scatter rugs are dangerous, as they can cause falls.
draperies	Have them dry-cleaned periodically.	
chairs and couches	Have them reupholstered when needed. Launder slip covers.	Dirty, frayed upholstery and slip covers create a bad impression of the practice.
tables and desk tops counter tops lights file cabinets telephones typewriters books	Wipe off with bactericidal or bacteriostatic agent.	Counter top items are best placed on trays or on paper. Typewriters should be serviced routinely. File drawers should be kept closed at all times.
wastepaper baskets ashtrays	Empty throughout the day.	Wastepaper baskets with lids and foot peddles are the safest. Line all wastepaper baskets with plastic liners.
sinks toilets	Scrub daily or more frequently with a bactericidal agent.	
cabinets	Clean inside and outside with a bactericidal or bacteriostatic agent.	Before cleaning cabinets, remove all materials from the shelves. Be sure that shelves are dry before returning materials.

Care of Equipment

Items	Tasks	Special Comments
glassware specimen bottles jars trays	Wash with soap and water. Sterilize by autoclaving.	A bottle brush is helpful.
Monel or enamelware	Wash the equipment with soap and water before sterilizing. Sterilize by autoclaving, dry heat, or boiling.	

Items	Tasks	Special Comments
examining tables	Change the paper after each patient. Wash the tabletop if necessary.	The examining table should be checked after each patient.
counter tops in examining rooms	Remove any soiled or used items, and wipe off the counter top if needed.	Counter tops should be checked and cleaned after each patient.

Care of Instruments

Items	Tasks	Special Comments
EKG machine X-ray machine microscope otoscope ophthalmoscope sigmoidoscope	Wipe off daily with a bactericidal or bacteriostatic agent.	Individual removable components should be sterilized after each use.
stainless steel, plastic, and plated instruments	Boil, disinfect, or autoclave to sterilize.	Clean all instruments thoroughly before sterilizing; pay attention to grooves and crevices. Open all instruments before sterilizing. Place instruments separately into the sterilizer. Stainless steel may tarnish. Wipe plastics with alcohol, as soaking them for long periods can discolor them. Plated metal will rust unless an antirust cleaning solution is used.
sharp-edged instruments	Sterilize with dry heat to avoid dulling the edges.	Avoid chemical disinfectants which will dull the cutting edges.
lens mountings in instruments	Autoclave these, but be sure to read the brochure that goes with each instrument before attempting to clean it.	Common sterilizing and disinfecting procedures can harm lenses.
syringes, nondisposable	Take them apart. Wash them under cold running water. Use a small bottle brush to clean inside them. Sterilize them by autoclave or dry heat.	

Care of Supplies

Items	Tasks	Special Comments
needles, disposable	Place disposables in a special container.	Break the needle at the hub.
needles, nondisposable	Clean nondisposables immediately after use by forcing cold water through them. Push the stylet through the needle from the hub end. Sterilize by autoclave or dry heat.	Check needles occasionally for sharpness. Check for burrs.

Items	Tasks	Special Comments
rubber goods	Rinse in cool water. Soak in a disinfectant.	When drying, inside surfaces should not touch each other. Fill with air or sprinkle with powder.
tubing	Be sure that the cleansing solution is run through the lumen of the tubing.	Hang tubes over two pegs so as to avoid bends in the tubing.
gloves	Gloves can be autoclaved.	Check gloves for punctures by filling them with water.
linens	Store in dust-free cabinets.	Restock cabinets by bringing the old supplies forward and by placing the new supplies in the back.

MORNING ROUTINES

Every office, regardless of its size, has daily routines designed to make the work progress more smoothly. In this regard, the medical assistant needs to develop sound task fulfillment habits. The most important tasks are outlined below.

Opening the office   Arrive at the office in plenty of time to attend to your own tasks before the workday begins. If you don't, the chances are that you'll be rushed for the rest of the day. Begin by calling the answering service to obtain all messages. Doing this will also alert the service that the office has been opened for the day and that all further calls can be put through to it.

Prepare each room in an organized way for the day's activities. Turn on the lights and adjust the heat or the air conditioning. Keep the inner offices a few degrees warmer than the outer rooms, since patients in the examining rooms are often undressed. Damp-dust the furniture, empty and reline the wastepaper baskets, empty and wash the ashtrays, and wipe the surface area of all machinery. Check each piece of electrical or battery-operated equipment to see that it is working correctly. Return to their proper places all instruments that have been soaking overnight. Restock cabinets and shelves with the necessary supplies. Prepare any special equipment that will be needed during the day.

Mail handling   The medical assistant or secretary must process both incoming and outgoing mail efficiently. Incoming mail can be expeditiously processed if it is sorted into piles before it is opened. When sorting the mail, use the following categories: (1) first class (2) second class (newspapers and magazines) (3) third class (circulars, booklets, catalogs, and other printed materials) (4) fourth class (domestic parcel post) (5) priority mail (air parcel post) (6) telegrams, and (7) international mail.

Letters marked *personal* or *confidential* should not be opened by the assistant unless special authority to do so has been delegated by the physician. (If you open a letter unintentionally, you should mark the envelope "Opened by Mistake," initial it, and reseal the envelope with tape.) Second and third class mail should be opened neatly: remove all protective covers and flatten any rolled items.

Before opening the envelopes, tap the bottom edges to ensure that the contents are not at the top. Checks and other important items have been damaged through neglect of this procedure. First, open all envelopes by slitting the top edges with a letter opener or by using an automatic letter-opening machine. Carefully remove all contents from the envelopes and attach them to the letters with paper clips or staples. Check the enclosure notations on letters to be sure that nothing is missing. If an enclosure is missing, you should make a note of this fact on the letter.

Some offices require that envelopes be fastened to letters. When this is not the practice, the assistant should check to see if the sender's address is on the letter before throwing away the envelope. Some experienced secretaries save all the envelopes for the day in order to recheck for missing enclosures, addresses, or other items.

Use a hand or automatic date stamp to record the date and, if needed, the time when the mail is received. If mechanical devices are not available, write "Received" and the date on the letter. Checks should be immediately stamped "For Deposit Only."

Mail placed on the physician's desk typically includes:

1. mail marked *personal* or *confidential*
2. letters from other professional persons
3. announcements of professional or other meetings
4. professional journals.

When placing correspondence on the physician's desk, you should also provide any additional information needed to respond to the letters. The file of previous correspondence may be particularly helpful.

The medical assistant handles the following mail:

1. letters from patients (except those requiring the physician's attention)
2. letters dealing with statements or accounts (except those requiring the physician's attention)
3. payments on accounts
4. letters soliciting contributions
5. invoices for medical or business supplies
6. monthly statements for office bills
7. magazines for the reception room
8. reports from health services or professional laboratories (except those requiring the physician's attention).

(See also Chapter 15, section 15.9, for a full discussion of letters composed by the medical assistant for the physician.)

Outgoing mail is checked for the following points before being mailed:

1. that the data on the inside address is the same as on the envelope;
2. that any notations such as *confidential, personal, certified mail,* or *special delivery* are typed on the envelope;
3. that the proper signature appears on the letter;
4. that all enclosures cited in an enclosure notation at the bottom of a letter have been included in the envelope with the letter.

The mail can skip an entire sorting operation at the post office if you separate it into categories such as *local* and *out-of-town.* The mail is usually bundled with an identifying label indicating the applicable category. Large mailings (such as patient bills) can be expedited further by sequencing the mail according to ZIP Code number if 10 or more pieces are destined for a single zone. The Postal Service suggests early mailings to alleviate the usual congestion at the close of the day. If possible, mailings should be made throughout the day to avoid one large mailing at the end of the day.

Mail received during a vacation period must be carefully discussed with the physician. Questions that need to be answered are:

1. Will personal mail be forwarded unopened?
2. Will personal mail be opened and a photocopy sent?
3. Can the medical assistant decide which mail needs to be sent to the physician?
4. Can the medical assistant answer any of the correspondence?
5. Can the letters wait until the physician returns?

When you are unable to forward mail to the physician, write a brief acknowledgment to the sender. State in the note that the physician is out of town and will attend to the correspondence upon returning to the office. (See Chapter 15, section 15.9, for a sample acknowledgment letter.)

If the entire office is to be closed for a period of time, make arrangements with the post office to forward the mail to a specific address. If this is impossible, then you can have the post office hold the mail to prevent the loss of important items. Allowing undeliverable mail to pile up outside the office door is a good indicator to a would-be thief that the office is closed.

Periodic straightening of the reception area   Throughout the day, you ought to make periodic checks of the reception room. Straighten the magazines and clean the ashtrays as necessary. Discard worn, tattered, or outdated magazines. In a pediatric office, toys need to be returned to the toy box.

Magazine subscriptions   Select magazines that are appropriate for the predominant patient population, keeping in mind such factors as age, sex, and ethnic background. For example, children and teenagers have reading interests that differ from those of adults. Many magazines are published with special interest groups in mind. Controversial literature should be avoided. If health care magazines are to be made available for reading, the physician should select the titles to be included in the reception area. Although you cannot subscribe to all magazines, you nevertheless ought to have a variety available. Better rates can be obtained by subscribing to magazines rather than by purchasing them at local newsstands.

Cleaning examining rooms after each patient   Allow yourself enough time between patients to clean the examining rooms. Change the paper on the examination table. (This paper is usually on a roll located at the head of the table.) Pick up all instruments and place them in the utility room to soak. Wipe off all used equipment with a bacteriostatic or bactericidal solution. While the wastepaper basket does not need to be emptied after each patient, you nevertheless should not let it overflow. Any medications that have been used need to be returned to their proper places. Collect any used linens and put them in hampers. Discard used paper gowns and drapes. In short, the examining room should not retain any evidence of a former patient when a new patient enters it.

EVENING ROUTINES

The medical assistant is responsible for closing the office at the end of the day, even if the physician remains. If the telephone method for appointment reminders is used, this is a good time to try to reach the patients you were unable to call in the morning. Notify the answering service that you are closing the office. Take any specimens with you that have to be delivered to a laboratory. Just as you have established a morning routine, so should you develop an evening routine for the final cleaning and securing of the office.

Final cleaning of the office   Give a final straightening to the reception room. Return all equipment left in the examining rooms to the proper place. Unplug all electrical equipment. Soak all instruments in disinfectant or prepare them for sterilization. Return to the files all patient records left in the secretarial work station. Clear the top of your desk of work materials.

Securing supplies and locking cabinets   Lock all cabinets—and particularly those containing medications, syringes, needles, and solutions. Some staffs also lock valuable equipment in closets or cabinets. Lock the filing cabinets and your desk drawers to secure confidential information about patients contained in those areas. Check all windows to see that they are locked. Adjust the heat and/or air conditioning for the night. Leave a light burning in the reception room or in the hallway or in both places. This procedure can deter a potential thief. As you leave, lock all doors that provide access to the office from the outside.

7.2

SUPPLIES

Supplies fall into two categories: business and clinical. Business supplies consist of all those materials and devices essential in the operation of the business/administrative side of the practice. Clinical supplies comprise all the materials used by the physician in treating the patients.

Choosing suppliers   Business supplies can be obtained from business supply houses or from stationers. Clinical supplies and equipment are ordered from medical supply houses. (Medications are acquired from pharmaceutical firms, of course.)

The decision to do business with a particular supply house rests with the physician. However, it is the assistant's responsibility to establish and maintain good credit and good business relationships with the designated suppliers. Likewise, it is prudent to continue to deal with the established supply houses and not to move from one to another without good reason. Most houses will try to please their long-time customers by expediting orders. If you have been dealing with a particular supplier on a regular basis, the supplier will often allow your office to test certain new products before they are purchased.

Stocking business and clinical supplies   First of all, you should decide how low the inventory of a particular item can get before it must be reordered. In making this decision, you should consider how often the item is used as well as the length of time required for placing and receiving the order. It is wise to set up a simple inventory control system which will assist you in controlling and ordering supplies. You can do this by first straightening up all business and clinical supplies, then counting the number of items in each category that are on hand, and finally noting on file cards or on inventory control sheets those requiring replenishment. You can group like items together for added convenience; for instance, all disposables from a single supplier can be listed sequentially on cards or can be listed together on one sheet so that you can determine at a glance what items must be reordered from a single firm.

The maintenance of the card or sheet system of inventory control is important because one cannot trust one's memory regarding many amounts, types, and stock numbers. If you choose the card system, put the following data on the top part of each card: (1) the name of the item (2) the identification or stock number (3) the firm's name and address (4) the quantity ordered (5) the reorder point, and (6) the price. In the remaining space on the card, record: (1) the date ordered (2) the quantity or amount ordered (3) the date on which the order was received, and (4) the date on which payment was made. See the next illustration.

Sample File Card

Item *patient gowns - paper*   ID # *456 A*
Firm *R. C. Downs Co.*
Address *100 West Lee Highway, Jonesville, ST 12345*
Quantity Ordered *200*   Reorder Point *75*
Price *$15.00/100*

Date Ordered *2/17/77*   Quantity Ordered *200*
Date Received *3/10/77*   Payment ✓ *3/12/77* On Account _____

If you decide to use the inventory control sheets, you should set up the following columns on every sheet:

Manufacturer's Name
Stock Number
Description of the Item
Size of the Item
Amount of the Usual Order
Minimum Order Required by Your Office
Date(s) of Inventory
Amount or Quantity Ordered
Date(s) of Order
Date(s) Received
Date(s) of Payment

Legal pads turned sideways are useful in constructing inventory sheets. Use a pencil to fill in the data, because the material on the sheets may change from time to time.

Bear in mind that for either system to work properly, you must count your supplies on a regular basis. The number of times that you must count certain items varies according to the nature of the individual item and the rate at which it is usually consumed. For instance, if you know that some items (as disposable needles and gowns) are used up rapidly, you may wish to make weekly or twice-weekly counts. (Your reorders will be large, too.) But for other items that are not consumed so rapidly, you may wish to make monthly counts.

Cost effectiveness   Economical and efficient organizational planning for the use and maintenance of equipment and supplies is the responsibility of the medical assistant. Waste is expensive. It is impractical to order materials in bulk if large quantities are beyond the reasonable needs of the practice. Consider the following questions:

1. Will the quantity be used within a reasonable time?
2. Will deterioration or spoilage take place before the items are used?
3. Can the supplies be stored conveniently within the space available?
4. Is there a chance that the physician will discontinue using the product before the existing supply has been consumed?

It is a myth that money can be saved by purchasing items from cut-rate or unknown suppliers. These kinds of houses very often do not provide for the servicing of equipment or the exchanging of defective supplies. Furthermore, the materials ordered may not be of top quality in the first place.

RECEIVING SUPPLIES FROM COMPANIES

Immediately check any supplies received against the original order and the invoice. (An invoice is a statement from the company listing the items shipped, the price, and the terms of sale.) Make sure that the listed items and the amounts are correct. Ensure that no part of the shipment has been damaged. If a mistake has been made, notify the supply house. Be prepared to provide the firm with the following information: (1) the invoice number (2) the date of the order (3) the name of the manufacturer, and (4) the complaint. After you have returned the defective items to the supplier, you will usually receive a credit slip stating that the items have been received. Put this slip into the current file for that company.

BUSINESS SUPPLIES

The following chart lists the essential business supplies needed in a typical medical office. The chart can be used in setting up your own inventory file card or control sheet system.

Business Supplies

Category	Item
furniture and equipment	desk lamp(s)
	desk(s)
	chair(s)
	telephone(s)
	intercom(s)
	dictation/transcription equipment
	recording media
	photocopier
	adding machine or minicomputer
	typewriter(s)
	file cabinets
	IN-OUT file boxes
	clock
	wastepaper basket(s)
books	dictionaries: medical, general
	procedures manual
	medical secretarial handbook
	office ROUTINES for transcription formats
	Physician's Desk Reference (PDR)
paper goods	prescription pads
	preprinted referral pads
	preprinted telephone message pads
	business cards
	appointment book(s)
	appointment cards
	patient reminder cards
	patient instruction forms
	insurance forms
	chart forms
	patient file folders
	billing cards
	cash receipt book
	ledger book
	checkbook
	shorthand pads
	stationery (letterhead, continuation sheets, envelopes)
	plain typing paper
	carbons

Category	Item
miscellaneous	Scotch tape
	paper clips
	file folder ID tabs
	file folder stick-on labels
	pens, pencils, and pencil sharpener
	ruler
	scissors
	blotters
	thumbtacks
	rubber bands
	letter opener
	stapler
	calendar
	typewriter ribbons
	typewriter erasers, correcting fluid, or correcting tape
	typewriter cleaning brush
	rubber stamp(s)
	postage stamps

CLINICAL SUPPLIES, EQUIPMENT, AND INSTRUMENTS

The clinical supplies, equipment, and instruments found in the office vary according to the nature of the practice and the preference of the physician(s). Furthermore, the quantities and the types of medications stored in the office vary according to the type of practice and the individual doctor's wishes. For example, many doctors prefer to keep the medication inventory to a minimum, especially if they are conveniently located near a pharmacy. But other doctors, and especially those in rural locations, may prefer to keep a large supply of medications on hand. Still other physicians rely heavily on free samples dispensed by drug salespeople. Medication supplies therefore are not discussed here.

With today's trend toward the use of disposables whenever possible, the quantity of permanent items (as nondisposable syringes and linen goods) kept on hand in the clinical areas of the office has markedly decreased.

Keeping in mind the above limitations and variations, see the following chart outlining some but certainly not all of the clinical supplies, equipment, and instruments needed in a typical nonspecialty practice. It is hoped that the chart will be useful to the assistant who has to set up an inventory of clinical items. Assistants employed in specialty practices should be briefed on the items they are responsible for inventorying, ordering, and reordering; the methods of caring for the items; and the nature and function of each item.

Clinical Supplies, Equipment, and Instruments – A General Overview of Essentials

Category	Item	Use
supplies	tape	securing dressings
	adhesive and nylon	
	size ½″, 1″, 2″	
	bandages	
	Kling	wrapping and securing dressings
	4x4s	dressing wounds
	gauze, sterile	dressing wounds
	gauze, unsterile	wrapping and securing dressings
	Band-Aids	dressing minor wounds
	Ace	providing support to an injured body part (as a sprained ankle)

Category	Item	Use
supplies	cotton balls	cleaning a body part or a wound
	cotton swabs	treating throat disorders and applying liquid medications to body parts
	tongue depressors	depressing the tongue in throat examinations
	lubricants	decreasing body surface friction during examinations
	gloves, sterile disposable and/or nondisposable	wearing during sterile procedures
	masks, sterile disposable and/or nondisposable	wearing during surgical procedures
	surgical gowns, sterile	wearing during surgical procedures
	drape sheets unsterile	covering a patient during an examination
	sterile	creating a sterile field or covering a sterile tray
	examining gowns disposable and/or nondisposable	wearing by patients during examinations
	table paper	covering examining table surfaces
	disposable diapers	absorbing body wastes (as with infants)
	sanitary napkins and tampons	absorbing especially blood
	plaster of Paris	constructing casts
	cast padding	cushioning casts
	tubular stockinette	protecting the skin under a cast
	crutches	aiding in the support and locomotion of a patient having hip, knee, leg, or ankle injuries
	slings	supporting an injured arm or wrist
	splints	immobilizing and supporting injured body parts
	rib belts	supporting the chest wall of a patient having broken or cracked ribs
	cervical collars	immobilizing and supporting an injured or a broken neck
	antiseptic cleansers	scrubbing hands before and after procedures
	powder	aiding in the donning of rubber gloves
equipment	examining table, chair	positioning and supporting patients during examinations
	scale and measuring rod	obtaining weight and height of children and adults
	baby scale	weighing infants
	tape measure	measuring the length and the head and chest circumferences of infants and young children
	Mayo stand	holding instruments during surgery
	sterile trays	carrying sterile items
	closed cabinets	storing supplies and instruments

Category	Item	Use
	eye test poster	testing vision acuity
	pediatric urine collection unit	obtaining urine specimens
	emesis basin	collecting and holding waste materials
	specimen containers	collecting urine and stool samples for lab analysis
	culture tubes	taking nose, throat, ear, and wound drainage or secretions as samples for lab analysis
	assorted glass and metal containers	storing sterile and unsterile items
instruments	EKG unit	recording changes of electrical potential during heartbeat and diagnosing irregularities of heart action
	stethoscope	listening to and studying chest and abdominal sounds
	otoscope	examining the ears
	ophthalmoscope	examining the eyes
	sphygmomanometer	measuring blood pressure
	thermometers rectal, oral	measuring and recording body temperature
	flashlight and batteries	providing small field of direct light during examinations
	neurological hammer	testing reflexes
	proctoscope, sigmoidoscope	examining the sigmoid colon
	vaginal speculum small, medium, large	visualizing the cervix and the vaginal wall
	cervical biopsy punch	obtaining cervical tissue for diagnostic examination
	cervical tenaculum	raising the cervix for better visualization
	pessaries	positioning a tipped uterus
	cervical dilators	enlarging the cervical os
	nasogastric tube	collecting gastric secretions, introducing matter into the stomach, and emptying the stomach
	syringes 1 cc, 2 cc, 5 cc, 10 cc, 50 cc	administering medications
	needles 16, 18, 19, 22, 25 gauge	injecting IM, IV, and SC medications
	scalpel	making surgical incisions
	small retractors	holding edges of wounds apart
	Kelly clamps	clamping large blood vessels
	hemostats	clamping small blood vessels
	needle holders	holding needles during suturing
	sutures nylon; silk; plain or chromic gut	closing wounds
	suture removal set	removing sutures and changing dressings
	forceps	picking up sterile and unsterile items
	transfer forceps	moving sterile items from storage to sterile field

Category	Item	Use
instruments	scissors	cutting (as bandages and dressings)
	cast cutter	cutting plaster casts in preparation for removal
	cast spreader	separating edges of casts for easy removal

Basic Laboratory Equipment, Instruments, and Supplies

Category	Item	Use
equipment	Bunsen burner	heating materials during testing
	refrigerator	storing materials requiring cold environments
	autoclave	sterilizing materials
	sterilizer	sterilizing materials
	incubator	cultivating microorganisms for testing and study
	centrifuge	separating substances of different densities
instruments	microscope	studying and identifying microorganisms
supplies	pipettes	transferring and measuring liquids by suction
	glassware (as test tubes)	holding liquid materials before, during, and after tests
	Tes-tape	testing urine for sugar
	Clintest tablets	testing urine for sugar
	Ketostix	detecting ketone bodies in urine
	Acetest tablets	testing urine for presence of acetone
	culture media	growing cultures for analysis and study

STORAGE OF SUPPLIES

The shelf lives of supplies can be maintained and even extended if proper storage procedures are followed. Supplies must be protected from damage caused by exposure to excessive heat and moisture and, in some cases, light. Many drugs, for example, must be kept in dark areas or in dark containers or they must be refrigerated. Furthermore, some items such as needles and syringes and some medications such as controlled substances require extra security precautions. (As an example, federal law requires that narcotics be kept in locked cabinets.)

If the physician keeps medications in the office, all of them ideally should be stored in one area having inside components capable of satisfying the diverse storage conditions required. You can organize the central storage area by drug and/or substance classification. Typical classifications might be: ANTIBIOTICS, DIURETICS, VITAMINS, and so on. If the physician chooses to keep medications in the examining rooms, they should be stored in locked cabinets, especially if patients are left unattended at any time in the rooms. This rule should also apply to other items (as drug samples, IUDs, birth control pills, and so on).

X-ray materials, if used in the office, also need special storage attention. Film must be kept in a cool, dry place, preferably in a lead-lined box. X-ray developer solutions have to be stored in a cool, moisture-free location, too.

Paper products (such as disposable gowns, masks, and drapes) should be stored in a cabinet or cabinets that will keep them dust-free, as opposed to storage on open shelves. Cleaning supplies should never be stored with other supplies. Separating them will eliminate any danger of their becoming mixed up with medications or other clinical items.

In general, you ought to organize the storage shelves by placing all like items together. When restocking the shelves, you should move the older supplies forward and place the newer supplies in the back. In this way you will ensure that older supplies will not be left unused to deteriorate.

LABELING ITEMS

Medications and solutions may be used only if they are in labeled containers. Since the original labels are the most informative, you must take care that they are maintained in the most readable condition possible. Always pour a liquid from the side of the bottle opposite its label so that any liquid running down the side of the bottle will not soil or obliterate the label. Discard medications immediately if their labels are illegible or lost. Discard a medication if you have any doubts whatsoever about the contents of the bottle in which it is stored. Do not rely on your memory as to the locations of any medication bottles because someone else may have moved them around without your knowledge. Do not rely on your sense of smell in identifying unmarked medications: for instance, water, silver nitrate, magnesium sulfate, and some disinfectants all are clear, odorless liquids.

Labels on bottles containing solutions such as alcohol or disinfectants can at times become soiled or torn. In such cases, you should type a new label neatly and accurately, following the exact information provided on the original. It is good practice to have the substitute label checked by someone else in the office before you affix it to the bottle.

EQUIPMENT REPAIR

It is safer and more economical to maintain all equipment in good working order. Follow the preventive maintenance procedure outlined in the printed literature accompanying all products. Have the equipment serviced at once when failures do occur. Following these procedures often postpones a need to replace the equipment. Bear in mind that replacement of defective equipment sooner than expected is very inconvenient, not to mention unnecessarily expensive.

Legal precautions   The medical assistant is accountable to the public who expect that health care services will be provided with skill and sound judgment. Defective and/or contaminated equipment and supplies can cause injury to a patient and when these conditions are known to exist, the medical assistant can be held liable for resultant injuries. Potential hazards include frayed cords, cords running across walking areas, broken plugs, loose electrical connections, poor electrical contact, overloaded plugs, outdated medications, incorrectly marked or unclearly marked medications, incorrect or insufficient sterilization, and a mixing up of solutions. (See Chapter 3.)

7.3

TASK PLANNING

Coordination of office activities among staff members is another responsibility of the medical assistant in larger practices. To have a smoothly run office, one must know one's responsibilities and the work expectations of one's employer (see also Chapter 6, section 6.1, for detailed discussion of staff interactions). Procedures manuals and tickler files are two devices useful in task planning.

A PROCEDURES MANUAL

A procedures manual is a guide establishing how secretarial and clinical routines are to be carried out. It provides each member of the office team with a written explanation of what is expected for each procedure. It is a helpful format for orienting a newly hired employee or a temporary employee.

Setting up a looseleaf binder for procedures The looseleaf format allows you to add or delete procedures as necessary. Generally, the procedures manual is organized with major headings on individual tabular dividers so that the headings can be read easily. Arrange the material in alphabetical order within each category. An alphabetical index should be provided at the end of the manual for quick reference. Individual manuals for secretarial procedures and for clinical procedures are handy because each manual can be located in the appropriate work area. However, if you decide to combine the two manuals, place a divider between the two sections to indicate the separation clearly.

A SECRETARIAL PROCEDURES MANUAL

A secretarial procedures manual is concerned with (1) job descriptions (2) general office policies (3) administrative procedures, and (4) samples of forms. A job description is a detailed outline of a particular position (see Chapter 14, section 14.1 for a sample job description for medical office transcription). Each staff position should have its own outline stating (1) the job responsibilities (2) the educational requirements for it (3) the hours of work, and (4) the promotion guidelines.

General office policies to be outlined in the manual usually include: (1) the office hours (2) the sick leave policy (3) the vacation and holiday policy, and (4) the physician's professional fee schedule.

Essential administrative responsibilities that should be covered in any secretarial procedures manual are shown in the following list. Individual physicians will, of course, include discussion of other responsibilities depending on their own personal preferences, the size of the office staff, and the kind of practice:

1. Scheduling of appointments
2. Billing and collection procedures
3. Banking procedures
4. Filing procedures
5. Financial record-keeping
6. Housekeeping tasks
7. Accident and health insurance
8. Correspondence formats and letter-writing techniques
9. Library responsibilities
10. Processing of incoming, outgoing, and vacation mail
11. Ordering of supplies
12. Telephone practices.

The next illustration exhibits two administrative procedures typewritten for a typical procedures manual.

Under the heading "Forms" in the manual, you should include one copy of every current form used in the office. Ideally, the forms all should be filled in with sample material to illustrate typewriting formats. This is especially important for long typewritten clinical résumés, operative reports, and other matter set up on preprinted sheets. You may wish to arrange the pages in the "Forms" section in the same order as those in the section devoted to administrative procedures. Miscellaneous forms can be grouped together to conclude the section.

An Example of an Administrative Procedure

BILLING

PREPARING MONTHLY STATEMENTS

All statements will be typewritten.

From the patient's ledger card head the statement with the patient's name, address, and today's date.

Begin the statement by entering: the previous balance, any cash payment and the date, and the current charges itemized and dated.

Itemize all charges in the column headed "Professional Services" according to the following categories: office call, house call, office procedure, and diagnostic test.

Before totaling the statement, verify the above information for the correct name, address, and services rendered against the medical record.

Total the statement.

CYCLE BILLING

Office policy is to cycle bill patients as follows:

A - F bill on the 5th of the month

G - L bill on the 10th of the month

M - R bill on the 15th of the month

S - Z bill on the 20th of the month

A CLINICAL PROCEDURES MANUAL

A nurse and/or the physician should develop the content of the clinical procedures manual; however, the medical assistant ought to be responsible for organizing, entering, and typing the procedures within the manual. Organize the manual by first determining the major category headings. Some examples of major headings are:

1. Clinical procedures
2. Diagnostic tests
3. Laboratory procedures
4. Sterilization techniques
5. Administration of medications.

Then typewrite the procedures within the headings exactly as dictated. Use capital letters to introduce the name of each procedure (as URINE ANALYSIS FOR SUGAR AND ACETONE). Use flush-left sideheads to introduce major segments of each procedure. Example:

Purpose:
Materials needed:
Procedure:

Typewrite the individual steps in the procedures exactly as dictated and align them vertically. The steps may be introduced with Arabic numerals. Skip at least two lines between major segments of procedures.

USING A TICKLER FILE

A tickler file is a device that can be used to remind you of your upcoming daily, weekly, monthly, and yearly tasks. Examples of typical reminders to be included in a tickler file are: (1) regular meetings attended by the doctor; these are also included on the doctor's desk calendar (2) housekeeping tasks (3) ordering of supplies (4) follow-up items excluding correspondence, and (5) paying bills such as those for rent, society dues, and journal subscriptions.

Assemble a 3x5 card file with two sets of blank tabular index cards—one set for each month of the year, and the other for each day of the month (1-31). Refer to the next illustration to see how a typical tickler file can be set up. The notations on the card should contain all necessary information to communicate the task to others who might be using the file. Tasks that are performed more than once a year or more than once a month are moved ahead in their respective files.

By using the tickler file and the other procedures and devices discussed in this chapter, the medical assistant can better organize the daily, weekly, and monthly tasks as well as the tools used in fulfilling these tasks. As a result, the practice will be better organized adminstratively.

Sample Tickler Card

Reminder: *Monthly Medical Meeting*
Date: *1st Wednesday of the month*
Amount:
Firm:
Address: *Conference Room, Hospital*
Brief Description:

8

CHAPTER EIGHT

APPOINTMENTS

CONTENTS

8.1

TIME MANAGEMENT

Time is a commodity that is easily wasted. Obviously the physician's time is valuable and so is yours. Indeed, the success of any practice depends largely on how well the physician's and the staff's time is appropriated. You, as a medical assistant, can work toward efficient time use by planning appointments sensibly, by organizing the general work flow in the office, and by doing more than a bare minimum in achieving positive results from established plans.

BASIC PRINCIPLES OF TIME MANAGEMENT

It is vital that you understand these two managerial principles and that you apply them every day:

1. Definite plans based on the objectives, policies, standards, and work procedures previously defined by the physician must be formulated and implemented.
2. All staff and patient activities must be arranged so that responsibility and authority for specific duties are delegated to particular staff members.

Plan for consistent routines designed to fulfill specific tasks. Strive for integration and coordination of all office staff activities. Work to achieve economies. Your adherence to set objectives, policies, standards, and procedures will be the basis of your planning decisions. And once any plan has been developed, it will be successfully implemented only insofar as its activities and its participants are well organized. Otherwise, chaos will result. As suggested above, good office management depends on the proper assignment of responsibility, the granting of enough authority to carry out the assigned responsibility, and the expectation of accountability by those responsible for the results of their actions.

APPOINTMENTS IN TIME MANAGEMENT

The appointment system, if used properly, is a planning device very effective in maintaining a well managed medical office. If not used sensibly, however, it can spell organizational disaster. At the least, the assistant will have to deal with angry patients; at the worst, the physician can face a fast dwindling patient population.

The following paragraphs discuss and illustrate ways by which you can better plan appointments for the sake of a smoothly run office.

The need for appointment keeping A good appointment keeping system will utilize the physician's time efficiently and will decrease the patients' waiting time. The daily work load can be anticipated and structured in an orderly way and more patients can be seen, thereby minimizing costs through it. It also enables activities throughout the organization to be coordinated, with all necessary materials, supplies, and equipment made available as needed. Confusion will thus be decreased, and the general office atmosphere will tend to be easier and more relaxed.

Work flow (time organization) Four components are necessary for effective time organization: (1) understanding (2) planning (3) anticipating the future, and (4) recording the plan. As a medical assistant, you need a clear understanding of what duties, responsibilities, and authority you have. You must become familiar with office policies and practices. You must have the knowledge and skills necessary to function within the office setting.

Planning is a continuous mental process necessary for determining in advance what needs to be done. The following six questions can be asked during the planning stage. (These are illustrated in the next table.)

Planning by Asking Questions of Oneself

1. What... needs to be done? provides me with a total overview of the day's work?
2. Why... is something being done? (My answer will indicate the order in which certain tasks will be carried out.)

NOTE: Determining the answers to the above two questions will aid in determining priorities.

3. When... do things need to be done? and in what order should I set up my work schedule?
4. How... are things done? (My answer will determine which procedures manual and/or what reference material is needed.)
5. Where... are the available space and facilities?
6. Who... will carry out a particular responsibility—a Nurse-Practitioner, the doctor, or I?

Once you have organized the known activities, be aware that unusual events are likely to occur. Try to anticipate these as often as possible and allow yourself options by which you can handle such situations with a minimum of confusion and rearrangement of schedules. Specific ways to accomplish this are discussed later in the chapter.

It is never wise to trust your memory with the complex activities of a medical office. Put your plans in writing. One useful technique is the appointment book; another, the desk calendar; and a third, the planning sheet.

Estimating time requirements Imagine a physician's having to wait 10 minutes for the next patient in a busy office. This should not happen. Lost time will be minimized if you know the approximate amount of time required for the different tests, examinations, and treatments carried out during a normal day. The next chart, "Estimated Time Requirements for Procedures," derived from experience and discussions with medical office personnel, cites some time estimates. It may be useful as you begin to develop for your own reference a list of time requirements according to the physician's practice and preferences. When a patient calls to make an appointment, refer to your list for the expected amount of time and then block the appointment book appropriately. Keep in mind that the patient's time is as valuable as yours.

Heavy vs. light work load   Most people function best earlier in the day. As the day continues, the body begins to become more tired. It is therefore recommended that patients requiring more concentrated attention be scheduled earlier in the day with a gradual trend toward booking the patients requiring less concentration at the end of the day. However, some physicians may have other preferences that you would respect, of course.

Estimated Time Requirements for Procedures

Medical Specialty	Procedure	Time in Minutes
surgery	suture removal	10–20
ophthalmology	eye examination	30
	treatment for	
	conjunctivitis	15
orthopaedic surgery	cast change	20–30
	X ray	10–15
allergy and	sensitization testing	30
immunology	desensitization shots	5–10
internal medicine	physical examination	30–45
family practice	with electrocardiogram	+15
	with sigmoidoscopy	+15
	hypertension follow-up	+5–10
	teaching session	30
obstetrics and	prenatal care	15–25
gynecology	teaching (midwife)	30–45
	postpartum visit	30
	Papanicolaou smear	10–15
pediatrics	well-child conference	30
	teaching	15–30

8.2

SCHEDULING APPOINTMENTS: Specific Techniques and Situations

This system of organization promotes the best use of time. Studies have shown that more patients can be seen under less pressure when appointments are scheduled and adhered to. An awareness of the general guidelines provided in the next paragraphs will assist you in handling the task.

THE PHYSICIAN'S PREFERENCE AS TO SCHEDULES
Every physician has preferences that determine how the office is to be managed. Some physicians set aside specific times or even block several days for certain activities. For example, an office of internal medicine may perform physical examinations only on certain days. An office of ophthalmology may see only school children for routine eye examinations during school vacation periods. It is also common for physicians to leave time at the end of the day for the working person. The medical secretary must be familiar with these preferences.

In addition to knowing the physician's particular preferences, you certainly do need to know the physician's schedule for repeated tasks such as:

1. hospital rounds
2. routine meetings
3. class times, if the physician holds a faculty position
4. office hours

Block out these times in the appointment book so that no confusion will arise as to when the physician will be available.

Also be aware that physicians occasionally alter their routines. For example, most physicians affiliated with hospitals have medical meetings on a monthly or a bimonthly basis. If the first Wednesday of the month is set aside for the medical staff meeting from 8:00–10:00 a.m. and the physician normally makes hospital rounds during that time, you would have to plan for the rounds to be made after the meeting. Consequently, office hours would not begin until afternoon on that day. The physician may present a paper at a conference or attend a workshop, thus causing the regular schedule to be altered. Noting these variations in the appointment book will serve as a reminder for both you and the physician.

Additional points to consider when blocking out unavailable time would be vacations, holidays, free time periods planned during the day, and lunch breaks. Some physicians may wish to have notations made in their appointment books when they have professional or personal evening engagements. Notations of these activities indicate that patients should not be booked right up to the last minute.

EVALUATING PATIENT NEEDS AND UNDERSTANDING THE NATURE OF EACH VISIT

People express their needs in various ways when asking for appointments. Some people play down the need to be seen by the doctor, while others seem to feel that they should be seen immediately. Talking a little with each individual can help you in assessing the nature of any distress and in planning the appointment to fit the specific needs of the patient within the available time. The following two hypothetical conversations illustrate the point:

Patient: I have been having a great deal of pain.

You: Where is the pain?
Can you describe it for me?
[*then* after the patient answers]
How long have you had the pain?
What have you been doing for it?

Patient: I received your notice that I am due for my annual physical.

You: Have you been experiencing any particular problems?

As the patient answers the above questions, you may be better able to assess his or her appointment requirements.

Estimating the time required and considering the facilities available It is your responsibility to assess the amount of time needed for the appointment. It is by this means that the patient work load is controlled. The chart "Examples of Estimated Time Requirements" presented earlier in the chapter illustrates examples of the estimated time required for particular situations.

The physical facilities have considerable influence on how the office is managed. If you are employed in a multiple-physician office, do not schedule two physicians for the same examining room at the same time. Also be sure that two patients requiring services available only in a single examining room are not scheduled simultaneously.

The same principle applies to the use of equipment or instruments. Remember that you may need to allow extra time for cleaning or sterilizing them between appointments. However, if duplicate sets of instruments or other sets of equipment are available, the time allowance need not be as great. Nevertheless, you should always plan your time wisely.

ADVANCED BOOKINGS

Decide how far in advance the bookings will be made—three months, six months, or longer—and select an appointment book that reflects this decision. Make a point to mark off in advance *all* unavailable time as previously described. When making advance bookings, schedule the appointments consecutively but leave some unfilled time so that openings will be available for patients needing appointments at the last minute. In the beginning, you might find it helpful to keep records detailing the number of emergency patients or patients urgently requiring attention who regularly need appointments each week. In this way, you will be able to estimate more accurately the amount of open time that must be reserved each week.

THE FALLACY OF DOUBLE BOOKINGS AS TIME-SAVERS

It is a misconception to think that it is more efficient to schedule a number of people for the same time block. A physician must see them in order, one person at a time. A waiting patient will quickly realize that other people (sometimes three or more) are expecting to see the physician at the same time. This can create negative feelings since each patient likes to feel that the physician is concerned solely about him or her.

When there are several physicians or Nurse-Practitioners in the office, it is obvious that a number of patients will be seen by these individuals at the same time. When you call each patient into the examining room, you can say the following:

"Mrs. Jones, Dr. Smith will see you now. Would you follow me, please."

"Mrs. Day, the nurse will see you and your baby. Would you please follow me."

APPOINTMENT PROBLEMS: The General Practitioner's Office and the Specialist's Office

Every office will have problems regardless of how well you have planned. One cannot plan for the patient who needs a longer than expected time with the physician. Patients sometimes need additional counseling, emotional support, or detailed explanations of how to carry out procedures at home. Also, patients occasionally will arrive late for their appointments. If a person is repeatedly late for appointments, a polite reminder about the importance of promptness is appropriate. But of course all emergencies are disruptive.

Some offices have built-in problems due to the nature of the medical specialty. An assistant in an obstetrician's office is aware that babies do not wait to be born during convenient breaks in the appointment schedule. In a surgeon's office, the physician may be on the way to the hospital to perform emergency surgery just as the waiting room starts to fill. A psychiatrist's schedule may be more reliable, but interruptions in the form of telephone calls from anxious patients nevertheless need to be managed. With experience, you will begin to identify the typical situations that are likely to occur from day to day in your employer's office.

SCHEDULING CHILDREN

When children are the patients, it is helpful to discuss with the physician any scheduling preferences. Some physicians like to block out school holidays, vacation periods, or Saturdays for children. (But remember also that many people find Saturday a convenient time to schedule their appointments. Therefore, you should plan some of the time blocks for adult patients.) After-school hours are other good times for children's appointments. It is beneficial to obtain a list of holidays, vacation periods, and school hours from the local school system. You should also know the school policies regarding excusing children for medical appointments. When scheduling appointments for children, obtain each child's name, his or her age, and the name and address and telephone number of the person who is responsible for the child.

In a pediatric office, preschool children should be scheduled before noon since they often nap in the afternoon. When their needed rest is interfered with, it can lead to fussiness which is, of course, disruptive to the entire office. When possible, arrange the children's appointments by these age groups: infants, toddlers, pre-schoolers, and school-agers. The reason for this pattern is that children of the same age tend to occupy each other better.

APPOINTMENTS MADE IN PERSON AND ON THE TELEPHONE

Appointments made in person are usually made as the patient leaves the office following a visit. It is best to offer an appointment rather than to ask when the individual would like to come. Imagine the following situation:

You:	The doctor would like to see you in about a month to check the incision. Is late in the day still a good time for you?
Patient:	No, mornings would be better because I've been changed to the evening shift.
You:	Oh, is it a permanent change?
Patient:	Only for three months.
You:	Would Wednesday, April 4th, at 11:30 a.m. be convenient for you?
Patient:	It would be all right but a little later in the day would be better.
You:	How much later?
Patient:	About 1:30?
You:	Dr. Smith can see you at 1:45 on Thursday, April 5th.
Patient:	That would be fine.

When making appointments over the telephone, follow the telephone techniques presented in Chapter 5, section 5.1. Remember that you are the first person with whom the patient comes in contact; thus, it is you who establish the initial impression of the whole office. The patient should feel that you are pleasant, interested, and willing to help.

If you are not at your desk when you take the call, explain this fact to the patient, tell the patient that you must push the HOLD button (never neglect to say this!), put the caller on HOLD, return to your desk, and get the appointment book. Pick up the telephone immediately upon returning to your desk and continue the conversation. People will not mind waiting if the wait is not unduly long and if you have explained the necessity for the delay ahead of time. Always bear in mind that to a caller waiting on HOLD, one minute seems endless.

End all telephone conversations with a pleasant "thank you," and repeat the appointment data to the patient. Something like the following might be said:

"Thank you for calling, Mrs. Jones. Dr. Smith will see you on Wednesday, April 4th, at quarter-of-two in the afternoon. Good-bye."

APPOINTMENTS FOR NEW AND RETURNING PATIENTS

When the appointment is for a new patient, obtain complete information on the individual. This is necessary in order to initiate the patient's medical record and the billing record. The following information is collected:

1. first name, middle initial, and last name
2. spouse's name, if applicable

3. home address: street, town, state, ZIP Code
4. home telephone number
5. mailing address, if different from the above
6. business address or spouse's business address
7. business telephone number
8. age
9. referred by whom
10. reason for visit

If the appointment is for a returning patient, check the patient's file to see that the information therein is correct. In this situation, you are most concerned with obtaining: (1) the patient's name (2) the correct address (3) the correct telephone number, and (4) the reason for the visit. If any changes have occurred since the file was originally begun, update the patient's record.

PATIENT REMINDER SYSTEMS

With today's fast-paced society, a system or a combination of systems for reminding patients of appointments can be beneficial. A reminder system is used to inform someone that an appointment needs to be made in the first place and also to remind someone of the specific date and time of an appointment. Three methods can be used: the appointment card reminder, the telephone reminder, and the mailed reminder card.

The appointment card   This card is given to the patient when he or she leaves the office. It should include (1) the person's name (2) the date of the appointment (3) the time of the appointment, and (4) the doctor's name, address, and telephone number. Various types of appointment cards can be chosen for different purposes, as shown in the next illustrations. Appointment cards can be obtained from business supply houses or from local stationery stores.

When a patient is going to make a series of visits, you should schedule all of them at once in the appointment book. If possible, it is wise to schedule the same time and the same day of the week for each appointment in the series. This practice helps establish the appointments in the individual's mind. Even though a complete series of visits may have been booked, you nevertheless should place *only* the upcoming appointment on the card. When numerous cards have to be saved for long periods of time, they can easily be lost. Sometimes patients like a listing of all the appointments so that they can record them on their calendars. Even in these cases, the patients should be given a separate card only for the next appointment, and this procedure should be repeated after each of the scheduled visits.

The telephone reminder   Telephone the patient the day before the scheduled visit. Mornings or late afternoons are often the best times to reach people at home. In some instances, it may be necessary to call the person at work, but you should do this only if the individual has indicated that calls may be received there.

Keep the telephone reminder simple. Identify your office and yourself, and mention the patient, the date, and the time of day of the appointment. Example:

"This is Dr. Jone's office, Mrs. Smith calling. We'd like to remind you of your appointment at 11 o'clock tomorrow morning." After the patient has indicated understanding of the message, you can say, "Thank you and good-bye."

The mailed reminder card   This method can be used either to remind someone that a certain amount of time has passed since the last appointment or to remind the person about an upcoming visit. When it is being used to remind a person that a certain amount of time has passed, the card is sent out in advance of the present

Sample Appointment Cards

Face

TELEPHONE 287-0505

FRANCISCO J. MARASIGAN, M.D.
ERLINDA R. MARASIGAN, M.D.

OFFICE HOURS   810 NORTH CENTRAL AVENUE
BY APPOINTMENT   CHICAGO, ILLINOIS 60651

Reverse

APPOINTMENT

FOR M_s._ *Janice Smythe*

Tues., May 13 AT *3:00* O'CLOCK

IF UNABLE TO KEEP APPOINTMENT KINDLY GIVE 24 HOURS NOTICE.

All Data on Face of Card

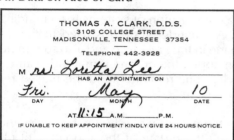

THOMAS A. CLARK, D.D.S.
3105 COLLEGE STREET
MADISONVILLE, TENNESSEE 37354

TELEPHONE 442-3928

M _rs._ *Loretta Lee*
HAS AN APPOINTMENT ON

Fri.   *May*   *10*
DAY   MONTH   DATE

AT *11:15* A.M. _____ P.M.

IF UNABLE TO KEEP APPOINTMENT KINDLY GIVE 24 HOURS NOTICE.

Multiple Appointments

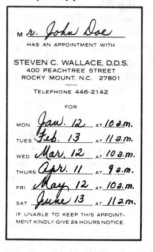

M _r._ *John Doe*
HAS AN APPOINTMENT WITH

STEVEN C. WALLACE, D.D.S.
400 PEACHTREE STREET
ROCKY MOUNT, N.C. 27801

TELEPHONE 446-2142

FOR

MON.	*Jan. 12*	AT *10 a.m.*
TUES.	*Feb. 13*	AT *11 a.m.*
WED.	*Mar. 12*	AT *10 a.m.*
THURS.	*Apr. 11*	AT *9 a.m.*
FRI.	*May 12*	AT *10 a.m.*
SAT.	*June 13*	AT *11 a.m.*

IF UNABLE TO KEEP THIS APPOINT-
MENT KINDLY GIVE 24 HOURS NOTICE.

Reprinted by permission of The Colwell Company.

booking schedule. If the person's year ends in March and you are now booking appointments two months in advance, send the card at the end of December or at the first of January. Then when the patient calls for an appointment, you can provide one for March.

When the mailed card serves as a reminder for an upcoming visit, allow enough time for the card to arrive at the address. Mail it three to five days ahead of the appointment, depending on mail service. See the illustrations of mailed reminder cards.

8.3

EXCEPTIONS TO THE SCHEDULE

Interruptions in the work schedule can come about in several ways. Some of the most common interruptions are emergency patients, physician referrals, cancellations, and special visitors (such as other physicians, salespeople, and insurance representatives). You will never be able to anticipate and plan for all possible unexpected visitors, but the following points may be helpful.

Mailed Reminder Cards

Recall Visit Reminders

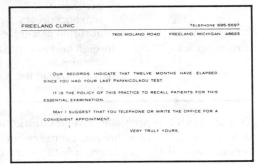

NICHOLAS S. GORDON, D.D.S.   TELEPHONE 893-8338
          318 SOUTH GARRARD   RANTOUL, ILLINOIS 61866

WHEN I EXAMINED *Richard Collins*
IN MY OFFICE, I SUGGESTED THAT (HE/SHE) COME IN AGAIN AT
A LATER DATE. IT IS NOW TIME FOR THIS RECALL VISIT.
          PLEASE CALL MY OFFICE FOR AN APPOINTMENT, IF YOU
DESIRE THIS SERVICE. THANK YOU.

FREELAND CLINIC   TELEPHONE 695-5597
          7605 MIDLAND ROAD   FREELAND, MICHIGAN 48623

OUR RECORDS INDICATE THAT TWELVE MONTHS HAVE ELAPSED
SINCE YOU HAD YOUR LAST PAPANICOLAOU TEST.
          IT IS THE POLICY OF THIS PRACTICE TO RECALL PATIENTS FOR THIS
ESSENTIAL EXAMINATION.
          MAY I SUGGEST THAT YOU TELEPHONE OR WRITE THE OFFICE FOR A
CONVENIENT APPOINTMENT.
                    VERY TRULY YOURS.

Dental Checkup Reminders

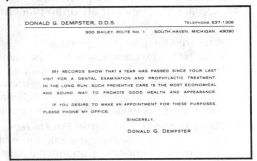

WALLACE B. THOMPSON, JR., D.D.S.   Telephone MA2-6661
          119 HERKIMER STREET   BROOKLYN, NEW YORK 11216

WE ARE REMINDING YOU THAT IT IS TIME FOR YOUR DENTAL CHECK-
UP AS WE HAVE DISCUSSED, PERIODIC EXAMINATIONS ARE NECESSARY
TO PROTECT YOUR INVESTMENT IN GOOD HEALTH KINDLY CALL THE
OFFICE TO ARRANGE AN APPOINTMENT
                    THANK YOU.

DONALD G. DEMPSTER, D.D.S.   TELEPHONE 637-1306
          900 BAILEY, ROUTE NO. 1   SOUTH HAVEN, MICHIGAN 49090

MY RECORDS SHOW THAT A YEAR HAS PASSED SINCE YOUR LAST
VISIT FOR A DENTAL EXAMINATION AND PROPHYLACTIC TREATMENT.
IN THE LONG RUN, SUCH PREVENTIVE CARE IS THE MOST ECONOMICAL
AND SOUND WAY TO PROMOTE GOOD HEALTH AND APPEARANCE.
          IF YOU DESIRE TO MAKE AN APPOINTMENT FOR THESE PURPOSES,
PLEASE PHONE MY OFFICE.
                    SINCERELY,
                    DONALD G. DEMPSTER

Reprinted by permission of The Colwell Company.

SCHEDULING EMERGENCY PATIENTS AND ACUTELY ILL PATIENTS

Sometimes it is difficult to differentiate between a patient with an emergency condition and one who is acutely ill. Nevertheless, you ought to try to do so, for this knowledge will assist you in determining when the person ought to be seen. An emergency is a serious, life-threatening situation and as such it *must* receive priority attention. On the other hand, an acutely ill person ordinarily would present a serious, though not life-threatening, condition. The next chart, "Examples of Emergency vs. Acutely Ill Patients by Medical Specialty," provides some insight into the differences between the two conditions.

Examples of Emergency vs. Acutely Ill Patients by Medical Specialty

Medical Specialty	Emergency Patient	Acutely Ill Patient
internal medicine family practice	heart attack (myocardial infarction) respiratory obstruction	strep throat
allergy and immunology	anaphylactic reaction acute allergic manifestations	sudden onset of severe hives
ophthalmology	foreign body in eye laceration of eye	corneal abrasion acute conjunctivitis
psychiatry	suicidal behavior rape	anxiety neurosis
pediatrics	poisoning burns	high fever

Medical Specialty	Emergency Patient	Acutely Ill Patient
obstetrics and gynecology	ectopic pregnancy complications of pregnancy: placenta previa abruptio placentae	vaginitis pelvic inflammatory disease
otolaryngology	foreign bodies obstructing the airway hemorrhage in the nasopharynx	tonsillitis

Discuss with the physician which emergencies will be treated in the office and which will be treated in the hospital emergency department. As a guide for assessing the seriousness of the situation, a list of questions for the patient should be developed with the physician's help. The following three examples illustrate the various types of questions that could be asked of a patient suspected of suffering from a heart attack, placenta previa or abruptio placentae, or poison ingestion.

1. **Heart Attack**
   When did the pain start? (suddenly)
   What were you doing just before the pain began? (variable response)
   How would you describe the intensity of the pain? (unbearable)
   Does it radiate down your left arm? (usually)
   Are you perspiring profusely? (yes - clammy skin)
   Are you experiencing any nausea or vomiting? (yes - common response)

2. **Placenta Previa or Abruptio Placentae**
   How would you describe the amount of bleeding? (severe)
   Are you experiencing any abdominal pain or discomfort?
      (no - placenta previa; yes - abruptio placentae)
   Would you describe your abdomen as rigid or soft?
      (soft - placenta previa; rigid - abruptio placentae)

3. **Poison Ingestion**
   What was the name of the product ingested? (name is very important)
   How much would you estimate was taken?
      (as accurate an amount as possible is essential)
   How long ago was the ingredient ingested? (time is important)
   How is the person acting now? (alert, lethargic, vomiting)

The emergency situation *always* takes priority. If the patient is to be seen in the office, give instructions for him or her to come there immediately. Inform the physician of the circumstances and the expected arrival time of the patient. Prepare an examining room with the necessary equipment so that there will be no delay once the person has arrived.

Acutely ill patients need to be seen as soon as possible during the day. When a free time period has been prearranged within the schedule, have the patient come then. If none is available, schedule the patient at a time estimated to be the least congested.

PHYSICIAN REFERRALS

Referrals from other physicians fall into two categories: those cases that need to be seen immediately and those cases that need to be seen as soon as possible. *Immediately* would indicate that the patient needs to be seen within the same day or on the next day, whereas *as soon as possible* could indicate an appointment for the patient within a week. The seriousness of the situation determines which type of referral it is. A woman having a lump in her breast that was discovered during a physical examination would be referred to a surgeon immediately. On the other hand, if the same woman needed to have a nonproblematic mole removed, the referral would indicate that she make as appointment as soon as possible.

A reciprocal understanding exists among physicians to accept referred patients outside of the regular scheduling. Most physicians understand the importance of maintaining a schedule and will not be overly demanding as long as judgment is used in giving their patients appointments. (See also Chapter 5, section 5.2, for a discussion of telephone referrals.)

HOW TO FIT REFERRALS INTO THE APPOINTMENT SCHEDULE

One device useful in fitting interruptions into the schedule is the sensible use of the free time period. Leave a 15- or 30-minute block of free time twice during each day if possible. This procedure not only will allow you to fit unexpected patients into the schedule, but also will provide you with valuable catch-up time in which other tasks can be performed.

Another method is to schedule expected patients for a certain number of hours during the day, while at the same time leaving the rest of the available hours for unexpected patients. This plan works most beneficially when a large portion of the patient population is inclined to be emergency, acutely ill and requiring urgent attention, or physician-referred. Of course, the amount of time needed in reserve for unexpected patients will vary according to the medical specialty and the nature of the practice.

If you find that you are unable to use a particular plan for certain interruptions, try to handle the situation calmly and pleasantly. People usually understand emergencies if they are offered a polite explanation.

PHYSICIAN DELAYS, PHYSICIAN AND/OR PATIENT CANCELLATIONS, AND FAILED APPOINTMENTS

These problems—difficult as they are—need working out so that a minimum of time is wasted. If the problem becomes apparent early in the day, there will usually be time for you to make the necessary corrective arrangements. In any case, however, you are expected to handle the situation when it occurs.

Physician delays   There are times when the physician will be delayed in reaching the office. The reasons for such delays can vary. For example, a patient may develop complications during surgery, a meeting may run longer than expected, or hospital consultations may cause the physician to arrive late at the office.

When you know in advance that the physician will be delayed, call the individual(s) involved and suggest other appointments, preferably for later that day. When you know that the delay will be brief, telephone the individual(s) and ask them to come 15 or 30 minutes later than planned. If you know that the delay will be extremely short, it may be wiser to have the patients wait in the office. When patients do wait in the office, explain that the physician has been detained but will arrive shortly. Apologize for the inconvenience.

Physician and/or patient cancellations   Illness or being called out of town for professional or personal reasons also can cause the physician to cancel appointments. In some offices (such as those of obstetricians or surgeons), it may be necessary to cancel appointments for the whole day due to emergencies. Patients who have been scheduled for appointments during this time need to be informed. People usually will understand such occurrences if you take the time to explain the situation.

Occasionally, a patient may have to cancel an appointment. The probability of such a cancellation increases when many appointments are made far in advance. However, the patient who habitually cancels appointments needs to be gently persuaded to keep the appointments. The medical assistant should be tactful but firm when suggesting another appointment. (Also, it is important to determine why the patient continually breaks the appointments in the first place.)

Once people start feeling better, they frequently feel that they no longer need to see the physician. An explanation of the importance of a follow-up visit to their full recovery often will prevent a cancellation. In other instances, patients may feel that they cannot afford the visits. However, satisfactory financial arrangements usually can be made (see Chapter 12, section 12.2). Fear is still another reason that people frequently cancel appointments. Having an open honest discussion with such patients regarding their fears may help to alleviate their anxieties.

Appointments canceled by either the office or the patient should be recorded in the patient's medical record and in the appointment book. The usual policy is not to charge a patient for a canceled appointment.

Failed appointments   When a person neglects to keep an appointment and does not notify the office, it is termed a *failed appointment*. Anyone can accidently forget an appointment. If it is a particularly busy day, you might consider the extra time as a blessing. When you get the opportunity, though, call the person at the end of the day or the next morning, determine the reason for the failure, and reschedule the appointment.

The person who habitually forgets appointments may need a special reminder. One approach is to call the individual on the morning of the appointment. This type of reminder can be more effective than sending a reminder card; however, use of the card *and* the call will serve as a double reminder. If the individual is a business person, suggest that the appointment be scheduled with the individual's secretary. In addition, you may have patients who continually fail to keep appointments as well as those who habitually cancel them for the same reasons discussed earlier. Handle these situations as indicated in the previous subsection.

Note the occurrence of a failed appointment in the patient's medical record. In addition, inform the physician so that the seriousness of the situation can be assessed. If the patient is seriously ill, the physician may wish to call him or her.

The physician can legally charge a patient who has not notified the office regarding the cancellation of an appointment. However, few physicians elect to do so because of the bad feelings it can create.

RESCHEDULING APPOINTMENTS
Contact the patient as soon as possible to reschedule an appointment. From the patient's problem and its seriousness the medical assistant can determine how long the person can wait to be rescheduled. In rescheduling appointments, follow the same principles used when scheduling the original ones.

FITTING OTHER PATIENTS (STAND-BYS) INTO OPEN TIME AT THE LAST MINUTE
The use of a waiting list is useful for quickly filling vacant time when you have had a cancellation. When you know in advance of a vacancy in your daily schedule, turn to the waiting list. Sometimes patients prefer to be placed on the waiting list instead of being given regular appointments. In this way, if a cancellation occurs, an individual who could not have had a regular appointment before several months had elapsed can see the physician earlier.

WAYS TO INFORM PATIENTS OF AN ANTICIPATED PHYSICIAN CANCELLATION
The method you choose to notify a patient of a cancellation by the physician will depend on how much advance notice you yourself have. When you know about it well in advance, write a short note informing the patient of the cancellation and

requesting that the individual call to reschedule the appointment. It is not always necessary to reveal the nature of the physician's absence, but it is important to include the date on which the physician will be returning to the practice. You can also provide the name and address of the other doctor(s) to whom the physician is referring patients during the absence. However, whether you do this or not will be determined by the physician as the two of you discuss the patient load. (See Chapter 15, section 15.9, for a model letter of appointment cancellation due to the physician's absence.)

When you have little advance notice of a physician cancellation, the most expeditious procedure would be to call the individual(s). State that an unexpected situation has developed requiring a rescheduling of the appointment(s). Although the explanation need not be detailed, it does need to be stated clearly.

If, as it sometimes happens, you are unable to reach the person or you did not know of the cancellation until the last minute and the patient has arrived at the office, explain the situation. A polite explanation and a simple apology showing that you understand the inconvenience will usually be satisfactory to the patient.

FITTING ADDITIONAL VISITORS INTO THE PHYSICIAN'S SCHEDULE
At times, people other than scheduled patients wishing to see the physician arrive at the reception desk. These people should be treated according to office policy.

Patients without an appointment   If the individual requires immediate attention, then an adjustment must be made in the schedule. Ask the person to be seated and explain that the physician will be available shortly. If the problem does not need immediate attention, then schedule a regular appointment. Make it clear to both kinds of visitors that the office runs on appointments and then request that they call for one in the future. Explain that the physician is able to give more attention to a person having a scheduled appointment than to a person not having one.

Some offices have a policy called *Open Office Hours.* A couple of hours each afternoon or on certain afternoons of the week are set aside for patients without appointments. This system nicely accommodates the individual who is unable to make an appointment.

Another physician   Regardless of your schedule, medical etiquette dictates that a visiting physician should not be kept waiting. If your employer is with a patient, tell the incoming doctor that, and ask the doctor to wait in your employer's private office. Immediately inform your employer that another physician is waiting in the office. You can best communicate this type of message by way of a note or a prearranged telephone code signal (as two short buzzes). In this way, the patient being seen by the doctor will not feel rushed or unimportant.

Salespeople   Salespeople from medical and business supply houses and pharmaceutical firms frequently stop in unannounced. Your role is to screen these people. Be sure that the equipment and/or pharmaceutical supplies being sold are used in your employer's medical specialty. Know which sales representatives the physician wishes to see and which ones you may talk to. Sometimes salespeople can be persistent in their demands to see the physician. You need to be diplomatic but firm in responding to their demands. Suggest that the individual leave the literature for the physician to look at. This strategy implies that the physician will contact the representative, but it does not commit the physician to do so. Usually, certain salespeople are regular visitors. You will quickly become familiar with them. If you are not familiar with a sales representative, ask to see indentification. (See also Chapter 6, section 6.2, for further discussion of medical office diplomacy.)

8.4

THE APPOINTMENT BOOK

The selection of an appointment book is an individual matter. It has to be a book that will work well for you and one that will meet the needs of the particular office. Consider the following aspects before choosing a book:

1. Is yours a single- or multiple-physician office? Is the staff large?
2. How far in advance do you book appointments—a month, three months, or an indefinite period of time?
3. Do you prefer to see a weekly schedule or a daily schedule at a glance?
4. Does the book contain adequate space to record the necessary information?
5. Does it satisfy your personal preferences?

FACSIMILE OF A TYPICAL APPOINTMENT BOOK PAGE

It is important to have a formal rather than an informal or offhand system for recording appointments. Appointment books can be looseleaf or bound. They can be purchased from business supply houses or from local stationers. Most firms have samples of the various styles to help you in the selection. The next illustration is a facsimile of a typical appointment book page.

Typical entries   The four important elements to include when scheduling an appointment are:

1. the patient's name	Use the full name since it is not uncommon for a person's last name to have two elements or for more than one person to have the same last and first name.
	Spell the name correctly. Ask the person to spell the name for you if you are unsure of it.
2. the patient's telephone number	Know where and how the person can be reached —both at home and at work.
	Although the telephone number is on the medical record, this procedure will expedite your getting in touch with the individual.
3. the reason for the appointment	Using a code system, state the reason briefly.
4. the time	Block out the correct amount of time by drawing a line through the needed amount.

Canceled appointments   Draw a line through the appointment or write the word *canceled* across it. Record the cancellation in the patient's medical record along with the date, the hour, and the reason for the cancellation. Omission of this information could have legal implications since medical records can be taken into court to show that the care provided did meet medical and legal standards.

HELPFUL HINTS FOR KEEPING ORDERLY APPOINTMENT BOOKS

Since the appointment book is not a legal document, use a pencil instead of a pen when making entries in it so that any mistakes or changes can be erased. An untidy appointment book can lead to confusion and error. Plan the appointments so that unused time can be filled easily, as illustrated below:

A patient requires a 45-minute appointment.
The morning hours between 9:00 and 12:00 are open.
Offer the time from 9:00 to 9:45 or from 11:15 to 12:00 rather than from 10:00 to 10:45.

Typical Appointment Book Page

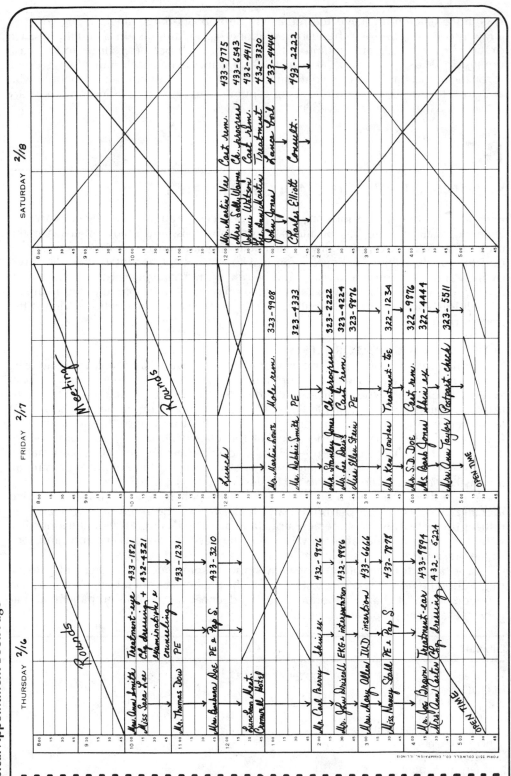

THURSDAY 2/16

Rounds

8:00		
9:00		
9:30		
10:00	Mrs. Ann Smith Treatment-eye	433-1821
	Miss Sara Lee Chg. dressing +	432-4321
	examination &	
	counseling	
11:00	Mr. Thomas Dow PE	433-1231
	Mrs. Barbara Doe PE & Pap S.	433-3210
12:00	Luncheon Mtg.	
	Carmel Hotel	
1:00		
2:00	Mr. Carl Perry Skin jr.	432-9876
	Mrs. Sue Driscoll EKG & interpretation	432-9896
3:00	Mrs. Mary Allen IUD insertion	433-6666
	Miss Nancy Stahl PE & Pap S.	433-7878
4:00	Mrs. Joy Brown Treatment-ear	433-7894
	Miss Ann Carter Chg. dressing	432-6224
5:00	OPEN TIME	

FRIDAY 2/17

Meeting

Rounds

8:00		
9:00		
10:00		
11:00		
12:00	Lunch	
1:00	Mrs. Martin Lowe Note renew.	323-9908
	Mr. Debbie Smith PE	323-1333
2:00	Mr. Stanley Jones Ck. progress	323-2222
	Mr. Joe Rois Cast renew.	323-4224
	Miss Ellen Stein PE	323-9876
3:00	Mr. Ken Towler Treatment-toe	322-1234
4:00	Mr. S.D. Doe Cast renew.	322-9876
	Mr. Barb Jones Skin jr.	322-4441
	Mrs. Ann Taylor Postpart. check	323-5511
5:00	OPEN TIME	

SATURDAY 2/18

8:00		
9:00		
10:00		
11:00		
12:00	Mrs. Martin Vee Cast renew.	433-9775
	Miss Sally Wayne Ck. progress	433-6543
	Johnnie Watson Cast renew.	432-4411
	Mr. Smith Martin Treatment	432-3330
1:00	John Jones Lance boil	432-4444
	Charles Elliott Consult.	492-2222
2:00		
3:00		
4:00		
5:00		

FORM 5517 COLWELL CO., CHAMPAIGN, ILLINOIS

Reprinted by permission of The Colwell Company.

It is more efficient to leave the remaining time in one large single block so as to allow more latitude for scheduling additional appointments. In a multi-physician practice, have a separate column in the book for each person in order to decrease confusion. Thus, you will be able to tell at a glance what each individual is doing throughout the day. It is less confusing when you limit the number of people who are given the responsibility for booking appointments. In a large office, one secretary is usually assigned this responsibility.

8.5

SETTING UP OUTSIDE APPOINTMENTS

Every community has various supporting resources to augment its health care: for example, visiting nurses' associations, clinics, hospitals, and many others. It is the medical assistant's responsibility to schedule appointments with these services for patients needing them. Become familiar with the patient acceptance system used by the various community services and by other physician specialists to whom your office refers its patients. Know what information is required before referring a patient. In addition, know whether the patient needs to receive any instructions prior to the appointment.

SCHEDULING LABORATORY TESTS

Your office will use either a hospital laboratory or a private laboratory for diagnostic tests. Some laboratories use the appointment system while others use a walk-in system for patients. When patients are scheduled by appointment, contact the laboratory and find out the available times. Call for the appointment before the patient leaves your office. Discuss the time with the patient and book the appointment. Provide the laboratory with the name of the diagnostic test(s), the name of the patient, and the name of the referring physician as well as any other information they may require. Provide the patient with a card stating the time of the appointment, any instructions, and directions to the facility.

When the walk-in method is used, give the patient a written statement that identifies the test to be performed and the name of the referring physician. The patient then presents this statement upon arrival at the facility. Provide the individual with the hours that the laboratory is open, any needed instructions, and directions to the facility.

Laboratory tests are often done early in the morning because eating and drinking might alter the reliability of the tests. To gain the patient's cooperation, clearly explain this fact. The next chart, "Laboratory Tests," delineates common outpatient laboratory tests and the preparations necessary for them.

Laboratory Tests

Test	Preparation
BLOOD	
complete blood count	none
red blood cell count	
white blood cell count	
hemoglobin	
hematocrit	
differential count	
sedimentation rate	none

Test	Preparation
prothrombin time	none
partial thromboplastin time	none
sequential multiple analysis (SMA–12)	nothing by mouth (NPO) after midnight
uric acid	
inorganic phosphorus	
cholesterol	
lactic acid dehydrogenase	
total protein	
albumin	
urea nitrogen	
glucose	
calcium	
bilirubin	
alkaline phosphatase	
glutamic oxaloacetic transaminase	
enzymes	nothing by mouth (NPO) after midnight
creatine phosphokinase (CPK)	
lactic dehydrogenase (LDH)	
glutamic oxaloacetic transaminase (SGOT)	
glutamic pyruvic transaminase (SGPT)	
electrolytes	nothing by mouth (NPO) after midnight
potassium	
sodium	
chloride	
carbon dioxide	
acid phosphatase	none
alkaline phosphatase	none
lipoproteins	
cholesterol	water only nothing by mouth (NPO) one hour before drawing specimen no alcohol 48 hours before test
triglycerides	water only for 14 hours before test
phospholipids	
URINE	
phenolsulfonephthalein (PS)	light breakfast with one glass of water no tea or coffee (Certain drugs should be avoided for 24 hours.)
glucose tolerance test	water only after midnight normal diet for three days prior to test free of acute illness for a minimum of one week
24 hr urine collection	first specimen (prior to collection of 24-hr sample) to be discarded all urine for 24 hours (including the first specimen the next day) to be saved

Test	Preparation
routine urine analysis	none
MISCELLANEOUS	
stool specimen	none
sputum specimen	specimen to be collected by patient upon rising
	material deep within lungs to be expectorated
gastric analysis	
tubeless	nothing by mouth (NPO) after midnight

SCHEDULING SURGERY, HOSPITALIZATION, X RAYS, PHYSICAL THERAPY, OCCUPATIONAL THERAPY, AND RESPIRATORY THERAPY

Surgery   Arrangements for hospital surgery are made directly with the head nurse of the Surgical Department (Operating Room) or with the admitting officer. Give this individual a description of the type of surgery to be performed; the date and the time of day that the doctor would like to perform the surgery; and the amount of time the doctor will require (this may already be standardized by the hospital). Once the patient has been scheduled, the hospital will need to know the name and age of the patient and any special requirements (such as diagnostic tests and units of blood to reserve). In your appointment book, state the name of the patient and the type of surgery and then block out the amount of time required.

Hospitalization   Call the hospital's Admitting Department to make the arrangements. Provide the admitting officer with the patient's name and age, the diagnosis, the physician's name, and the patient's status. Usually the patient's status is defined as either *emergency, urgent,* or *elective.* Emergencies are usually admitted the same day, while urgents and electives are placed on a waiting list. The hospital will inform the patient of the exact admitting date and the time when the patient is expected to arrive.

   While your responsibility really ends at this point, you nevertheless can decrease the patient's anxiety if you tell the patient what to expect upon arriving at the hospital. A person from the Admitting Department will usually greet the patient and after some questions have been asked, he or she will show the patient to the appropriate nursing floor. Once the patient has been brought to the nursing unit, the staff there will make the patient comfortable and will answer any further questions.

X rays for patients   It is common to have X-ray examinations performed on an outpatient basis either by a private radiologist or by the hospital X-ray Department. When making the arrangements, furnish the name of the patient, the name of the referring physician, and the type of X-ray study that is to be performed. Some X rays require special patient preparation the night before and/or the morning of the examination. It is important to know the particular requirements for the various X rays. Refer to the chart, "X-ray Examinations," for common examinations and their preparations.

X-ray Examinations

Examination	Preparation
computerized axial telemetry (CAT scan)	none
skull series	none
abdominal X ray	none

Examination	Preparation
chest X ray	none
intravenous pyelogram (IVP)	laxatives or enemas the night before exam nothing by mouth (NPO) for eight hours prior to exam

laminography
   tomography
   planography
	none

pulmonary scintiphotography lung scan	none
barium enema	enemas till bowels are clear the evening before nothing by mouth (NPO) after midnight rectal suppository in the morning

radioisotope scanning
   liver
   brain
   bone
	none

upper gastrointestinal series	nothing by mouth (NPO) after midnight
gallbladder series	low-fat evening meal Telepaque tablets the evening before nothing by mouth (NPO) after midnight

ultrasound
   gallbladder
   pregnancy
   abdomen
	none

When preparing a patient for an X ray, go over the instructions orally and then provide the patient with written directions to be taken home. Since oral directions can be easily forgotten, written instructions are essential. Printed cards are frequently used for this purpose. It is common to find the patients preoccupied, fearful, or embarrassed. Consequently, you ought to be aware of their nonverbal cues and you should try to answer their unasked questions. A repeat X-ray examination required because of poorly given or misunderstood instructions is an unnecessary expense.

Physical therapy, occupational therapy, and respiratory therapy   Physical therapy is concerned with the rehabilitation processes of patients suffering from a wide range of problems. A physicial therapist uses light, heat, cold, water, electricity, and mechanical devices in managing the disease process. The occupational therapist is concerned with the restoration of physical functions with regard to the patient's development of work tolerance, socioeconomic adjustment, and prevocational testing. Occupational therapy attempts to restore activity. The respiratory therapist performs diagnostic pulmonary function examinations and administers respiratory treatments to people suffering from pulmonary disorders.

    All of these people are associated with physicians, are associated with hospitals, or are in private practice. When scheduling appointments for any of the above services, provide the office with the patient's name, the type of therapy required, the referring physician's name, and any information about the patient that you believe would increase the therapist's ability to provide the best treatment.

SCHEDULING CONFERENCES WITH NUTRITIONISTS, NURSE-PRACTITIONERS, AND PHYSICIANS' ASSISTANTS

Today, health needs can often be met by health care providers other than the physician. These professionals include Nutritionists, Nurse-Practitioners, and Physicians' Assistants.

Nutritionists   A Nutritionist is concerned with the dietary requirements of patients. When a patient needs dietary counseling, schedule an appointment with a Nutritionist. The Nutritionist will be able to give you some idea of how much time is needed for various types of dietary counseling. Schedule the time as for any other appointment. It is not uncommon for the Nutritionist to be employed by the hospital and not by the office. In this case, a referral is made. The Nutritionist will need to know the name of the patient, the type of diet needed, the medical diagnosis, and the name of the referring physician.

Nurse-Practitioners   A Nurse-Practitioner assesses the physical and psychosocial status of patients through interviewing, history taking, physical examination, and diagnostic testing. This individual interprets data, develops and implements therapeutic plans, and follows through on the continua of care for patients. A Nurse-Practitioner is usually employed by a physician and interdependently provides care to many patients while often working closely with the physician in the joint management of other patients. Schedule a patient for the Nurse-Practitioner according to regular office policy.

Physicians' Assistants   A Physician's Assistant (usually not a nurse) is qualified by academic and practical training to provide patient services under the supervision and direction of a licensed physician. The Physician's Assistant is an "extension" of the physician and so implements the physician's plan of care. The Physician's Assistant might perform treatments such as suture removal, dressing changes, and physical examinations.

8.6

HOUSE CALLS

Although fewer house calls are made today than in the past, they still require certain tasks on the part of the medical assistants working for physicians who make the calls.

SCHEDULING SET HOURS FOR HOUSE CALLS

When house calls are a regular part of the office routine, the medical assistant working in conjunction with the physician should block time for them. Frequently, physicians prefer to make house calls following hospital rounds. Another common time is after office hours when the doctor is on the way home. Some physicians make house calls only in emergencies; in this instance, you ought to find out from the physician when the call will be made and then schedule it in the appointment book.

SETTING UP A BOOK FOR PHYSICIAN HOUSE CALLS

In addition to recording the house calls in the regular appointment book, you ought to keep and annotate a small looseleaf notebook for house call appointments. Record the following information for each call in the notebook: (1) the name and address of the patient (2) the patient's telephone number (3) directions for reaching the home (identify some landmarks or streets) (4) the reason for the visit, and (5) the name of the person who made the appointment. This notebook will be carried by the doctor. (See the next illustration.)

You should keep a carbon copy of each notebook page. The carbon copy is your record of the appointment. It serves as a reminder to record the visit in the patient's medical record. It is also a reminder for you to obtain follow-up information from the physician. The copy will serve as a record for billing purposes, too.

Sample House Call Notebook Page

Tuesday, May 25

1- Mrs. Elizabeth Colgate
42 North St. (2 houses past school
336-1234   on rt, white house)

Catheterization -
husband called

2- James Baker
9½ Mullen Hill (5th house on left, going
336-4321   up the hill)

fainting spells & vomiting -
Temp. 103 F.
wife called

KNOWING THE WHEREABOUTS OF THE PHYSICIAN
In an emergency, you must be able to reach the physician. Your appointment book should reflect whether the physician is in a hospital, at a clinic, on a house call, or at a meeting. If the physician is between house calls, telephone ahead and leave a message for the doctor to call the office. At times, you may decide to have patients who call contact the physician directly, but usually you will get in touch with the physician yourself. The patients will feel more at ease if you are able to tell them where the physician is and when they might expect to have their calls returned.

THE PHYSICIAN'S BAG
The physician's bag contains items (e.g., instruments, supplies, and medications) needed to treat patients. Take time to familiarize yourself with its contents. Make a list of the items usually kept in the bag. Check the bag daily to be sure that all needed items are there. At the same time, add any special items that the physician will require on a particular day. Remember that the doctor relies on the medical bag when seeing patients. It must contain the appropriate types and amounts of supplies and medications.

Supplies in the medical bag should be given the same care as those kept in the office. The bag itself should be completely cleaned periodically and all nondisposable equipment should be sterilized after each use. Regularly check the dates on items that deteriorate and change them if necessary. Return all materials to the same location in the bag. People have their own systems for organizing. It can be disconcerting to discover that the location of an item has been changed. When you have to substitute items, tell the doctor about it.

The following is a list of supplies commonly contained in the medical bag:

Instruments

sphygmomanometer
stethoscope
thermometers (oral and rectal)
flashlight and batteries
percussion hammer
otoscope

ophthalmoscope
scissors
sterile suture set
scalpel and blades
probe
forceps
tuning fork

Accessories

tongue depressors
cotton-tipped applicators
cotton balls
4x4 gauze
Band-Aids
adhesive tape
safety pins

sterile gloves
specimen containers
culture material
prescription pads
pen
syringes
needles

Medications

epinephrine
narcotics: codeine, morphine
antibiotics
sedatives
digitalis
diuretics

spirits of ammonia
normal saline
alcohol swabs
lubricating jelly
antiemetic
tranquilizer

9

CHAPTER NINE

MEDICAL RECORD ADMINISTRATION SYSTEMS

CONTENTS

9.1

INTRODUCTION

Medical record administration is concerned with the development, implementation, maintenance, and management of systems in order to capture, use, store, retrieve, and release patient health information effectively. The procedures and practices of medical record administration are quite similar in all health care settings, although the ones used in the office of a physician in a single practice are less complex than those used in large medical centers. This chapter guides the medical assistant in the establishment of appropriate systems for capturing, using, storing, retrieving, and releasing patient health information in the single and the group practice settings. Health information systems maintained by hospitals are discussed only when they relate to medical record administration systems appropriate for the single or the group practice.

RECORD MANAGEMENT

Information is the basis for all decision-making and planning. No organization can grow and prosper without adequate records. *Record management* is commonly defined as the systematic control over the creation, maintenance, retention, protection, and preservation of records. The efficient and economical handling of records is the primary objective of any record management program. Record managers function by controlling the creation of records and their subsequent processing.

The record manager, the medical assistant, and the medical record administrator all follow similar practices in maintaining, retaining, protecting, and preserving records. The role of the health care information manager is a critical one in health care facilities because the data handled are of a very personal nature. Also, the absence of needed data may jeopardize appropriate patient care. Not only do medical record administrators serve as health record managers, but also they use patient care information to meet the many needs of patients, physicians, and regulatory and accrediting agencies.

THE MEDICAL RECORD

The medical record is a compilation of knowledge concerning the patient and his or her care. It is an orderly report providing a total picture of the patient's health status. Subjective information such as the patient's complaint is supported by objective physical findings and diagnostic test data. The diverse information in the medical record serves as a channel of communication between those involved in caring for the patient. Records remember what patients and health care providers forget. The medical record identifies: (1) who the patient is (2) what care or procedures were administered (3) who provided the care (4) where and when the care was given, and (5) how the patient responded to the care.

Every health care provider must maintain adequate records to: (1) afford continuity of patient care (2) document that quality care has been rendered (3) justify payment for services rendered (4) serve as a defense against malpractice suits, and (5) function as a basis for submitting required reports to appropriate government agencies.

The medical record facilitates continuity of patient care by providing data on earlier illnesses—data that may supply the key to a patient's current medical problems. The patient's response to treatment is noted so that the treatment may be adjusted accordingly. Diagnostic test results may be compared over a particular time period, with improvement or lack of improvement noted.

The medical record can document that quality care was rendered in a certain case by demonstrating the physician's logic in collecting a data base and efficiently applying it to manage the patient's ongoing care. The medical record may be reviewed by the physician's peers to evaluate the appropriateness of the care. The medical record also provides proof that specific services charged to a patient or a third party were actually rendered, for the findings and/or results of these services are noted in that record. The patient's record can be the most important evidence in any medical professional liability suit regardless of the factual issues involved. Detailed office records ordinarily prevail with a jury as opposed to a patient's recollections. Juries often assume that good records indicate good care, while inadequate records imply substandard care. The physician's office records also provide the documentation that the medical assistant needs to complete various reports required by law—reports on gunshot wounds, reports on communicable diseases, death certificates, and others.

Maintaining good medical records requires expenditures of time and money. However, the physician's productivity and collection rates can be improved through the availability of complete, orderly, and legible medical records.

9.2

PATIENT RECORDS AND CASE HISTORIES

Licensure laws and accrediting agencies impose many requirements on the record-keeping practices of hospitals and other health care facilities, but physicians in single or in group practice are free to choose any record system appropriate to their needs. Therefore, the records maintained by an individual health care provider usually reflect the patient care goals and the philosophy of the provider. A health care provider offering comprehensive care to a rather stable patient population requires a more detailed record system than the one used by a practitioner offering episodic care to a transient patient population. As an example, the records maintained by a family practitioner often provide health data on an individual from infancy to adulthood. However, the records of many specialists focus narrowly on a specific problem and describe a few brief episodes of care. Physicians in single practice usually make fewer demands on their record systems than those in group practice because group practice records must be comprehensive enough to permit another member of the group to take over the care of any patient when necessary.

Although single-physician practices are free to establish their own record systems, the documentation needs of today's medical practices nevertheless cannot be met by maintaining each patient's record on a 5 x 8-inch card. All information about a patient should be centralized in a single file folder. This file is known as the patient's medical record or case history, and it usually contains medical and administrative data on the patient. Data related to the patient but not necessarily to his or her care (e.g., carbons of insurance reports) may be included in the same folder with the information about the care. However, accounting records should not be maintained in the patient's medical record, because outside auditors legally accessing accounting records do not have the right to see medical information.

The following patient care data are normally collected by single and by group practices:

1. Identifying information
2. Historical data
3. Physical examination findings
4. Results of various diagnostic procedures and special examinations
5. Records of treatment
6. Immunizations and medications administered and/or ordered
7. Reports of the patient's progress in response to therapy
8. Summaries of treatment rendered by outside consultants or institutions
9. Consents for treatment and release of information.

MEDICAL RECORD FORMS

We live in a forms-oriented society. It seems that every significant event in our lives is controlled by forms such as birth certificates, diplomas, licenses, and death certificates. However, forms are indispensable information processing tools that help physicians and their office staffs provide continuous quality patient care with minimal expenditures of money, time, and effort. Effective office records are kept concise but not at the expense of necessary information. Forms themselves do not guarantee accurate and adequate medical recording. However, forms providing for the notation of essential data facilitate the capture of requested information. Commercial form companies offer varied forms which the physician may purchase for office use. Many physicians, however, prefer to design their own forms and have them printed locally. The medical office assistant therefore should be familiar with the basic principles of forms design.

A Medical Record

REGISTRATION FORM

Patient Name	Austin, Jane Marie		Phone	829-2956

Address	2400 Lakeview, Chicago, IL 60614

Date of Birth	2-10-33	Sex	F	Marital Status	Single	Social Security #	123-45-6789

Occupation of Patient	Secretary	Employer	First National Bank	Address	1 North LaSalle, Chicago

Name of Nearest Relative	Elizabeth Austin	Sister	Phone	528-1774

Address of Above	2626 Lakeview, Chicago, IL 60614

Insurance Company Name	Blue Cross-Blue Shield, 1 North Wacker

Address	Chicago, IL 60606	Policy #	23257 Group

RECORD INDEX

VISIT DATE	SERVICES RENDERED	CODE

00-45-20

PATIENT'S NAME Austin, Jane

FORMS DESIGN

The following queries may be used to evaluate the appropriateness of commercial forms or self-designed forms:

1. What purpose will this form serve? Do we really need such a form? Why?
2. Does the form contain all necessary information and no unnecessary information?
3. Is there wasted space on the form? Could this form be combined with another one?
4. Will the form save time for the data recorder and retriever?
5. Is the content logically organized? Are terms and symbols clear and unambiguous?
6. Is the format appropriate? Are the data arranged so as to permit continuous recording from left to right and from top to bottom?
7. Is related information grouped together? If more than one person is responsible for entering data on the form, are the blocks for these data arranged in sequence?
8. Is the form identified with an appropriate title briefly but clearly indicating the function and purpose of the form?
9. Has the data entry method (i.e., handwriting vs. typing) been considered in determining the appropriate size of the spaces for entering the information?

New forms should not be initiated until there is a demonstrated need for them and unless alternative means for meeting that need have been considered. For example, a rubber stamp providing spaces for the entry of new data may be affixed to an existing form in order to meet new information requirements. One should also determine the anticipated use of every piece of information requested on a form. Since it costs money to acquire information, one must guard against the dangers associated with collecting nice-to-know but unessential data.

When designing or evaluating commercial forms, one's appraisal cannot be limited just to content because physical form characteristics also play an important role in determining whether a form is appropriate for a specific practice. Whenever possible, medical record forms should be of the standard 8½ x 11-inch size so as to reduce paper and printing costs as well as to achieve economy of space.

Factors to be considered in selecting the weight of the paper include (1) the writing method used (2) the amount and kind of handling involved (3) the way in which the records are filed and stored, and (4) the required retention period. Heavier weight paper such as bond must be used for records that are handwritten, extensively handled, and unprotected by folders; as well as for those intended to be retained for many years. (Pulp and sulfite papers are less expensive and less durable than papers of rag content.)

Color may be used on forms to assist in the rapid identification of specific sections of a record. The most practical approach is to use a colored edge or band. It should be remembered, however, that forms printed on colored paper may not microfilm well, especially if a dark color is used on them.

One should always consider printing medical record forms on both sides in order to conserve storage space and reduce bulk. The type of record binding or fastener used will also be a determining factor in planning printed forms. If a top binding is chosen, those forms using both the front and reverse sides of the pages must have the printing on the reverse sides tumbled (i.e., printed foot to head). Sufficient margins must be allowed for binding. Side binding may offer more convenient retrieval since most users are accustomed to reading side-bound books.

CAPTURING MEDICAL RECORD DATA

The most common medical record forms used to capture patient care information in the physician's office include: (1) a registration or encounter form (2) a history and physical examination form (3) diagnostic and therapeutic procedure report forms (4) progress note forms, and (5) consent forms. Remember that it is most important for every form to be dated when the information is first entered on it, and for every note thereafter to be dated.

The registration or encounter form   This form, completed on the patient's first visit to a health care provider, initiates that patient's medical record. As a minimum, the following identifying information should be collected: (1) the patient's full name (2) the patient's address (3) the patient's telephone number (4) the patient's date of birth (5) the sex of the patient (6) the patient's marital status (7) the patient's occupation (8) the name and address of the patient's employer (9) the patient's Social Security number, and (10) the name, address, and telephone number of the patient's nearest relative or friend. Information on insurance or other sources of payment also should be recorded on the registration form. Care should be exercised in acquiring this information and in verifying its accuracy. In fact, the continuing accuracy of the identifying information should be verified by the assistant each time the patient returns to the office. Some physicians may elect to gather additional information such as a referral source, the number of family members, the place of employment of the patient's spouse, and other data.

A portion of the registration form may function as an index to the patient's record. An index can be very useful especially for patients with lengthy records. Ordinarily the index is a listing of visit dates with a brief statement explaining the purpose of each visit. For example, one might record "physical exam," "dressing change," "prenatal visit," or "influenza."

History and physical examination   The history is largely subjective information obtained from the patient. The following items should be included:

1. Chief complaint—in the patient's own words, the reason(s) that the care was sought
2. Present illness—a detailed description of the patient's illness from the appearance of the first symptom to the present time
3. Past history—summaries of all previous illnesses, accidents, operations, allergies, drug reactions, and other such incidents
4. Family history—the health status of immediate relatives including their ages at death and the causes of death
5. Review of systems—a systematic series of questions for the purpose of revealing information about the various body systems (cardiac, genitourinary, gastrointestinal, etc.) which may or may not be related to the present illness, but which could be important to the patient's overall well-being.

The physical examination report identifies the physician's findings following a complete assessment of all body systems. The information obtained from an adequate history and physical aids the physician in establishing a diagnosis on which to base subsequent care and treatment. Historical and physical examination data may be recorded in several formats: checkoff, structured, or outline.

Historical data is often collected by way of checkoff forms or questionnaires. The patient is asked to answer an extensive series of questions to provide information about past and present illnesses. Occasionally the checkoff format is used also for recording physical examination findings. Specialists are more likely to use checkoff physicals, while internists or family practitioners often prefer to prepare records to fit the patients rather than try to have the patients fit the forms.

Although structured forms offer more flexible recording than checkoff forms, they nevertheless impose limits on the amount of information about particular body systems that can be recorded.

On the other hand, the outline form places no limits on the amount of recordable information. This format features a reminder listing so that the physician will not forget essential factors.

Registration Form

REGISTRATION FORM

Patient Name	Phone
Austin, Jane Marie	829-2956

Address
2400 Lakeview, Chicago, IL 60614

Date of Birth	Sex	Marital Status	Social Security #
2-10-33	F	Single	123-45-6789

Occupation of Patient	Employer	Address
Secretary	First National Bank	1 North LaSalle, Chicago

Name of Nearest Relative	Phone
Elizabeth Austin Sister	528-1774

Address of Above
2626 Lakeview, Chicago, IL 60614

Insurance Company Name
Blue Cross-Blue Shield, 1 North Wacker

Address	Policy #
Chicago, IL 60606	23257 Group

RECORD INDEX

VISIT DATE	SERVICES RENDERED	CODE
2-3-78	1st visit - sore throat - culture -	
	R PCN IM Ret. 2d.	
2-10-78	cult. - Beta hem. strep.	
	Rx continue p.o. PCN x 8d.	
	Ret. 3 wks.	
3-6-78	No complications - UA ok.	
	Ret. for complete Hx & PE.	

Medical Questionnaire

Name _____ Age _____ Single / Married   Divorced / Widow(er)   Date _____

Occupation _____ All previous occupations _____

Birth Place _____ Birthdate _____   List all States in which you have lived _____

Education: _____ years High School   _____ years College   _____ years Post Grad.

Date of last physical examination _____

P.I. Please do not write in this space.

Please list all Symptoms

1. _____
2. _____
3. _____
4. _____
5. _____

Routine check-up—no symptoms ☐

	If Living Age	Health	Age at death	If Deceased Cause	Has any blood relative ever had:	Please encircle no or yes	Who
Father					Cancer	No Yes	
Mother					Tuberculosis	No Yes	
Brother or Sister 1.					Diabetes	No Yes	
2.					Heart Trouble	No Yes	
3.					High blood pressure	No Yes	
4.							
5.					Stroke	No Yes	
Husband or Wife					Epilepsy	No Yes	
Son or Daughter 1.					Insanity	No Yes	
2.					Suicide	No Yes	
3.							
4.							
5.							
6.							

NOTE: This is a confidential record of your medical history and will be kept in this office. Information contained here will not be released to any person except when you have authorized us to do so.

PERSONAL HISTORY

ILLNESSES: Have you ever had

PLEASE ENCIRCLE ALL ANSWERS

	No Yes	
Measles	No Yes	
German Measles	No Yes	
Mumps	No Yes	
Chicken Pox	No Yes	
Whooping cough	No Yes	
Scarlet fever or Scarlentina	No Yes	
Diphtheria	No Yes	
Smallpox	No Yes	
Pneumonia	No Yes	
Influenza	No Yes	
Pleurisy	No Yes	
Rheumatic fever or heart disease	No Yes	
Arthritis or Rheumatism	No Yes	
Any bone or joint disease	No Yes	
Neuritis or neuralgia	No Yes	
Bursitis, Sciatica or Lumbago	No Yes	
Polio or Meningitis	No Yes	
Nephritis	No Yes	
Gonorrhea or Syphilis	No Yes	
Gallbladder disease	No Yes	
Anemia	No Yes	
Jaundice	No Yes	
Bladder disease	No Yes	
Epilepsy	No Yes	
Migraine headaches	No Yes	
Tuberculosis	No Yes	
Diabetes	No Yes	
Cancer	No Yes	

High or low blood pressure _____ No Yes
Colitis or other bowel disease _____ No Yes
Hemorrhoids or any rectal disease ____ No Yes
Nervous breakdown _____ No Yes
Food, chemical or drug poisoning _____ No Yes
Hay fever or Asthma _____ No Yes
Hives or Eczema _____ No Yes
Frequent infections or boils _____ No Yes
Any other disease _____ No Yes

ALLERGIES: Are you allergic to
Penicillin or Sulfa _____ No Yes
Aspirin, Codeine, or Morphine _____ No Yes
Mycins or other Antibiotics _____ No Yes
Merthiolate or Mercurochrome _____ No Yes
Any other drug _____ No Yes
Any foods _____ No Yes
Adhesive tape _____ No Yes
Nail polish or other cosmetics _____ No Yes
Tetanus Antitoxin or Serums _____ No Yes

INJURIES: Have you had any
Broken or cracked bones _____ No Yes
Sprains _____ No Yes
Lacerations _____ No Yes
Dislocations _____ No Yes
Concussion, or head injury _____ No Yes
Ever been knocked unconscious _____ No Yes

WEIGHT: now _____ one year ago _____
Maximum _____ when _____

TRANSFUSIONS: Have you ever had
Blood or Plasma transfusion _____ No Yes

SURGERY: Have you had
Tonsillectomy _____ No Yes
Appendectomy _____ No Yes
Any other operation _____ No Yes
Type _____ Year _____
Type _____ Year _____
Type _____ Year _____

Have you ever been advised to have any surgical operation which has not been done _____ No Yes

Have you been hospitalized for any illness _____ No Yes

Give details:

FORM 9878 COLWELL CO., CHAMPAIGN, ILLINOIS

DO YOU NOW HAVE OR HAVE YOU HAD WITHIN THE PAST YEAR:

Frequent or severe headaches _____ No Yes
Fainting spells _____ No Yes
Dizziness on change of position _____ No Yes
Unconscious spells _____ No Yes
Blurred vision _____ No Yes
Double vision _____ No Yes
Spots before eyes _____ No Yes
Infected eyes _____ No Yes
Pain behind eyes _____ No Yes
Any change in vision _____ No Yes
Do you wear glasses _____ No Yes
   When were they last checked _____
Earaches _____ No Yes
Discharge from ears _____ No Yes
Ringing in ears _____ No Yes
Decrease in hearing _____ No Yes
Recurrent nose bleeds _____ No Yes
Recurrent head colds _____ No Yes
Sinus trouble _____ No Yes
Hay fever _____ No Yes
Strange persistent odors _____ No Yes
Strange taste or loss in taste _____ No Yes
Persistent hoarseness _____ No Yes
Difficulty swallowing _____ No Yes
Enlarged glands _____ No Yes
Recurrent sore throats _____ No Yes
Recurrent sores in mouth _____ No Yes
Soreness or bleeding of gums on brushing _____ No Yes
Chest pain _____ No Yes
Angina pectoris _____ No Yes
Coughed up blood _____ No Yes
Pain in arm(s) _____ No Yes
Night sweats _____ No Yes
Chronic or frequent cough _____ No Yes
Chronic or frequent cough on laying down _____ No Yes
Wake up night short of breath _____ No Yes
How many bed pillows do you use _____ No Yes
Shortness of breath on
   Walking several blocks _____ No Yes
   One flight of stairs _____ No Yes
   On laying down _____ No Yes
Purple lips or fingers _____ No Yes
Palpitations or fluttering of heart _____ No Yes
High blood pressure _____ No Yes
Swelling of hands, feet or ankles _____ No Yes
   At what time of day _____
Leg cramps on walking or at night _____ No Yes
Enlarged veins in legs _____ No Yes
Recurrent stomach pain _____ No Yes
Belching or heartburn _____ No Yes
   Relieved by food or medication _____ No Yes
Appetite — Good ☐   Fair ☐   Poor ☐
Nausea or vomiting _____ No Yes
Vomited blood _____ No Yes
Avoid some foods _____ No Yes
   What kinds _____
Avoid spices _____ No Yes
Abdominal cramping _____ No Yes
Color of bowel movement _____
Any blood in BM _____ No Yes
Rectal pain with bowel movement _____ No Yes

DO YOU NOW HAVE OR HAVE YOU HAD WITHIN THE PAST YEAR:

Change in size, shape or texture of BM _____ No Yes
   Describe _____
Pain on urinating _____ No Yes
Difficulty in starting urination _____ No Yes
Do you get up at night to urinate _____ No Yes
   How many times _____
Urinate more than before _____ No Yes
Urinate less than before _____ No Yes
Any blood in urine _____ No Yes
How many times per day do you urinate _____
Full feeling of bladder, but only small
   amount of urination _____ No Yes

Lose urine on coughing or sneezing _____ No Yes
Discharge from penis _____ No Yes
Recurrent back pains _____ No Yes
Backaches _____ No Yes
Joint pains _____ No Yes
Swelling of any joints _____ No Yes
Redness or heat of any joint _____ No Yes
Tingling or weakness of hands or feet _____ No Yes
Muscle spasms _____ No Yes
Loss or change in sensation of hands or feet _____ No Yes
Trembling of any extremity _____ No Yes
Growth in neck or throat _____ No Yes
Hot flashes _____ No Yes
Tiredness without apparent reason _____ No Yes
Brittleness of nails _____ No Yes
Dryness of skin _____ No Yes
Easy bruising _____ No Yes
Inability to stand heat _____ No Yes
Inability to stand cold _____ No Yes
Change in hair texture _____ No Yes
Change in skin texture _____ No Yes
Any skin rash _____ No Yes
X-RAYS Have you ever had x-rays of
   Chest _____ No Yes
   Stomach or colon _____ No Yes
   Gall bladder _____ No Yes
   Extremities _____ No Yes
   Back _____ No Yes
   Teeth _____ No Yes
   Other _____ No Yes
EKG Ever had an electrocardiogram? _____ Yes No
IMMUNIZATIONS Have you had
   Smallpox vaccination within last 7 years _____ Yes No
   Tetanus shots (not antitoxin which lasts only 2 weeks) _____ Yes No
   Polio shots within last 2 years _____ Yes No

DRUGS Laxatives: never ☐   occ. ☐   freq ☐   daily ☐
   Vitamins: never ☐   occ. ☐   freq ☐   daily ☐
   Sedatives: never ☐   occ. ☐   freq ☐   daily ☐
   Tranquilizers: never ☐   occ. ☐   freq ☐   daily ☐
   Sleeping pills, etc. never ☐   occ. ☐   freq ☐   daily ☐
   Aspirin, etc. never ☐   occ. ☐   freq ☐   daily ☐
   Cortisone, Acth. never ☐   occ. ☐   freq ☐   daily ☐
   Thyroid: never ☐   yes, in past, none now ☐
         daily ☐   now on _____gr daily
   Appetite depressants. never ☐   occ. ☐   freq ☐   daily ☐
   Have you ever been treated for drug habits _____ No Yes
   Have you ever taken Insulin or tablets for diabetes _____ No Yes
   Have you ever taken Hormone tablets or injections _____ No Yes
SEX — Entirely satisfactory? _____ Yes No

WOMEN ONLY — MENSTRUAL HISTORY

Age at onset _____
Regular?   Yes ☐   No ☐   Varies
Cycle _____ days (from start to start)
Flow   Heavy ☐   Medium ☐   Light ☐
Number of pads used per period _____
Any clots passed _____ No Yes
Pains or cramps _____ No Yes
Date of last period _____
Date of last pelvic exam _____
Date of last Pap test _____
   Results   Neg. ☐   Pos. ☐
Any discharge from vagina _____ No Yes
   If so, color _____
   amount _____
Any itching of vaginal area _____ No Yes
Do you take birth control pills _____ No Yes
   How long have you taken them _____
Pregnancies:
   How many children born alive _____
   How many still births _____
   How many premature births _____
   How many Cesarean Sections _____
How many miscarriages _____
Any complications with pregnancy _____ No Yes
   Describe _____
Other _____

Reprinted by permission of The Colwell Company.

Structured Physical

PHYSICAL EXAMINATION

NUTRITION & GENERAL APPEARANCE _____

_____

_____

HEAD & NECK _____

_____

_____

EENT _____

_____

_____

BREASTS _____

_____

_____

CARDIO-RESPIRATORY _____

_____

_____

_____

GASTROINTESTINAL _____

_____

_____

_____

NEUROMUSCULAR _____

_____

_____

_____

BONES, JOINTS, & SKIN _____

_____

_____

_____

GLANDS _____

_____

_____

_____

PROVISIONAL DIAGNOSIS _____

1. _____
2. _____
3. _____
4. _____

                              Signed: _____MD

Outline History

PATIENT

HISTORY

ORDER OF RECORDING
1. Chief Complaint
2. History of Present
   Illness
3. History of Past
   Illness
   a) Child
   b) Adult
   c) Operations
   d) Injuries
4. Family History
5. Social History
6. Systemic Review
   a) General
   b) Skin
   c) Head—Eyes—
      Ears—Nose—
      Throat
   d) Neck
   e) Respiratory
   f) Cardio-
      vascular
   g) Gastro-
      intestinal
   h) Genito-
      urinary
   i) Gyneco-
      logical
   j) Locomotor
   k) Neuro-
      psychiatric
7. Signature

Since many physicians do not like to be restricted by standard forms, they may decide to use blank or ruled forms for recording histories and physicals. If the physician plans to dictate the histories and physicals, blank forms are preferable. However, ruled forms should be used if the physician prepares handwritten histories and physicals.

Complete information should be recorded regardless of the format chosen for the history and physical. Completeness is especially important for legal reasons when checkoff or structured forms are used. (For example, in litigation a jury might feel that the physician had committed an error of omission simply because a particular entry had not been made in one section of a form.) When questionnaires are used, the physician must read the information generated, amplify the data when indicated, and integrate these data with any other information accrued. The citation of any negative facts is important. For example, if a patient first seen for abdominal pain develops a mass in the right upper quadrant, it would be significant that an examination two weeks earlier had revealed "no masses or organs palpable."

The maintenance of complete office records may reduce the physician's record-keeping responsibilities when patients are admitted to the hospital. The Joint Commission on Accreditation of Hospitals allows that a copy of a history and a physical examination performed in the physician's office one week prior to hospital admission be entered into the hospital record, provided that no change has occurred in the patient's condition subsequent to the examination and provided that any change which did occur is recorded at the time of admission.

Forms designed for recording histories and physical examinations in various specialties are available from professional societies and commercial form companies. The prenatal record is an example of a commonly used special history and physical examination form. This form is initiated by the physician at the time a pregnancy is confirmed. Many hospitals furnish the physician with prenatal forms to be completed in duplicate. Another method is for the physician to forward a durable legible photocopy of the prenatal record to the hospital shortly before the expected delivery.

Diagnostic and therapeutic procedures   Physicians often order these procedures to assist in establishing a diagnosis or to help in evaluating the ongoing treatment. The kind and number of procedures vary, depending on each patient's problem and the physician's specialty. Laboratory tests, X rays, and electrocardiograms are common diagnostic procedures.

Laboratory tests may indicate the diagnoses for some patients. In other situations, laboratory tests are used to screen a patient for unspecified disease. Blood, urine, feces, spinal fluid, exudates, tissues, or virtually any part of the body may be examined in the laboratory. All laboratory tests have a normal range. The normal range establishes the limits within which one may say with confidence that no pathologic condition exists. Normal ranges are established for every laboratory on the basis of their equipment and procedures. Many physicians routinely perform blood counts and urinalyses on their patients because these simple procedures may offer evidence of unsuspected disease.

Physicians who emphasize preventive medicine frequently order blood chemistry screening procedures. A laboratory instrument called the SMA (sequential multiple analysis) permits multiple automated tests. This device can be used to test the following in one blood sample: (1) uric acid (2) inorganic phosphorus (3) cholesterol (4) lactic dehydrogenase (5) total protein (6) albumin (7) urea nitrogen (8) glucose (9) calcium (10) bilirubin (11) alkaline phosphatase, and (12) glutamic oxaloacetic transaminase.

Laboratory test procedures vary from one physician's office to another. They may be performed in the office, specimens from the patient may be transmitted to an outside laboratory for analysis, or the patient may be given a requisition and instructed to go to an outside laboratory or hospital to have the test performed.

Laboratory reporting mechanisms for tests performed in the physician's office may differ from those used for tests performed in an outside laboratory. In the office of a single practitioner, the medical assistant may perform some routine laboratory tests and simply note the results in the patient's medical record. In this setting, laboratory summary sheets with an appropriate section for recording each specific test are often used. A laboratory summary sheet permits the rapid comparison of new test results with previous data.

If laboratory tests are performed by an outside laboratory or hospital, the results are often reported on a snap-out form serving as a requisition to the laboratory, as a charge slip, and as a report for the medical record. These reports range in size from about one-quarter to one-half a standard page. When reports of this nature are received in the physician's office, they should be attached flat to a backing sheet. A separate backing sheet should be used for each test so the physician can rapidly compare new test data with previous test results (as when monitoring the blood sugar of a diabetic patient or the hematocrit of an anemic patient).

Radiological procedures expose body parts to X rays in order to create films which, when interpreted, frequently assist the physician in establishing a diagnosis. Because radiological equipment is very sophisticated and expensive, most physicians requisition X-ray examinations from outside sources such as local hospitals. However, larger group practices or single-physician practices located in rural areas may perform some X rays in their offices.

X rays are normally interpreted by a radiologist who then dictates the findings and radiological diagnosis. X-ray reports should be filed in one section of the medical record. If these reports constitute less than a full page, they should be attached to a backing sheet. An X-ray report should always be prepared, even if the X rays are interpreted by a physician other than a radiologist. Failure to enter X-ray results in a medical record could be interpreted as failure to use that evidence for the patient's benefit.

Electrocardiograms provide a graphic tracing of heart action and are an important aid in the diagnosis and management of heart disease. This procedure is used by some physicians as a routine screening mechanism for patients over 40 years old. An electrocardiogram report includes electrocardiographic tracings and an interpretation by a cardiologist or other physician. A variety of techniques are used for filing electrocardiogram tracings in the medical record. The electrocardiogram equipment manufacturer can provide assistance in developing a technique appropriate for a specific practice. Electrocardiographic reports received from hospitals or outside laboratories should be chronologically filed in the medical record.

Progress notes   Having obtained the history, the physical findings, and data from diagnostic examinations, the physician normally enters a diagnosis or an impression of the patient's condition in the progress notes. This notation is usually followed by the physician's treatment plan and/or instructions to the patient. The progress notes also are used to add information to the medical record after each follow-up visit by the patient. Objective data about the patient's own subjective report are noted there.

The nature of a patient's complaint often determines how detailed a particular record should be. Patients seen for self-limiting problems (such as a lacerated finger or an immunization injection) do not require detailed records like those that are necessary for monitoring cardiac, hypertensive, and diabetic patients. The office records of practitioners primarily offering episodic care may consist almost entirely

Laboratory Summary

PATIENT *Jane Austin*

EXAMINATION	NORMAL	DATE OF RESULT					
HEMATOLOGY		2-3-78	3-3-78	4-3-78			
Hemoglobin							
Hematocrit	40 - 45	35	37	39			
WBC	6,000-9,000	13,000	4,000				
Segs./Bands		40/20	55/5				
Lymph/Mono.		30/5	33/2				
Eos./Baso		3/2	3/2				
RBC							
Sed. Rate							
COAG. & IMMUN.							
P R O T Patient Seconds							
Patient %							
Control Seconds							
URINE ANALYSIS		2-3-78					
Specific Gravity	1.010 - 1.025	1.015					
Reaction (pH)	4.5 - 7.5	6.0					
Albumin	none	none					
Sugar	none	none					
Acetone							
Hemoglobin							
Microscopic							
Miscellaneous		2-3-78	3-3-78	4-3-78			
cholesterol	150 - 250	370	350	340			

LABORATORY   Administrative Supervisor *Paul Door*

of progress notes. The complaint and relevant details of the patient's illness, the significant physical and diagnostic findings, the treatment, and the patient's response to the treatment should be recorded for each episode.

Most physicians record medications and immunizations in their progress notes. However, some physicians prefer to use special forms for noting immunizations and medications. Pediatricians usually find it easier to monitor a child's immunizations if these data are maintained in one table in the record rather than being scattered throughout the progress notes. Special printed immunization forms may be used, or a rubber stamp providing space for immunization data may be affixed to the folder or to another designated area within the record.

Medications ordered should be entered in detail with the name, strength, and amount of medication prescribed and instructions given to the patient. Although this information may be entered chronologically within the progress notes, a special listing of medications nevertheless alerts the physician to the medications that the patient is currently taking. In this way, additional medications that may be contraindicated will not be ordered. Maintaining a special medication list also facilitates prescription renewals.

Medication List

MEDICATION LIST					
MEDICATION	DATE STARTED	DATE STOPPED			
Digoxin 0.25 mg (100) one daily	2-3-78				
Ferrocholinate (60) 330 mg. twice daily	2-3-78				
Polycillin 250 mg. (30) 4 X a day	2-5-78	2-12-78			

Consent forms   Documentary evidence of the informed consent process is provided by consent forms, which are legal documents permitting the physician to render a specified type of treatment, perform a specific procedure, or release medical information to a specific individual or agency. Consent forms must be completed properly and must be signed by the patient or by a responsible representative of the patient. All consent forms should be filed in one section of the medical record.

DOCUMENTATION RESPONSIBILITIES

Notations should be made in the office records about every visit, prescription, or telephone call for advice. (The last applies to every telephone call to the doctor by a patient and every call to a patient by the doctor in which medical advice is requested and given.) The medical assistant should make appropriate notations on the records of patients who cancel appointments, fail to show for appointments, and so on. Records indicating that a particular patient was to return for further treatment but failed to do so can serve as an adequate defense against that patient's allegation that the treatment received was not beneficial or was harmful. The physician should enter notations regarding authorized prescription refills and treatment recommendations provided on the telephone. In short, every physician and every staff member should be responsible for including all pertinent information in the patient's record. All entries should be dated and signed by the individuals making them.

When patients are referred to a consulting physician for special procedures or examinations, the consulting physician, as a matter of professional courtesy, should send a report of the findings to the referring physician. This report may follow a special format in some instances, or the consultant's findings may be outlined in a letter (see also Chapter 15, section 15.9). Reports summarizing examinations or treatment rendered elsewhere should be filed in the appropriate section of the office record.

Discharge summaries of hospital treatment also should be included in the physician's office record. Most hospitals routinely provide admitting physicians with copies of the hospital discharge summaries for office use. These summaries may be filed in a specific section of the patient's record or they may be entered chronologically in the progress note section of the patient's office record. However, if a hospital discharge summary is filed in a special section, a cross-reference should be entered on the progress notes so as to maintain a chronological picture of the patient's illness.

In order to obtain a complete history for a particular patient, the medical assistant may have to request medical information from other care providers who previously treated the patient. To obtain this information quickly, the assistant should ask the patient to complete a release of medical information request specifically describing the desired data. Physicians and hospitals normally provide this type of information without charge. However, when many records have been requested, some health care providers may assess photocopying charges.

9.3

OBTAINING DATA FOR RECORDS FROM PATIENTS

The medical assistant plays a very important role in obtaining data from the patients treated in a single or a group practice. The assistant's specific responsibilities depend on (1) the specialty of the physician (2) the nature of the practice (3) the staffing of the practice, and (4) the preference of the physician(s) in the practice. Some practices maintain large paramedical staffs who are expected to relieve the physicians of many data collection responsibilities. In these practices, the medical assistants collect identifying information from the patients; take medical histories; and enter physical and diagnostic data such as weight, blood pressure, and temperature into the patients' records. In other practices, the medical assistants may only obtain identifying information and data on follow-up visits by the patients.

INTERVIEWING PATIENTS

Although the amount of data that the medical assistant must collect varies from one practice to another, the methods used in data collection are similar in all settings. The interview is the most common method of obtaining patient care information. On the patient's first visit, the assistant interviews the patient so as to initiate a medical record by way of a completed registration or encounter form. The interviewing of patients should be done in a private area: people do not like to reveal personal data in front of strangers. The interviewer should explain in a friendly way to the patient that certain data must be gotten for the office records. Questions should be expressed clearly, and great care should be exercised in recording the patient's responses. The spelling of names should be verified. If possible, the assistant ought to copy Social Security and insurance numbers directly from the patient's cards in order to verify that the patient has provided the correct identification. It is also efficient to ask the patient questions and to type the information onto the permanent record simultaneously. In some settings, the medical office assistant may be expected to obtain historical data from the patient during the interview. If privacy cannot be assured for these interviews, you ought to ask the patient to complete a registration form. If the registration form is attached to a clipboard, it will be easier for the patient to fill in.

SELF-ADMINISTERED HISTORIES

Many physicians and group practices use self-administered histories—i.e., histories completed by the patients themselves. Patients may complete these histories in several ways. For example, a patient may complete a questionnaire, sort a set of cards, or respond to questions generated via a computer terminal. The data obtained through any of these approaches can then be processed by a computer and an optical scanner. Cathode ray terminals offer the greatest capability for entering detailed information into computerized systems. Input may be made by a light pen or by keyboarding. Each method requires that the information be entered into the computer in quite a structured format to afford maximum use of the computer's information processing and display capabilities.

Minicomputers have made special-purpose information systems obtainable and cost-effective even for the smallest of group practices. However, since many physicians are unwilling to use computer terminals, their assistants are responsible for transcribing the handwritten information from the physical examination into the computer.

DICTATED REPORTS

Many physicians prefer to collect historical data personally by questioning their patients and then dictating the histories and physical examination results for later transcription by their medical assistants. The dictating of histories, physical examinations, and progress notes saves time for the physician and increases the quality of the record in that most physicians tend to include more detail in their records when they dictate them. In addition, the dictated records are more legible when transcribed. (See also Chapter 14 for a full discussion of medical dictation and transcription.)

CORRECTING MEDICAL RECORDS

Occasionally, the medical assistant may have to make corrections in medical records. It is not permissible to use ink eradicator or an eraser on a legal document. Errors should be struck out first by drawing a line through the incorrect information and then by entering the correct information above or immediately following the entry. The word *error,* the signature of the person making the correction, and the date should be entered. This procedure applies to corrections occuring in handwritten documents or in final copies of typed documents. Errors found by the assistant while typing the record are corrected in the usual way (e.g., by erasing or by using correction fluid or tape).

ORGANIZING MEDICAL RECORDS

Medical record information kept in a folder can be highly organized by stapling separate pages together in a prescribed order. On the other hand, the material can be simply dropped into the correct folder without using a particular order. Most physicians and assistants prefer some sort of order even though they may not use fasteners and dividers to produce a bound file folder that is truly systematic. But in most practices, the records can be organized effectively by adopting a specific filing arrangement and then by stapling the pages together. The latest information accrued is usually placed on the top since it is of greatest significance to the patient's care. Reports appearing on small sheets should be affixed to standard pages.

The following three formats are commonly used in organizing medical records: the source oriented format, the integrated format, and the problem oriented format. These formats are appropriate for records maintained by all types of health care facilities including single and group practices, hospitals, health maintenance organizations, and mental health centers.

The source oriented format   This format compartmentalizes data according to origin; hence, all X rays are filed together, all laboratory reports are filed together, and so forth. Each type of report is filed chronologically within each specialty. However, the bulk of the record is increased by use of this format. Also, one must search through the entire record to locate all data related to a specific episode of care. When source oriented records are used for patients having multiple complaints, it can be very difficult for health care practitioners to keep track of all the information and to remember which test and treatment relate to a given complaint.

For example, with a patient having pneumonia, the physician's notes on the complaints and physical findings will appear in the history and physical if it is a first encounter with the patient. However, the complaints and physical findings will appear in the progress notes if the individual is a continuing patient. The chest X-ray data will be in the X-ray section of the record. The culture reports on the infecting organism will appear in the laboratory section of the record.

Integrated format   With the integrated record, the data are arranged in strict chronological order so that all information about a specific episode of care is recorded as the care occurs. For example, a physician following the integrated format would record data about the patient's complaints, the physical findings on examination, and the treatment orders. The medical assistant would file the chest X ray and the culture reports in the record immediately following the physician's notes. The physician's notes on follow-up visits, repeat chest X rays, and laboratory results would also be entered in strict chronological order.

Advantages of the integrated medical record format are that (1) the chronology of an illness can be read quickly by each individual caring for the patient (2) meaningful and concise recording is encouraged (3) important observations are unlikely to be overlooked, and (4) the number of differing record forms within the total record is reduced, thus decreasing overall bulk.

Disadvantages of this format are that (1) only one person at a time can use the record (2) one cannot turn quickly to a specific section to locate the latest report, and (3) one must be careful to note the credentials of the health care provider associated with each entry because the observation and treatment notes of physicians, nurses, and allied health practitioners appear in sequence on one page.

The integrated record format may be used effectively by many single practices or group practices. It is particularly appropriate for general and family practitioners, pediatricians, and internists. Specialists in ophthalmology, otorhinolaryngology, and orthopaedics may wish to modify the integrated format with some special forms. These specialists often use specific printed forms for recording examinations of the eyes and ears or of the musculoskeletal system.

9.4

THE PROBLEM ORIENTED RECORD (WEED SYSTEM)

The problem oriented system of patient care, devised by Lawrence L. Weed, MD, is outlined in his book *Medical Records, Medical Education and Patient Care* (Chicago: Year Book Medical Publishers, 1970). The Weed system provides for four essential components of data organization in medical records: (1) the data base (2) the numerical problem list (3) the initial plans, and (4) the progress notes.

The problem oriented record system emphasizes content and structure rather than specific forms. The assistant can maintain very satisfactory problem oriented office records by use of a simple ruled form for acquiring the data base, a problem list, and a general flow sheet.

THE DATA BASE
The data base is the initial information gathered about the patient. The following components are included in it:

1. Chief complaint—a statement in the patient's own words about the problem causing him or her to seek medical care
2. Patient profile—a description of the way that the patient spends an average day; also related social data
3. Present illness or illnesses—the relevant facts about a problem or a series of problems
4. Past history, family history, and systems review—the patient's answers to a series of explicit questions
5. Physical examination—a report that is defined, explicit, and thorough enough to uncover significant problems
6. Diagnostic procedures—laboratory test data and other diagnostic procedures (such as a Pap smear or tonometry)

THE NUMERICAL PROBLEM LIST
This list is prepared when the patient first visits the physician. In this context, a *problem* may be defined as anything that concerns the patient and/or the physician. The numerical problem list is updated on subsequent visits as new problems are identified and others are clarified or resolved. The problem list should be placed conspicuously within the record so as to remind health care providers of each problem on subsequent visits by the patient. In this way the tendency to treat an individual problem out of context can be avoided. The problem list is often kept on the inside cover of the record folder. The list also serves as a useful index to the record, for most office records have no summary from which one can readily identify all the problems that have caused a patient to seek care in the first place. As the patient's problems are clarified, altered, or delineated further, the original problem list is modified accordingly. To modify the list, one does not erase material; one inserts an arrow followed by the new diagnoses or by the terms *dropped* or *resolved*. All such changes should be dated. If two problems turn out to be separate manifestations

Patient's Problem List

PROBLEM NO.	DATE ENTERED	PROBLEM LIST	PROBLEM RESOLVED	DATE RESOLVED
1.	2-3-78	Hypochromic anemia		
2.	2-3-78	Arteriosclerotic heart disease		
3.	2-3-78	Bronchopneumonia	X	3-3-78
4.				
5.				
6.				
7.				
8.				
9.				
10.				
11.				
12.				
13.				
14.				

PROBLEM NO.	TEMPORARY PROBLEM LIST (ACUTE–LIMITED)	DATES OF OCCURRENCES		

of a single problem and have been assigned different numbers, they may be grouped together, with the first number and postion being used for both. In this situation, the second number is never reused. It is often desirable to divide the list into active and inactive problems so that those of immediate concern are immediately discernible. At the same time, the complete list serves as a compact medical history of the patient. If the data base is incomplete, problem #1 will be annotated as "Incomplete data base." The records of patients who seek care only for episodes of illness may show this problem unresolved for long periods of time. Some health care providers modify the list to afford space for recording acute self-limiting problems like "influenza," "sore throat," and so on, in a special section of the list.

The degree of completeness in the problem list is determined by the degree of thoroughness exercised in establishing the data base. The more questions one asks, the more information one will collect. Comprehensive patient care is not possible unless a complete problem list emerges from an adequate data base. However, not every patient wants or can afford to have a complete data base collected. Many patients see single practitioners only for treatment of a specific complaint.

INITIAL PLANS
Each problem is addressed by its own correspondingly numbered plan so that all individuals caring for a particular patient will know the purpose of the tests performed and the medications administered. The plans may be modified as additional data are collected during subsequent office visits.

THE PROGRESS NOTES
The progress notes serve as follow-ups for each problem. Various test data and the patient's response to treatment should be entered in the progress notes. Each note is preceded by the number and title of the appropriate problem. Progress notes should be structured according to the SOAP Format:

S   Subjective—statements revealing how the patient feels about the problem and the symptoms

O   Objective—laboratory results, X rays, and physical findings

A   Assessment—interpretation and coordination of the above information to formulate a diagnosis or a description of the problem

P   Plan—statements dealing with the results of assessments and describing additional treatment or a workup to be performed; also instructions to the patient.

With certain problems such as diabetes, it is difficult to evaluate progress by narrative notes; hence, flow sheets should be used. Flow sheets are plain forms having squares where parameters can be shown for the interrelated and changing variables associated with a particular problem.

THE ADVANTAGES AND DISADVANTAGES OF THE PROBLEM ORIENTED MEDICAL RECORD
The problem oriented record format has the following advantages: (1) it facilitates retrieval of all information relating to a specific complaint (2) it permits evaluation of the physician's logic in assessing patients' conditions (3) it places less reliance on the physician's memory, thus decreasing the chance of error, and (4) it enables continuous care to be given in a more efficient way. Disadvantages of this format are that development of the initial problem list is time-consuming, and repetitious recording is necessary because one must title and number every entry.

The problem oriented medical record is a systematic and oganized tool which can help health care practitioners render quality care to the patients they serve. It is more often adapted by physicians who are involved in primary care than by others.

SOAP Progress Note

PATIENT *Jane Austin*	**PROGRESS NOTES**

4-3-78 #1 Urinary tract infection

S Patient complaining of low back pain, burning, urgency, and frequency of urination.

O Physical examination reveals temperature 100°. Urinalysis reveals numerous white cells, no red cells.

A Probably acute pyelonephritis.

P Culture taken. Explained to patient no treatment will be given until culture results available.

Jane Lord, M.D.

9.5

THE DAILY PAGE

This document itemizes the activities occurring on a particular day in a given practice. In a group practice, a separate page is usually maintained for each associate physician. The daily page summarizes the physician's professional and financial affairs including hospital visits, operations performed, and telephone consultations. Commercial form companies sell bound books with standard daily pages. However, many medical assistants prefer to design forms that meet their specific needs. These forms can be filed in a looseleaf notebook.

MAINTAINING THE DAILY PAGE

Effective methods of acquiring information on the physician's activities outside the office must be developed to ensure that all such activities are recorded on the daily page. Physicians often carry small notebooks in which they enter notations regarding hospital and other outside activities. Data about hospital admissions and discharges may be available routinely from the hospital, but procedures also must be developed and followed in order to collect data regarding services rendered by the other staff members in the practice. These data would include records of laboratory tests performed, immunizations given, and injections administered. Each individual rendering services to patients should keep a daily log or should complete individual charge slips for these services. The data then can be collated on the daily page. The medical assistant must ensure that all activities of the practice are recorded on the daily page, because unreported services represent lost revenues.

The daily page can function as a control for maintaining the medical record and billing systems. The assistant should routinely cross-check the medical records and billing forms against the daily page to make sure that the appropriate notations have been made. For instance, it is very easy to forget to make a charge slip or to record a notation in the medical record of a patient who requests a dressing change on a busy day. However, if the daily page is routinely rechecked, any record deficiencies can be found and corrected.

A physician may get into serious legal difficulties with third-party payers such as Medicare and Medicaid if bills are sent to them for services for which there is no supporting medical record documentation. Therefore, the medical assistant must never return a medical record to its file without first ensuring that the appropriate billing support documentation exists in the record. Appropriate insurance or other billing forms can be completed when the daily page is checked against the medical and financial records before they are refiled, thus expediting collections and avoiding the necessity of pulling those records again.

The assistant ought to total and summarize each daily page in order to help the physician in maintaining a professional and financial profile of the practice. Data on the total number of office visits by patients, the total charges, the total number and amount of collections, the total number of hospital visits by the physician, and the total number of telephone consultations made by the physician can be obtained by adding up each section of the daily page. The physician also may wish to classify the reasons for patient visits so as to develop a professional practice profile. A standard list describing the treatment rendered by the practice each day can be developed. Examples are: (1) hospital visits (2) physical examinations (3) prenatal visits (4) obstetrical deliveries (5) postoperative visits (6) postpartum visits, and (7) prescription refills.

An Example of a Custom-designed Daily Page

MAY 2 • FRIDAY

OFFICE APPOINTMENTS

HOUR		NAME OF PATIENT	SERVICE RENDERED	CHARGE	RECD. ON ACCT.	BAL. DUE
9:30	1.	John Smith, III	stitches – Rt arm	10.00	10.00	
9:45	2.	Mary Aston	throat swabbed	5.00	5.00	
10:00	3.	Joshua Bales, Jr.	complete P.E.	15.00	15.00	
10:30	4.	Ann Lee	ear treatment	10.00	5.00	5.00
10:45	5.	Samuel Bronson	chg dressing	10.00	10.00	
11:00	6.	Martha H. Meyers	hospital	5.00	5.00	
11:15	7.	Ann T. Lawton	set fracture	40.00	10.00	30.00
1:00	8.	Marion Thomas	exam – Rx	10.00	5.00	5.00
1:30	9.	Thomas Martin	consult.	10.00	5.00	5.00
2:00	10.	Elisabeth Abbott	eye treatment	15.00	10.00	5.00
2:30	11.	Beth Watson	PE = Pap S.	20.00	10.00	10.00
	12.					
	13.					
	14.					
	15.					
	16.					
	17.					
	18.					
	19.					
	20.					
	21.					
	22.					
	23.					
	24.					
TOTALS				150.00	90.00	60.00

TELEPHONE CALLS

	NAME OF PATIENT	CHARGE
1.	Barbara Provo	5.00
2.	Sarah Daniels	8.00
3.	Albert Watson	5.00
4.		
5.		
6.		
7.		
8.		
9.		
10.		
11.		
12.		
13.		
14.		
TOTALS		15.00

HOSPITAL VISITS

	NAME OF PATIENT	CHARGE
1.	Porter Weeland	10.00
2.	Annabel Dav	10.00
3.	Daniel Thomas	10.00
4.	Martin Williams	10.00
5.	Susan August	10.00
6.		
7.		
8.		
9.		
10.		
11.		
12.		
13.		
14.		
TOTALS		50.00

USING THE *CURRENT PROCEDURAL TERMINOLOGY*

More detailed data may be compiled by using a standardized coding system such as *Current Procedural Terminology,* published by the American Medical Association. *Current Procedural Terminology* is a list of descriptive terms and identifying codes for reporting medical services and procedures performed by physicians. Each procedure or service is identified with a five-digit code that accurately designates medical, surgical, and diagnostic services. For example, code 90831 is assigned when the service rendered is "telephone consultation with or about patient for psychiatric therapeutic or diagnostic purposes." *Current Procedural Terminology* provides a uniform language serving as a nationwide communication tool among physicians, patients, and third parties. The comprehensive *CPT* coding system gives code numbers for services rendered by various specialists in the office, in the home, in a long-term care facility, in the emergency room, and in the hospital.

AUTOMATED BILLING SERVICES

A physician may have an automated billing service to complete insurance forms, to collect all receivables, and to maintain data on services rendered. When an automated billing service is used, a master patient source document is filed with the service bureau on the patient's first visit to the doctor. This information is computerized by the billing service so that on subsequent visits by the patient, only one special charge slip need be completed for that patient. This slip gives the date, the appropriate diagnostic code numbers, the service codes, and the charges. If a physician uses an automated billing system, the assistant must routinely cross-check the daily page against the charge slips to see that every medical service is reported to the billing service. Automated billing services may also provide statistics on medical services rendered by the practice and may prepare diagnostic or problem profiles of the practice.

9.6

FILING SYSTEMS

Filing is the arrangement and storage of recorded information according to a simple and logical sequence so as to facilitate future retrieval. A filing system is effective only when all required information can be located promptly. Indexing is a way of classifying items so that they can be retrieved when needed. The two basic classification methods are alphabetical and numerical. Medical records may be classified, arranged, and stored by either method. The assistant can also use derivations and combinations of the basic alphabetic and numeric methods.

ALPHABETICAL FILING

Alphabetical filing follows the sequence of letters in the alphabet and the sequence of letters in patients' names. In alphabetical files, the needed information can be retrieved by direct references without the use of a separate index. However, errors in alphabetizing and misspelled names can often cause retrieval problems.

It is difficult to plan for the expansion of alphabetical files because one cannot accurately predict where the expansion will occur. It is therefore helpful to assign space within alphabetic files by way of a Table of Name Frequencies. For example, the following table suggests that 10% of the available filing space should be assigned to patients whose names begin with *S*.

Classification Division Frequencies in Filing Names

Letter category	Frequency	Letter category	Frequency
A	3.15	N	1.72
B	9.46	O	1.43
C	7.40	P	4.90
D	5.17	Q	.18
E	1.94	R	5.14
F	3.58	S	10.03
G	4.92	T	3.31
H	7.74	U	.22
I	.39	V	1.09
J	2.84	W	6.26
K	3.91	X	less than 0.005
L	4.69	Y	.49
M	9.57	Z	.47

(In communities with large ethnic populations, these frequencies may not prove totally accurate.)

Phonetic classification   Phonetic classification systems have been developed to overcome the difficulties associated with misspelled names in alphabetical filing. Phonetic classification systems are based on a numerical code that represents consonant sounds. Vowel sounds are ignored. Each name is reduced to one letter and three digits. For example, in a phonetic file, the names *John Smith* and *Jon Smythe* would be filed together. The main advantages of phonetic filing are: (1) similar sounding names are grouped together (2) silent letters and double consonants are disregarded, thus reducing retrieval time, and (3) duplicate entries are avoided because names that may have been spelled incorrectly or that contain typographical errors still can be filed correctly. A disadvantage of the phonetic filing system is that special training is needed before one can use the system. Also, filing errors can occur when more than one person is responsible for coding, filing, and retrieving from a phonetic file.

NUMERICAL FILING

With the numerical filing system, each new patient is assigned a sequential number. Although numbers are easier for some people to remember than names, the maintenance of numerical files is still time-consuming because additional filing procedures are required. For example, a separate alphabetical index file must be maintained. This file must be consulted to locate the record of a specified patient. Nevertheless, the advantages of the numerical filing system are that (1) orderly expansion is possible, thus eliminating the shifting of files (2) the number of misfiles is reduced, and (3) speedy retrieval is possible because it is unnecessary to search through several files labeled with the same name in order to find the right name.

The three basic methods of numerical filing are the straight numerical, the middle digit, and the terminal digit. In straight numerical filing, consecutively numbered folders are filed in exact numeric order. Anyone who can count can become proficient in filing with the straight numerical method. However, errors can occur in large files because all digits of the record number must be considered at one time, thus making the inadvertent transposition of numbers common.

In middle and terminal digit filing, the number of a given folder is divided into groups of two for filing. For example, folder 12-34-56 is filed first by 34 in middle digit filing and by 56 in terminal digit filing. The sequence of numbers in each type of file is as follows:

Middle Digit Files	Terminal Digit Files
12–34–56	12–34–56
12–34–57	13–34–56
....	....
12–34–99	99–34–56
13–34–00	00–35–56
....	....
13–34–99	99–35–56
14–34–00	00–36–56
....	....
99–34–99	99–99–56
00–35–00	00–00–57

Middle digit and terminal digit filing can eliminate traffic jams in the files because each file section contains recently assigned numbers, and the new folders do not become backed up at the end of the files. Responsibility for a specific file section also may be assigned to one clerk, thus promoting more accurate work. Sorting of the records before filing them is facilitated because two digits are sorted at a time. The chief disadvantage of middle digit and terminal digit filing is the need to give special training to the staff filing the records. Although most employees are able to learn terminal digit filing rapidly, it is difficult for them to learn how to file accurately with the middle digit system because the filer first must read the middle of a number and then move to the far left and finally to the right.

The terminal digit system is considered the most effective numerical method of filing for organizing, storing, and retrieving medical records. This method offers a virtually perfect distribution of folders throughout the file. It also greatly increases filing speed and retrieval because the filer works with only two numbers at a time.

COLOR-CODING

A system of color-coded folders is highly desirable in extensive files or in situations when more than one person has regular access to the files. There are many color-coding systems available which provide immediate visual recognition of errors. Filing errors are therefore reduced and the time needed in finding misfiles is minimized. Color-coding may be used with the numerical or the alphabetical filing systems, but it proves most beneficial when it is used with terminal digit filing. The simplest system requires colored folders. Ten colors indicate the numerals 0 thru 9. In straight numerical files, the third digit from the right is coded since it is where most filing errors in straight numerical files occur. In alphabetical files, colored folders can also be assigned to certain letters of the alphabet.

Alphabetical Color-Coding

Alphabet Designation	Folder Color	Folder Name
ABCD	yellow	Carson
EFGH	blue	Thomas
IJKL	purple	Clark
MNOP	orange	Morris
QRST	green	Brown
UVWXYZ	red	Owens

With the color-coded alphabetical filing method, the second letter of each patient's last name is color-coded, since the first letter is rarely misfiled. With terminal digit files, many variations of color-coding can be used including tinting and blocking and the use of preprinted colored labels. Extensive color-coding systems necessitate the purchase of preprinted folders. Companies that sell such folders may offer assistance in the selection of the most appropriate color-coding method for the particular practice.

SELECTING A FILING SYSTEM

In choosing a medical record filing system for a single or group practice, one should analyze the size and the nature of the practice and its staffing patterns. An alphabetical filing system will usually meet the needs of single and small group practices. The alphabetical method satisfies physicians who sometimes find it necessary to retrieve records in minimally staffed practices. On the other hand, numerical files are more satisfactory when the volume of records is large and when many individuals file and retrieve the material. The numerical filing system also provides the extra privacy that may be desirable in a psychiatrist's office, for instance. It is also important to remember that in pediatrics and family practice it is common to file the charts of all members of the same family in a single folder.

FILING PROCEDURES

To have an effective system, one must develop and carefully follow specific procedures for maintaining and using the filing and indexing systems. Records must be labeled correctly at the time they are created. In an alphabetical filing system, each folder should be labeled with the patient's name (last name first) and with another identifier. The patient's birth date is usually the most appropriate secondary identifier because it, unlike the patient's address, cannot change. In a numerical filing system, the record should be labeled clearly with the patient's name and number. Labels should be typed and placed on the folder in a standard position (e.g., on the folder tab). Labels of different colors may be used to distinguish the patients of different doctors in an association.

Creating an index   If a numerical filing system is used, an alphabetical index card must be created for each patient folder. This typewritten card should contain at least the name, address, birth date, and file number of the patient. Additional information such as visit dates and billing information may be listed on the index card in order to increase its utility. Use of a single card for billing and for alphabetical indexing sharply reduces the time required in maintaining numerical files. The presence of an informative alphabetical patient index also may make it unnecessary to pull a patient's entire medical record just to handle some requests for information. A good index also facilitates rapid record retrieval but requires no more effort to maintain than its use warrants.

Guides   To expedite the filing and retrieving of records, the assistant should place guides throughout the files to separate the cards or folders into groups. One guide for every 50 folders is adequate unless the records are very thick. With card files, one guide should be placed for every 25 cards—a procedure that will facilitate quick retrieval.

When purchasing guides, the assistant should remember that durability and visibility are the most important considerations. The tab on each guide should project far enough beyond the record folders to ensure complete visibility. With straight numerical files, new guides must be added constantly, but with terminal digit and alphabetical files, the guides are usually permanent. Guides should be made of pressboard or vinyl. Pressboard is preferable for patient records because heavy guides are needed to help support the records. Vinyl guides are very satisfactory for card files. Since guides are sold in sets based on the size of the files, potential growth within the office files must be considered when the guides are purchased.

Filing rules   For the sake of accuracy, written filing rules should be prepared, and new staff members should be instructed thoroughly in file maintenance procedures. Appropriate rules for arranging alphabetical files are as follows:

1. Alphabetize the names of individuals by surname + given name + middle name or initial. Example: *Jones, Mary Ann*

2. Arrange all cards and folders in alphabetical order letter by letter to the end of the surnames, then the given names and initials. For example, these names would be filed in the following order: *Morison, John A.; Morison, John Thomas; Morrison, John Andrew*

3. Treat hyphenated or compound names as one word. Example: *Fitz Smith, Patrick; Foster-Brown, James.*

4. During alphabetizing, disregard titles such as *Dr., Mrs., Captain* or *Senator.* However, these designations may be used to provide additional identifying information. Example: *Nyhus, Lloyd (Dr.); Smith, Walter (Senator).*

5. Disregard religious titles (such as *Reverend* and *Sister*) in filing. File the material according to the patients' last names. Example: *Raphael, Mary (Sister); Smith, John (Reverend).*

6. Alphabetize abbreviated prefixes such as *St.* according to the complete spelling *Saint.* Example: *St. Peter, Joanne* is filed as if it were written *Saint Peter, Joanne.*

7. Disregard designations such as *Jr., Sr.,* or *2nd* in filing. Examples: *Smith, John T. (Sr.); Smith, John Thomas (Jr.)*

8. Consider the legal signature of a married woman in filing. Her husband's name may be cross-referenced if desired. Example: *Jones, Mary Ann (Mrs. John).*

9. File "nothing" before "something" if initials are used for a given name. For example, these names would be filed in the following order: *Peters, J.; Peters, J.G.; Peters, John.*

10. Arrange surnames having the prefixes *de, La,* and *Mac* just as they are spelled. For example, these names would be filed in the following order: *MacDougal, John; Mbasdeken, Joan; McDover, Mary.*

11. File as written those surnames in which it is impossible to determine the given name, or middle name. Examples: *Chin Sing Hop, Osak Wong,* and *Hope Big Feather* should be filed in this order: *Chin Sing Hop; Hope Big Feather; Osak Wong.*

Number accession register   With numerical files, adequate controls must be established to ensure that a patient's number can be located and that two patients are not given the same number. The assistant can control number allocation by maintaining an accession register which is a written and bound record of regular entries. A register differs from an index in that it is usually arranged chronologically. Registers describe events (as births or deaths) in the order of their occurrence. (However, registers do not identify how a record is to be filed.) Only three columns are required in a number accession register. These are a list of numbers in numerical order, the name of the person to whom each number has been issued, and the date of issue

The number accession register may be used in searching for a patient's number when the index card cannot be located if the patient can provide an approximate date of registration with the physician. One may also keep track of the next unused number by purchasing prenumbered folders and matching prenumbered index cards.

Misfiles   Filing and indexing errors can be minimized by using standardized procedures, by carefully orienting and training the staff, and by limiting access to files and indexes. However, since occasional misfiles are inevitable, the following hints for conducting a search are useful:

1. Think of alternate ways that the patient's name might have been spelled.

2. Search for transposed letters due to typographical errors.

3. Check the folder just before and after the one that is needed: the one you want may have been put into another folder rather than between two folders.

4. Look for transposition of the last digits of the number or the hundred or thousand digits.

5. Look for misfiles that may have been caused by unclear numbers; for example, look for a missing *3* under *5* or *8,* and a missing *1* under *7,* and vice versa.

Number Accession Register

NUMBER ACCESSION REGISTER

NUMBER	PATIENT'S NAME	DATE
2340	Jones, Ann	4 - 3 - 78
2341	Peters, Paula	4 - 3 - 78
2342	Martin, James	4 - 3 - 78
2343	Sontag, Betsey	4 - 3 - 78
2344	Petersen, Patrick	4 - 4 - 78

6. Check for a missing number in the hundred group just preceding or following it; for example, look for *288* in the *188* and in the *388* sequences.

7. Look next to the folders of patients seen on the same day as that of the one whose record is lost.

SPECIAL INDEXES

Although the daily page is sufficient for most practices, some single physicians and group practices may wish to maintain special indexes designed to provide a detailed profile of the care they render. Ambulatory care records may be indexed by using the *Current Procedural Terminology* (described in section 9.5) or the *International Classification of Problems in Primary Care (ICPPC)*. The American Hospital Association published *ICPPC* in 1975 for use by physicians in general practice and family practice. The *ICPPC* is designed to classify morbidity information for statistical purposes and to offer a way of indexing ambulatory care records according to diagnoses and problems. It has three- and four-digit codes that can be assigned at the time of each encounter with a patient. For example, a patient seen for influenza would be assigned the code 470, while an infant having a feeding problem would be assigned code 2699. The appropriate code for the condition may be assigned by the physician, or the medical assistant may learn the coding and do it for the physician.

The index format is determined by the particular classification system used. Indexes may be manual or may be computerized in conjunction with an automated billing system. When a manual indexing system is used, one must decide what data will be put into the index. Only two items of information are required: the code number and a patient identifier (number or name). Other information which can be added includes: (1) the patient's age (2) the patient's sex (3) the physician's name, and (4) the date of the visit. Appropriate index cards can be purchased from medical form companies, or self-designed cards may be used. Index cards are always filed by code number in numerical order.

ICPPC Index Card

ICPPC INDEX	Code No. 470	Title Influenza		Year 1978	Card No. 1
Patient's Name			Patient's Name		
Stroud, Mary					
Peters, Eliza					
Little, Aileen					
Jones, Sally					

To ensure that every record is indexed, some controls must be set up. First of all, the coding and indexing activities can be conveniently completed right after the medical records are checked against the daily page. The code numbers may be entered directly on the record beside the physician's entry describing the diagnosis or the problem treated during the patient's visit. An alternative procedure is to enter the code numbers on the problem list. When this code number has been posted in the index, a check mark should be placed beside the number. All index entries should be made in ink. At the end of each calendar year, a line should be drawn after the last entry on each card and the entries totaled. A very specific summary of the physician's professional yearly activities can be compiled from these totals.

9.7

HANDLING MEDICAL RECORDS

Patients have the right to expect that physicians will safeguard their medical records against loss and against unauthorized use or disclosure of information. Therefore, the medical assistant must develop appropriate procedures for the release of medical information to outside users and for the internal handling of medical records.

RELEASE OF MEDICAL INFORMATION
The doctrine that a physician may not reveal the confidences entrusted to him or her in the course of medical attendance was originally espoused in the Hippocratic Oath and is currently embodied in the American Medical Association's Principles of Medical Ethics (see Chapter 4, section 4.2). In addition, many state statutes specify that information acquired in a doctor-patient relationship constitutes a confidential or privileged communication and therefore may not be disclosed by the physician except with the consent of the patient or as required by law.

The medical assistant is responsible for making sure that no unauthorized person ever removes, reads, copies, or otherwise tampers with any record in any way at any time. However, some individuals are authorized to receive medical information, and it must be made available to them. Information may be released from the records maintained by a physician upon receipt of a written authorization from the patient for the release, in response to a court order or subpoena, or as required by statute. The greatest number of requests for the release of information come from the patients themselves or from other physicians. Requests also come from the patients' employers, government agencies, or insurance companies.

LEGAL RESTRICTIONS

The legal requirements and restrictions regarding the release of medical information vary from state to state. For this reason, the medical assistant must be familiar with the statutes that apply to the state in which the practice is located. For example, physicians in some states are responsible for reporting suspected cases of child abuse to appropriate authorities. Consequently, the laws in those states authorize the release of this information. On the other hand, when an employer arranges for the medical care of employees or agrees to pay for that care, the confidential relationship between the patient and the physician is not waived. In some states, the employer may be entitled to medical information under the Workers Compensation Act if the employee was injured at work. This legislation guarantees that an employee injured in the course of employment will have an adequate means of support during the period he or she is unable to work. The medical bills of employees injured on the job are paid even if their carelessness may have contributed to the injury. Some statutes require the physician to submit a treatment report to the employer and to the appropriate state agency within specified time limits. The requirements of the various state workers compensation laws differ, so the medical assistant has to be familiar with the laws of the state in which the practice is located.

CONSENT TO RELEASE MEDICAL INFORMATION

The signed consent to release medical information may be given by (1) the patient (2) a legally qualified representative (such as a parent or guardian) of the patient (3) an executor or administrator of an estate, or (4) an agency designated by the court as a guardian. A valid consent to release medical information must fulfill the following requirements:

1. It should be directed to the doctor or group practice.
2. It should specify what information is to be released.
3. It should indicate the period of care for which the information is being requested.
4. It should specify to whom the information will be released.
5. It should be dated within a 90-day period prior to the request but subsequent to the treatment.
6. It should be signed by the patient or by a legally qualified representative of the patient.

A consent to release medical information should be obtained when that information is requested by other doctors and institutions, insurance companies, government agencies not entitled to access by law, attorneys, and the media (i.e., publishers, radio stations, and television stations). No consent is necessary for releasing medical information to a health care facility to which the physician has arranged admission for a patient. By the same token, no consent is required prior to releasing follow-up medical information to such an institution for the maintenance of its tumor registry.

POLICIES AND PROCEDURES

The medical assistant should develop written policies and procedures for handling inquiries concerning the release of medical information to the patient, the patient's family, other physicians, hospitals and nursing homes where the physician sees patients, attorneys, government agencies, social agencies, life insurance companies, and third-party payers. These policies and procedures should cover requests made by telephone, in person, and by mail. The policies and procedures should be approved by the physician(s) in the practice and/or the attorney for the practice.

Telephone requests for medical information should be discouraged. The assistant can suggest that the callers make their requests in writing. Or if the callers are current patients, the assistant can suggest that they discuss their requests with the physician. On some occasions, another physician or a hospital emergency room may need information immediately in order to treat a patient. These requests should be honored by a prompt call-back to verify the identity of the person requesting the information. Many physicians prefer to handle this type of request personally.

If a record is personally reviewed in the office, the person inspecting it should show identification and should sign and date the authorization. The assistant should verify the identity of the reviewer. The person also should be observed during review to ensure that the record is not being altered.

Upon receipt of a written request for medical information, the medical assistant should compare the signature on the release form with a signature in the medical record to determine its authenticity. (However, this step is not necessary if the signature on the release is notarized.) If the authorization carries the appropriate signature, the assistant should prepare and forward the requested information promptly. Only that information specifically covered by the release authorization should be provided. Release authorizations may be limited to a specific time period or to a certain kind of information (such as an electrocardiogram report).

Techniques that may be used to release information include (1) completing the form presented by the patient (2) abstracting the information onto a standard form, or (3) photocopying pertinent sections of the record. A carbon or other copy of any completed forms should be retained in the patient's record with the consent to release the medical information. When photocopies of portions of the record are sent to the individual or the institution requesting the data, a notation should be entered on the release listing the forms sent.

Many requests that the medical assistant handles are from third-party payers. The request forms ask for minimal medical information and usually contain an information release permitting disclosure of the information necessary to pay the claim. Extreme care should be used in completing insurance forms because payment delays occur when they have not been filled in properly. Standard forms and/or photocopies of pertinent documents are usually used in providing information to life insurance companies, social agencies, government agencies, and attorneys.

Physicians usually prefer to respond personally to inquiries from patients and their families about current illnesses. Most physicians recognize that informed patients are more cooperative in following treatment plans. The courts are also recognizing the patients' rights of access to the information in their own medical records if the information is desired for legitimate purposes. Statutes in several states give patients the right to view and copy their hospital medical records. For these reasons, many physicians provide patients with summaries of their records for their own use, or they permit patients access to their own records on request.

The medical records of patients treated for psychiatric problems, alcoholism, or drug abuse should have special handling. Many state laws accord privileged status to psychiatric records. This status gives a psychiatrist the opportunity to refuse to release a record because the patient may or may not be competent to determine whether others should examine the record. The *Code of Federal Regulations* (Part 2, Title 42) governs the confidentiality of patients suffering from alcohol or drug abuse. The *Code* should be consulted prior to disclosing any information about such patients, including the fact that treatment was rendered for disabilities covered by the regulations therein.

MEDICAL ETHICS IN RECORD MANAGEMENT

The privacy of medical records has been a keystone of medical ethics for many years. The physician is responsible for the consequences of any action of any assistant acting within the scope of established duties. The physician-employer may be subject not only to professional embarrassment but also to a lawsuit for invasion of privacy if the assistant violates the principles of medical ethics especially as to confidentiality. These principles apply to formal and informal requests for medical information. Thus, it is a good idea to leave all information about patients at the office and to avoid discussing patients with anyone outside the work situation. You also should refrain from answering questions about the details of illnesses of neighbors, friends, and others. To avoid direct or indirect disclosure of information, you should be silent when others discuss patients. You can simply express your sympathy over the other person's illness, or you can indicate that all patients are entitled to privacy.

Obviously medical information must be handled carefully within a practice. The office staff should not gossip about the patients' conditions. Staff members should not be granted access to any records that they do not need to see in fulfilling their responsibilities. The physician should insist that contracts for outside services (such as computerized billing) include a statement specifying that the company providing the services is responsible for maintaining the confidentiality of all medical information processed by it.

INTERNAL HANDLING OF MEDICAL RECORDS

Patient records must be accessible at any time in order for the doctor to provide continuous care to the patients. Therefore, some controls must be used whenever several individuals use the files. The easiest method of controlling the files is to insert a lightweight cardboard OUT guide slightly larger than the folder in place of the withdrawn record. If access to the files is limited only to four or five individuals, a different colored guide may be assigned to each individual using the files. In this way it will not be necessary to write on the OUT guides in numerical files. Staff members will therefore know that guides of one color indicate records pulled for one doctor, while guides of another color indicate records pulled for still another doctor (or a nurse), and so on. When many individuals have access to the files or when alphabetical files are used, OUT guides should be employed to record the name of the patient, the name of the staff member using the record, and the date on which the record was pulled. Staff members should make every effort to return records to the files promptly, because filed records are more easily located than those scattered about the office. In addition, filed records are less accessible to other patients, the cleaning staff, and other unauthorized persons. Records removed from the files should always remain in their folders because they protect the records from prying eyes and accidental damage. If possible, the office should be arranged in such a way that patients do not have access to the record storage area. Physicians and office staff also should not leave records lying on desks where patients and other visitors can read them.

The extra expense of locked files for record storage is not always justified since most staff members leave the files unlocked during the day. However, locked files may be entirely justified especially in a psychiatrist's office. The medical assistant also may wish to keep the records of public figures or those of patients involved in malpractice litigation in special locked files. If the physician decides to use locked files, make sure that they are secured properly at the end of each working day.

9.8

RECORD RETENTION, TRANSFER, AND DISPOSAL

Patients' medical records should be preserved for four reasons: (1) to secure continuity of patient care (2) to serve as evidence in possible future litigation (3) to fulfill research and educational needs, and (4) to fulfill statutory or regulatory requirements. The necessity of retaining records to meet each of these needs must first be evaluated before any decision can be made about establishing retention schedules.

An effort must be made to decide whether or not a particular record is likely to be of future medical, economic, or social benefit to the patient. Experience demonstrates that a medical record documenting a prolonged period of care will be needed in the future to help provide the patient with appropriate care or to establish the presence or absence of disability. However, records documenting care for minor self-limiting problems are not likely to be of future benefit to the patient or the physician.

Records may be required as evidence in future litigation if a patient brings a lawsuit alleging improper treatment against a physician. The period of time during which a patient may file suit is specified in various statutes of limitations. This time period varies from one state to another and from one type of lawsuit to another. For example, in Illinois a suit may be filed against a physician any time within a two-year period subsequent to an alleged malpractice act, but the statute of limitations for breach of contract is five years. Minors in most states may file suit after they achieve majority (i.e., ages 18–21). Recent court decisions have also upheld in some cases (i.e., those usually involving foreign objects left in the body during surgery) the patient's right to file a malpractice suit after discovery of the injury. Discovery of this type of injury can occur as long as from 10 to 20 years after surgery.

Nowdays, office records are assuming even more importance in teaching and in research. For instance, recent research reveals that the incidence of cancer has increased in individuals treated with neck radiation and in the female offspring of mothers having received diethylstilbestrol 20 years ago. These kinds of data attest to the research potential of office records in identifying and documenting long-term sequelae of accepted treatment methods.

Very few statutory or regulatory requirements apply to records maintained by physicians' offices. However, the Medical Practice Act of the state in which a specific practice is located should be reviewed to determine whether it imposes any record-keeping requirements on physicians. Medical records for patients whose care has been financed by government programs should be maintained for a minimum of five years to protect the physician from fraud charges.

RETENTION SCHEDULES

Because it is very difficult to say that a medical record will *not* offer the physician legal protection and will *not* be of future benefit to the patient, most physicians adopt schedules requiring permanent retention of their medical records. Others permanently retain the majority of their records, but destroy those records relating to single episodes of care after 10 years have elapsed. In some practices, only an index card is maintained after 10 years. (The index card summarizes the care rendered and indicates that the record has been destroyed.)

A retention schedule should specify the following for each type of document being evaluated: (1) its active life—the period during which it should be readily accessible in its original form (2) its inactive life—the period during which it should be retained but transferred to storage or microfilm, and (3) its destruction—the point when further retention is not justified by usage or law.

INACTIVE MEDICAL RECORDS

After a retention schedule has been adopted, a definite plan should be developed for handling the inactive medical records. Physicians' offices typically file medical records according to three classifications: active, inactive, and closed. Active records are those for patients who have been seen within the past year, while inactive records belong to patients who have not returned for care during that period. Records are pulled from the inactive files and are returned to the active section when the individuals return for care. Closed files are records of patients who have terminated their relationship with the physician, have died, or have moved away.

Maintaining three separate file sections is a time-consuming practice which should not be followed unless an acute shortage of record storage space mandates the rapid transfer of active files to inactive status. One reason why two instead of three sets of files should be kept is that many patients feel that they have an active physician-patient relationship although they have not had to see their physician for several years. Thus, if space permits, it is more efficient to maintain only two sets of files—active and inactive. The active files contain the records of all patients who have consulted the physician within a five-year period. All other records are then considered inactive.

RECORD TRANSFER

A notation of each year that a patient is seen in the office should be made on the outside of the folder. This will facilitate later transfer of records to inactive status. The assistant can make the notation by stamping each record with the appropriate year the first time a patient is seen. Or, if preprinted folders are used, years can be printed on the folder with a line being drawn through the appropriate year the first time a patient is seen. One can determine by either method without opening the folder whether the record is active or inactive. And either method facilitates record inventory and clearance. (Each year, the files must be emptied of the records of patients not seen within the specified retention period.)

RECORD STORAGE

If office space is scarce, inactive records may be placed in storage. File storage boxes may be purchased from most stationery supply houses. These boxes are available with lift-off lids or drawers. Ordinarily the drawer models are preferable because they afford access to the records when the boxes have been stacked. Each box should be clearly labeled so that needed records can be retrieved rapidly. These boxes can be kept in the office if space is available, or they can be stored commercially. When it is necessary to store records outside the practice, a list of the contents of each box should be kept in the office. A firm specializing in record storage should be used, if possible, because this type of firm can assure confidentiality and can promptly produce requested records. For many practices, microfilming rather than storage may be a more feasible solution to the space problem, because continuous and indefinite storage of records in their original form often cannot be maintained. (Microfilming is discussed in more detail in section 9.9.)

DISPOSAL OF RECORDS

When a retention schedule calls for the destruction of records, the material must be burned or shredded to maintain confidentiality. If it is necessary to close the practice, each patient should be informed of the fact and should be given the opportunity to have his or her records forwarded to another physician. When a practice is purchased by another physician, the same procedure should be followed. A physician purchasing a practice is entitled to receive only the records of those patients who elect to transfer their records and become patients of the new physician. The remaining records should be stored or microfilmed. Some local medical societies store the records of their deceased members. In order to protect the physician or an estate from legal claims, all patients' written requests to forward medical records to another physician (or to other physicians) should be retained.

9.9

FILING EQUIPMENT AND SUPPLIES

Adequate record storage space rarely exists in a single or group practice because: (1) the space needs for patient care receive priority (2) record storage needs are often underestimated (3) inappropriate record storage equipment is selected, and (4) the file area layout is less than desirable. This situation need not exist, however, if the physician and the assistant plan carefully and select appropriate equipment. The following suggestions are intended to give some guidance in this area.

ESTIMATING STORAGE NEEDS

A fairly accurate estimate of the amount of record storage space that will be needed in a given practice can be established first by measuring the number of records that can be filed per filing inch and then by multiplying that figure by the number of new records initiated each year. About four to six records can be filed per inch, but the situation can vary according to the nature of the practice. For instance, a family practitioner with a stable patient population may have thicker records than those of a specialist with a referral practice. To estimate the number of records that will be initiated by a physician in a year, count the new patients for a month and multiply this number by 12. Divide the number of records initiated per year by the number of records filed per inch to obtain an estimate of the number of inches of filing space required per year. Filing space should be considered in terms of estimated practice growth over 10 years.

FILING SUPPLIES

To maintain an efficient and economical filing system, an effort should be made to standardize both supplies and equipment. Every patient record should be maintained in an individual file folder unless family folders containing several individuals' records are kept. Four types of materials are commonly used for constructing folders:

1. Manila—the most common and least expensive folder material. It is available with wax or Mylar coating for extra durability and it is available in multiple colors.
2. Kraft—heavier and darker in color than manila. It is quite durable and does not soil easily, but it is more expensive than manila and should be used only for folders subjected to much wear and tear.
3. Pressboard—expensive heavy-duty material. It is more suitable for guides than for folders.
4. Vinyl or other plastic—very durable but quite expensive. The texture is very smooth; hence, folders are slippery and do not stack well. Vinyl and other plastics are available in a variety of colors.

Folders may be purchased with or without protruding tabs at the tops or sides of the backs. Although tabs often appear to facilitate filing, they soon become worn and tattered, so it is better to use straight-cut folders with rounded corners. Rounded corners retain their appearance better and are less likely to cause paper cuts. Prenumbered and preprinted folders are also available, but such folders are expensive. A variety of color-coded folders may be purchased commerically.

Although a wide variety of commercial folders can be purchased for filing patient records, ordinary manila folders are adequate in most single and group practices. Manila folders are inexpensive and durable enough to stand the wear encountered in most physicians' offices. Labels or tapes are easily affixed to manila folders for indexing and color-coding if desired. Manila folders are also available with pronged fasteners. The purchase of the color-coded printed folders mentioned earlier is economically feasible only when a practice initiates 20 or more new patient records per day.

RECORD STORAGE EQUIPMENT

Patient records may be stored in vertical or lateral metal filing cabinets, on open shelves, or in electrically powered files. In most physicians' offices, the common method of record storage is the five-drawer vertical file cabinet. File cabinets are available in standard letter, legal, and card sizes. Drawers should offer ball bearing roller suspension with compressors or follower blocks to support the records from the back because the drawers are very heavy. It is false economy to buy inexpensive file cabinets lacking ball bearings, because one must literally pick up such drawers in order to return them to file. If file cabinets are selected, plenty of aisle space must be allowed so that the work area will be adequate for the operator when the drawers are fully extended. File cabinets provide a neat method of storage, offer security and confidentiality, and provide protection from dirt and dust. However, they store about 50% less material per square foot of floor space than shelf files do. They can also be a safety hazard because if several drawers are extended at the same time, the cabinets may tip over.

Open shelves or lateral files are preferable to vertical file cabinets because they offer space savings and flexible layouts. With lateral files, the length of each cabinet is against the wall and the drawers extend only about one foot toward the operator. In a lateral file, the front of each folder faces the side of the drawer instead of the front of the file.

Horizontal open shelf filing units are available in a variety of styles. Some open shelf units may contain doors that slide out to protect the contents and that serve as work shelves, while other units contain glide-out drawers or removable file boxes. Open shelf filing has the following advantages: (1) reduced equipment costs (2) savings in time and energy because the opening or closing of drawers is unnecessary (3) the creation of a quiet working environment, and (4) fast retrieval of records. There are disadvantages as well, however. These include: (1) reduced record security (2) minimal protection from dirt and dust, and (3) less orderly files.

Movable open shelf units mounted on tracks or electrically powered file units are also available. They offer additional space conservation but dramatically increase filing equipment costs. For this reason, movable open shelf units are rarely installed in single-physician or even many group practices unless the patient population is exceedingly large. This equipment is more appropriate for institutional settings.

Filing equipment should be standardized, of course. If shelf filing is going to be used for the storage of records, then only shelves should be used. It is not efficient to mix file cabinets and shelf units because the design of vertical and lateral filing supplies differs.

The most efficient space-saving arrangement for storing medical records is the use of open shelves or lateral files with pairs of units back to back in long rows with 36-inch aisles. However, only large group practices or hospitals need to consider this type of layout. The record storage needs of most physicians and small group practices can be met by placing lateral files or open shelf file units against one wall of the medical assistant's office. At the rate of 4 records per inch, an open file unit containing seven 36-inch shelves will hold 1000 records, while a five-drawer vertical filing cabinet will hold 720 records.

CARD STORAGE EQUIPMENT

A single or group practice requires card storage equipment. Three types of equipment are commonly used:

1. Vertical file cabinets—hold 3 x 5, 4 x 6, or 5 x 8-inch cards. The drawers are usually partitioned to hold two or three rows of cards. The quality of this equipment varies, but only metal cabinets with ball bearings and compressor blocks should be used.

2. Visible file cabinets—contain horizontal trays of cards held in paper pockets with one line of information visible through a celluloid tab. Entries can be made without removing the cards from their pockets.

3. Electrically powered files—automatic retrieval units. At the touch of a button, needed information is brought from storage to an operator in a stationary position.

Vertical card file cabinets or electrically powered files ordinarily are used for maintaining the patient index and/or billing records. Visible files may be used for maintaining diagnostic or procedural indexes. Visible files are expensive and require quite a lot of space, so they are not suitable for large files unless one's objective is rapid retrieval of one line of information. Power files are rarely found in the office of a single practitioner or in a group practice because the record volume does not justify the high cost of the equipment. Large group practices may use power files for the patient index and/or microfilm storage. However, most physicians' offices contain only vertical file cabinets for card storage.

MICROFILMING

Physicians' offices with record storage problems should microfilm inactive records; otherwise, the volume of stored records and storage costs will continually increase. Microfilming is a method for miniaturizing records on film. Medical records are usually filmed on 16 mm film at a reduction ratio of 24:1. This means that an 8½ x 11-inch page is reduced to 11/32 x 7/16 of an inch. Microfilm lasts 100 years and burns no more freely than paper. The cost of microfilming is approximately equal to that of storing a record in an inactive filing area for approximately 10 years.

Medical records can be microfilmed in a variety of formats:

1. Roll film—documents are filmed sequentially in alphabetical or numerical order on a 100-foot roll of film.

2. Microfiche—a single sheet of film is used and a number of images are exposed onto the sheet (available in 3 x 5, 4 x 6, or 5 x 8-inch sizes).

3. Jackets—roll film is converted to flat film by cutting the roll and inserting each patient's record into a separate jacket.

The advantages of microfilming medical records are that: (1) record storage space requirements are reduced by 90% to 98% depending on the microfilming format used (2) retrieval time spent going to secondary storage areas is eliminated (3) protection against record loss or misfiling is provided with roll film, and (4) record content alterations are eliminated. The disadvantages of microfilming are that: (1) a special viewer is required to read the microfilm (2) microfilm files containing handwritten documents are hard to read (3) it is difficult to update microfilmed patient records, and (4) it is expensive to produce paper copies from the film.

If a decision is made to use microfilm, the records should be sent out to a commercial microfilm service with a staff trained in filming medical records. A written agreement documenting the proposed microfilming methods and the costs as well as written assurance of confidentiality and a written promise to destroy the medical records after filming should be obtained from the microfilm service. Microfilming charges are usually based on a set fee per 1000 images.

It should be pointed out that the decision whether or not to microfilm medical records would be made by the physician.

9.10

QUALITY ASSURANCE IN AMBULATORY CARE

Every physician is responsible for providing quality care and for preparing an adequate medical record documenting that quality care has been rendered to each patient seen. Although current techniques for measuring whether health care providers really do offer quality care are very imprecise, medical records are still perhaps the best measure of the actual quality of the care given. The medical assistant can help the physician to offer good care by maintaining proper surveillance over the data flowing into the medical records.

RECORD REVIEW

The assistant should routinely review for completeness and accuracy the medical records of all patients receiving care on a particular day. The assistant must ensure that each record contains an appropriately dated note describing all services received by a patient. There must be notations describing the results or findings of each test or procedure for which the patient has been billed. Medical record entries must be accurate; for example, one entry cannot indicate that "sutures were removed from a wound of the left arm," if a previous note about the same injury indicates that "the right arm was sutured." The assistant is responsible for identifying such omissions and discrepancies in office records and for seeing that they are corrected by bringing them to the attention of the appropriate staff member.

The medical assistant should also develop follow-through procedures for pending reports when patients are scheduled for laboratory tests, X rays, or consultations with other physicians. These reports must be obtained, evaluated, and entered in the proper records. The physician should initial each such report as proof that the results have been seen. In some instances it may be necessary to inform patients that further care is required. Notations to this effect should be entered in their records. Methods usable as follow-ups on reports not yet received include holding the patient's medical record in a pending file until all outstanding reports have been received or returning the record to the file and maintaining a tickler card file that identifies pending reports. Regardless of the method used, a regular follow-up is necessary to ensure that test results have been received on a regular basis. One cannot assume that outside laboratories, hospitals, or consultants will automatically forward the appropriate reports to the physician's office. Quality health care demands constant vigilance. For example, if a throat culture report revealing the presence of some types of *streptococci* is delayed, the physician may not realize that antibiotic therapy is called for and the patient may develop rheumatic fever as a result.

On some occasions, the assistant may have to contact a hospital for a copy of a discharge summary. In order to assure continuity of care, the discharge summary should be in the patient's office record when the patient returns to the physician for follow-up care. In an obstetrician's office, the providing of continuous care requires that all prenatal records be forwarded to the appropriate hospital prior to the patient's delivery date. These forms may be mailed to the hospital, or the patient may be given a copy to present to the hospital at the time of admission.

PATIENT CARE AUDIT

Some physicians and group practices have attempted to ensure that patients receive quality care by auditing the care that they render. Good records play an important role in patient care audits. In some instances outside auditors or consultants are employed to assess the treatment of specific problems. Other audit methods are used to compare the appropriateness of the data base and treatment plan for a particular problem or diagnosis with specified criteria. Additional research is needed to develop cost-effective methods for auditing the care rendered in physicians' offices.

REGULATORY DEVELOPMENTS
The physician's office has traditionally been viewed as the physician's workroom, and the activities performed there have not been subject to outside scrutiny. However, just as the involvement of government and third-party payers in the financing of health care has grown, so has the demand for accountability. For example, two federal laws regulating physicians' office activities have been passed. These statutes created Professional Standards Review Organizations and Health Systems Agencies endowed with broad authority.

Professional Standards Review Organizations   A Professional Standards Review Organization (PSRO) is a nonprofit professional association made up of licensed physicians organized to perform professional reviews of the medical care provided under federally financed programs. Initially, the review efforts of the PSROs concentrated on institutional services provided by physicians and other health care providers. After experience was gained in reviewing institutional care, the PSROs reviewed noninstitutional services including care rendered in physicians' offices. PSROs are responsible for determining whether the services rendered are medically necessary, are of the quality to meet professionally recognized standards of health care, and are provided in the least expensive setting consistent with the provision of appropriate medical care. Although some PSROs are currently trying to develop appropriate methods for examining ambulatory care, office-based care may not be widely reviewed for many years.

Health Systems Agencies   The legislation with regard to Health Systems Agencies is designed to coordinate existing health resources and to provide for future development of necessary resources. It assigns each Health Systems Agency primary responsibility for effective health planning in a designated geographic area. Each agency is responsible for preparing and implementing plans to improve the health of the residents of its health service area; to increase the accessibility, acceptability, continuity, and quality of health services in its area; to restrain increases in the cost of providing health services; and to prevent unnecessary duplication of health resources.

One of the major activities of a local Health Systems Agency is the collection and analysis of data on current patterns of health care delivery within that area. Traditionally, very little information has been available on care rendered in physicians' offices, even though ambulatory care accounts for most of the medical profession's efforts and the majority of the population's encounters with the health care system. The government has conducted some studies estimating the number of physician visits each year, but effective mechanisms for collecting data on all visits to physicians' offices are not in existence at the present time. In the future, Health Systems Agencies may require the submission of uniform data on each ambulatory care encounter in order to help them plan effectively to meet the health care needs of the populations that they serve.

THE FUTURE
Although the full regulatory impact of Professional Standards Review Organizations and Health Systems Agencies will not be apparent for many years, the health care industry will soon face additional government regulations. Legislation regulating clinical laboratories is expected to become law soon, and some form of national health

insurance is anticipated within three to five years. Physicians engaged in single and group practices can no longer expect to avoid outside scrutiny of their activities, for the future will be characterized by a pattern of increasing regulation with its attendant paperwork. Many physicians view PSROs and Health Systems Agencies as unnecessary intrusions by government into the practice of medicine that threaten the sanctity of the physician-patient relationship and the confidentiality of medical records.

The role of the medical assistant in the future will be to keep up-to-date regarding the constraints that changing government regulations will continue to impose on the private practice of medicine and to help the physician obtain, store, retrieve, and release patient health information in an appropriate manner.

10

CHAPTER TEN

INSURANCE

CONTENTS

10.1

INTRODUCTION: Insurance and Public Programs

Several types of private insurance and public programs are concerned with paying the costs of medical care and the replacement of income lost as a result of disability. The medical assistant should have a general understanding of these kinds of financial protection. They involve total or partial payment of the fees of physicians or other health professionals. They affect the nature and the content of the billings sent to the patients or to the various other payers. They have a significant relationship to medical record maintenance and to the confidentiality of those records. They also require the filling out of claim forms and the submitting of supporting information to verify the cause and the degree of disability.

Therefore, familiarity with insurance and public programs is important to the medical assistant in fulfilling the duties of the position. In fact, dealing with insurance matters is a <u>major</u> segment of the assistant's responsibilities and is important to the patient and the physician.

The medical assistant also should be familiar with all of the insurance that the physician must or should have, i.e., the insurance that is directly related to the conduct of professional practice.

This chapter is intended for two broad groups of readers—the inexperienced who wish to familiarize themselves with health insurance in general as well as with the mechanics of claims handling, and the experienced who need quick answers to specific questions in on-the-job situations. Sections 10.2 through 10.6 and section 10.10 (i.e., those sections providing overviews of private health insurance, disability income insurance, workers' compensation, government-sponsored plans such as Medicare and Medicaid, CHAMPUS and FEHB, and physicians' insurance) are addressed primarily to the first group. Sections 10.7 through 10.9 (i.e., those sections offering routines for fast and accurate claims processing, medical history handling, and answers to questions often asked by patients about insurance) are intended not only for the first group but also for the second group: the format of these latter sections has been designed to afford the reader maximum information with a minimum amount of time-consuming searching. The final subsection at the end of this chapter provides a list of useful publications having to do with health insurance.

10.2

PRIVATE HEALTH INSURANCE: An Overview of Group and Individual Plans

In the United States, three general types of private health insurance plans provide protection against the costs of medical care. Over 165 million persons under age 65 have this protection. In addition, some 11.6 million persons of age 65 and over who are covered by the Medicare program also have private health insurance protection. One type of health insurance is provided by insurance companies covering over 50% of the people with private health insurance protection. Another kind of insurance is provided by the Blue Cross and Blue Shield plans giving coverage to over 30% of those persons having private insurance protection. A third type of insurance is offered by the prepaid group practice plans or health maintenance organizations (HMOs) and labor-union or employer health centers providing prepaid medical care for the remaining percentage of the population having private insurance protection. In addition, some employers and other organizations make health insurance available to groups of people on a self-insured basis.

The medical assistant should be aware of the existence of varying deductible amounts and of coinsurance paid by patients having certain types of health insurance coverage since partial payments on bills may come to the physician's office from several sources. For this reason, deductibles and coinsurance are mentioned but are not discussed in any detail in this chapter.

INSURANCE COMPANY COVERAGES
Insurance companies provide health insurance coverages on a group basis and on an individual policy basis. The benefits are on a cash indemnity basis payable to the covered person or to his or her assignee. Except where otherwise required by law or by the dictates of competition, each insurance company can determine the types of benefits that it will make available.

Group insurance   Group insurance is the means by which the majority of coverages are offered to over 80 million persons. No individual evidence of insurability is required from the person covered. The insured group is made up primarily of the employees (and their dependents) of a common employer. The premiums are more and more often being paid by employers, although in some instances employee contributions are required. Group insurance is also written on trade associations of employers in a common business, on the members of various types of professional associations, on multiple-employer trusts for small-business employers and their employees, and on trusteed health and welfare funds. It is important to recognize that the group insurance purchaser determines the nature, content, and scope of the benefit pattern, frequently dictated by union collective bargaining agreements. As a result, group insurance benefits vary from group to group. With group insurance, the protection may be continued during periods of work shutdown or strike. Upon leaving the insured group, the individual—subject to certain conditions—can convert to individual insurance without giving evidence of insurability.

Group health insurance benefits assume two broad patterns: basic health insurance and major medical expenses insurance coverages. Basic health insurance coverages provide benefits for hospital care, surgery, physicians' services, and certain forms of out-of-hospital care rendered in the outpatient department of a hospital or at the office of a physician. Hospital care benefits are most usually for the full cost of a semiprivate room for a specified number of days, which might range from 21 to 120 days or to 365 or more days. The coverage also includes charges for miscellaneous services and supplies such as the operating room, the intensive care unit, anesthesia, dressings, and casts. Alternately, the coverage might provide a flat per diem benefit (as $70) plus miscellaneous charges. A third alternative provides for the payment of a specified amount for each day of hospitalization regardless of the charges, up to a specified number of days. The surgery benefit might pay the usual, reasonable, and customary charge for the services provided, or it might pay maximum amounts for each type of surgical procedure up to $500 as provided in a schedule of benefits. These amounts may be based on a Relative Value Study. The surgery might be performed in a hospital or in a physician's office. The benefit usually provides for the costs of an assistant surgeon and for anesthesia. The benefits for physician services, often called *regular medical benefits*, pertain to services performed in the hospital, in the physician's office, or at the patient's home. The benefits might provide for the payment of reasonable and customary charges, or might offer a specified amount per visit with an overall maximum amount of benefit, such as $500. In some instances, the coverage may include diagnostic tests, laboratory work, or X rays performed by the physician or done by order of the physician. Also, hospital outpatient services are usually covered for diagnostic tests and X rays, radiotherapy, or the emergency treatment of an injury. The benefits for this care might be the actual charge up to a maximum amount (as $150), or they might be based on a maximum scheduled amount for each service.

Major medical expense insurance coverages assume two forms. The first, comprising about two thirds of all the major medical coverages, is known as "supplemental," since it supplements the basic benefits that might be provided by insurance companies or Blue Cross-Blue Shield plans. The second form, known as *comprehensive major medical,* is used in cases where no basic benefits apply. Whether supplemental or comprehensive, major medical expense insurance provides benefits for practically all types of medical care performed in or out of a hospital including the reasonable, customary, and necessary charges for hospital care and for a semiprivate room; for surgery; for physicians' services in the hospital, in the office, or at the home of the patient; for private-duty nursing by a Registered Nurse or a Licensed Practical Nurse; and for physiotherapy, anesthesia, oxygen, blood transfusions, prescribed drugs, laboratory tests, or X rays administered in or out of the hospital. In some instances, the costs of care in a skilled nursing home or an extended-care facility are included if the care follows hospitalization. Sometimes an additional per diem amount is paid if a private room in the hospital is necessary. In any case, the costs of casts, braces, crutches, and artificial limbs and other prosthetic devices, the rental of medical equipment, and ambulance charges are covered. Major medical expense insurance establishes a variable deductible amount that must be paid by the patient.

Commonly excluded from group health insurance coverages are medical charges resulting from an act of war, charges for which workers' compensation benefits are payable, and services provided without charge to the patient by public facilities or public financing programs. Also usually excluded from the coverages are the costs of hearing aids and cosmetic surgery unless the surgery was necessitated as the result of an accident. Medical care charges resulting from preexisting conditions are also excluded from some policies written on small groups of employees. Routine dental care, routine vision care, and routine periodic physical examinations are also excluded but can be made available under separate coverages or by special provisions.

Special aspects of these insurance coverages are also important since they are variations of the coverage patterns discussed previously. One such variation has to do with maternity coverages. Under the basic benefit plans, the costs of maternity care including hospitalization, delivery, performance of a caesarean section, related abdominal operations, and miscarriage are covered—usually on a scheduled basis with the amount of benefits for the various procedures specified. (In some plans, however, a maximum lump sum benefit is provided for all necessary expenses.) Charges resulting from complications are often paid for on the basis of any other illness. In a minority of coverages, *all* maternity costs are paid as for any other covered illness. Some plans also cover the full cost of prenatal care. In most of the coverages, maternity benefits also apply to unwed mothers if they are employees in the insured group. However, major medical expense insurance most often does *not* cover maternity costs except in cases where there are complications.

Coverage for the medical care of newborn infants is usually provided from birth, although some coverages do not become applicable until the fourteenth day after birth. In some instances, certain costs of well-baby care are included in the coverage.

In a few situations, the costs of family planning services—including prescribed contraceptives, voluntary sterilization, and abortion—are covered, sometimes on the same basis as other coverages and at other times with a maximum amount of coverage (such as $300).

Another variation involves care provided in skilled nursing homes. If such care is covered, it usually must follow hospitalization within a 7- to 14-day period. A dollar limit is typically established for each day of this care: it might be stated as a specified amount or as one-half the rate payable for hospital care. The number of days of care that is covered may range from 30 to 200. (Custodial care is excluded.)

Home health care services prescribed by a physician and provided by a licensed agency following hospitalization may or may not be covered in the insurance benefits. When covered, home health care can include services such as care by a physician, a physical therapist, a part-time nurse, or a home health aide. The services might be provided in the residence of the patient or in a hospital outpatient clinic. The coverage would most often provide for a deductible amount (such as $50) and for coinsurance. The coverage could be limited to a maximum number of days of care—a time period that might range from 40 to 270 days or more. Excluded from coverage are custodial care, the preparation of meals, general housekeeping services, and services whose purpose is personal comfort.

The treatment of venereal disease may or may not be included in the coverage, regardless of whether the treatment is administered in a hospital, at a clinic, or in a physician's office. If coverage of such treatment is included, the benefits would usually not differ from the other benefits covered in a particular plan.

Another variation in medical care coverage concerns the treatment of mental disorders. In most group health insurance policies, the treatment of mental, nervous, emotional, or personality disorders is covered to some extent. The costs of hospitalization (except in public hospitals) are usually covered just as they are for the treatment of any other condition. Under major medical expense insurance, the benefit typically has special limitations for out-of-hospital treatment, such as 50% coinsurance, a limit of 50 visits a year to a psychiatrist, and a limit on the amount payable per visit (such as $20). A special maximum of benefits (as $500 a year or $10,000) might be established for this type of treatment.

The treatment of alcoholism—considered a disease by the American Medical Association, the American Hospital Association, and the American Psychiatric Association—is included in most group health insurance coverages, although it is still excluded from some others. When it is included, there are usually special coverage limitations. For example, in some plans the coverage is limited to hospital care, while in others the coverage might include care administered in special facilities for the treatment of alcoholism. Most of the time, coverage is limited to from 60 to 89 days of care, although some benefits extend for 180 days or longer. A special maximum amount of benefit (as $5,000) might also be established.

Insurance benefits for preventive health services are generally available but are seldom purchased. These benefits might include the cost of periodic health examinations or multiphasic health screening, diagnostic tests, immunization, or well-baby care. These special benefits might be limited to a fixed amount (such as $50) a year. On the other hand, the benefits might pay the full cost on a reasonable and customary charge basis. Also, there might be a schedule of benefits payable which could range from about $25 to about $200. Physical examinations are most often limited as to frequency; frequency, in turn, is age-related. Thus, persons under age 40 might be covered for one examination every 2 to 5 years, while persons over age 40 would be covered for an annual examination or for one examination every other year. Well-baby care might be limited to six visits for those children under six months of age, to four visits for those between six months to two years of age, and to one visit a year for those aged two to five years.

Certain rehabilitation services might be included in the group health insurance coverage, limited in some cases to special amounts of benefits. These services can include physiotherapy, speech therapy, artificial limbs, and other prosthetic appliances or devices. Vocational rehabilitation is not covered, since this service is provided by the states.

Blanket insurance   Blanket insurance is also provided by some insurance companies. This insurance—essentially similar to group insurance—might cover groups such as passengers of a common carrier, employees who are subject to special hazards (such as those of travel), students, newspaper carriers, members of an athletic team or a sports group, campers at a camp, or members of an association of persons (such as a volunteer fire department, a first aid or a civil defense group, or Boy and Girl Scout troops) having a common interest. Blanket insurance benefits normally include medical expense protection and might also include disability income insurance or accident, death, and dismemberment benefits.

Individual insurance   Individual health insurance policies are also available. This kind of insurance is particularly important to those persons not having group insurance: professionals, small-business people, unemployed persons, casual workers, persons (such as service or farm workers) employed where group insurance protection is not available, and some sales personnel. Individual health insurance can also be appropriate for those who wish to supplement other forms of health insurance such as group insurance or Blue Cross-Blue Shield coverages. As with group insurance, the dependent spouse or children can be included in the individual health insurance coverage.

In the main, individual health insurance policies follow the same benefit patterns as those of group insurance. It is difficult, however, to generalize about the benefit patterns of individual health insurance policies due to the extreme variety of available coverages. A few points can be made here, though. Most individual policies are hospital-surgical policies. They commonly cover the cost of hospital-ization, surgery, physician in-hospital services, care in an extended-care facility, and outpatient diagnostic X-ray and laboratory services. The amounts of the benefits and the limits on them can vary according to the insured individual's own selection. The hospital expenses covered can be the actual charges up to a maximum daily limit. Some policies contain added benefits for intensive care unit charges ranging from 7 to 14 days. The hospital benefit can be limited to a period of from 30 to 365 days of care. The costs of miscellaneous hospital care are usually covered, including the costs of X-ray and laboratory services, drugs, dressings, the operating room, ambulance services, and the fees of hospital-based professionals such as patholo-gists, radiologists, and anesthetists—all subject to a maximum amount which can currently range from 10 to 25 times the daily hospital benefit. (Note: Some policies limit the maximum amount to be paid for each of the miscellaneous services.) A maternity hospital benefit is commonly included subject to a variety of limitations. Surgical benefits are frequently limited to maximum amounts for each type of surgical procedure. These amounts may depend on Relative Value Studies es-tablished by medical societies. The surgery may be performed in a hospital or in a physician's office. The physician's visits to the hospital also are covered by the benefits subject to a maximum amount for each visit (a typical range is from $3 to $10). The daily charge for care in an extended-care facility or in a skilled nursing home might also be covered subject to a maximum amount per diem and a maximum number of days of care which can range from 30 to 100 days. Some individual policies also contain a benefit for diagnostic X-ray and laboratory services performed out of the hospital (including services performed in the physician's office) subject to a maximum amount (such as $50 or $100) for any one sickness or injury. Individual hospital-surgical policies may or may not provide for a deductible amount before the benefits begin. Common exceptions to individual health insurance coverages are medical expenses caused by war or those occurring while the insured person is on active military duty, self-inflicted injuries, or those injuries covered by workers' compensation. The treatment of psychiatric disorders also may be excluded from the coverage, may be limited to certain types of treatment such as hospital care, and may be limited to a maximum amount of benefits.

Also available are major medical expense insurance policies covering types of care such as house calls and office visits, private-duty nursing, and drugs, supplies, and medical equipment prescribed and/or ordered by the physician. The benefits are based on reasonable and customary charges. A maximum limit on the benefits is also established with the limit ranging from $10,000 to $100,000. Certain maximum amounts of benefits might be established for specific types of services, too.

SELF-INSURANCE
Some large employers provide health insurance benefits on a self-insurance basis. With this arrangement, the benefits and details are similar to those described for

group insurance coverage. The major difference between the two is that with self-insurance, the employer finances the program internally without insurance company involvement. In such cases, the employer either administers the program or obtains the services of a consulting firm specializing in such matters. The employer might finance the program alone or the employees might be required to contribute to the cost of the program.

BLUE CROSS-BLUE SHIELD PLANS

Blue Cross-Blue Shield plans provide coverages which are generally similar to those made available by the insurance companies. Each plan is an autonomous organization determining its own benefits, which are then made available to its subscribers. Each plan makes more than one type of benefit option available. Each plan is confined to a specified geographic territory—most often a state or a specific area within a state—although the plans have national organizations to enable the coverage of multistate groups such as large employers or labor unions. In many geographic areas, the Blue Cross-Blue Shield plans are combined into what is called a "joint plan." The coverages are sold largely on a group basis with most of the individual coverages resulting from an insured person's conversion to that coverage after he or she has left a group plan. Unlike insurance company benefits which are paid on a cash indemnity basis to the insured person or to his or her assignee, Blue Cross-Blue Shield benefits are referred to as *service benefits*. The plan pays the benefits directly to the provider of care, with the provider then billing the patient for those services not covered by the plan benefits. The plan has contractual arrangements with member hospitals, member physicians, and other care providers.

Blue Cross   Blue Cross plans—nonprofit organizations offering health care benefits to their subscribers—are often called *prepayment plans* since the subscribers pay in advance for the health care that they might need in the future. Blue Cross plans provide coverage for the full cost of semiprivate hospital care which might range in time from 21 to 365 days. Some plans, in addition to full coverage for a limited time period (such as 21 days), provide coverage for half the cost for an additional time period (such as 180 days). The coverage is for hospital costs such as room and board and miscellaneous expenses such as the operating room, laboratory tests and X rays, drugs, oxygen, blood transfusions, anesthesia, dressings, casts, and radiation therapy. Maternity costs are usually limited to a fixed sum or to a limited time (such as eight days of hospitalization). Complications in pregnancy, however, are covered under the usual benefit structure. If the patient is confined in a hospital not having a contract with a Blue Cross plan, the benefits are limited to a specific dollar amount. In addition, hospital outpatient services for emergency accident care or for diagnostic tests and X rays are covered in full but can be limited to a specific number of visits a year (such as 30). Exclusions to the coverage might be those costs covered under workers' compensation, care provided in public institutions, or in-hospital care for purely diagnostic purposes.

Blue Shield   Blue Shield plans are also *prepayment plans*. Blue Shield coverage pertains mainly to surgery and physicians' services. The surgery might be performed in a hospital or in a physician's office, although some plans limit the surgery benefit to that performed in a hospital. Payment for physicians' services might be limited to in-hospital visits or might include both home and office visits. There also might be a limit on the number of such visits, either per year or per illness. In-hospital consultation is usually covered, as is the cost of an assistant surgeon. In addition, the costs of emergency services for accidental injuries, anesthesia, X rays, diagnostic tests, EKGs, laboratory tests, and radiation treatment are typically covered. Some

Blue Shield plans provide for the payment of benefits on a cash indemnity basis, with the payment being made in accordance with a schedule of allowances for the care administered and with the patient being required to pay the physician directly any difference between the schedule payment and the actual charge. In other instances, the Blue Shield plan pays the physician on a schedule basis in relation to the care provided, the physician agreeing to accept the schedule benefit as full payment. However, the most common practice is a combination of these two approaches with the full payment approach applying to persons below a specified income level and the cash indemnity approach applying to persons above that income level. Usually excluded from Blue Shield coverages are the care covered by workers' compensation benefits, publicly provided care, and care administered for purely cosmetic reasons.

Blue Cross-Blue Shield plans also offer major medical expense coverages which might alternatively be called "extended benefits" or "catastrophe benefits." These benefits are supplemental to the basic benefits discussed previously. The coverage applies to the costs of hospital care, surgery, care in the physician's office or elsewhere, home care, and auxiliary costs such as those for diagnostic tests, medical devices, and equipment. There is a deductible amount (such as $100) which must be paid by the patient, there is a provision for coinsurance under which the patient pays 20% of all charges, and there is a maximum amount of benefits.

Coverage of nervous and mental disorders   A majority of the Blue Cross plans currently make benefits available that cover the treatment of nervous and mental disorders. In-hospital care may be limited to a specified time span (such as 30 or 120 days or more). Certain other services are covered by most of the plans for care such as partial hospitalization on a day or night basis. Some plans exclude care in a private psychiatric hospital while other plans limit this care to 30 days of coverage. (Most Blue Cross plans do not cover care provided in a public mental hospital or facility.) Most of the Blue Shield plans also provide for the treatment of nervous and mental conditions by a physician, with some of the plans limiting the coverage to 10 visits a year to a physician. Some Blue Shield plans also provide benefits for outpatient care such as psychotherapy, psychological testing, psychotropic drugs, and the services of psychiatric social workers. The treatment of alcoholism in specified alcoholism treatment centers is also covered by some Blue Cross-Blue Shield plans.

Blue Shield Permanent Reciprocity Program   The Blue Shield Permanent Reciprocity Program is a means by which out-of-area claims can be paid by the Blue Shield plan in the particular locale where the medical services are performed. The medical assistant should be aware of the existence of this Program and should be able to recognize the identifying symbol borne on the ID cards of the Blue Shield subscribers having Reciprocity Program coverage. All such patients' ID cards show a double-ended red arrow containing the letter N followed by three digits (as N 987). All other data on these patients' ID cards relevant to the Reciprocity Program are outlined in red. (See also section 10.7 for the procedures to be followed in billing under this Program.)

HEALTH MAINTENANCE ORGANIZATIONS (HMOs)
Prepaid group practice plans and health maintenance organizations—called HMOs—provide medical care to their members at established centers on a prepaid basis. The care is usually quite comprehensive and includes physical examinations, preventive dental care for children, health education, prenatal and postnatal care, immunization, and other preventive health services. Psychiatric care, dental services, vision care, and prescribed drugs are sometimes included in the services.

Copayments by the patients may be required. HMO sponsors can be employers, labor unions, cooperatives, insurance companies, or Blue Cross plans.

In 1973 the Health Maintenance Organization Act was passed by the Congress to stimulate the development of HMOs by making funds available for the organization and the initial period of operation of an HMO. According to the law, employers who offer health insurance as a fringe benefit and who have more than 25 employees must pay either for their workers' enrollment in an HMO or for their own company-offered health insurance plan. Today, some four to five million persons receive their health care principally through HMOs. The physician providing the care may be employed by the HMO on a salary basis but may also conduct private practice on a part-time basis. If a member of an HMO chooses to receive care elsewhere, he or she is responsible for the payment for that care.

Closely related to the HMOs are certain employer plans or labor union programs which, while not based on a prepayment system as such, nevertheless do provide medical care to some extent. Today, a great many of the larger employers have established industrial health programs that provide, to varying extents, care for their employees and, if necessary, referral to other sources of care. Many such programs also provide preemployment and periodical physical examinations. These plans also conduct health education programs and work toward the elimination of hazards on the job. As suggested earlier, the plans vary considerably. In some instances, smaller employers hire a physician or a nurse on a part-time basis or function cooperatively with other employers through various types of health centers. Programs of this kind have been encouraged by congressional enactment of the Occupational Safety and Health Act (OSHA) in 1970. Many labor unions have also established health centers to provide care for their membership. The care provided varies from the quite comprehensive to the very limited. In either instance, referrals can be made to private practicing physicians. (The medical assistant should therefore be aware of these kinds of referrals.) Referrals would come to private practicing physicians from physicians connected with the individual programs. The referring physicians would, of course, follow up on the progress of the referred cases. Payment to the private physician would be made on a fee-for-service basis. This fee would be paid by the HMO, the employer, the union or through any related health insurance benefits.

SPECIAL TYPES OF INSURANCE

In addition to the foregoing types of insurance, other coverages for special forms of health care, vision care, and prescribed drugs are available. This insurance is usually underwritten on a separate basis.

Dental care insurance   Dental care insurance customarily covers the costs of oral examinations, X rays, cleaning, fillings, extractions, inlays, bridgework, and dentures, as well as oral surgery, root canal therapy, and, in some instances, orthodontia. In the majority of cases, coverage is based on scheduled amounts payable for specific procedures. In the remainder of the cases, the coverage reimburses reasonable and customary charges subject to the payment of a variable deductible amount. Dental care insurance is made available by insurance companies largely on a group insurance basis, by certain Blue Cross-Blue Shield plans, and by dental service corporations currently operating in over 30 states. (Dental service corporations are the dental equivalents of Blue Shield plans.) Some union self-insured trusts provide dental care through their own clinics or health centers. (Two completed attending dentists' statements are shown in section 10.7.)

Vision care insurance   Vision care insurance is yet another form of insurance made available by private health insurers, most often on a separate basis. *Vision care* has been defined by the American Optometric Association as all of the professional services that an optometrist may render including eye examinations and refraction and the materials found to be necessary— principally eyeglasses and contact lenses. Vision care is distinguished from surgical or medical eye care in that the latter is performed by an ophthalmologist and is typically covered under the health insurance plans described earlier. In several states, vision care services plans— essentially similar to Blue Shield plans—have been established. Labor-union clinics or health centers may also provide vision care to their members. In addition, certain prepaid group practice plans or HMOs might include aspects of vision care in the services provided to their enrollees. Some insurance companies also make vision care benefits available on a group basis. These coverages may provide a schedule of benefits to be paid for each type of service or might provide for the payment of reasonable and customary charges for vision care subject to a deductible amount and coinsurance by the patient. The coverage might be limited to one set of lenses per year and one set of frames every two or three years. Coverage might exclude contact lenses, sunglasses, and special types of frames.

Prescription drug insurance   Prescription drug insurance is at times provided on a separate basis, although most insurance for the costs of prescribed drugs is included in the more general forms of health insurance. Separate coverages vary considerably and assume no discernible pattern. The drug coverages are offered by several insurance companies which at times underwrite programs established by pharmacists in several localities. This type of coverage is also provided by several Blue Cross-Blue Shield plans, by certain prepaid group practice plans or HMOs, and by prepaid prescription plans established by some pharmacists. They are essentially similar to Blue Shield plans. The insurance approaches to prescription drug coverage usually involve a deductible amount (such as $2 per prescription or $25 a year) to be paid by the patient, a coinsurance amount (usually 20%) to be paid by the patient, and a maximum amount of benefit (typically ranging from $50 to $2,000) per year per family. Drugs excluded from the coverage may include contraceptives, anti-obesity drugs, multiple vitamins, or psychotropic drugs. There may be a limit on the dosage of a prescribed drug which will be covered by the insurance. Also, drugs covered by the particular program may be limited to generics or to those contained in an established formulary.

THE PHYSICIAN AND HEALTH INSURANCE

Attending physicians have a basic and significant role with respect to health insurance, excluding the coverages provided by salaried physicians under prepaid group practice plans or HMOs. For billing purposes, the physician and/or the assistant should make certain that the patient has health insurance protection in the first place. If the protection is provided by a group plan, the physician can then determine the validity, the nature, and extent of the coverage by contacting the employer, the insurance company, or Blue Cross-Blue Shield. The physician and/or the medical assistant can obtain the necessary claim forms from these sources or from the patient. In preparing the bill for services rendered, the physician should state the diagnosis, the treatment provided, and the charges for the services rendered. If the services are beyond any limits in the insurance coverages, or if deductible amounts or coinsurance are provided for, the patient is responsible for the payment of those amounts. This situation indicates the importance of maintaining complete and understandable medical records (see Chapter 9). In turn, the records should be kept on a confidential basis except when different procedures are required by law or when the patient authorizes release of information. Health insurance benefits payable by insurance companies can be assigned by the patient to the provider(s) of service. The Uniform Health Insurance Claim Form for private health insurance benefits developed by the American Medical Association is shown in section 10.7. Since the proper completion of this and other such forms is extremely important to both the patient and the physician, the assistant should examine carefully the completed form shown in 10.7.

COST CONTROL

Today there is considerable interest in controlling the costs of medical care. While much interest centers around the Medicare and Medicaid programs and considerations of a system of national health insurance, the principles of cost control also influence and affect the various forms of health insurance currently in use. Concern about cost control assumes several forms, all of which are directly related to the physician.

One approach to medical care cost control has been the development of Professional Service Review Organizations (PSROs) encouraged by the Social Security Act Amendments of 1972 in regard to Medicare and Medicaid. For many years the concept of peer review by and of physicians has been advocated and urged both by medical societies and by insurers. The purpose of the PSRO is to develop a way of determining the medical necessity of institutional care and a method of reviewing and evaluating ambulatory health services. Today, over 100 PSROs are operational or are being planned. They may operate locally or they may function through state councils. In order to eliminate unnecessary tests and excessive forms of treatment, the full cooperation of the physicians is requisite.

Another approach to cost control, and one that is a forerunner of the PSRO concept, is the medical care foundation which functions through the physicians in a particular area. The first such foundation was formed in 1968 in San Joaquin, California. Its purpose was to monitor health services, to evaluate the care rendered, and to engage in claim surveillance. Wasteful practices were identified and discouraged. Experience has shown that foundations have the ability to generate savings, a fact that has been demonstrated by the Foundation for Health Care Evaluation in the Twin Cities.

Yet another approach to cost control that is attracting considerable interest is the requiring of a second opinion before surgery is performed. In some instances, Blue Cross-Blue Shield plans have adopted this requirement, with the plan paying for the additional costs involved, including diagnostic tests. The purpose of the second opinion is to eliminate any cases of unnecessary surgery while at the same time recognizing that professional opinions on such matters can often differ.

Still another approach to the reduction of hospital costs is the utilization review. The purpose of a utilization review is the reduction of unnecessary hospital care principally by reducing the length of a hospital stay to no more than what is dictated by the particular circumstances of a case. Some savings do result from this approach, although a 1970 Senate Committee on Finance report stated that utilization review requirements have generally been perfunctory. More recently it has come to be recognized by many that the traditional approach to hospital reimbursement does not provide any incentive to contain the cost of this form of care. The solution proposed is referred to as a system of "prospective rating" which in turn would subject hospital financing to public accountability. Under such a system, hospitals would have to justify in advance before a state rate review commission any increases in their rates and would have to furnish a certification of need for any rate increase. The objective is to bring about increased efficiency, to limit plans for expansion or modification in plant or services to those consistent with community needs, to discourage the duplication of expensive equipment and services, and to bring about equality of charges to all patients. Since the implementation of this idea is so recent, its effectiveness cannot yet be proved. In some states, the law applies only to certain patients (such as those whose expenses are carried by Medicaid).

The process of comprehensive community or area-wide health planning, encouraged by the Partnership for Health Act of 1967, is also supportive of cost control. In 1974, the National Health Planning and Resources Development Act, providing assistance to state and local health planning agencies, was passed. The purpose of the Act is to impede unnecessary hospital construction while at the same time assuring the availability of needed health care facilities.

All such approaches containing the costs of medical care serve to make the physician more publicly accountable respecting his or her practice, decisions, and charges. While such approaches are now essentially experimental, they will become more important in the years ahead, and particularly so if a system of national health insurance becomes law. The well-informed medical assistant should have general knowledge of the issue of cost control.

10.3

DISABILITY INCOME INSURANCE: Group and Individual Plans

Disability income insurance that pays benefits during periods of disability is made available in varying degrees through both private and public sources. In either instance, the attending physician or other health professional can be called on to verify the existence of the disability and to fill out the necessary claim forms for the patient. As a medical assistant, you should have a general understanding of what this insurance is.

Disability income insurance is offered by many insurance companies on either a group or an individual basis. It is an important form of protection for employees, self-employed persons, and professionals who may become disabled as a result of illness or injury. Because workers' compensation provides disability benefits for income lost as a result of occupational injuries and diseases, disability insurance usually covers only disability from causes not covered by workers' compensation. There are exceptions particularly with group disability insurance for long-term disabilities. In such cases, however, the benefit is usually reduced in proportion to any benefit received under workers' compensation or under the Social Security Disability Insurance program. (This reduction is termed an *offset*.)

GROUP DISABILITY INCOME INSURANCE
Group disability income insurance takes essentially two forms: short-term and long-term disability protection.

Short-term disability income insurance   Short-term disability income insurance is limited typically to disabilities resulting from nonoccupational illnesses or injuries. The time period for which the benefits are payable is most often 26 weeks, although some plans are limited to 13 weeks and others extend to 52 weeks. Benefits usually begin with the eighth day of disability, although many plans begin benefits on the first day if the employee is hospitalized or if the cause of disability is an accident. The amount of the benefit is always wage-related, and it usually ranges from 50% to 80% of the insured person's wages up to a stated maximum dollar amount which can vary considerably. Some group short-term disability insurance at a place of employment is limited to certain types of employees (as nonoffice workers), usually because other employees are entitled to salary continuance benefits. Benefits are typically payable when the employee is totally and continuously disabled and therefore cannot perform the duties of his or her occupation.

Today, more and more group short-term disability insurance programs are providing benefits for disabilities resulting from pregnancy and childbirth. The benefit is usually limited to six weeks of disability, although some groups provide longer benefits. Many group plans, however, do not contain this coverage. Group short-term disability plans also provide disability benefits resulting from the treatment of alcoholism, so long as the treatment is administered under medical supervision. The benefit commences when the alcoholic employee begins the treatment. The benefit continues for as long as the treatment continues, subject to the overall limits of the particular coverage.

Long-term disability insurance   Long-term disability income insurance has grown rapidly in the past decade. Today, about 18 million employed people are estimated to have this form of protection. The protection is in effect regardless of whether the disability results from nonoccupational or occupational diseases or injuries. Where occupational hazards are covered, an offset is provided for against workers' compensation payments. Whether the cause was occupational or not, an offset is provided for against any payments made under the Social Security Disability Insurance program. Some long-term disability programs exclude certain worker categories (as hourly employees). Under most programs, the long-term disability benefits begin after six months' disability or upon the cessation of short-term disability insurance benefits or benefits under a salary continuance program. The benefits usually continue to age 65. The length of time that the benefits are payable typically ranges for as short a period as 52 weeks or for as long a period as up to age 65, depending on the employee's length of service. Under some programs, however, the benefits continue for life. The amount of benefit payable under long-term disability programs varies considerably. While most programs provide benefits for an established percentage (usually 60%) of average wages, others have a maximum monthly amount payable. Still others increase the amounts payable as the period of disability increases. Other plans' benefits vary with the employee's length of service.

The conventional definition of *disability* is as follows: the inability to engage in one's occupation for one or two years, and thereafter the inability to engage in any gainful occupation for which one is reasonably fitted by education, training, or experience. Long-term disability benefits at times exclude disability resulting from preexisting conditions; or disability resulting from psychiatric disorders, alcoholism, or drug addiction unless the employee is confined to a hospital or other institution specializing in the medical care and treatment of these disorders. The role of disability insurance in aiding the rehabilitative processes of a disabled employee should be noted. It is a general procedure to continue the payment of benefits in whole or in part during a period when the insured employee returns to work on a full-time or part-time basis—provided that the individual is undergoing formal rehabilitation in which employment plays a definite therapeutic part and provided that the program has the approval of the attending physician. The Universal Health Insurance Claim Form shown in section 10.7 can be used for short- and long-term disability claims.

Temporary disability benefits Temporary disability benefits are compulsory in a few states. The laws pertain primarily to nonoccupational disability since occupational disabilities are provided for under workers' compensation. The benefits for disabled eligible employees are a proportion of average pay rates for a maximum of 26 weeks following a 7-day waiting period. In a few states, the disability benefit is allowed for pregnancy; in a few others, a small hospital benefit is paid for up to 20 days of hospitalization. The benefits are financed by employer-employee contributions.

Disability insurance under Social Security The disability insurance program under the Social Security system was established in 1956 by the Congress to provide basic income benefits for totally and presumably permanently disabled persons of age 50 and over until age 65. In 1960, the 50-years-of-age limitation was removed, and in 1965 the definition of *disability* was changed to the inability to engage in any substantially gainful activity by reason of any medically determinable physical or mental impairment which can be expected to result in death or has lasted or can be expected to last for a continuous period of not less than 12 months. Eligibility for the benefits under the disability insurance program depends on work experience, but some employed people such as farm workers, domestic workers, employees of nonprofit organizations, public employees, and some self-employed persons are not covered under the program.

Each year, the cases eligible for benefits are reexamined. Monthly payments similar to Social Security benefits are payable after disability has continued for five months. An offset is provided for if workers' compensation disability benefits are payable. Since 1973, disability insurance beneficiaries have been eligible for hospital and medical care benefits under the Medicare program. The program is administered by the Social Security Administration.

The Railroad Retirement Act The provisions of the Railroad Retirement Act are directly related to the disability insurance program. According to this act, permanently disabled railroad workers who have had 10 years of railroad service are entitled to a total disability annuity. The amount of the benefit depends on the employee's average wages and his or her number of years of service. The program is administered by the Railroad Retirement Board. All employers are insured through a government fund financed by a payroll tax paid by the employer.

Workers' compensation Workers' compensation provides disability benefits for various types of disabilities resulting from occupational injuries or diseases. (See section 10.4 for full discussion.)

Veterans Administration The Veterans Administration program also provides disability benefits for service-connected disabilities. The benefit is related to the degree of impairment and, in certain instances, added benefits are provided if there are dependents. (See also section 10.5 for a discussion of veterans' benefits.)

Assistance to the Permanently and Totally Disabled The program entitled Assistance to the Permanently and Totally Disabled (APTD), administered by the Social Security Administration, is another public program providing income benefits to eligible persons who are in financial need, regardless of whether they have any work experience and regardless of whether they qualify for the Social Security Disability Insurance program. A program similar to APTD is Aid to the Blind, which also provides public assistance.

10.4

WORKERS' COMPENSATION

Workers' compensation—the most important of all coverages written to protect people against medical costs sustained as the result of industrial accidents—has been established by law in all states and by the federal government for longshoremen, harbor workers, railroad workers, and employees of the District of Columbia. Specifically, the legislation deals with occupational accidents and diseases occurring at the workplace or in the course of task fulfillment away from the workplace. It provides that certain benefits are to be paid. Over 80% of the work force is protected by such legislation today. (Originally designated "workman's compensation," the appellation has been changed recently to "workers' compensation" to avoid sexist connotations.)

Because the individual state laws differ, only generalizations can be made here concerning the details of workers' compensation legislation and benefits. Individuals interested in the details of the legislation in a particular state should contact the workers' compensation board in that state. Included in the differences among the state laws are the compulsory or elective nature of the programs, the types of employees covered, the benefits provided, and the types of insuring mechanisms employed.

COVERAGE

In 19 states, the coverage is elective on the part of the employer; in the remainder of the states, it is compulsory. None of the state workers' compensation laws cover all employees. Most often exempt from the coverage are the following people: farm workers (who are only covered in about half of the states), domestic employees (who are covered in only a few states), casual workers, and those persons working for small-business employers (i.e., those employers retaining less than three, four, or five workers) depending on the state.

BENEFITS

Workers' compensation benefits pertain to occupational accidents and occupational diseases, although in four states the coverage applies only to certain specified diseases. The benefits for the hazard covered differ from state to state. The benefits are essentially of three types, but only the first two of them are of interest to medical assistants:

1. **Medical care benefits to defray the cost of the treatment of occupational injuries and diseases** Included are the costs of hospitalization, surgery, and medical care. These benefits are payable from the date of the occurrence of an injury or from the date of discernment of an occupational disease. Most states provide for the payment of all reasonable and necessary costs of this care without limitations or exceptions for as long as is required to complete the necessary treatment. For physicians and other health professionals, payment is made on a fee-for-service basis. In five states, however, there are some limitations to these benefits. The regulations might limit the amount of payable benefits to a specified maximum amount, or they might limit the duration of time over which the benefits are payable, or both.

2. **Disability benefits to partially replace income lost as a result of an occupational injury or disease** The benefits differ as to the degree of disability. *Disability* can be classified according to the following degrees: temporary total disability (most workers' compensation claims are based on this degree), temporary partial disability (or impairment of a temporary nature), partial disability (or impairment of a permanent nature for which a flat sum payment is usually provided, depending on the nature of the impairment), and

total and permanent disability. Disability benefits vary among the states but typically provide for the payment of 60% or 67% of the worker's average wages subject to maximum and minimum weekly limits. Benefits commence after a waiting period which varies among the states from two to seven days. In some states, the total number of weeks for which benefits are payable is limited. For example, the number of weeks for the payment of permanent disability benefits might be limited to 330 or 550 weeks. However, most states provide that the payment of benefits for permanent total disability be for life. Only a few states provide for any adjustment in the disability benefits to cover the effects of economic inflation.

3. **Survivor benefits and burial expense benefits**   These benefits are important but have no effect on the work of the medical assistant.

Workers' compensation benefits are directly related to the rehabilitation of the disabled worker, because the purpose of the benefits is to restore the disabled worker to useful and remunerative employment through prompt treatment and therapy and the provision of psychiatric and social services as well as vocational counseling and training, if needed. As a consequence, some states provide additional benefits under the medical payments benefit structure particularly in cases where amputation, injury to the central nervous system, burns, blindness, loss of hearing, severe deformity, speech impairment, or injury to the back or spinal cord are involved. The courts have expanded workers' compensation to include occupationally related mental disorders possibly caused by the work performed or those mental disorders resulting from a traumatic injury suffered during employment.

The physician, hospital, or other medical care provider can determine the patient's status under workers' compensation by contacting the patient's employer. Claim forms can be obtained from the employer, from the insurance company, or from the state fund, and payment is made by those sources depending on where the insurance responsibility lies. In section 10.7, an illustration of the United States Department of Labor claim form is found. (Claim forms, however, differ from state to state.) In the last analysis, the responsibility for claims administration rests with the workers' compensation boards or commissions in the individual states, and any necessary appeals should be presented to those sources. Bills for services rendered must be complete as to diagnosis and treatment rendered and the charges for the services provided. Furthermore, the physician can be called on to verify the occurrence of any resultant disability. Another point to remember is that individual states differ as to the *selection of the physician* who will treat the disabled worker; in some states, the worker does not have first choice since the decision regarding physician selection rests with the employer or the insurer.

10.5

GOVERNMENT-SPONSORED PLANS: Medicare, Medicaid, and Others

Several types of government-sponsored programs have come into existence to pay the costs of medical care in whole or in part or to provide such care with or without charges to the patients. These programs can have differing relationships to private physicians or other health professionals depending on the nature of the particular government-sponsored plan as well as on the type and location of the practice.

MEDICARE
In 1966 the Medicare program was instituted to finance the costs of medical care within limits for most persons aged 65 and over. In 1973 the program was extended

to include the totally and permanently disabled under the age of 65 who are eligible under the Social Security Disability Insurance program. The Medicare program was also extended to include persons under the age of 65 while undergoing kidney dialysis or transplants. Medicare is part of the Social Security system and is provided for in Title XVIII of the Social Security Act.

The Medicare program is composed of two parts: Part A, a compulsory program, and Part B, a voluntary program. Under Part A (Hospital Insurance), benefits are paid for hospital care, care provided in extended-care facilities, and home health care. (Custodial care is not covered by the program.) The hospital care includes a semiprivate room and other necessary services in a hospital approved by the program for 90 days per incidence of illness. The patient is responsible for the initial payment of a deductible amount which increases periodically, and he or she must share in the costs of care after 60 days of hospitalization. A maximum lifetime reserve of 60 days of hospitalization is also provided for, with the patient sharing the costs. Psychiatric hospitalization is limited to 190 days of care in the person's lifetime. After 3 days of hospitalization, the patient is covered for up to 100 days of care in an extended-care facility, with the patient sharing the cost after the first 20 days of such care. The home health care benefit is limited to 100 visits by health care professionals such as visiting nurses and physical therapists employed by an approved health care program, following discharge of the patient from the hospital. A physician's home visits are not covered under Part A of Medicare.

Part B (Supplementary Medical Insurance) covers the care provided by physicians or surgeons in hospitals, in outpatient clinics, at their offices, or in the patients' homes. The reasonable or customary charge is paid by the program subject to its being commensurate with the prevailing fees for such services in the particular geographic area. The patient is responsible for the payment of an initial deductible amount which increases periodically and for 20% of all charges thereafter. For psychiatric care, however, the patient must pay half the charges in a calendar year. Home health care visits by a physician are covered under Part B of the program to the extent of 100 visits per incidence of illness. Prior hospitalization is not required for this benefit. The services covered include diagnostic tests and X rays, surgical dressings, braces, artificial limbs, splints, casts, medical equipment rental, and ambulance services. Prescribed drugs out of the hospital are not covered, nor are routine physical examinations, private-duty nursing, vision care, hearing aids, personal comfort services, or dental care other than oral surgery. The Medicare program does not cover care paid for by workers' compensation benefits.

The administration of the Medicare program rests with the Secretary of Health, Education and Welfare through the Social Security Administration, which determines the rate of payment for care that is to be paid for under the program. In turn, fiscal intermediaries are designated to conduct the actual administration of the program. Under Part A, each institution for health care makes its own selection of the intermediary, with 60% of them having selected the Blue Cross plans and the remainder having selected insurance companies. Under Part B of the program, the Social Security Administration assigns an intermediary in each state or locality. Under either Part A or B, prepaid group practice plans function directly with the Social Security Administration.

The Medicare patient can be identified by the Medicare Health Insurance identification card indicating whether the patient is covered under Part A or under both Part A and Part B. Any question as to whether the deductible amount has been satisfied can be answered by the designated fiscal intermediary in a particular locality or by the Social Security Administration. Claim forms are readily available from the same sources, and billing is made to them for the covered amounts and to the patient for the amounts not covered by the program. The billing should specify the diagnosis, the services provided, and the charges. A copy of the Uniform Health Insurance Claim Form developed by the American Medical Association is shown in section 10.7. The Request for Medicare Payment form is also illustrated in section 10.7. [HEW Publication No. (SSA) 77–10050 entitled *Your Medicare Handbook* is a useful document to have on hand. It is especially helpful in answering patients' questions about Medicare.]

Medicare carriers   The following is an alphabetical state-by-state list of the names and addresses of organizations selected by the Social Security Administration to handle medical insurance claims. When corresponding with these organizations be sure to include *Medicare* in the carrier's envelope address.

Alabama
Medicare
Blue Cross-Blue Shield of Alabama
930 South 20th Street
Birmingham, Alabama 35205

Alaska
Medicare
Aetna Life & Casualty
Crown Plaza
1500 S W First Avenue
Portland, Oregon 97201

Arizona
Medicare
Aetna Life & Casualty
Medicare Claim Administration
3010 West Fairmount Avenue
Phoenix, Arizona 85017

Arkansas
Medicare
Arkansas Blue Cross and
Blue Shield
P.O. Box 1418
Little Rock, Arkansas 72203

California
Counties of Los Angeles, Orange,
San Diego, Ventura, San Bernardino,
Imperial, San Luis Obispo,
Riverside, Santa Barbara
Medicare
Occidental Life Insurance Co. of
California
Box 54905
Terminal Annex
Los Angeles, California 90051

Rest of State
Medicare
Blue Shield of California
P.O. Box 7968, Rincon Annex
San Francisco, California 94120

Colorado
Medicare
Colorado Medical Service, Inc.
700 Broadway
Denver, Colorado 80203

Connecticut
Medicare
Connecticut General Life
Insurance Co.
200 Pratt Street
Meriden, Connecticut 06450

Delaware
Medicare
Blue Cross and Blue Shield of
Delaware
201 West 14th Street
Wilmington, Delaware 19899

District of Columbia
Medicare
Medical Service of DC
550 - 12th St., SW
Washington, DC 20024

Florida
Counties of Dade, Monroe
Medicare
Group Health, Inc.
P.O. Box 341370
Miami, Florida 33134

Rest of State
Medicare
Blue Shield of Florida, Inc.
P.O. Box 2525
Jacksonville, Florida 32203

Georgia
The Prudential Insurance Co. of
America
Medicare Part B
P.O. Box 95466
Executive Park Station
Atlanta, Georgia 30347

Hawaii
Medicare
Aetna Life & Casualty
P.O. Box 3947
Honolulu, Hawaii 96812

Idaho
Medicare
The Equitable Life Assurance
Society
P.O. Box 8048
Boise, Idaho 83707

Illinois
Cook County
Medicare Part B
Illinois Medical Service
P.O. Box 210
Chicago, Illinois 60690

Rest of State
Medicare
CNA Insurance
Medicare Benefits Division
P.O. Box 910
Chicago, Illinois 60690

Indiana
Medicare Part B
120 West Market Street
Indianapolis, Indiana 46204

Iowa
Medicare
Iowa Medical Service
636 Grand
Des Moines, Iowa 50307

Kansas
Counties of Johnson, Wyandotte
Medicare
Blue Shield of Kansas City
P.O. Box 169
Kansas City, Missouri 64141

Rest of State
Medicare
Kansas Blue Shield
P.O. Box 239
Topeka, Kansas 66601

Kentucky
Medicare
Metropolitan Life Insurance Co.
1218 Harrodsburg Road
Lexington, Kentucky 40504

Louisiana
Medicare
Pan-American Life Insurance Co.
P.O. Box 60450
New Orleans, Louisiana 70160

Maine
Medicare
Union Mutual Life Insurance Co.
Box 4629
Portland, Maine 04112

Maryland
*Counties of Montgomery, Prince
Georges*
Medicare
Medical Service of DC
550 - 12th St., SW
Washington, DC 20024

Rest of State
Maryland Blue Shield, Inc.
700 East Joppa Road
Towson, Maryland 21204

Massachusetts
Medicare
Blue Shield of Massachusetts, Inc.
P.O. Box 2194
Boston, Massachusetts 02106

Michigan
Medicare
Blue Shield of Michigan
P.O. Box 2201
Detroit, Michigan 48231

Minnesota
*Counties of Anoka, Dakota,
Fillmore, Goodhue, Hennepin,
Houston, Olmstead, Ramsey,
Wabasha, Washington, Winona*
Medicare
The Travelers Insurance Company
8120 Penn Avenue South
Bloomington, Minnesota 55431

Rest of State
Medicare
Blue Shield of Minnesota
P.O. Box 8899
Minneapolis, Minnesota 55404

Mississippi
Medicare
The Travelers Insurance Company
P.O. Box 22545
Jackson, Mississippi 39205

Missouri
*Counties of Andrew, Atchison,
Bates, Benton, Buchanan, Caldwell,
Carroll, Cass, Clay, Clinton,
Daviess, De Kalb, Gentry, Grundy,
Harrison, Henry, Holt, Jackson,
Johnson, Lafayette, Livingston,
Mercer, Nodaway, Pettis, Platte,
Ray, St. Clair, Saline, Vernon,
Worth*
Medicare
Blue Shield of Kansas City
P.O. Box 169
Kansas City, Missouri 64141

Rest of State
Medicare
General American Life
Insurance Co.
P.O. Box 505
St. Louis, Missouri 63166

Montana
Medicare
Montana Physicians' Service
P.O. Box 2510
Helena, Montana 59601

Nebraska
Medicare
Mutual of Omaha Insurance Co.
P.O. Box 456, Downtown Station
Omaha, Nebraska 68101

Nevada
Medicare
Aetna Life & Casualty
4600 Kietzke Lane
P.O. Box 7290
Reno, Nevada 89510

New Hampshire
Medicare
New Hampshire-Vermont
Physician Service
Two Pillsbury Street
Concord, New Hampshire 03301

New Jersey
Medicare
The Prudential Insurance Co.
of America
P.O. Box 3000
Linwood, New Jersey 08221

New Mexico
Medicare
The Equitable Life Assurance
Society
P.O. Box 3070, Station D
Albuquerque, New Mexico 87110

New York
*Counties of Bronx, Columbia,
Delaware, Dutchess, Greene, Kings,
Nassau, New York, Orange,
Putnam, Richmond, Rockland,
Suffolk, Sullivan, Ulster,
Westchester*
Medicare
Blue Cross-Blue Shield of
Greater New York
P.O. Box 458
Murray Hill Station
New York, New York 10016

County of Queens
Medicare
Group Health, Inc.
P.O. Box 233—Midtown Station
New York, New York 10018

*Counties of Livingston, Monroe,
Ontario, Seneca, Wayne, Yates*
Medicare
Genesee Valley Medical Care, Inc.
41 Chestnut Street
Rochester, New York 14647

*Counties of Allegany, Cattaraugus,
Erie, Genesee, Niagara, Orleans,
Wyoming*
Medicare
Blue Shield of Western
New York, Inc.
298 Main Street
Buffalo, New York 14202

*Counties of Albany, Broome,
Cayuga, Chautauqua, Chemung,
Chenango, Clinton, Cortland,
Essex, Franklin, Fulton, Hamilton,
Herkimer, Jefferson, Lewis,
Madison, Montgomery, Oneida,
Onondaga, Oswego, Otsego,
Rensselaer, Saratoga, Schenectady,
Schoharie, Schuyler, Steuben, St.
Lawrence, Tioga, Tompkins,
Warren, Washington*
Medicare
Metropolitan Life Insurance Co.
276 Genesee Street
P.O. Box 393
Utica, New York 13503

North Carolina
The Prudential Insurance Co.
of America
Medicare B Division
P.O. Box 2126
High Point, North Carolina 27261

North Dakota
Medicare
Blue Shield of North Dakota
301 Eighth Street, South
Fargo, North Dakota 58102

Ohio
Medicare
Nationwide Mutual Insurance Co.
P.O. Box 57
Columbus, Ohio 43216

Oklahoma
Medicare
Aetna Life & Casualty
1140 NW 63rd Street
Oklahoma City, Oklahoma 73116

Oregon
Medicare
Aetna Life & Casualty
Crown Plaza
1500 SW First Avenue
Portland, Oregon 97201

Pennsylvania
Medicare
Pennsylvania Blue Shield
Box 65 Blue Shield Bldg.
Camp Hill, Pennsylvania 17011

Rhode Island
Medicare
Blue Shield of Rhode Island
444 Westminster Mall
Providence, Rhode Island 02901

South Carolina
Medicare
Blue Shield of South Carolina
Drawer F, Forest Acres Branch
Columbia, South Carolina 29260

South Dakota
Medicare
South Dakota Medical Service, Inc.
711 North Lake Avenue
Sioux Falls, South Dakota 57104

Tennessee
Medicare
The Equitable Life
Assurance Society
P.O. Box 1465
Nashville, Tennessee 37202

Texas
Medicare
Group Medical and Surgical Service
P.O. Box 22147
Dallas, Texas 75222

Utah
Medicare
Blue Shield of Utah
P.O. Box 30270
2455 Parley's Way.
Salt Lake City, Utah 84125

Vermont
Medicare
New Hampshire-Vermont
Physician Service
Two Pillsbury Street
Concord, New Hampshire 03301

Virginia
Counties of Arlington, Fairfax,
Cities of Alexandria, Falls
Church, Fairfax
Medicare
Medical Service of DC
550 - 12th St., SW
Washington, DC 20024

Rest of State
Medicare
The Travelers Insurance Company
P.O. Box 26463
Richmond, Virginia 23261

Washington
Medicare
Washington Physicians' Service
Mail to your local
Medical Service Bureau.
If you do not know which bureau
handles the claim, mail to:
Medicare
Washington Physicians' Service
220 West Harrison
Seattle, Washington 98119

West Virginia
Medicare
Nationwide Mutual Insurance Co.
P.O. Box 57
Columbus, Ohio 43216

Wisconsin
County of Milwaukee
Medicare
Surgical Care—Blue Shield
P.O. Box 2049
Milwaukee, Wisconsin 53201

Rest of State
Medicare
Wisconsin Physicians Service
Box 1787
Madison, Wisconsin 53701

Wyoming
Medicare
The Equitable Life
Assurance Society
P.O. Box 628
Cheyenne, Wyoming 82001

Puerto Rico
Medicare
Seguros De Servicio De Salud De Puerto Rico
P.O. Box 3628
104 Ponce de Leon Avenue
Hato Rey, Puerto Rico 00936

Virgin Islands
Medicare
Seguros De Servicio De Salud De
Puerto Rico
P.O. Box 3628
104 Ponce de Leon Avenue
Hato Rey, Puerto Rico 00936

American Samoa
Medicare
Hawaii Medical Service Assn.
P.O. Box 860
Honolulu, Hawaii 96808

Guam
Medicare
Aetna Life & Casualty
P.O. Box 3947
Honolulu, Hawaii 96812

MEDICAID

The Medicaid program, established by the federal government, became effective in 1966 via Title XIX of the Social Security Act. Under this program, the federal government provides monetary assistance (ranging from 50% to 83% of the costs) to the states to finance medical care for needy persons. By July 1977 all states and the District of Columbia had established Medicaid programs. The eligibility of medical care recipients under the Medicaid program is determined by the states, although recipients of the federal assistance programs for the blind (AB), the totally and permanently disabled (APTD), the aged (OAA), and families with dependent children (AFDC) must be included. Beyond those recipients, each state establishes its own financial levels of eligibility. Thus, persons receiving cash welfare payments or those able to meet normal living expenses with the exception of their medical bills (a situation often called *medical indigency*) might be covered by the program.

The states also determine the types of medical or psychiatric care for which payment is made under the Medicaid program. However, inpatient and outpatient hospital care, laboratory and X-ray services, skilled nursing home care for persons over the age of 21, physicians' services, and home health services must be included. The treatment of psychiatric disorders is covered in quite a few states, although in some instances the care provided in state mental hospitals, nursing homes, community mental health centers, or freestanding clinics might be excluded. In some states the program also covers within certain limitations other services such as dental care, pharmaceutical services, private-duty nursing, vision care, diagnostic and preventive health services, and transportation costs.

With these considerable variations among the states, it is only possible to generalize about the Medicaid program. Each hospital, physician, or other provider of care must determine the pertinent details that apply to the particular state where the care is provided. Providers of care, however, are free to accept or reject Medicaid patients.

Administration of the Medicaid program at the federal level is by the Social and Rehabilitation Service of the Department of Health, Education and Welfare. At the state level, Medicaid is administered by whatever department or agency is designated—most usually the state department of welfare. A few states, however, have contracted the administration of the program out to Blue Cross-Blue Shield plans, insurance companies, or prepaid group practice plans.

In providing care for Medicaid patients, physicians must determine from the local administrative office the kinds of care covered by the program and the extent to which they are covered, the eligibility of individual patients for Medicaid benefits, the manner in which bills are to be presented, and the claim forms to be filled out. See section 10.7 for the Universal Health Insurance Claim Form that can be used for Medicaid patients.

A Medicaid card (plastic or paper) or, in some states, a coupon is usually issued to the beneficiary on a monthly basis although the issuance dates vary from state to state. In any case, the card should show the bearer's eligibility for the month during which the medical services are being provided. The physician bills either the appropriate fiscal intermediary or the local Department of Social Services, depending on the state where the practice is located.

VETERANS ADMINISTRATION PROGRAMS
The Veterans Administration offers medical care and disability compensation for veterans of the armed services. To be eligible a veteran must have a service-connected disability or must need economic assistance. Medical or psychiatric care is provided principally in hospitals, outpatient clinics, and domiciliary institutions established by the Veterans Administration, although the services of private physicians or other health professionals are employed at times under what is called the "home town" program. Care provided under the VA program is unlimited, and no patient payments are permitted under the law. Should a physician or other health professional have a patient referred to him or her by the VA, the bills for the services provided should be sent to the VA source of referral and under the conditions established by VA. (See also the discussion of CHAMPVA at the end of section 10.6.)

PUBLICLY PROVIDED CARE
There are many types of publicly provided medical care. Publicly provided care is funded by municipal, county, state, and federal governments. Institutions offering such care include hospitals; health centers; clinics; and resource centers for immunization, maternal care, prenatal and postnatal care, and the treatment of alcoholism and drug addiction. Also included are mental hospitals, institutions for the mentally retarded, child guidance clinics, community mental health centers, and various other types of clinics for the treatment of psychiatric disorders. Physicians and other professionals in private practice customarily have little if any relationship with these publicly provided forms of care except in the case of referrals.

The national health insurance question   The matter of national health insurance in the United States is not new: in fact, the question of establishing a national health insurance program here was first raised in 1912. Although there had been spurts of interest in it from time to time since then, it was only in 1967, after the enactment of Medicare, that a truly broad interest in the subject developed. A host of proposals for differing types of national health insurance was placed before the Congress. These proposals were sponsored by many groups and individuals. Since 1967 each session of Congress has received many more proposals for national health insurance or amendments to original proposals. The subject became a prime issue in the 1976 Presidential campaign, and in 1977 the President indicated that full consideration of the matter would be forthcoming in 1978. What the various proposals have in common is that each would establish a program whereby almost all persons would be eligible to varying degrees for coverage of most health care expenditures. According to some of the plans, the program would be administered by the federal government; according to other proposals, the program would be administered by private insurers. In either case, the private insurers could supplement the national program. Some proposals provide for financing by federal taxation of employers, employees, and the general taxpayer; others provide for the payment of premiums by the employer and the employees, supplemented by federal tax funds. The benefits for the treatment of physical or mental illnesses differ among the various proposals. Likewise, the benefits for various forms of preventive medicine (including well-child care, prenatal care, immunization, eye and teeth examinations, and periodic health examinations) differ from proposal to proposal. The degrees to which the patient would share in the costs of care also differ. However, most of the proposals make some provision for controlling or containing health care costs and for improving the availability and distribution of health care services.

State health insurance programs currently in existence   It should be mentioned in passing that by 1977 four states (Rhode Island, Hawaii, Connecticut, and Minnesota) had enacted programs to ensure that all employees had some form of health insurance benefits. The programs differ from state to state. The Rhode Island plan, for example, features a state pool providing catastrophe health insurance benefits up to $10,000 with 20% coinsurance and a $100 deductible amount after an uninsured individual has paid $5,000 and/or 50% of his or her income for medical expenses, or after an individual has used $500 and/or 10% of his or her income for medical expenses following the exhaustion of any other insurance benefits. Claim forms for these state programs are similar to the ones customarily used by other insurers.

10.6

CHAMPUS AND FEHB

Two types of health benefit programs have been developed by the federal government for its own employees and their dependents: CHAMPUS (the Civilian Health and Medical Program of the Uniformed Services) and FEHB (the Federal Employees' Health Benefits Program). The relationship of physicians and other health professionals to these programs is essentially the same as their relationship to the insurance plans already discussed.

CHAMPUS
The Civilian Health and Medical Program of the Uniformed Services finances the cost (or, in some cases, part of the costs) of civilian-provided medical care (including the treatment of mental illness) for dependents of active-duty and retired members of the armed forces (i.e., the United States Army, Navy, Air Force, Marine Corps, and Coast Guard) as well as dependents of members of the Commissioned Corps of the United States Public Health Services and the Commissioned Corps of the National Oceanic and Atmospheric Administration. The care is provided by civilian physicians, psychiatrists, and other individual CHAMPUS-authorized health professionals or by civilian CHAMPUS-authorized hospitals and other institutions when it cannot be provided by government personnel or by uniformed services facilities. CHAMPUS is administered jointly by the Secretary of Defense and the Secretary of Health, Education and Welfare. It functions through CHAMPUS contractors—organizations that process claims for professional medical care that has been received by CHAMPUS beneficiaries.

The following individual professional providers may be called on to treat CHAMPUS patients: physicians (MDs and DOs), dentists (DMDs and DDSs), doctors of podiatry, and clinical psychologists. These individuals must be CHAMPUS-authorized—i.e., they must meet specific requirements outlined in the *CHAMPUS Regulation* DoD 6010.8–R. In addition, the following persons can be CHAMPUS-authorized to provide care if the patient is referred to them by a supervising physician: registered nurses, licensed practical nurses, licensed vocational nurses, licensed midwives, licensed registered physical therapists, psychiatric and clinical social workers, and marriage and family counselors. Institutional medical care providers may be CHAMPUS-authorized if they meet the standards set forth in the *Regulation*. These providers include: short-term general and special care hospitals, long-term hospitals, psychiatric hospitals, skilled nursing facilities, college and university infirmaries, residential treatment centers for emotionally disturbed children and adolescents, and special treatment facilities.

Coverage and restrictions to coverage Specifically covered by CHAMPUS are spouses and dependent children of uniformed services personnel. If the service person dies while on active duty, the spouse and/or the dependent children continue to be eligible for benefits. (NOTE: dependent parents and parents-in-law are not eligible under CHAMPUS.)

By law, retirees and their dependents as well as spouses and children of deceased active-duty and retired personnel who become eligible at age 65 for Medicare Part A (i.e., hospital benefits) lose their eligibility for all CHAMPUS benefits. Retirees and their dependents as well as spouses and children of deceased active-duty and retired personnel who are enrolled in another health benefits plan provided by law or through employment must use the benefits of that program before they turn to CHAMPUS. (Examples of health plans provided by law are Medicare and VA benefits.) In addition, some insurance policies held by CHAMPUS beneficiaries have exclusionary clauses prohibiting payment if the beneficiary is covered by a federal plan. In spite of this, CHAMPUS will not pay until the benefits of the other plan are used. Refer patients with exclusionary clause problems to the CHAMPUS contractor in the state where the care was rendered. Still other CHAMPUS patients may hold private health insurance whose payments are made directly to the care provider. These payments will *not* be duplicated by CHAMPUS. CHAMPUS will pay only the difference between the amount charged by the physician or other care provider and the amount paid directly by the private insurance—up to the amount that CHAMPUS would ordinarily pay if the patient did not have the private insurance.

Covered care includes a semiprivate hospital room (or a private room if medically dictated), board (including special diets), surgery, operating room and recovery room, treatment rooms, services provided in a hospital outpatient facility, acute medical care, obstetrical and maternity care, treatment of acute mental disorders, and diagnostic tests. Also included in the benefits are the costs of prescribed drugs, blood and plasma, anesthesia and oxygen, IV injections, renal dialysis, shock therapy, and private-duty nursing if ordered by the physician, immunization if required as part of medical treatment or for duty-related travel abroad, physical examinations related to duty-related travel abroad, radiation therapy, chemotherapy, and the cost of nongovernment ambulances. Maternity and infant care as well as family planning services are also included in the benefits. The costs of artificial limbs or eyes, the costs of orthopaedic braces and crutches, and the rental of necessary medical equipment are covered too. Physical therapy and dental care are covered if they are a necessary part of the medical treatment. The treatment of mental disorders is covered on the same basis as the costs of treating other diseases. The cost of the services of clinical psychologists is also covered. The cost of organ transplants is covered if the recipient is a CHAMPUS beneficiary; this coverage also includes the donor's costs. However, if the CHAMPUS beneficiary is a donor, the costs are not covered. If the required care is beyond the capability of the uniformed services facilities, the patient is released for civilian care under the CHAMPUS benefits. If professional opinion differs between a uniformed services physician and a civilian physician and the beneficiary elects to use the civilian physician's services, a Nonavailability Statement (DD Form 1251) may be issued.

The CHAMPUS benefits do not cover routine physical examinations, immunization, well-baby care, abortions or sterilization procedures unless medically dictated, vision care, hearing aids, orthopaedic shoes, and domiciliary or custodial care.

Eligibility: specific categories of patients   The following categories of persons are eligible for CHAMPUS benefits:

1. spouses of active-duty members of the uniformed services
2. dependent children of active-duty members
3. retirees from the uniformed services
4. spouses of retirees
5. dependent children of retirees
6. unremarried widowers and widows of deceased active-duty members and retirees
7. dependent children of deceased active-duty members and retirees.

CHAMPUS identification cards and claim forms   ID cards are issued to persons covered by CHAMPUS as evidence of their status as beneficiaries. The form DD 1173 is for dependents of active-duty personnel, and the form DD2 (Ret.) is for retirees. Cards are usually not issued to dependent children under age 10. The identification of such a child is the responsibility of the parent, legal guardian, or acting guardian. The spouse's, retiree's, or active member's ID card is sufficient identification for a child under age 10.

Claim forms generally follow the pattern of private health insurance forms. You should keep a supply of the CHAMPUS form 500 on hand in the office. They can be obtained from the nearest CHAMPUS Advisor/Health Benefits Advisor (located at a uniformed services medical facility), from a CHAMPUS contractor (see the list of names and addresses by state of CHAMPUS contractors at the end of this subsection on CHAMPUS), or from OCHAMPUS, Denver, CO 80240.

Completed claim forms are to be sent to the CHAMPUS contractor in the state where the care was rendered. The claim form must include full information: the name and address of the patient, his or her relationship to the sponsor, the Social Security number of the sponsor, a designation of the sponsor's active or retired status, the diagnosis, the care provided, the dates on which the care was provided, and the charges for the services. Claims are settled on the basis of reasonable and customary charges in the geographic area where the care was provided. NOTE: Guidelines to the completion of CHAMPUS forms are given in section 10.7 where the form 500 is illustrated.

Nonavailability Statement (DD 1251)   The Defense Department Form DD 1251 entitled "Nonavailability Statement Dependents Medical Care Program" may be issued by commanders of uniformed services hospitals or by their lawful representatives to CHAMPUS beneficiaries who live within 40 miles of a uniformed services hospital but who wish to obtain medical care as inpatients at a civilian hospital. The dependent must give the form DD 1251 (signed by the hospital commander) to the civilian care provider. If you are working in a civilian hospital, you should attach this form to the CHAMPUS claim form before submitting it to the CHAMPUS contractor. NOTE: DD 1251 is not required in emergency situations.

Hospital commanders may issue DD 1251 when an expectant mother lives more than 30 miles from a service hospital, when an individual who has been an outpatient at a civilian hospital requires hospitalization preferably at the same civilian facility, when the local service hospital is full, when local conditions are such that excessive and/or unreasonable cost or hardship are involved in transporting the patient to the nearest service facility, or when the local service hospital's facilities are inadequate for the treatment of a particular complaint.

CHAMPUS contractors   The following is a list of the names and addresses of organizations that process claims for professional medical care received by beneficiaries of CHAMPUS. These organizations are called *CHAMPUS contractors:*

Alabama
Mutual of Omaha Insurance Co.
3301 Dodge Street
Omaha, Nebraska 68131

Alaska
Dikewood Industries, Inc.
1009 Bradbury Drive, SE
University Research Park
Albuquerque, New Mexico 87106

Arizona
Blue Shield of California
Post Office Box 85019
San Diego, California 92138

Arkansas
Arkansas Blue Cross/Blue Shield, Inc.
Post Office Box 2181
Little Rock, Arkansas 72203

California
Blue Shield of California
Post Office Box 85020
San Diego, California 92138

Colorado
Mutual of Omaha Insurance Co.
Post Office Box 31700
Omaha, Nebraska 68131

Connecticut
Blue Shield of Massachusetts, Inc.
Post Office Box 2194
Boston, Massachusetts 02111

Delaware
Blue Shield of Pennsylvania
Blue Shield Building
Box 65
Camp Hill, Pennsylvania 17011

District of Columbia
Blue Cross of Southwestern Virginia
P.O. Box 13828
Roanoke, Virginia 24034

Florida
Blue Shield of Florida, Inc.
Post Office Box 2170
Jacksonville, Florida 32203

Georgia
Medical Association of Georgia
938 Peachtree Street, NE
Atlanta, Georgia 30309

Hawaii
Hawaii Medical Service Assn.
Post Office Box 860
Honolulu, Hawaii 96808

Idaho
Dikewood Industries, Inc.
1009 Bradbury Drive, SE
University Research Park
Albuquerque, New Mexico 87106

Illinois
Mutual of Omaha Insurance Co.
3301 Dodge Street
Omaha, Nebraska 68131

Indiana
Wisconsin Physicians' Service
P.O. Box 7942
Madison, Wisconsin 53701

Iowa
Blue Shield of Iowa
636 Grand Avenue
Des Moines, Iowa 50309

Kansas
Wisconsin Physicians' Service
P.O. Box 7934
Madison, Wisconsin 53701

Kentucky
Wisconsin Physicians' Service
P.O. Box 7925
Madison, Wisconsin 53701

Louisiana
Blue Cross/Blue Shield of Mississippi
P.O. Box 3500
Jackson, Mississippi 39207

Maine
Blue Shield of Massachusetts, Inc.
Post Office Box 2194
Boston, Massachusetts 02111

Maryland
Blue Cross/Blue Shield of Maryland
700 East Joppa Road
Baltimore, Maryland 21204

Massachusetts
Blue Shield of Massachusetts, Inc.
Post Office Box 2194
Boston, Massachusetts 02111

Michigan
Blue Cross & Blue Shield of Michigan
600 Lafayette East
Detroit, Michigan 48226

Minnesota
Blue Cross and Blue Shield of Minnesota
P.O. Box 3357
St. Paul, Minnesota 55165

Mississippi
Blue Cross and Blue Shield
of Mississippi, Inc.
Post Office Box 3500
Jackson, Mississippi 39207

Missouri
Dikewood Industries, Inc.
1009 Bradbury Drive, SE
University Research Park
Albuquerque, New Mexico 87106

Montana
Dikewood Industries, Inc.
1009 Bradbury Drive, SE
University Research Park
Albuquerque, New Mexico 87106

Nebraska
Mutual of Omaha Insurance Co.
3301 Dodge Street
Omaha, Nebraska 68131

Nevada
Blue Shield of California
Post Office Box 85023
San Diego, California 92138

New Hampshire
Blue Shield of Massachusetts, Inc.
Post Office Box 2194
Boston, Massachusetts 02111

New Jersey
Blue Cross of Rhode Island
One Weybosset Hill
Providence, Rhode Island 02903

New Mexico
Blue Shield of California
Post Office Box 85021
San Diego, California 92138

New York
Blue Cross of Rhode Island
One Weybosset Hill
Providence, Rhode Island 02903

North Carolina
Blue Cross and Blue Shield of North Carolina
Post Office Box 35
Durham, North Carolina 27702

North Dakota
Blue Shield of North Dakota
301 Eight Street South
Fargo, North Dakota 58102

Ohio
Mutual of Omaha Insurance Co.
3301 Dodge Street
Omaha, Nebraska 68131

Oklahoma
Wisconsin Physicians' Service
P.O. Box 7936
Madison, Wisconsin 53701

Oregon
Dikewood Industries, Inc.
1009 Bradbury Drive, SE
University Research Park
Albuquerque, New Mexico 87106

Pennsylvania
Blue Shield of Pennsylvania
Blue Shield Building
Box 65
Camp Hill, Pennsylvania 17011

Rhode Island
Blue Cross and Blue Shield of Rhode Island
One Weybosset Hill
Providence, Rhode Island 02903

South Carolina
Blue Cross and Blue Shield of North Carolina
Post Office Box 35
Durham, North Carolina 27702

South Dakota
South Dakota Medical Service, Inc.
711 North Lake Avenue
Sioux Falls, South Dakota 57104

Tennessee
Blue Cross/Blue Shield of Tennessee
801 Pine Street
Chattanooga, Tennessee 37402

Texas
Mutual of Omaha Insurance Co.
3301 Dodge Street
Omaha, Nebraska 68131

Utah
Dikewood Industries, Inc.
1009 Bradbury Drive, SE
University Research Park
Albuquerque, New Mexico 87106

Vermont
Blue Shield of Massachusetts, Inc.
Post Office Box 2194
Boston, Massachusetts 02111

Virginia
Blue Cross of Southwestern Virginia
Post Office Box 13828
Roanoke, Virginia 24034

Washington
Dikewood Industries, Inc.
1009 Bradbury Drive, SE
University Research Park
Albuquerque, New Mexico 87106

West Virginia
Medical-Surgical Care, Inc.
Post Office Box 1948
Parkersburg, West Virginia 26101

Wisconsin
Wisconsin Physicians' Service
Post Office Box 1787
Madison, Wisconsin 53701

Wyoming
Dikewood Industries, Inc.
1009 Bradbury Drive, SE
University Research Park
Albuquerque, New Mexico 87106

Canada
Mutual of Omaha Insurance Co.
3301 Dodge Street
Omaha, Nebraska 68131

Mexico
Mutual of Omaha Insurance Co.
3301 Dodge Street
Omaha, Nebraska 68131

Puerto Rico
Mutual of Omaha Insurance Co.
3301 Dodge Street
Omaha, Nebraska 68131

CHAMPVA   The Civilian Health and Medical Program of the Veterans Administration is a medical benefits program similar to CHAMPUS. The Department of Defense and the VA use OCHAMPUS in Denver and the CHAMPUS contractors to process and pay CHAMPVA claims. (The CHAMPUS form 500 is used for claims processing.) Beneficiaries of CHAMPVA are the spouses and dependent children of veterans suffering total, permanent, service-related disabilities and the surviving spouses and dependent children of veterans who have died as a result of service-related disabilities. Beneficiaries carry special ID cards headed "VETERANS ADMINISTRATION CHAMPVA." Benefits and cost-sharing are the same as those for CHAMPUS beneficiaries.

FEHB
The Federal Employees' Health Benefits Program (FEHB) is a program of health insurance protection for active and retired federal civilian employees and their dependents. Included in it also are the surviving widows and/or dependent children of deceased federal employees. The program is administered by the Civil Service Commission, which arranges with private insurers to provide the insurance and pay

the claims. The majority of the insurance is written by Blue Cross-Blue Shield plans under the Government-wide Service Benefits Plan. The remainder is provided by employee organizations or union health centers and by several prepaid group practice plans.

FEHB coverage and benefits   The program provides two benefit levels—with the choice of benefits to be made by the individual employee who volunteers to enroll in the plan: (1) the low option, which provides fewer benefits, a higher deductible amount, and a greater percentage of coinsurance, and (2) the high option, which provides greater benefits.

The benefits under the Government-wide Service Benefit Plan (the predominant form of coverage) are categorized as basic benefits, maternity benefits, and supplemental benefits. With the basic benefits, protection is provided without any deductible amount to be paid by the patient for hospital services, surgery, in-hospital physician care, and certain other physician services. There is no maximum lifetime dollar amount of the benefit. Under the high option, 365 days of hospital care are covered for each confinement; under the low option, however, the limit is 30 days. Hospital care includes room and board in semiprivate accommodations, use of the operating room, intensive care, drugs and other medications, dressings and casts, X rays, laboratory examinations, electrocardiograms and similar procedures, radiation and physical therapy, anesthetics, injections, and renal dialysis. Outpatient hospital benefits cover services for an accidental injury or a medical emergency, surgery, X rays, laboratory services, various tests, radiation therapy, cast and suture removal, and rabies shots. Surgical care, including oral surgery and an assistant surgeon (if required), is covered. In-hospital physician medical care including psychotherapy is covered up to 365 days under the high option and up to 30 days under the low option for each confinement. Other physician services covered under the program's basic benefits include consultations, anesthesia, emergency treatment (including emergency dental care), radiation therapy, electroshock or physical therapy, removal of casts or sutures, X rays, and laboratory services performed out of the hospital (exception: allergy tests).

The maternity benefits under the high option include normal maternity care. Both the high and the low options cover the costs of maternity care involving complications. The services covered are hospitalization and physician services including prenatal and postnatal care, consultations, X rays, laboratory services, necessary tests, and anesthetics.

Supplemental benefits   Supplemental benefits include: (1) hospitalization, physician services in the hospital or in the office or at home, surgery, and consultations (2) anesthetics, oxygen, radiation therapy, blood transfusions, X rays, laboratory services, and various tests (3) ambulance services (4) physical therapy (5) required medical devices and equipment, and (6) any necessary private-duty nursing. The costs of treatment for nervous or mental disorders—covered when treatment is administered under the direction of a physician—include day-night hospital care; family therapy; and the services of a psychologist, a psychiatric nurse, or a psychiatric social worker. With the supplemental benefits to FEHB coverage there is a variable deductible amount of money which must be paid by the patient first.

Exclusions to FEHB benefits   Excluded from the FEHB program benefits are the following: (1) any services or supplies furnished without charge or for which there is no obligation to make payment (2) care paid for under workers' compensation (3) care required as the result of an act of war (4) periodic physical examinations (5) immunization (6) care provided in connection with uncomplicated obesity

(7) convalescent care or rest cures (8) custodial care (9) travel even if prescribed by the physician (10) certain types of therapy such as speech, occupational, educational, or group therapy (11) self-care (12) care not deemed medically necessary (13) eyeglasses or hearing aids (14) air conditioners or dehumidifiers (15) tonsorial services (16) use of the radio, television, or telephone (17) removal of corns or calluses, and (18) cosmetic care unless the care is directly related to an accidental injury. The cost of hospitalization is not covered when it is primarily for diagnostic purposes, physical therapy, or rehabilitation. Dental care is generally excluded unless it is required as the result of an accident; however, oral surgery is generally covered. The benefits under the other forms of coverages are essentially similar, although there are some differences in detail.

FEHB identification, billing, and claims   Identification cards are made available to the insured persons by the carriers of the insurance. These cards should be presented to the hospitals and/or to the physicians providing the care. (A sample FEHB ID card is shown at the end of this subsection.) The hospital or the physician should have the necessary claim forms filled out in detail and accompanied by itemized bills for the services rendered. The itemized bills must show the name and address of the provider of service, the name of the patient, the dates the services were performed, the types of services performed, and the charge for each service. Bills for prescribed drugs must show the prescription numbers. Bills for the services of a private-duty nurse must show whether the nurse was a Registered Nurse or a Licensed Practical Nurse. If the private-duty nursing services were performed in a location other than a hospital, the bills must be accompanied by a statement from the attending physician that the nursing was medically necessary. Claims for the services of a member of a mental health team (e.g., a psychologist, a psychiatric nurse, or a psychiatric social worker) must be accompanied by a statement from the attending physician saying that the services were performed under his or her direction and supervision. The claims should be sent to the insurance carrier. If the claimant is over the age of 65, the claim form should also show the Medicare identification number. In such cases, the Medicare benefits pay first. Claim payments are based on the usual, customary, and reasonable charges of the provider of care.

Government-wide Indemnity Benefit Plan ID Card (FEHB)

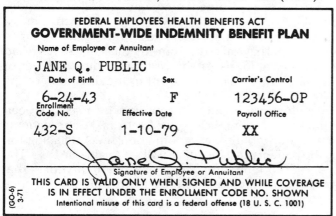

Having overviewed health insurance from the standpoint of benefits, coverage, eligibility, and types of plans, this chapter now discusses health insurance claims processing.

10.7

INSURANCE CLAIMS: Routines for Accurate, Fast Processing

The completion of insurance forms has become an increasingly important aspect of administrative work in medical offices because more and more people are now covered by private, group, or government insurance. These forms are indicative of a major source of income for the physician regardless of whether the benefits are paid to the patient or whether they are paid on an assignment to the physician. Prompt submission of completed forms by the medical office will result in more expeditious processing by the insurance carrier and thus will entail fewer follow-up procedures by the medical office staff.

OFFICE POLICY

Each medical office has to establish a policy and routine for completing insurance forms. The office procedures manual should have a separate section outlining this policy in detail. How these claims are handled will depend primarily on the preference of the individual physician. However, several other factors influencing the manner in which claims are processed are given below. Certainly, the nature of the practice plays a major part in the routine followed in claims handling. For example, a surgeon will be inclined to secure assignments routinely on all claims. But in a family practice having continuing contact with entire families, it may not be as desirable to secure assignments unless the patient/subscriber so desires. Volume is also a deciding factor in claims handling. For the group practices or clinics generating large volumes of insurance claims, computer systems capable of completely itemizing insurance forms are now available. These systems also have the capacity to print out diagnoses as well as the codes for each procedure.

Charging fees for completion of insurance forms   The American Medical Association publication *Judicial Council Opinions and Reports* (1977) states that it is the physician's ethical duty to complete the necessary insurance forms for the patient without levying an extra charge for the service. However, the proliferation of insurance forms and the introduction of government programs with all of their rules and regulations have increased the work load for the physician's staff. Many times a physician is required to hire staff members to deal exclusively with insurance matters. In order to cover the additional payroll costs, some medical offices have *had* to charge fees for completing insurance forms. The decision regarding whether or not to charge fees for this service is one that has to be left to the discretion of the individual physician.

   Once the office policy regarding the handling of insurance forms has been established, it is the responsibility of the medical assistant to make the patients aware of the policy. Preparing and distributing an information sheet detailing the procedures to be followed by the patients and the office will save valuable time. The patients will have the data to refer to long after they have forgotten your verbal explanation. Don't forget that patients who are informed of the policy in advance will be more cooperative.

FILE RETENTION

Develop a method of file retention that will afford maximum efficiency with minimum effort in storage and retrieval. The next paragraphs discuss one method that can be adapted to accommodate the needs of various types of medical offices.

Keeping an alphabetical file of all copies of the completed insurance forms is advantageous whether the material is photocopied from the completed original or whether it is a duplicate supplied by the insurance company. Separate insurance files make the patients' charts less bulky. This type of file is also a ready reference for all claims completed. Furthermore, with the use of a separate file financial considerations are no longer part of the patients' medical records. Finally, the alphabetical insurance file will be available for follow-up procedures even when a patient's chart is out of file.

A hanging file located in or near the desk or a conventional file drawer near a desk and set aside for insurance paperwork will be advantageous to you. The following are the three main file categories:

1. A holding or pending file
2. A completed file: Active
3. A completed file: Inactive

A holding or pending file   It is usually not possible to complete all insurance forms on the date of receipt: the treatment may not be completed yet, surgery may have to be scheduled, or the current load of outstanding insurance forms may be heavy. Therefore, all forms should be dated when received and should be placed in the holding or pending file.

A completed file: active   It is advisable to maintain more than one file category due to the diverse requirements of the insurance plans and the necessity for frequent follow-up procedures on files having to do with government programs. The completed file is for the duplicate copies of the insurance forms that have been submitted to the insurance companies.

You should periodically discard those insurance forms that are no longer of use. This should be done every three to four months. However, do not forget that the retention time for Medicare and Medicare/Medicaid claims is stipulated in the government regulations; thus, these claims may not be discarded until the retention time has expired. These and other claims that cannot be discarded are transferred to the inactive file described below.

Follow-up procedures will be more easily accomplished when the forms in the completed file are additionally categorized and filed under separate headings. You may wish to add to the following suggested headings so that they will accommodate the forms that you handle most often.

1. **Private insurance and group plans**   This would be an alphabetical file using the names of the patients for filing.
2. **Medicare claims**   This file would contain only those forms that are submitted to Medicare. Offices that complete large volumes of Medicare claims may find it beneficial to maintain them in a separate alphabetical file. However, in other offices where the volume is light, Medicare claims can be interfiled easily with the private plan forms.
3. **Medicaid and Medicare/Medicaid claims**   Twelve folders used for this subheading—one for each month of the year—will serve as a revolving file and will prove most useful to you. As the forms are completed and submitted each month, they are filed in alphabetical order in the folder for that particular month. These claims are seldom paid in full and will frequently require follow-up procedures—more so than any other claims. Delays in payment beyond 60 days should prompt an inquiry by the medical office. The delay may be due to the fact that the fiscal intermediary has referred the claim to a claims consultant for review. Equally it may be due to the combination claims of Medicare/Medicaid. With combined claims two processing procedures are involved. The fiscal intermediary for Medicare determines the allowable charges and forwards the payment for the Medicare portion of the claim to the physician. The claim is then routed to the fiscal intermediary for the Medicaid program, and this fiscal intermediary forwards the payment for the balance of the allowable charges.

A patient who is a recipient of Medicaid must present proof of eligibility for the month in which the medical care is received. Therefore, such claims are submitted on a monthly basis. Payment by the fiscal intermediary can only be made for the month in which proof of eligibility accompanies the claim. When payment has been received for all claims in a particular month, the forms may be removed and placed in an inactive file where they will be retained until the expiration of the retention time stipulated by the regulations governing these programs.

4. **Civilian Health and Medical Program of the Uniformed Services and Civilian Health and Medical Program of the Veterans Administration (CHAMPUS/CHAMPVA)**   The necessity for a separate file will depend on the volume of claims handled in the office.

5. **Workers' Compensation**   The necessity for a separate file will depend on the volume of these claims handled in the office.

A completed file: inactive   This file is for the forms that are no longer needed for follow-up procedures but that you might need to use for reference when subsequent claims are filed for continuing conditions. It would also be used for the Medicare and Medicare/Medicaid forms that must be kept for a specified time, as previously explained.

CODING SYSTEMS FOR INSURANCE FORMS: Standard Nomenclature

The publications used in the coding of medical procedures and diagnoses are the Relative Value Studies (RVS), *Current Procedural Terminology* (*CPT*), and the *International Classification of Diseases, Adapted* (*ICDA*). The RVS and the *CPT* contain five-digit codes and two-digit modifiers for identifying and reporting medical procedures. The *ICDA* contains code numbers for identifying and reporting diagnoses. Each book contains detailed instructions for its use which the medical assistant should read. However, since some background is helpful in understanding why the books are used, each one is discussed briefly below.

Relative Value Studies (RVS)   One original purpose of the RVS was to establish standard nomenclature for medical procedures with code numbers which could be used for submitting insurance claims. Another purpose of the RVS was to examine the complexity of procedures used by physicians and the time involved for their performance and to establish from that analysis a relativity between the various procedures performed: hence, the designation "Relative Value Studies." Unit values assigned to the procedures indicated the relative value of a procedure when it was compared with other procedures. The RVS was not designed as a fee schedule per se and was never intended to be used as one. However, some insurance companies use the RVS in the assigning of arbitrary conversion factors during the writing of policies for different levels of medical insurance coverage and also during the processing of claims. The California Relative Value Studies, published in 1956, was updated thereafter with new procedures added and the unit values reevaluated. The RVS was not widely used until 1966 after the 1965 enactment by the federal government of Title XVIII (Medicare—medical care for the aged), Title XIX (Medicaid—medical care for the needy), and Title XXII (the enabling act for Medicaid). Many states adopted the CRVS (or a similar RVS developed independently) for fiscal intermediaries to use in the facilitation of claims processing. The procedure numbers in the RVS were a ready-made mechanism for computer processing. By 1977, nineteen states had implemented the use of the CRVS. Thirteen states had adopted and published an RVS system, and another 13 states were using the *Current Procedural Terminology* (*CPT*) published by the AMA. In some instances, a combination of the RVS and the *CPT* was used.

In 1975 the Federal Trade Commission (FTC) started to investigate certain specialty societies and medical associations regarding the use of the RVS. The FTC maintained that the use of an RVS constituted fee fixing. The California Medical Association (CMA), the primary publisher of this type of code book, entered into an agreement with the FTC to cease publishing and circulating all editions of the RVS. In the meantime, the CMA decided to publish a procedural terminology manual devoid of unit values. The future use of Relative Value Studies is somewhat doubtful even though the RVSs are still being used by the fiscal intermediaries for the government programs as well as by other insurance companies for claims processing.

Current Procedural Terminology (CPT)   The *Physicians' Current Procedural Terminology* published by the American Medical Association is essentially the same as the RVS insofar as procedure numbers are concerned, with the exception that the *CPT* does not contain the controversial unit values. The *CPT* lists descriptive terms and identifying codes that are used in reporting services and procedures performed by doctors. The book provides its users with a uniform language to designate accurately medical, surgical, and diagnostic services. The book is updated at intervals. Each office should have at least one current edition of the *CPT*.

International Classification of Diseases, Adapted (ICDA)   The *ICDA*, a two volume publication of the Department of Health, Education and Welfare, has been widely used in the classifying of morbidity and mortality information for statistical purposes and in indexing hospital records according to diseases and operations for data storage and retrieval. Although it was originally developed for the reasons given above, the *ICDA* now is being used by many insurance companies and especially the fiscal intermediaries for the Medicare program in order to code diagnoses.

***ICDA* Volume 1 Tabular List**   This is a numerical list that can be used to retrieve the alphabetically listed nomenclature when the diagnoses have been coded without their descriptive terms having been entered.

***ICDA* Volume 2 Alphabetical Index**   The Index gives the diagnoses in an alphabetical sequence using standard nomenclature. The appropriate code numbers follow the descriptive terms. This volume also contains several useful appendices. In order to use the *ICDA* effectively one must have both volumes at hand.

STANDARD INSURANCE FORMS
To ease the burden created for health care providers by the many different required health insurance claims and report forms, the Health Insurance Association of America (HIAA) inaugurated its Standard Forms Program many years ago. The Standard Forms Committee of the Consumer & Professional Relations Division developed and promoted the use of standard forms to expedite the payment of insurance benefits and to simplify insurance paperwork for health care providers. The forms developed by this committee are reviewed and revised periodically to reflect changes in the provision of health care and in insurance claims administration as well as the development of new coverages.

Many of the forms discussed in the following paragraphs are available from the individual insurance carriers if the physician wishes to maintain a supply of the forms in the office. However, the majority of group and private insurance carriers furnish the forms directly to the patients since the patients are required to fill out portions of the forms before delivering them to the physicians for completion. The forms most often kept on hand in the medical office are those used for the various government programs such as Medicare, Medicaid, worker's compensation, and CHAMPUS. Blue Cross and Blue Shield also furnish forms directly to physicians.

(These organizations are now converting to the Uniform Health Insurance Claim Form.) Some insurance forms also can be secured from local printers supplying medical forms. The Uniform Health Insurance Claim Form can be purchased from the American Medical Association as well as from local suppliers. (When ordering the forms in bulk from the AMA, use this address: AMA Order Handling, P.O. Box 821, Monroe, Wisconsin 53566.)

Hospital form   The Uniform Hospital Billing Form was approved by the American Hospital Association (AHA) in 1975, although many insurance companies had been using the form as early as 1970. Insurance companies were requested to observe certain rules in developing their group or individual forms and to use the approved components if they wished to identify their forms as "approved" by affixing the Health Insurance Council (HIC) seal and the AHA statement of approval to them. These forms are not used in the medical office and therefore are not illustrated here.

Dental form   Shortly after the development of dental insurance, the HIAA Standard Forms Committee worked closely with the American Dental Association to develop the jointly approved Attending Dentist's Statement (ADS 75). This form was released in 1967. A revision was approved in 1975 by all involved organizations. There are special requirements for the completion of dental forms. These requirements are given along with illustrations of two attending dentist's statements at the end of section 10.7, in the subsection entitled "Completing Dental Insurance Forms."

Medical office form   The AMA in cooperation with the HIAA Standard Forms Committee developed a Uniform Health Insurance Claim Form, approved by the AMA in 1974. Insurance companies are gradually converting to the use of the AMA approved form, and those which have not already done so will often accept this form when it is attached to the form that they supply. Companies adopting the Uniform Health Insurance Claim Form have been urged to adhere to the specifications established by the Committee. A completed form is illustrated at the end of section 10.7.

Workers' compensation   The two forms most frequently used for workers' compensation coverage are the Doctor's First Report of Work Injury and the Doctor's Final (or Monthly) Report and Bill. Supplementary report forms are frequently necessary; however, these are mailed to the physician by the insurance carrier at the time they are required and are self-explanatory. Examples of these two forms are illustrated at the end of section 10.7.

Medicare forms   The Medicare form currently being used is the Request for Medicare Payment (1490A). The fiscal intermediaries in each area of submission supply the patient or the physician with these forms on request. The AMA is negotiating with the federal government in an effort to have the Uniform Claim Form adopted for Medicare claims. The Medicare claim form is illustrated at the end of section 10.7.

CHAMPUS/CHAMPVA forms   Several forms are used for submitting CHAM-PUS/CHAMPVA claims; however, the ones that the medical assistant sees most often are the Nonavailability Statement (DD Form 1251) that the patient must obtain and give to the physician, and the Services and/or Supplies Provided by Civilian Sources, Except Institutions (claim form 500). Samples of forms used in processing CHAMPUS claims can be found in *A Guide for Physicians and Other Providers of Care under the Civilian Health and Medical Program of the Uniformed*

Services. The *Guide* is provided by the Office of CHAMPUS in Denver, Colorado. Its address is given at the end of this chapter in the section headed "Publications." (A sample CHAMPUS claim form with detailed instructions regarding its completion is found at the end of section 10.7.)

Other forms   Several other forms have been developed by the HIAA, the AMA, and in the case of dental insurance, the ADA. These forms, also accepted for universal use, include: (1) the Long-Term/Permanent & Total Disability Form (2) the Vision Insurance Claim Form (3) the Medical Expense Insurance Duplicate Coverage Inquiry, and (4) the Dental Expense Insurance Duplicate Coverage Inquiry.

REASONS FOR CLAIM DELAYS

It is important to know some of the key reasons for delays in the payment of claims before you begin the process of claims completion. Unfortunately, the primary reasons for processing and payment delays by the carrier are the fault of the medical assistants who completed the forms in the first place. Any one of the following very common errors will result in processing and payment delays:

1. Incorrect identification of the member and incorrect group numbers
2. Spelling errors, especially with respect to the patients' and subscribers' names
3. Incorrect addresses for the patients and/or physicians
4. Missing information (such as a missing operative report)
5. Insufficient information (such as an inadequate description of a procedure)
6. Inadequate itemizations of fees
7. Use of codes (such as RVS and *CPT* codes) that do not correspond with the procedures described.

Always proofread the completed forms to check their accuracy before you put them on the physician's desk. Be sure that all data have been included. Make certain that all substantiating documents (such as operative reports) are attached. Make sure that the fee has been fully and correctly itemized. Finally, see that the correct codes for procedures have been used. The medical assistant should not use ditto marks for the dates or for the services performed. It is also a good practice to insert *DNA* (*does not apply*) or *N/A* (*not applicable*) rather than to leave blanks. When the forms are returned to you for mailing, you should check one more time before mailing them to be sure that all of the required documents are still attached to the forms.

There is also a potential for error on the part of the insurance company. One cause for delay may be that the person inputting the data into the computer may strike an incorrect key so that the claim is kicked out for review and reprocessing. In addition, heavy claims volume can create backlogs for insurance companies just as it can for medical offices.

COMPUTER PROCESSING OF INSURANCE FORMS

Hospitals, clinics, group practices, and many smaller offices are now using computers for the processing of insurance forms. In this procedure a computer company is engaged to store and retrieve all essential information such as the appropriate code numbers and the corresponding procedural terminology as well as the necessary patient identifying data and the diagnoses. At the time the computer service is contracted and the terminals installed, the company instructs the medical assistant in the techniques used to input the data into the computer. The process involves the completion of charge slips in the medical office. The charge slips show the coded information that is to be used as computer input for the later completion of the printouts requested by the office. The computer company usually supplies the medical office with two copies of the insurance form.

THE PEGBOARD SYSTEM FOR FILING INSURANCE CLAIMS

One of the most widely used methods of billing patient accounts is the pegboard system (see also Chapter 11, section 11.2 for full discussion of the pegboard system.) With this system you can post the day sheet, the account card, the statement, and the patient's receipt at one writing. The procedure code numbers and their descriptors are printed on the statements. A space is provided for entering the necessary identifying information and the diagnosis. The statement can be attached to the company insurance form either by the patient or by the medical assistant. Thus, there is no need to complete the physician's portion of the company's form.

In the event that certain procedures are not printed on the statement because they are performed infrequently, it would be necessary to add these onto the statement or to complete an insurance form. Also, complicated procedures would require that additional information be given. Generally, this type of insurance billing is not practical for surgical procedures calling for lengthy and individualized definition in order for the office to secure reimbursement commensurate with the time and complexity of the procedure performed.

TELEPHONE DICTATION FOR INSURANCE FORMS

Some insurance companies now provide telephone service for direct dictation of claims information. While telephone dictation may eliminate some of the paperwork, it still requires the time of office personnel. Since most insurance companies want the signature of the physician on the insurance form, the dictation method may not fulfill the companies' requirements. Additionally, the medical office would not have a copy of the completed form for reference purposes and for use in connection with any necessary follow-up procedures.

BASIC REQUIREMENTS FOR COMPLETING INSURANCE FORMS

1. **Patient information section** Establish a general procedure that requires and encourages the patients to complete their portion of the claim forms first.

2. **Assignments and release of information** Assignment of benefits is frequently desirable, depending on the established policy of the office. Assignments are executed by the policyholder (subscriber). A Release of Information authorization is signed by the patient, parent and/or guardian.

3. **Identifying information** All patient identifying information should be accurately recorded. This is especially important on any form used as an attachment to a company form. Identifying information could include:

   a. Name and address of the insurance company
   b. Policy and/or Group number
   c. Name and address of the employer
   d. Social Security and/or ID number of the employee
   e. Name and address of the subscriber/employee
   f. Full name and birth date of the patient
   g. Relationship of the patient to the subscriber/employee.

4. **One patient, one claim** Information for only *one* patient is entered on a claim form. Even though some policies are written for a combined family deductible, services for each patient are filed on *separate* forms.

5. **Diagnosis** The following considerations apply:

   a. As a general rule, enter only one diagnosis per claim: however, list concomitant conditions for same dates. Major Medical claims do allow the listing of more than one diagnosis on a single claim.
   b. The diagnosis must be complete and must be phrased in standard nomenclature.

The use of either "no diagnosis established" or "for diagnostic purpose" is unacceptable. It is preferable to give a chief complaint if no diagnosis has been confirmed. Some insurance companies now write policies including coverage for annual physicals. These are the exceptions to the rule of completeness, and may be filed with the simple statement "annual physical examination."

c. On a claim filed for continuing treatment where a previous claim for the same diagnosis has been filed, state in parentheses after the diagnosis, "continued treatment: see previous report dated --------," and give the exact date.

d. *International Classification of Diseases, Adapted (ICDA)* codes are used by many computer systems. Always use the proper codes together with the diagnoses to ensure that the computer processing will be accurate.

6. **Procedures**   The following considerations apply:

a. Record one procedure per line.

b. Use procedure codes, if applicable in your area.

c. If injections have been administered, state the injectable used, the amount given, and the manner of injection.

d. If surgical trays and supplies have been used, itemize them and then give the separate fee (if any) for the surgical trays and for supplies (such as cast materials).

e. If multiple visits occurred on the same date, state the time of day for each visit so that the claims clerk will know that separate procedures were performed at separate times.

7. **Special procedures**   The following considerations apply:

a. Detention time—state the length of time and validate the reason for detention. If the patient is in critical condition, this condition should be noted.

b. Indicate when any after-hours procedures (such as those occurring late at night, on Sundays, or on holidays) have been performed

8. **Referrals**   Whenever a patient is referred for laboratory work, for X rays, to another physician, or to a facility for special services, state it. Likewise, when the physician treats a patient who has been referred for a consultation and/or further treatment, the name of the referring physician should be entered on the form. This notation will establish a continuity of claims and will serve to validate claims for the referral treatment.

9. **Concurrent treatment**   Many times patients are concurrently treated for a medical as well as a surgical condition. In such a case, state that the presurgical or postsurgical care is for the medical diagnosis as opposed to the surgical procedure. In most cases, payment will be made.

10. **Place and time of service**   Record where the procedure was performed—at the office, at the patient's home, in an outpatient facility, in an inpatient hospital, in an extended-care facility, or in a nursing home.

11. **Reports**   Attach a copy of any hospital summary or operative report that will assist the company in processing complicated claims. It is advisable to attach operative reports to *all* claims for surgery. Even a short report on an office surgical procedure will secure better payment for the patient. This also saves some time. The insurance company will probably request the operative report anyway.

12. **Fees**   The following considerations apply:

a. On all claim forms regardless of the source, give the physician's usual, customary, and reasonable (UCR) fee. Do this regardless of the expected amount of payment. In the presence of contracts with the physician for a specific fee schedule, this is the UCR for those patients.

b. Some policies provide for an inclusive fee and others also pay for additional services performed before and after the surgical care. Since you will have no way of knowing what provisions will be made, it is advisable for you to record all pre- and postoperative care. This will aid the claims clerk in evaluating the claim.

c. *Never* bill one fee to the insurance company and a different fee to the patient.

13. **Discrepancies** *Never,* for any reason, alter a claim as to the service performed, the fee established, or the date of service. For example: the patient tells you that the insurance coverage will not take effect until next week and wants you to change the date of the service to one that is after the start of coverage. You must not do this. *Never* submit a claim form for a patient if the services were actually performed for someone else. Such discrepancies constitute fraudulent claims.

14. **Filing claims promptly** File a claim form when asked to do so, even though you might think there is no coverage, unless the patient accepts your tactful suggestion that there is no coverage. (An official rejection from the patient's insurance company will work wonders for the next time.)

15. **Physician identification** All forms require physician identification in addition to the doctor's name and address. Other identification includes the physician's state license number, Social Security number, federal ID used for reporting, or provider number assigned the physician by the insurance company.

16. **Signature** Unless the physician has legally authorized someone else to sign insurance forms, these forms *must* always be signed by the physician.

BLUE SHIELD PERMANENT RECIPROCITY PROGRAM: Billing

Follow these guidelines in billing for services rendered to patients covered by the Blue Shield Permanent Reciprocity Program discussed earlier in this chapter:

1. Note the number (such as N 987) in the double-ended red arrow identification symbol indicating on the patient's ID card that he or she is covered by the Permanent Reciprocity Program.
2. Include the above number on the local Blue Shield claim form.
3. Also include on the local Blue Shield claim form the patient's ID number (such as N 987 678–90–1234) which appears in a red box on the patient's Blue Shield ID card. These numbers will differ for each subscriber and for each plan.
4. Bill the local Blue Shield plan on the local Blue Shield claim form. The doctor will then receive from Blue Shield his or her usual, customary, or reasonable fee payment for the services rendered.

If your physician treats an out-of-town Blue Shield subscriber whose ID card does *not* identify him or her as a Permanent Reciprocity beneficiary, you should file that patient's claim with his or her home plan.

Medicare Permanent Reciprocity Program beneficiaries Recipients of Medicare who also are Blue Shield Permanent Reciprocity beneficiaries carry both a Medicare ID card and a Blue Shield ID card, the latter of which bears the distinctive double-ended red arrow. When the medical services have been rendered, include the numbers shown in items 1 and 3 in the above list in the appropriate space on the Medicare Part B Request for Payment form. Forward this form to your local Blue Shield office if your local Blue Shield plan is the Medicare Part B carrier.

If your local Blue Shield plan is not the Medicare Part B carrier, you should instead send the completed Request for Payment form to the Part B insurance company-carrier. Your office and the patient in question will then receive an Explanation of Medicare Benefits (termed *EOMB*) from the commercial carrier.

Universal Health Insurance Claim Form

**HEALTH INSURANCE
CLAIM FORM**
READ INSTRUCTIONS BEFORE COMPLETING OR SIGNING THIS FORM

TYPE OR PRINT   [ ] MEDICARE   [ ] MEDICAID   [X] OTHER

PATIENT & INSURED (SUBSCRIBER) INFORMATION

1. PATIENT'S NAME (First name, middle initial, last name)	2. PATIENT'S DATE OF BIRTH	3. INSURED'S NAME (First name, middle initial, last name)
Elizabeth A. Harding	06 | 07 | 55	Elizabeth A. Harding

4. PATIENT'S ADDRESS (Street, city, state, ZIP code)	5. PATIENT'S SEX	6. INSURED'S I.D. MEDICARE AND/OR MEDICAID NO. (Include any letters)
17 White Avenue Anywhere, USA 00000	MALE [ ] [X] FEMALE	000-00-0000

| TELEPHONE NO. 123-4567 | 7. PATIENT'S RELATIONSHIP TO INSURED: SELF [X] SPOUSE [ ] CHILD [ ] OTHER [ ] | 8. INSURED'S GROUP NO (Or Group Name) 34567810 |

9. OTHER HEALTH INSURANCE COVERAGE - Enter Name of Policyholder and Plan Name and Address and Policy or Medical Assistance Number

None

10. WAS CONDITION RELATED TO:
A. PATIENT'S EMPLOYMENT   YES [ ] [X] NO
B. AN AUTO ACCIDENT   YES [ ] [X] NO

11. INSURED'S ADDRESS (Street, city, state, ZIP code)

12. PATIENT'S OR AUTHORIZED PERSON'S SIGNATURE (Read back before signing)
I Authorize the Release of any Medical Information Necessary to Process this Claim and Request Payment of MEDICARE Benefits Either to Myself or to the Party Who Accepts Assignment Below

SIGNED *Elizabeth A. Harding*   DATE 5/1/78

13. I AUTHORIZE PAYMENT OF MEDICAL BENEFITS TO UNDERSIGNED PHYSICIAN OR SUPPLIER FOR SERVICE DESCRIBED BELOW

SIGNED *Elizabeth A. Harding* (Insured or Authorized Person)

PHYSICIAN OR SUPPLIER INFORMATION

| 14. DATE OF: 3/1/78 | ILLNESS (FIRST SYMPTOM) OR INJURY (ACCIDENT) OR PREGNANCY (LMP) | 15. DATE FIRST CONSULTED YOU FOR THIS CONDITION 4/14/78 | 16. HAS PATIENT EVER HAD SAME OR SIMILAR SYMPTOMS? YES [ ] [X] NO |

| 17. DATE PATIENT ABLE TO RETURN TO WORK N/A | 18. DATES OF TOTAL DISABILITY FROM N/A THROUGH | DATES OF PARTIAL DISABILITY FROM N/A THROUGH |

19. NAME OF REFERRING PHYSICIAN OR OTHER SOURCE (e.g., public health agency)

John Jones, MD

20. FOR SERVICES RELATED TO HOSPITALIZATION GIVE HOSPITALIZATION DATES
ADMITTED N/A   DISCHARGED

21. NAME & ADDRESS OF FACILITY WHERE SERVICES RENDERED (If other than home or office)

22. WAS LABORATORY WORK PERFORMED OUTSIDE YOUR OFFICE? YES [X] NO   CHARGES

23. DIAGNOSIS OR NATURE OF ILLNESS OR INJURY. RELATE DIAGNOSIS TO PROCEDURE IN COLUMN D BY REFERENCE TO NUMBERS 1, 2, 3, ETC. OR DX CODE

ICDA CODES
1. 250.9   Diabetes Mellitus
2. 517   Fibrosis, Pulmonary, Interstitial
3. 279   Hyperglyceridemia, Ess. Carbohydrate Induced
4.

Outside Laboratory:
Give name and address.

24. A DATE OF SERVICE	B PLACE OF SERVICE	C PROCEDURE CODE (IDENTIFY CPT)	FULLY DESCRIBE PROCEDURES, MEDICAL SERVICES OR SUPPLIES FURNISHED FOR EACH DATE GIVEN (EXPLAIN UNUSUAL SERVICES OR CIRCUMSTANCES)	D DX CODE (ID ICDA)	E CHARGES	F
4/14/78	0	90020	New patient/ Complete history and physical	above 279	200 00	
4/14/78	0	82947-90	Glucose	250.9	3 05	
4/14/78	0	99000	Collection and Handling	250.9	5 00	
4/14/78	0	81000	Urinalysis	250.9	5 00	
4/14/78	0	82465-90	Cholesterol	250.9	9 00	
4/14/78	0	71020	PA & Lateral Chest Xray	517	30 00	
4/28/78	0	90050	Limited Service	as above	20 00	

**All fees are fictitious

25. SIGNATURE OF PHYSICIAN OR SUPPLIER
(I certify that the statements on the reverse apply to this bill and are made a part hereof.)

SIGNED *John Jones, M.D.*   DATE 4/30/78

32. YOUR PATIENT'S ACCOUNT NO.
57834

26. ACCEPT ASSIGNMENT (GOVERNMENT CLAIMS ONLY) (SEE BACK) YES [ ] NO [ ]

30. YOUR SOCIAL SECURITY NO.
000-00-0000 or

33. YOUR EMPLOYER I.D. NO.
Employer ID if Clinic   I.D. NO.

| 27. TOTAL CHARGE 272 05 | 28. AMOUNT PAID -0- | 29. BALANCE DUE 272 05 |

31. PHYSICIAN'S OR SUPPLIER'S NAME, ADDRESS, ZIP CODE & TELEPHONE NO.
444-5555   John Jones, MD
25 Main Street
Anywhere, USA 00000

* PLACE OF SERVICE CODES

1—(IH) —INPATIENT HOSPITAL	4—(H)—PATIENT'S HOME	7—(NH) —NURSING HOME	0—(OL) —OTHER LOCATIONS
2—(OH) —OUTPATIENT HOSPITAL	5— DAY CARE FACILITY (PSY)	8—(SNF) —SKILLED NURSING FACILITY	A—(IL) —INDEPENDENT LABORATORY
3—(O) —DOCTOR'S OFFICE	6— NIGHT CARE FACILITY (PSY)	9— AMBULANCE	B— OTHER MEDICAL/SURGICAL FACILITY

APPROVED BY AMA COUNCIL ON MEDICAL SERVICE 6-74

Courtesy of the American Medical Association.

Doctor's First Report of Work Injury (Workers' Compensation)

DOCTOR'S FIRST REPORT
OF WORK INJURY

FILL OUT AND
FORWARD 1 COPY
IMMEDIATELY AFTER
FIRST SEEING
PATIENT

ALSO, Immediately after first examination mail one copy directly to the Division of Labor Statistics and Research
Failure to file a report with the Division is a misdemeanor.
Answer all questions fully.

Do not write
in this space

1. **EMPLOYER** _Jones Hardware_
2. Address (No., St. & City) _750 Tenth Street, San Francisco, CA 94120_
3. Business (Manufacturing shoes, building construction, retailing men's clothes, etc.) _Retail store_

SOCIAL SECURITY NO.

4. **EMPLOYEE** (First name, middle initial, last name) _John J. Doe_   _000-00-0000_
5. Address (No., St. & City) _234 Eleventh St., San Francisco, CA 94119_
6. Occupation _Clerk_   Age _40_   Sex _M_
7. Date injured _October 13, 1977_ Hour _3_ P.M Date last worked _same_
8. Injured at (No., St. & City) _750 Tenth Street, San Francisco_   County _San Francisco_
9. Date of your first examination _10/13/77_ Hour _5_ P.M Who engaged your services? _Employer_
10. Name other doctors who treated employee for this injury _None_

11. **ACCIDENT OR EXPOSURE:** Did employee notify employer of this injury? _Yes_   Employee's statement
of cause of injury or illness:

Fell from ladder distance of four (4) feet to floor.
Twisting injury to right ankle.

12. **NATURE AND EXTENT OF INJURY OR DISEASE** (Include all objective findings, subjective complaints, and diagnoses.
If occupational disease state date of onset, occupational history, and exposures.)

Simple fracture lateral malleolus rt. ankle - undisplaced.

13. X-rays: By whom taken? (State if none) _St. Martha's Hospital_
Findings:
As above

14. Treatment:
Short leg cast applied - no anesthesia
15. Kind of case (Office, home, or hospital) _Office_   If hospitalized, date _____ Estimated stay _____
Name and address of hospital _____
16. Further treatment (Estimated frequency and duration) _Weekly_
17. Estimated period of disability for: Regular work _3 months_ Modified work _6 weeks_
18. Describe any permanent disability or disfigurement expected (State if none) _None_

19. If death ensued, give date

20. **REMARKS** (Note any pre-existing injuries or diseases, need for special examination or laboratory tests, other pertinent information.)

N. B.—ONLY UNDER EXCEPTIONAL CIRCUMSTANCES WILL A HERNIA BE CONSIDERED DISABLING PRIOR TO OPERATION.
THE INJURED SHOULD BE ADVISED TO CONTINUE WORK, IF POSSIBLE, UNTIL NOTIFIED THAT HIS CLAIM IS ACCEPTED.

Name _Friend Hunton,_   Degree _M. D._ [PERSONAL SIGNATURE OF DOCTOR]
(Type or print)
Date of report _10/14/77_ Address (No., St. & City) _450 Sutter St., San Francisco,_   Tel. No. _473-1234_
FORM 10-LA   *Use reverse side if more space required*   CA 94128   21762-218 8-64 800M ① △ OSP

Doctor's Final (or Monthly) Report and Bill (Workers' Compensation)

DOCTOR'S FINAL (OR MONTHLY) REPORT AND BILL

Itemized bills, IN DUPLICATE, are to be submitted at the termination of the case.
Monthly statements are POSITIVELY required on cases under treatment.
Mail to .....USA Insurance Company.................Address .One Market St., San Francisco, CA
Services beginning late in month and extending into succeeding month may be itemized on one statement.

EMPLOYER .....Able Laundry Service...................... Case No. 1234
EMPLOYEE .....James Doe
DATE OF INJURY Nov. 1, 1977 SERVICES FOR MONTH OF .....November........., 19.77.

Patient refused treatment................., 19......   Patient able to return to work.....11/28/., 19.77.
Patient stopped treatment   Patient discharged as cured.........11/28/., 19.77.
    without orders................., 19......   Condition at time of last visit.....
Patient entered hospital.........11/1/..., 1977.

Any other charges authorized such as Drugs? .X.....Hospital? .X...
                              (Check)   (Check)

Code: O—Office; V—Home Visit; H—Hospital Visit; N—Night Visit; S—Operation; X—X-Ray.

Month	1	2	3	4	5	6	7	8	9	10	11	12	13	14	15	16	17	18	19	20	21	22	23	24	25	26	27	28	29	30	31
Nov $	H	H	O	O	O							O																O			

                     Admit to hospital: CPT CODES Totals *

First aid treatment (describe).Debridement wound and suture..........$
.............................palm of right hand - 3.0 cm. wound 12002   40.00
Office Visits............Five - limited service.............90050 $ 75.00
Home Visits.....................................$
Hospital Visits.One-admit/examination/history/records 90215 $ 50.00
Operations .....See above.............................$
MATERIAL (Itemized at cost).............................$
Hospital Visits - Two - limited service   90250 $ 50.00
                                               TOTAL $ 215.00

*All fees are fictitious.

Any charges shown above which are in excess of the minimum fee must be explained below regarding nature
of such services, indicating the date rendered.

Make check payable to:

Doctor .....Friend Hunton, M. D..............   Signature.............................M. D..
       450 Sutter Street
Address ...San Francisco, CA 94128.........   Date .December 28, 1977.............

Request for Medicare Payment

REQUEST FOR MEDICARE PAYMENT

MEDICAL INSURANCE BENEFITS—SOCIAL SECURITY ACT (See Instructions on Back—Type or Print Information)

Form Approved
Budget Bureau No.
72-RO730

NOTICE—Anyone who misrepresents or falsifies essential information requested by this form may upon conviction be subject to fine and imprisonment under Federal Law.

PART I—PATIENT TO FILL IN ITEMS 1 THROUGH 6 ONLY

When completed, send this form to:

Occidental Life Insurance Co. of California
Box 54905
Terminal Annex
Los Angeles, California 90054

Copy from your HEALTH INSURANCE CARD (See example on back) →

1 Name of patient

JOHN DOE

2 Health insurance claim number

6 6 6 4 4 8 8 8 8 8 Letter A

☒ Male ☐ Female

3 Patient's mailing address
One Main Street

City, State, ZIP code
Anywhere, USA   00000

Telephone Number
222-3333

4 Describe the illness or injury for which you received treatment (Always fill in this item if your doctor does not complete Part II below) Hypertensive heart disease (ICDA 401)

Ischemic heart disease (ICDA 412.0) Tachycardia (ICDA 427.9)

Was your illness or injury connected with your employment?
☐ Yes ☒ No

5 If you have other health insurance or if your State medical assistance agency will pay part of your medical expenses and you want information about this claim released to the insurance company or State agency upon its request, give the following information.

Insuring organization or State agency name and address

None

Policy No.
Medi-cal Identification No.
N/A

6 I authorize any holder of medical or other information about me to release to the Social Security Administration or its intermediaries or carriers any information needed for this or a related Medicare claim. I permit a copy of this authorization to be used in place of the original, and request payment of medical insurance benefits either to myself or to the party who accepts assignment below.

Signature of patient (See instructions on reverse where patient is unable to sign)

SIGN HERE ►

Date signed

5/1/78

PART II—PHYSICIAN OR SUPPLIER TO FILL IN 7 THROUGH 14

7

A. Date of each service	B. Place of service (*See Codes below)	C. Code surgical or medical procedures and other services or supplies furnished for each date given		D. Nature of illness or injury requiring services or supplies	E. Charges (If related to unusual circumstances explain in 7C)	Leave Blank
			Code CPT			
3/3/78	O	Examination – intermediate	90060	See above	$ 25.00	
3/3/78	O	Electrocardiogram with interpretation and report	93000		30.00	
3/4/78	O	Rhythm ECG with interpretation	93040		15.00	
		Patient referred to Cardiac Scan Service for 24 hr ECG-Holter Monitor-Hospital to bill separately				
		Name of Hospital Address of Hospital				

8 Name and address of physician or supplier (Number and street, city, State, ZIP code)

Give full name and address

Telephone No.

000-0000

Physician or supplier code

0000000

9 Total charges
$ 70.00

10 Amount paid
$ -0-

11 Any unpaid balance due
$ 70.00

12 Assignment of patient's bill (See reverse)
►
☒ I accept assignment   ☐ I do not accept assignment

13 Show name and address of facility where services were performed (If other than home or office visits)

14 Signature of physician or supplier (A physician's signature certifies that physician's services were personally rendered by him or under his personal direction)
►
PHYSICIAN MUST SIGN IF ACCEPTING ASSIGNMENT

☒ MD ☐ DO ☐ DDS
Other degree _____

Date signed

4/1/78

*O—Doctor's Office
IL—Independent Laboratory

H—Patient's Home (If portable X-ray services, identify the supplier)
IH—Inpatient Hospital

ECF—Extended Care Facility
OH—Outpatient Hospital

OL—Other Locations
NH—Nursing Home

FORM SSA-1490D(2)CA (10-69)

Department of Health, Education, and Welfare
Social Security Administration

Either you or the patient (but <u>not</u> both of you) should file the EOMB with Blue Shield. Again, the ID numbers mentioned in items 1 and 3 of the preceding list should be included on the EOMB. These numbers are also required when you file for supplementary benefits with your local Blue Shield plan. Your physician then should receive the appropriate payment for both Medicare Part B and Blue Shield's covered services.

If your physician does not accept assignment, you should encourage the patient to file his or her copy of the EOMB directly with Blue Shield. The patient also must include the two ID numbers mentioned above when submitting the EOMB.

COMPLETING MEDICAID FORMS

A Medicaid form is not illustrated here because the forms vary so much from state to state. Any one of the other forms that have been illustrated here can be used as a guide for completing the Medicaid form. You must remember to complete the section of the form provided for the recipient's identification number as well as to provide the necessary document showing evidence of the patient's eligibility for the medical service. The proof of eligibility document may also vary from state to state.

THE FILLING OUT OF CHAMPUS FORMS

The CHAMPUS/CHAMPVA form 500 is to be used when submitting bills for professional services under the CHAMPUS/CHAMPVA Program. Items #1 through #18 of a claim form 500 must be completed. Each medical bill must include the name and address of the source of care; the name of the patient; the nature of the illness; the date, charge, and description of each service; the name, strength, and amount of any drug and injection; related dates of hospitalization; any surgical procedure and the duration of anesthesia; and, for maternity care, the estimated or actual date of delivery. A claim form 500 must be completed for each patient.

Submission of patient reimbursement claims   Complete items #1 through #18 only on the CHAMPUS/CHAMPVA Form 500:

1. **Name**   Enter the patient's complete name (last, first, and middle initial, if any).
2. **Date of Birth**   Enter the patient's complete date of birth (month, day, year).
3. **Address**   Enter the patient's complete address (number and street, city, state, and ZIP Code). The patient's telephone number must be indicated on all claims.
4. **Patient's sex**   Check the appropriate box.
5. **Military/VA Identification Card**
   (a)   Dependent children 10 years old or over should use their own cards.
   (b)   Children under age 10 may use either parent's ID card.
   (c)   The issue date, effective date, and expiration date must be inserted on the form and should be present on the ID card.
6. **Patient's Relationship to Sponsor**   Check the appropriate box.
7. **Sponsor's Name**   Enter the sponsor's full name (last, first, middle initial, if any).
8. **Sponsor's Social Security Number or VA File Number**   Enter the sponsor's SSA number or VA file number for CHAMPVA beneficiaries.
9. **VA Station Number**   Indicate the three-digit VA issuing station number found on the ID card.
10. **Sponsor's Duty Station or Address for Retirees**   For active-duty dependents, enter the current assignment of the sponsor. If it is a ship, enter the home port. For retirees or CHAMPVA beneficiaries, state the home address and telephone number.
11. **Sponsor's Branch of Service**   Check the appropriate box.
12. **Sponsor's Grade/Rank**   Show the sponsor's rank/pay grade (e.g., O–7, E–5).

CHAMPUS Form

CHAMPUS/CHAMPVA CLAIM FORM

For services or supplies provided by civilian sources except Institutions

Read cover instructions and the back of this form before completing and signing!

Form Approved
OMB No.
022-RO382

Patient/Sponsor Information (Items 1 through 18 to be completed by the beneficiary/patient or sponsor)

1 PATIENT'S NAME (Last name, First name, Middle initial)

2 PATIENT'S DATE OF BIRTH
MONTH   DAY   YEAR

7 SPONSOR'S NAME (Last name, First name, Middle initial)

3 PATIENT'S ADDRESS (Street, city, state, ZIP code)

4 PATIENT'S SEX
☐ MALE   ☐ FEMALE

8 SPONSOR'S SOCIAL SECURITY NO. OR VA FILE NO.

9 VA STATION NO.

PHONE NO. (Include area code)

6 PATIENT'S RELATIONSHIP TO SPONSOR
☐ SELF
☐ NATURAL or ADOPTED CHILD
☐ SPOUSE
☐ STEPCHILD
OTHER (Specify):

10 SPONSOR'S DUTY STATION OR ADDRESS FOR RETIREES

5 MILITARY/VA IDENTIFICATION CARD

CARD NO.

ISSUE DATE
MONTH DAY YEAR

EFFECTIVE DATE
MONTH DAY YEAR

EXPIRATION DATE
MONTH DAY YEAR

15 IS CONDITION WORK RELATED?
☐ YES ☐ NO
MILITARY SERVICE RELATED?
☐ YES ☐ NO
AUTOMOBILE ACCIDENT RELATED?
☐ YES ☐ NO

PHONE NO. (Include area code)

11 SPONSOR'S BRANCH OF SERVICE
☐ USA ☐ USAF ☐ USMC ☐ USN
☐ USCG ☐ USPHS ☐ NOAA ☐ VA

12 SPONSOR'S GRADE/RANK

14. DO YOU HAVE OTHER HEALTH INSURANCE? ☐ YES ☐ NO
IF YES, ENTER NAME OF OTHER PLAN OR PROGRAM

13. SPONSOR'S STATUS
☐ ACTIVE DUTY   ☐ RETIRED   ☐ DECEASED

ADDRESS

CITY   STATE   ZIP

16. INPATIENT/OUTPATIENT CARE
☐ OUTPATIENT ☐ INPATIENT-EMERGENCY ☐ INPATIENT HOSPITAL-OUTSIDE 40 MILE RADIUS
☐ INPATIENT-SKILLED NURSING FACILITY ☐ INPATIENT-OTHER
☐ INPATIENT HOSPITAL-WITHIN 40 MILE RADIUS (ATTACH DD FORM 1251)

14a. TYPE OF COVERAGE:
☐ EMPLOYMENT (GROUP)   ☐ MEDICAID   ☐ STUDENT PLAN
☐ PRIVATE (NON-GROUP)   ☐ MEDICARE   ☐ OTHER

17. DESCRIBE CONDITION FOR WHICH YOU RECEIVED TREATMENT. IF AN INJURY, NOTE HOW IT HAPPENED.

14b. OTHER IDENTIFICATION NUMBER

14c. EFFECTIVE DATE
MONTH DAY YEAR

14d. OTHER PROGRAM THROUGH EMPLOYMENT?
EMPLOYER NAME:

18 SIGNATURE OF PATIENT OR AUTHORIZED PERSON. CERTIFIES CLAIM INFORMATION AND AUTHORIZES RELEASE OF MEDICAL OR OTHER INSURANCE INFORMATION. READ INSTRUCTIONS AND BACK OF THIS FORM BEFORE SIGNING

SIGNED   DATE

RELATIONSHIP TO PATIENT

Physician/Other Provider (Items 19 through 33 are to be completed by the physician or other provider.)

19. NAME, ADDRESS & PHONE NO. OF REFERRING PHYSICIAN

20 NAME & ADDRESS OF FACILITY WHERE SERVICES RENDERED (other than home or office)

☐ PRIVATE PRACTICE or ☐ UNIFORMED SERVICES

21. PROVIDER OF SERVICES
☐ ATTENDING PHYSICIAN
☐ OTHER

22. HOSPITALIZATION INFORMATION
MO DAY YEAR
ADMITTED

MO DAY YEAR
DISCHARGED

23. LAB WORK OUTSIDE YOUR OFFICE?
☐ YES ☐ NO CHARGES

24. DIAGNOSIS, SYMPTOM OR NATURE OF ILLNESS OR INJURY. RELATE DIAGNOSIS TO PROCEDURE IN COLUMN "D" BY REFERENCE TO NUMBERS 1, 2, 3, or DX CODE

1.
2.
3.

25. A DATES OF SERVICE MO/DAY/YEAR	B. PLACE OF SERVICE	C PROCEDURE CODE IDENTIFY:	D. DESCRIBE PROCEDURES/SUPPLIES FOR EACH DATE. SUBMIT REPORT EXPLAINING UNUSUAL SERVICES OR CIRCUMSTANCES	E DIAGNOSIS CODE	F CHARGES	LEAVE BLANK

26. PATIENT'S ACCOUNT NO.

29. PHYSICIAN'S OR OTHER PROVIDER'S NAME ADDRESS, ZIP CODE & PHONE NO. (INCLUDING AREA CODE)

G. TOTAL CHARGES
$

30 AMOUNT PAID BY BENEFICIARY
$

31 AMOUNT PAID BY OTHER INSURANCE
$

27. PROVIDER'S SOCIAL SECURITY NO.

32. AGREEMENT TO PARTICIPATE (READ BACK OF THIS FORM)
☐ YES   ☐ NO

28. PROVIDER'S EMPLOYER I.D. NO.

33. SIGNATURE OF PHYSICIAN OR OTHER PROVIDER (READ BACK OF THIS FORM BEFORE SIGNING)

PROVIDER NO.

SIGNED: DATE:

*PLACE OF SERVICE CODES
1 — (IH) — INPATIENT HOSPITAL
2 — (OH) — OUTPATIENT HOSPITAL
3 — (O) — DOCTOR'S OFFICE

4 — (H) — PATIENT'S HOME
5 — (DCF) — DAY CARE FACILITY (PSY)
6 — (NCF) — NIGHT CARE FACILITY (PSY)

7 — (NH) — NURSING HOME
8 — (SNF) — SKILLED NURSING FACILITY
9 — (AMB) — AMBULANCE
0 — (OL) — OTHER LOCATIONS

A — (IL) — INDEPENDENT LABORATORY
B — (OF) — OTHER MEDICAL/SURGICAL FACILITY
C — (RTC)— RESIDENTIAL TREATMENT CENTER
D — (STF) — SPECIALIZED TREATMENT FACILITY

CHAMPUS FORM 500 JUNE 1978

13. **Sponsor's Status** Check the appropriate box (e.g., active-duty, retired, deceased).

14. **Other Health Insurance** Indicate if the patient has other insurance. If so, check "yes" and give the name and address of the program. Fill in items 14a through 14d.

15. **Work-related Conditions** Indicate if the condition being treated is work-related, related to a service-connected injury or illness, or related to an auto accident.

16. **Inpatient/Outpatient Care** Check the right box according to the patient's status at the time that the care was rendered. DD Form 1251 (Nonavailability Statement) is required whenever nonemergency inpatient hospital services are provided for patients living within a 40-mile radius of a uniformed services facility. DD Form 1251 is not required for CHAMPVA dependents.

17. **Diagnosis or Condition** Indicate the diagnosis or condition for which treatment is provided. If the treatment is for an injury, indicate how the injury happened.

18. **Authorized Signature** Every CHAMPUS/CHAMPVA claim must be signed by the person receiving the care if 18 years old or over, by the parent of a minor child, or by the legal guardian of a mental incompetent.

Submission of provider payable claims Items #19 through #33 are to be completed by the provider of care. In addition to the above listed instructions on completing items #1 through #18 for patient reimbursement claims, the following are given in order to help medical assistants in completing items #19 through #33 when submitting claims using the CHAMPUS/CHAMPVA Form 500:

19. **Name, Address, and Telephone Number of Referring Physician** The name of the physician ordering the care must be present on all billings for consultations, nonphysician claims (e.g., medical supplies, allied scientists). Psychologists and optometrists can provide care without physican referral. Check the appropriate box for "private practice" or "uniformed services."

20. **Name and Address of Facility Rendering Services (other than home or office)** Enter the name and address of the facility rendering the services.

21. **Provider of Services** Check the appropriate box. If other, so specify: e.g., assistant surgeon, radiologist, consultant, etc.

22. **Hospitalization Information** Enter the admission and discharge dates of confinement whether this was the first confinement or a subsequent one for the same or a related medical condition.

23. **Laboratory Work outside your Office** Check the appropriate box. If "yes", indicate the lab charge and give the name and address of the outside lab. (Item 20 may be used to give the name and address of the outside lab.)

24. **Diagnosis, Symptoms, or Nature of Illness or Injury** Use standard nomenclature to list these. The use of ICDA codes should be consistent with the nature of the patient's illness.

25. **Services and Supplies** Enter only those services and/or supplies that are authorized for payment under CHAMPUS. All services and supplies must be itemized to ensure prompt/correct payment. Payment from the government to the source of services/supplies is normally based on the usual, customary, and reasonable (UCR) charges. However, should a physician, dentist, or other health professional expend unusual effort to care for the patient properly, he or she should submit a clinical résumé with the claim in support of a request for a special consideration of the amount payable for the services rendered.
    (a) Enter the date on which the care was provided.
    (b) Enter the Place of Service Code as indicated at the bottom of the claim form.
    (c) Give the appropriate procedure code for each procedure.
    (d) Give a description of each procedure or supply for each date.
    (e) Give the appropriate ICDA code.

(f)   Enter the UCR fee for each service.

(g)   Enter the total amount for all authorized charges.

26. **Patient's Account Number**   The provider's internal patient account number can be entered in this area of the form.

27. **Provider's Social Security Number**   Enter this number in the space available.

28. **Provider's Employer ID Number**   Enter the IRS number if applicable.

29. **Physician's or Other Provider's Name, Address, ZIP Code, and Telephone Number**   Indicate these data for the provider billing for the services.

30. **Amount Paid by Beneficiary**   Enter any amount that the patient has already paid toward this billing.

31. **Amount Paid by Other Insurance**   Enter any amount already paid by other insurance.

32. **Agreement to Participate**   By checking "yes" in item 32 and signing in item 33, the provider agrees to submit the claim as a participating provider and to accept the CHAMPUS-determined reasonable charge as the total charge for medical services and/or supplies listed on the form. The provider will accept the CHAMPUS-determined reasonable charge even if it is less than the billed amount, and also agrees to accept the amount paid by CHAMPUS combined with the cost-shared amount and deductible (if any) paid by or on behalf of the patient or the beneficiary as full payment for the medical services and/or supplies provided. The provider may not collect from the patient or beneficiary or sponsor amounts in excess of the CHAMPUS-determined reasonable charge. CHAMPUS pays directly to the provider of care. Any alteration of the Provider Participation Agreement by the provider may result in the claim being returned or processed as a nonparticipating claim with payment being made to the beneficiary instead.

33. **Signature**   Make sure that the physician or other care provider signs the form.

COMPLETING DENTAL INSURANCE FORMS

For the most part, an insurance company will not accept a dental insurance form that is not its own. However, the majority of the forms are modeled after the ADA official form. The dental assistant completing dental forms follows the same general procedures that have been given for completing health insurance forms. However, some requirements do set the dental form apart from the medical forms. These requirements are discussed in the next few paragraphs.

Preauthorization: predetermination of benefits   Nonemergency treatment, services that will be over $100, and gold or prosthetics usually require preauthorization or a predetermination of benefits. The preauthorization form is completed with a description of the service, the procedure number, and the pretreatment estimate of cost. The preauthorization form is also the one used for billing when the dental work has been completed. If the company requires X rays to be submitted with the preauthorization form, these should be labeled and staple-mounted to the upper right-hand corner of the treatment form. X rays are identified with the name of the patient, the name of the dentist, and the dentist's license number. In most instances, X rays are required for work over $100, for all inlays, for onlays, for individual crowns, for fixed bridges, for surgical extractions, for impactions, and for endodontic services. The office should expect the preauthorization to be returned within four weeks with the amount that the insurance company will pay indicated on it.

Tooth and surface identification   The dental form for the attending dentist features in one of its sections a diagram where all teeth are identified. You must also become familiar with the method of indicating the type of work to be done. This is drawn on the diagram. There is a column for listing the tooth number or letter and for

Attending Dentist's Statement

ATTENDING DENTIST'S STATEMENT

| 1. PATIENT NAME | James A. Jones | 2. RELATIONSHIP TO EMPLOYEE SELF / SPOUSE / CHILD / OTHER: X | 3. SEX M / F: X | 4. PATIENT BIRTHDATE MO. 5 DAY 3 YEAR 34 | 5. IF FULL TIME STUDENT SCHOOL | CITY |

| 6. EMPLOYEE NAME FIRST | NAME MIDDLE | LAST | Same | 7. EMPLOYEE SOCIAL SECURITY NO. 436-25-0832 | 9. NAME OF GROUP DENTAL PROGRAM Martin Machinery |

8. EMPLOYEE MAILING ADDRESS
9672 Torrance Blvd.
CITY STATE ZIP
Los Angeles, Calif. 90508

10. EMPLOYER (COMPANY) NAME AND ADDRESS
Martin Machinery-2289 Vermont Ave. L.A.

| 11. GROUP NUMBER 54695 | 12. LOCATION (LOCAL) L.A. | 13. ARE OTHER FAMILY MEMBERS EMPLOYED? YES ☐ NO X EMPLOYEE NAME N/A SOC. SEC. NO. | 14. NAME AND ADDRESS OF EMPLOYER IN ITEM 13. N/A |

15. IS PATIENT COVERED BY ANOTHER DENTAL PLAN? YES ☐ NO X | DENTAL PLAN NAME | UNION LOCAL | GROUP NO. | NAME AND ADDRESS OF CARRIER

I HAVE REVIEWED THE FOLLOWING TREATMENT PLAN. I AUTHORIZE RELEASE OF ANY INFORMATION RELATING TO THIS CLAIM.
James A. Jones
SIGNED (PATIENT, OR PARENT IF MINOR) DATE

I HEREBY AUTHORIZE PAYMENT DIRECTLY TO THE BELOW-NAMED DENTIST OF THE GROUP INSURANCE BENEFITS OTHERWISE PAYABLE TO ME.
James A. Jones
SIGNED (INSURED PERSON) DATE

DENTIST'S INFORMATION   PLEASE PRESS FIRMLY

16. DENTIST NAME
John Doe, D.D.S.

17. MAILING ADDRESS
36950 Crenshaw Blvd.
CITY STATE ZIP
Los Angeles, Calif. 90503

24. IS TREATMENT RESULT OF OCCUPATIONAL ILLNESS OR INJURY?	NO X	YES	IF YES, ENTER BRIEF DESCRIPTION AND DATES
25. IS TREATMENT RESULT OF AUTO ACCIDENT?	X		
26. OTHER ACCIDENT?	X		
27. ARE ANY SERVICES COVERED BY ANOTHER PLAN?	X		

| 18. DENTIST SOC. SEC. OR T.I. NO. 445-63-5520 | 19. DENTIST LICENSE NO. 63652 | 20. DENTIST PHONE NO. 378-6920 | 28. IF PROSTHESIS, IS THIS INITIAL PLACEMENT? | (IF NO, REASON FOR REPLACEMENT) | 29. DATE OF PRIOR PLACEMENT |

| 21. FIRST VISIT DATE CURRENT SERIES 2-8-78 | 22. PLACE OF TREATMENT OFFICE X / HOSP / ECF / OTHER | 23. RADIOGRAPHS OR MODELS ENCLOSED? NO / YES X / HOW MANY? 2 | 30. IS TREATMENT FOR ORTHODONTICS? X | IF SERVICES ALREADY COMMENCED, ENTER | DATE APPLIANCES PLACED | MOS. TREATMENT REMAINING |

TO THE DENTIST: PREDETERMINATION OF BENEFITS REQUIRED FOR CLAIMS IN EXCESS OF $100.00

CHECK ONE: X DENTIST'S PRE-TREATMENT ESTIMATE   ☐ DENTIST'S STATEMENT OF ACTUAL SERVICES

TOOTH # OR LETTER	SURFACE	31. EXAMINATION AND TREATMENT PLAN - LIST IN ORDER FROM TOOTH NO. 1 THROUGH TOOTH NO. 32 - USE CHARTING SYSTEM SHOWN DESCRIPTION OF SERVICE (INCLUDING X RAYS, PROPHYLAXIS, MATERIALS USED, ETC.)	DATE SERVICE PERFORMED MO. DAY YR.	PROCEDURE NUMBER	FEE	ADMINISTRATIVE USE
		Full mouth X-rays	2 8 78	0210	25 00	
		Prophylaxis	2 8 78	01100	20 00	
3	M	Amalgam		02140	15 00	
4	DO	Amalgam		02150	20 00	
8	M	Composite		02310	18 00	
10	ALL	Porcelain to Gold Crown		02750	170 00	
19	ALL	Full gold crown		02790	155 00	
18	MOD	Amalgam		02160	25 00	

32. REMARKS FOR UNUSUAL SERVICES

I HEREBY CERTIFY THAT THE PROCEDURES AS INDICATED BY DATE HAVE BEEN COMPLETED.
John Doe, DDS
SIGNED (DENTIST)   DATE 2/9/78

TOTAL FEE CHARGED	448 00
MAX. ALLOWABLE	
DEDUCTIBLE	
CARRIER %	
CARRIER PAYS	
PATIENT PAYS	

ELIGIBILITY CERTIFICATION
VALID ONLY WHEN THIS SECTION INITIALED AND DATED

ELIGIBILITY VERIFIED BY   DATE
VALID ONLY FOR 60 DAYS FROM ABOVE DATE. ANY EXTENSION MUST BE IN WRITING.   CLAIM NO

Occidental Life Insurance Company of California A Member of Transamerica Corporation

ADA ADS (75)

Form Approved by the Council on Dental Care Programs of the A.D.A. 1975

GML-643 ED. 8-75

Reprinted by permission of Occidental Life Insurance Company of California.

Attending Dentist's Statement

CONNECTICUT GENERAL LIFE INSURANCE COMPANY

ATTENDING DENTIST'S STATEMENT — Hartford, Connecticut, 06152

INSURANCE COMPANY USE ONLY	MAIL THIS FORM TO: CONNECTICUT GENERAL LIFE INSURANCE CO.

Acct. **0413994** Pol/ Plan **01** Div. ___ Eff. / /

Sex ___ Sched # ___ PTR ___ Clmt. ___

MAIL THIS FORM TO: **CONNECTICUT GENERAL LIFE INSURANCE CO.**
P. O. BOX 1776
SANTA MONICA, CA. 90406

Telephone : (213) 826-3574 Local calls. All other areas, collect.

PART I - TO BE COMPLETED BY EMPLOYEE

1. Patient Name **Mary Clark**

2. Relationship to employee: Self / Spouse / Child / Other — X (Spouse)

3. sex M, F — X (F)

4. Patient Birthdate Mo **4** Day **8** Year **35**

5. If full time student — School ___ City ___

6. Employee Name: First **Thomas** Middle **B.** Last **Clark**

7. Employee Social Security No. **545-33-9783**

8. Employee Mailing Address **3285 Artesia Blvd.**

City, State, Zip **Los Angeles, Calif. 90532**

10. Employer (Company) Name **CITY OF LOS ANGELES**

12. Location (Local) ___

13. Are other family members employed? ☐ Yes ☒ No — If yes, Employee Name ___ Soc. Sec. No. ___

14. Name and Address of Employer in Item 13 ___

15. Is Patient Covered ☐ Yes ☒ No by another Dental Plan? If yes, Dental Plan name ___ Union Local ___ Group No. ___ Name and Address of Carrier ___

AUTHORIZATION TO RELEASE INFORMATION — I hereby authorize any Dentist, Physician, Hospital, Insurance Company, Organization, or Employer to release any information to the Connecticut General Life Insurance Company, for any oral or dental observation, treatment, services or benefits rendered or payable to me or on my behalf. A photostat of this authorization shall be valid as the original.

SIGNED (PATIENT OR PARENT IF MINOR) *Mary Clark* DATE **1-9-78**

AUTHORIZATION TO PAY BENEFITS TO DENTIST — I hereby authorize payment directly to the below named Dentist of the Group Insurance Benefits otherwise payable to me.

SIGNED (INSURED PERSON) *Thomas B. Clark* DATE **1-8-78**

PART II - TO BE COMPLETED BY ATTENDING DENTIST

16. Dentist Name **John Doe, D.D.S.**

17. Mailing Address **23058 Western Ave.**

City, State, Zip **Los Angeles, Calif. 90534**

18. Dentist Soc. Sec. or T.I.N. **389-67-5249**

19. Dentist License No. **13245**

20. Dentist Phone No. **371-5200**

21. First visit date current series **1-9-78**

22. Place of treatment: Office **X** / Hosp / ECF / Other

23. Radiographs or Models enclosed: No ___ Yes **X** / How Many **FM**

24. Is treatment result of occupational illness or injury? No **X** Yes ___

25. Is treatment result of auto accident? No **X**

26. Other accident? No **X**

27. Are any services covered by another plan? No **X**

28. If Prosthesis, is this initial placement? No **X** — If no, reason for replacement **Worn out**

29. Date of prior placement **1969**

30. Is treatment for Orthodontics? No **X** — If services already commenced, enter Date appliances placed: ___ Mos. treatment remaining: ___

CHECK ONE: ☐ DENTIST'S PRETREATMENT ESTIMATE ☒ DENTIST'S STATEMENT OF ACTUAL SERVICES

Identify Missing Teeth With "X"

FACIAL / LINGUAL / UPPER / LOWER / RIGHT / LEFT / PERMANENT / PRIMARY / FACIAL

31. Examination and treatment plan-list in order from tooth No. 1 through tooth No. 32-use charting shown

Tooth # or Letter	Surface (i.e., M,O, D,B,L,A,I)	DESCRIPTION OF SERVICE (including X-rays, prophylaxis, materials used, etc.)	Date Service Performed Mo	Day	Year	Procedure Number	FEE	For Carrier Use Only See Reverse For Reason Explanation	R E A S O N	C O D E
3	All	Full gold crown	2	4	78	6790	155:00			
4		Porcelain w metal	2	4	78	6240	165:00			
5	All	Porcelain w metal	2	4	78	6750	170:00			
12	DO	Amalgam	2	21	78	2150	20:00			
13	MOD	Amalgam	2	21	78	2160	25:00			
19	MOD	Amalgam	3	5	78	2160	25:00			
19		Pulp Cap	3	5	78	3110	10:00			
24	F	Composite resin	3	12	78	2330	18:00			
28	L	Amalgam	3	19	78	2140	10:00			
30		Tri-rooted canal	3	19	78	3330	185:00			
30	All	Full gold crown	4	15	78	6790	155:00			

32. Remarks for unusual services

I hereby certify that the procedures as indicated by date have been completed.

SIGNED (DENTIST) *John Doe, D.D.S.* Date **4-16-78**

TOTAL FEE CHARGED **938:00**

MAXIMUM ALLOWABLE ___

Please Note: Pretreatment Review is not a guarantee of benefits payable.

This estimate advises you in advance of the amount of insurance benefits payable if the described procedures are performed during a period of the patient's eligibility.

Form Approved by Council on Dental Care Programs of the A.D.A. 1975   ADS (75)   CL 1928   REV. 10/77   CAT. # 214106

Reprinted by permission of Connecticut General Life Insurance Company.

indicating the surface involved as well as the description of the dental work to be performed. You use the following for identification:

1. Permanent teeth are identified by using the numbers *1* through *32*.
2. Primary teeth are identified by using the letters *A* through *I*.
3. Surface areas are identified by using the appropriate terms, such as *mesial, distal, occlusal,* and *incisal.*

Description of services and procedure codes   The description of services is illustrated in the sample of the ADA form at the end of this section. The procedure code numbers to be used are shown on the back of many of the forms supplied by the individual insurance companies. However, labor and trade unions require that you use their codes exclusively. (When no codes are provided on the form, you should use the ADA code numbers.)

Filing of the dental insurance forms   Due to the special requirements of dental insurance, it is to your advantage to retain the preauthorization in the patient's chart after you have received it from the insurance company with the work authorization. The dentist must refer to the form during the course of treatment. The claim cannot be submitted for payment until the work has been completed. The dentist can also note on the form any necessary changes in the original diagnosis. After the work has been completed and the claim submitted, the duplicate form can be placed in an alphabetical file for completed forms.

Fees   The dentist should always list the usual, customary, and reasonable (UCR) fee on the treatment form regardless of the insurance company's method of payment (such as a fixed fee schedule or UCR).

10.8

REQUESTS FOR MEDICAL HISTORIES: Routines and Legal Precautions

MEDICAL ETHICS

The Judicial Council of the American Medical Association under the direction and with the approval of the AMA House of Delegates has prepared a booklet entitled *Judicial Council Opinions and Reports.* This booklet is a compilation of interpretations, opinions, and statements concerning medical ethics and is used as a guide by physicians in these matters. It also reflects legal opinions and is revised from time to time to incorporate the decisions made by the judicial system that are relevant to medicine. In section 5.62 of *Judicial Council Opinions and Reports,* the Council has this to say about patient confidentiality with respect to the release of information:

Medical notes made by a physician in private practice are for his own use in treating a patient and belong to him. With the patient's consent, the record may be examined by an attorney, another physician engaged by the patient, or other party, but the patient has no legal right to its possession or ownership . . . the patient . . . has certain legal rights to the information contained in the record about the patient's diagnosis and treatment. The record is a confidential document involving the physician-patient relationship and should not be communicated to a third party without the patient's prior written consent, unless it is required by law or is necessary to protect the welfare of the individual or the community. Medical reports should not be witheld because of an unpaid bill for medical services. Simplified, routine forms can be prepared without charge, but a charge for more complex, complicated reports may be made in conformity with local custom.

The Judicial Council in section 5.61 of *Judicial Council Opinions and Reports* elaborates on releasing the patients' records to other physicians by stating that "it is unethical for a physician, who formerly treated a patient, to refuse for any reason to make his records of that patient promptly available on request to another physician presently treating the patient." However, the manner of transmitting the patient's record is left to the discretion of the physician.

PRIVATE INSURANCE COMPANIES
Patients frequently apply for new or additional coverage for which insurance companies require the clients' past medical histories. Medical offices receive these requests in varying ways. For example, the insurance company may employ a photocopy company to secure the information. A representative of the photocopy company may telephone or may suddenly appear in the office, requesting that he or she be allowed to copy certain patient records. Most often, however, these requests are mailed to the medical office. The company asks that a form be completed in which past treatment of the patient is given. The request may be for information regarding a specific condition, as well as for laboratory test results. As a general rule, the company is primarily interested in treatment administered or conditions occurring in the preceding five years; however, the request sometimes may be for data regarding all past and present conditions and treatment. It is customary for a physician to bill the insurance company for providing such services.

An insurance company processing a claim for medical bills may also initiate a request for additional information, either for data on the current treatment or for data on any past treatment that might have a bearing on the claim being submitted. This second request should present no problem since the physician's office will have obtained the necessary permission to release the information prior to filing the claim. (The section on insurance claims deals with this type of release.) It is customary for a physician to bill the insurance company if the client is not a patient of the physician for the condition being examined.

GOVERNMENT AGENCIES
The Federal Insurance Contribution Act (FICA) makes it possible for disabled persons to apply for disability compensation. In order to establish the beginning date and the severity of the disability, the Social Security Administration needs the patient's past medical history. A formal request is mailed to the physician's office along with a properly executed form for releasing this information.

Medicare, Medicaid, and Medicare/Medicaid fiscal intermediaries often require additional information to evaluate a claim. The Medicare Request for Medicare Payment incorporates this release in the statement that the patient signs when submitting the claim. Title XXII is the federal enabling statute for Medicaid with regard to fiscal intermediaries. It provides for the release of any information necessary in the processing of these claims.

A RELEASE-OF-INFORMATION DOCUMENT AND THE INFORMATION REQUESTED
Care must be exercised so as not to violate the confidentiality of the patient's medical record. Unauthorized release of a patient's medical record constitutes invasion of privacy. A request for medical information must always be accompanied by a valid release-of-information document. The four items constituting a valid release are discussed in the next few paragraphs.

Current release: no alterations The date on the release should not exceed six months prior to the date of receipt of the release by the physician's office. Inspect the document for alterations: there should be none. Return the request for information to the insurance company and ask that the company secure a new release from the patient if it exceeds six months' time and/or if alterations appear to have been made on it.

Signature(s)   The release must bear the signature of the patient. In the case of a minor or a legally incompetent adult, the release is to be signed by the patient's parent or legal guardian. A signature of the patient or of the patient's parent and/or guardian should be kept on file in the physician's office for checking the authenticity of these individuals' signatures on important documents. This procedure is an added safeguard both for the patient and for the physician.

An insurance company will sometimes secure the signature of only one spouse when writing a family policy. This release is valid only for the person signing the document and for any minor children. An additional release bearing the complete and proper signature will then be necessary since *only the patient* can release medical records.

Original and photostatic copy   The release must always be an original unless it bears the following kind of statement: "A photostatic copy of this release (authorization) shall be as valid as the original." Photostatic copies not bearing this or a similar statement are to be returned to the insurance company either for the original or for a new document with the required statement included in it.

Sample Release

I, the undersigned, hereby authorize and request any person to whom this is presented to furnish to a representative of _____ (insurance company's name) _____ any information or copies of any records concerning me or my dependents that such representative may desire and to permit him to read such records and copy any data he may require. A photostatic copy of this authorization shall be considered as effective and valid as the original.

Date _____   Insured's signature _____

Patient's signature _____

Information requested   Inspect the document to be completed for inclusion of the specific information that has been requested. Supply only the information that is requested on the form and that has been authorized for release by the patient. Remember that the patient also has the right to limit the release-of-information authorization to a specific time, condition, or accident.

METHODS OF RESPONSE

Telephone dictation   The company may attach instructions for dialing a toll-free number for the telephone dictation of the requested information. Assist the physician by preparing the information in the appropriate format ahead of time. This will enable the physician to make the call and dictate the data without too much interruption of the office schedule.

Typed information   The information also may be dictated by the physician as a narrative report or as fill-ins to be typed on the form supplied by the insurance company. A medical assistant having the capability to extract the necessary information is a valuable asset to the physician. However, this task is to be done only with the approval of the physician. The physician's personal signature is required by the insurance company and he or she should check the extracted data before signing the document.

Photostatic copy   It is also permissible to photocopy the information directly from the record. However, great care must be exercised so that irrelevant or unauthorized information is not inadvertently included. On the other hand, blocking out irrelevant information could give the appearance that vital data are being withheld. Thus, the alternate methods of response already given in the preceding paragraphs are preferable especially if there is a chance that irrelevant or unnecessary information might be included during photocopying.

The photocopy company requesting permission to copy records will bring its own equipment to be set up in the physician's office. Ask the company representative to make a definite appointment since the physician will want to review the chart beforehand. Also, the release must be inspected by the doctor before any copying can be done. In the event that space availability and patient scheduling would interfere with the office routine, the medical office itself may wish to copy the record and mail the material to the company. Establish the procedure to be followed and inform the company of it in the very beginning.

EXCEPTIONS
The two notable areas where exceptions are to be made when releasing information to private insurance companies are as follows: workers' compensation cases and Social Security Administration examinations or reports.

Workers' compensation   Treatment for work-related illness or injury is covered by workers' compensation insurance and is regulated by the legislature in each state. The history of and the treatment for these conditions are confidential to the employer, the insurance carrier, any other physicians treating the patient for the same condition, appeals boards, and the courts when the records are subpoenaed. The patient's release is tacit for these purposes when he or she is treated for a work injury. Requests from other agencies regarding such treatment are referred to the employer's insurance carrier.

Social Security Administration (SSA)   In order for the SSA to verify a disability and to establish a beginning date of eligibility, the agency will often require the attending physician to examine the applicant and submit a written report of the findings of that examination. However, the SSA may not need a recent examination and may only request a report of a past treatment. These findings and reports are confidential to the SSA. The SSA will send to the physician a form that has been signed by the patient/applicant to authorize the release of the information. Frequently, a report of an examination performed by another physician at the request of the SSA will be received by the attending physician. This copy will be marked "Confidential" and may not be released to other agencies without the written permission of the SSA.

RESPONSIBILITY TO RESPOND
One of the physician's responsibilities to the patient is to respond to requests by the patient for medical information. Statutes in some states set a time limit for such responses. In the absence of state laws regarding this, 10 days is considered a reasonable length of time for the doctor to respond to these requests. Suits have been brought against physicians for failure to comply with information requests made by patients. Lack of necessary information has been cited as a cause of denying insurance coverage in some instances. The following incident exemplifies this situation. A treating physician was held liable for damages resulting from his neglecting to fill out an insurance form, according to a Delaware trial court ruling. In this particular case, the patient had applied for health insurance following treatment

by her physician. A short form seeking information concerning the treatment was sent to the physician. The physician's long delay in completing the form resulted in the insurance policy's not being issued. The patient and her husband then sought to recover damages for the medical expenses that they had incurred during the interval when they had no medical insurance. The court held that filling out medical insurance forms is one of the duties owed to a patient by an attending physician. However, the court dismissed charges that the physician had interfered with contractual relations and had engaged in fraudulent practices because it was not shown that he had intentionally failed to fill out the form. The court did rule that he could be held liable for negligently causing the losses sustained if a physician-patient relationship could be proven in subsequent proceedings. [*Murphy v. Godwin*, 303 A. 2d 668 (Del. Super. Ct., Feb. 15, 1973)]

FEES
The physician is entitled to receive a fee for supplying reports or photocopies to an insurance company. The insurance company may attach instructions to its request for information that indicate how the payment will be made. The payment or the data regarding payment may be in the form of (1) a check attached to the request (2) a voucher on which the physician is to enter the charge, or (3) a statement that the physician is to bill the company for a reasonable fee. When no provision for reinbursement has been indicated by the company, a statement that is consistent with the complexity of the report may be rendered to the company by the doctor. Some physicians require that payment be made prior to their performing the service. This policy should be communicated to the insurance company as soon as such a request is received in the office. A form letter outlining the physician's fee policy can be written and used consistently. See Chapter 15, section 15.9.

CHART NOTATIONS: Permanent Record
Make a dated notation on the patient's chart to indicate the information that has been submitted when you forward photocopies of a record to an insurance company. A copy of a narrative report or information submitted on the company's form is also placed in the chart.

MEDICAL INFORMATION BUREAU (MIB)
Because of the importance of medical record confidentiality especially with the advent of computerization and subsequent widespread concern about computerized data access and information sharing, it is felt that you as a medical assistant should know something about the Medical Information Bureau (MIB) and its relationship vis-à-vis insurance companies and their clients who are, of course, your employer's patients. Of equal importance to the medical assistant is the fact that a patient may request data on himself or herself from the MIB. These data will be sent by the MIB to the patient's private doctor for explanation and interpretation. As a medical assistant, you may deal with MIB data, and you may be questioned by a patient regarding the functions of the MIB and its security arrangements for protecting patient record confidentiality.

The MIB is a nonprofit organization started in 1890, with its insurance company members sharing its information. The group was reorganized in 1902 under the control of the medical directors (licensed physicians) of the member companies. In 1947, it was again restructured—this time into a separate entity—but with the medical directors retaining a key role in its operations. Computerization of the MIB was accomplished in 1970. The data now contained in its computer bank are available for the exclusive use of the life insurance companies in the United States and Canada comprising its current membership.

Why is the MIB useful? Insurance companies often need MIB data (1) to determine the risk potential of a prospective policyholder (2) to help determine the amount of the premium on a particular individual's policy, and (3) to decide whether or not a policy should be issued in the first place.

Many patients worry about the confidentiality of computer-stored medical records. If you are queried with respect to the MIB record security safeguards, you can tell the patient or patients the following:

1. MIB data are *not* routinely disseminated among its member companies. Only authorized queries stemming from legitimate applications are accepted.
2. The medical director of each member company is directly responsible for the company's proper use of MIB data.
3. The MIB does *not* store complete medical records of patients nor does it store company files on patients; rather, the highlights of the records are recorded and encoded into three digits, the meanings of which are strictly confidential and are not available to insurance sales people.
4. Decisions made by companies regarding applicants (e.g., decisions as to whether or not policies should be approved) are not recorded by the MIB.
5. There is no interface between the MIB computers and outside computers.
6. Medical data are destroyed seven years after original input into the MIB system.

It is also important to know that applicant authorization must be obtained by a company prior to requesting data from MIB on the applicant. Applicants for insurance have the right to examine all information on themselves that is contained in the MIB bank. This information, as mentioned earlier, is sent by the MIB to the applicant's private physician for interpretation and explanation. If the physician, the applicant, or the company discovers an error in a record, the MIB will correct it.

With these points in mind, the medical assistant should be able to reassure any patient who is worried about the security of his or her medical records within the MIB system. A detailed treatment of this topic may be found in the 29 September 1975 issue of the *Journal of the American Medical Association.* The article, entitled "Medical Information Bureau," is written by Paul S. Entmacher, MD, and is found on pages 1370–1372.

AVAILABILITY OF INFORMATION TO OTHER PHYSICIANS

Patients frequently change physicians or see other physicians for a variety of reasons. When this occurs and the new physician of choice sends your physician's office a properly executed authorization for the release of the patient's records, your physician should promptly make the records available to the attending physician. This may be accomplished by permitting a personal inspection of the records, by preparing an oral report, or by writing a summary of the records. In some instances it might be appropriate for the former physician to *lend* the complete record to the new attending physician. It is important for the medical assistant to remember to make a record of where the chart is being sent and to make sure that it has been returned after a reasonable length of time.

10.9

HEALTH INSURANCE: Questions and Answers

Many of the questions about health insurance that are often asked of the medical assistant can be anticipated by use of a preprinted information sheet detailing the procedures to be followed by patients when they submit insurance forms to the physician's office. Some of the patients' questions may seem silly, unnecessary, and repetitive. However, if the patients do not understand what is to be done, then they will ask questions. At all times their queries deserve accurate and courteous replies. If you do not know the answer to a question, you can say so. Saying "I don't know the answer but I will find out for you," is much better than giving incorrect information to the patient. Bear in mind also that some questions are loaded; these should be referred to the appropriate insurance company for the correct answer.

The following are typical questions you can expect from the physician's patients. Guidelines for answering them are given below the questions.

1. **Here is my policy; how much will the insurance pay?**
   No matter how helpful you might wish to be, it is inadvisable for you to attempt to interpret a policy. A misinterpretation can backfire and can cause misunderstandings and possibly the loss of a patient for the physician. Policy interpretation queries should be referred to the agent who sold the policy. You can tactfully and courteously point out to the patient the need for such referral. However, this is not to say that you cannot be helpful enough to find a specific procedure on a fee schedule spelling out the exact amount of the coverage.

2. **Where can I get "good" medical insurance?**
   It is inadvisable to recommend a specific company for underwriting insurance policies. If the patient later should become dissatisfied with the payment received, the medical assistant could be blamed for recommending the company. Therefore, it is far better to tell the patient that no matter which company is selected, the agent should explain the coverage satisfactorily. Tell the patient to be sure that the agent explains what *full coverage* means within the limitations of the particular policy. The term *full coverage* is the most often misunderstood matter so far as patients are concerned. To patients, *full coverage* means that the insurance company pays all charges; however, to insurance companies, it means that they will pay a certain amount for each covered procedure.

3. **Why haven't I received payment from my insurance company? When did you submit the insurance form?**
   Even though you have no way of knowing what has delayed the payment of a claim, you will be asked about it when payment is not received as soon as a patient expects. There are two ways of handling the situation. If the responsibility for submitting claims has been placed with the patient, then you can suggest that the patient either call or write the insurance company and request that a tracer be placed on the claim. If your office files the claims and accepts responsibility for follow-up procedures regarding outstanding claims, then you can tell the patient that you will try to find out the reason(s) for the delay and that you will let the patient know what you have learned. (In the latter case, checking the duplicate form or the insurance submission notation made on the account card will readily give you the date of submission for the claim.)

4. **Will you please include my spouse's (or some other relative's) calls on my claim so that the insurance will pay more?**
   If you do this it will be a fraudulent claim and the physician could be prosecuted. You <u>must</u> tell the patient that this simply <u>cannot</u> be done under any circumstances. Although this request is seldom made, it will be heard once in a while; therefore, you should be alert so as not to compromise the physician.

5. **What does it mean when I sign the assignment on the insurance form?**
   Or: you accepted an assignment on my insurance, so why did I get a bill? The

answer to these two questions is the same. Patients often have misconceptions about their liability when they assign benefits to the physician. You should explain in advance that the assignment of benefits means that the insurance company will send the check to the physician for the amount that represents the company's coverage of the claim. You should also explain that the patient will receive billing from the physician for the full amount of the fee until the insurance payment has been received or until the bill has been paid in full by the patient. You should add, of course, that the patient is expected to remit what the insurance company did not pay.

6. **I paid my bill and submitted it to Medicare because you don't accept assignments. Why did they pay so little on my claim? What do they mean by** *disallowed?*
Even though Medicare patients receive a booklet detailing what the coverage will be, they often do not understand the material, or they do not take the time to read the booklet in the first place. Others simply cannot read the booklet because of failing eyesight. You should have the physicians' *Guide* for Medicare on hand, and you should be knowledgeable regarding the coverage. You ought to be able to explain that there is a deductible and that the insurance company (i.e., the fiscal intermediary) pays claims as directed by federal regulations. You should also become familiar with the *Explanation of Medicare Benefits (EOMB)* so that you can point out to the patient those instances when certain amounts were not paid because of their having been disallowed. Point out that *disallowed* means that the particular amount or service is not a covered item for Medicare. However, you should add that the term *disallowed* does not mean that an unpaid service was deemed medically inappropriate or unnecessary.

7. **If you don't accept assignments for Medicare, how do I get the needed forms and how do I submit my claim?**
The office may elect to stock the Request for Medicare Payment forms for the convenience of the patients. If so, offer the form and then indicate the portion to be completed by the patient. Tell the patient to be sure to attach the itemized statement to the form and then mail it to the company processing the claims in the area. Remember—when this claim submission method is used, the statement must be completely itemized and must have the diagnosis entered on it. Offices that do not stock the Medicare form will have to refer the patient to the insurance company or to the local Social Security Administration office to secure the form. Once a claim has been submitted and processed, the patient will receive another form to use when the check for the claim is mailed to him or her.

8. **I have other insurance to cover what Medicare does not pay. How do I submit a claim for that?**
This patient needs to be advised that the form for other insurance must not be submitted until after Medicare has paid its coverage. In some instances, the supplemental coverage company will pay the claim upon the receipt of its own form with the *EOMB* attached. However, others require that the physician complete the insurance form and attach the *EOMB* as well.

9. **Will you please explain what the difference is when the doctor does not accept assignment and when the doctor does accept assignment for Medicare?**
Assignment means that the doctor accepts the determination of the fee made by the fiscal intermediary as the total physician charge. However, *assignment* does not mean that the patient does not have to pay part of the bill. You must explain that patients are still expected to pay the deductibles and the 20% that Medicare

does not pay. Disallowed procedures that are not covered by Medicare in any way are also the patient's responsibility. For example, routine Papanicolau smears are not covered. General physicals without a diagnosis are also not covered, but elderly patients rarely have this kind of physical without a diagnosis. *Billing without assignment* means that the patient is liable for the entire bill regardless of what Medicare determines to be "allowable." You must point out to the patient that just because a procedure has been disallowed, it does not mean that the procedure was medically unnecessary. *Disallowed* is the term used by the fiscal intermediaries for those amounts or procedures not covered by Medicare (see also question 6).

10. When and where can I sign up for Medicare coverage?
Since this is a complex process, you should refer the patient to the nearest Social Security Administration office for complete details.

11. What is included in a general physical examination?
One of the questions most frequently asked concerns a general physical examination. Since many insurance companies write their policies to include the performance of an annual physical, the patient is anxious to know what is included in the examination and just how much the insurance will cover. A general physical differs from office to office, depending on the type of practice. It also varies for other reasons: How recently has the patient been seen? Is the patient new or established? What does the physician recommend? What does the patient elect to have done during the examination? A basic physical includes a review of the patient's family medical history, a review of the patient's medical history and a review of all systems. A review of all systems includes an examination of the heart with an electrocardiogram; of the lungs with a PA and lateral chest X ray; of the extremities; and of the eyes, ears, nose, and throat. Neurological, abdominal, and rectal examinations are also performed in a systems review. Special attention may be given to any symptoms described by the patient. Additionally, women have pelvic examinations with Papanicolau smears. Some physicians routinely perform the more thorough rectal examination—proctosigmoidoscopy. Basic laboratory work includes urinalysis, a complete blood count, or a basic health panel including several tests. Any other tests done would be those indicated by the individual patient's history and symptoms.

10.10

PHYSICIANS' INSURANCE

The Medical Assistant/Administrative should be aware of the several types of insurance which physicians and other health professionals usually carry. A prime responsibility of the assistant may be to see that the premiums are paid on time, since lapses in premium payment can result in the cessation of coverage—a situation that could have serious consequences. It is therefore a good idea to keep a tickler file of premium due dates if the task of paying insurance premiums has been delegated to the assistant. The following section gives a very brief summary of the various kinds of insurance coverage most often purchased by physicians today.

LIFE INSURANCE
Life insurance provides protection for the policyholder's family, and it can provide coverage for mortgages and other debts or obligations in the event of the policyholder's death. The amount of protection is determined by the individual policyholder. Physicians usually have available to them group term insurance—at times in large amounts. This insurance may be obtained through their professional societies. Term life insurance protects the policyholder against short-term obligations such as the education of children and may be held for varying periods of time (such as 10 or 12 years). Life insurance is also useful when physicians are involved with one or more other persons in partnerships or corporations. In a partnership or corporation, the death of one partner or associate can result in a joint financial loss; this type of loss can be prevented through the purchase of life insurance. Insurance can also be used to buy out the interest of a deceased partner, to reorganize the practice, to replace the services of a deceased partner, and, if necessary, to reestablish credit status.

DISABILITY INSURANCE
Physicians, and particularly surgeons, can become partially, totally, or permanently disabled from earning an income as a result of an accident or illness. Therefore, protection is usually sought by the purchase of disability or loss of income insurance. While the amount of protection is contingent on the income level of the individual, it nevertheless should include consideration of the overhead costs of maintaining the office during the period of disability. Group disability insurance for physicians can be purchased through the American Medical Association, through many state or county medical societies, or through many of the speciality societies.

HEALTH INSURANCE
Physicians and their families have traditionally received medical care without charge. Recently, however, hospitals have been discontinuing this practice. Depending on the circumstances in their communities, physicians can consider health insurance and particularly major medical expense insurance protection.

ANNUITIES
Physicians planning for their retirement income sometimes purchase annuities. *Webster's Third New International Dictionary* defines *annuity* as "an amount payable yearly or at other regular intervals (as quarterly) for a certain or uncertain period (as for years, for life, or in perpetuity)." To the extent that their practices or their savings and investments will not provide for an adequate retirement income, physicians as well as other health professionals often provide such protection for themselves by purchasing annuities to supplement their Social Security benefits.

WORKERS' COMPENSATION
Physicians and other health professionals must carry workers' compensation insurance according to the laws of the states in which they practice. Since individual state requirements differ, the physician should therefore determine whether he or she is required to carry this insurance for those employed by the practice. If workers' compensation is optional or voluntary in a state, the physician located there must decide whether or not to purchase the insurance or to be subjected to the possibility of employers' liability suits. The former course of action is, of course, advisable.

PUBLIC LIABILITY INSURANCE
A physician's place of practice, as with any other place of business or residence, can be subject to public liability suits for personal injury on the premises or on the

adjacent property (as outside steps, parking lots, and sidewalks). The amount of insurance is determined usually by the attitudes of the courts in the geographical location of the practice, the socioeconomic level of the particular area, and the income and financial resources of the physician—all of which can affect the amounts involved in potential suits.

FIRE AND THEFT INSURANCE
As with any business or residence, a physician's office is liable to the hazards of fire and theft. In fact, the vast majority of physicians' offices are subject particularly to theft because of the customary presence of expensive equipment and drugs there. Insurance is thus essential to protect the physician against such potential losses. The amount of insurance is determined by the value of the premises, by the worth of the supplies and equipment kept there, and by the amount of the financial loss which would result from theft or destruction or the loss of occupancy of the premises and the use of the equipment.

AUTOMOBILE INSURANCE
Most physicians require automobiles in the conduct of their practices. They are subject both to public liability suits and to property damage suits should an accident occur. Thus, insurance is carried to cover these liabilities.

PROFESSIONAL LIABILITY INSURANCE
The matter of professional liability has been discussed from the legal standpoint in Chapter 3, and in Chapter 9 the importance of maintaining clear and complete records has been discussed from the viewpoint of medical record administration. Both liability and the importance of accurate records management come into play with respect to professional liability insurance. Today, professional liability is a matter of great concern. Insurance protection against such liability is necessary, and, because of the adverse court decisions that have been handed down, this insurance is becoming more costly and difficult to obtain. Malpractice suits have attracted increasing publicity and have become more frequent.

Professional liability insurance has traditionally been made available to the medical profession by the insurance companies. Doctors as well as hospitals and other health care facilities have been so covered. Recently, however, the cost of this insurance—reflecting the awards handed down by a great many courts in malpractice litigation—has risen drastically. One consequence is that many insurance companies have stopped writing professional liability insurance, and some doctors have had to resort to boycotts as well as to dropping this insurance completely. This situation has led some state and county medical societies to make professional liability insurance available to physicians on a self-insurance basis. By 1977, there were 15 physician-owned medical liability insurance companies in existence. The cost of professional liability insurance differs according to factors such as the geographical location of the physician's practice, the size of the practice, and the nature of the specialty or specialties (if any).

The medical assistant should find out from the physician whether the assistant's name is included in the physician's medical professional liability insurance policy. If it is not, the assistant could be sued as an individual. Medical assistants as agents of physicians should be covered in the physician's policy.

Insurance record-keeping for the doctor   Your physician may ask you to assist in keeping his or her insurance current. One easy way of doing this is to set up an insurance card file containing a 5 × 8 card for each policy. The data to be inserted on each card are as follows:

the physician's name (if in a group practice)
the title of the policy
the policy number
the type of insurance coverage
the name of the insurance carrier
the carrier's address + the telephone number
the name of the agent + the telephone number
the dollar value of the policy
the effective date of the policy
the expiration date of the policy
the renewal date of the policy
the amount of the annual premium
the dates and amounts of all premium payments
the name of the beneficiary

It is wise to use pencil when inserting the above data on the cards, for mistakes can occur and changes sometimes must be made. If you need more space, you can staple a blank card to the face card for this purpose.

PUBLICATIONS
Additional information on health insurance can be obtained by writing to the following places:

Health Insurance Institute
1850 K Street, NW
Washington, DC 20006

Source Book of Health Insurance Data

Chamber of Commerce of
the United States
1615 H Street, NW
Washington, DC 20062

Analysis of Workers' Compensation Laws

Executive Director
OCHAMPUS
Denver, CO 80240

A Guide for Physicians and Other Providers of Care under the Civilian Health and Medical Program of the Uniformed Services

FS–3 *Claim Filing Procedures Under the Basic CHAMPUS Program*

FS–4 *CHAMPUS Eligibility and Identification*

FS–5 *Effect of Medicare on CHAMPUS Benefits*

FS–9 *Reasonable Charge—An Explanation*

FS–11 *CHAMPUS Contractors*

Superintendent of
Documents
U.S. Government Printing
Office
Washington, DC 20423

Your Medicare Handbook HEW Publication No. (SSA) 77–10050

CHAMPUS Regulation DoD 6010.8–R

Parts of sections 10.7, 10.8, and 10.9 have appeared in somewhat different form in a series of articles by Lorene Euler Berman published in *The Professional Medical Assistant,* the journal of the American Association of Medical Assistants. They are used here by permission of the AAMA.

11

BOOKKEEPING AND BANKING FOR THE PHYSICIAN

CONTENTS

11.1

INTRODUCTION

IMPORTANCE OF THE MEDICAL ASSISTANT

In no field except law is the assistant's position as a financial manager so important as it is in the practice of medicine. Most medical practices do not employ specialized business people but instead rely heavily on the medical assistant to fulfill these roles. A physician wants to practice medicine, not act as a business executive and therefore needs a secretary who is able to operate bookkeeping, billing, and collection systems with a minimum of supervision. The medical assistant must be competent in all areas of business that affect the doctor's practice: bookkeeping, banking, fee charging and the extension of credit, billing, and collections. If the assistant cannot perform well in these areas, it is likely that the physician's earnings will be adversely affected.

The medical assistant must maintain clear, up-to-date financial records. This is important for the control of patients' accounts and office expenditures. It is also essential for the preparation of tax returns and insurance forms.

IMPLICATIONS OF PROFESSIONAL INCORPORATION

The impact of professional incorporation on the medical assistant is minimal because the assistant's duties and responsibilities are similar to those in nonincorporated practices. Though physicians involved in professional corporations obtain substantial tax advantages, the main advantage to the medical assistant is the possible availability of a pension plan. If the incorporating physicians set up a retirement plan for themselves, they must also include their full-time employees. Restrictions as to which employees are eligible are allowed, as, for example, length of service; however, the pension plan must meet the standards for any qualified plan as stipulated by the government. The assistant has little to do with administration of a retirement plan.

Group vs. single-physician practices   The basic record-keeping differences between group- and single-physician practices lie in the complexity of the bookkeeping system. In a single-physician practice, there is no concern about a division of income. A group practice, on the other hand, involves several doctors who treat different patients or who share the treatment of the same patients. As a result, the division of net income must be agreed on and adequate records must be maintained.

The medical assistant in a group practice must be able to handle records for the group as an entity as well as for the individual doctors.

11.2

BOOKKEEPING SYSTEMS AND PROCEDURES

TYPES OF FINANCIAL RECORDS

The types of records kept by physicians are not specified by law. However, those records that are kept must be systematic, in that they must reflect accurately and permanently all transactions that occur. The records are kept not only for the physician's personal use, but also for the Internal Revenue Service and other government agencies. Under current income tax law, mere estimates of income, deductions, and other pertinent tax information are not acceptable, a fact which again emphasizes the need for accurate record-keeping.

Satisfactory records should be maintained for both practice-related and outside income. Though outside income may be secured from a variety of sources, physicians have had particular problems with keeping track of investment income and speaking and writing fees. A concerted effort must be made to record these items properly in order to avoid difficulty with tax agents.

Although there are a multitude of bookkeeping systems to choose from, they must all contain the following basic elements:

1. A daily record of charges (income) and payments (expenses).
2. A record of accounts receivable (amounts owed to a doctor by patients) that must be updated on a daily basis. This record is essential for accurate billing and collection of patients' charges.
3. A detailed breakdown of receipts and disbursements. This information is secured from the daily records for practice-related receipts and disbursements. In addition, the records may include outside income and expenses. These records are ongoing for a specific tax year and tax returns are prepared from them.
4. A patient's ledger card that is kept separate from the patient's medical records and represents a chronological history of the patient's account. All ledger cards should be updated daily to reflect the current position of the accounts.
5. Individual payroll records for employees. These records are essential for the proper withholding of taxes and for filing payroll tax forms.
6. A petty cash fund to record small expenditures.

COMMON BOOKKEEPING SYSTEMS USED IN MEDICAL OFFICES

Single-entry system   A single-entry bookkeeping system is one of the simpler methods for keeping records in a medical practice. It embodies all the essential elements for the physician's personal fiscal needs as well as for tax returns without employing the more complex records of the traditional double-entry system. Although no one system can meet the requirements of all medical practices, a good single-entry system includes the following:

1. **A daily log, also known as a day or appointment book or a charge journal**   The daily log should make provision for amounts received from or charged to specific patients and the treatment rendered. At the end of the day, the money columns are totaled and carried forward to the monthly summary of income, the business summary. It is important that all charges to or cash received from patients, including house calls and amounts received through the mail, be entered in the daily log. It may be necessary to set up a special system with the doctor(s) involved to ensure that all house calls are properly recorded. It is not necessary to enter charges or receipts on the patients' ledger cards immediately. However, when an entry is made to the appropriate card, a check mark should be placed in the daily log to show that the entry has been posted to the individual's card.

2. **A monthly summary of all practice-related income, known as a business summary**   The amounts entered are the totals from the individual daily logs. Any receipts (or disbursements) from outside sources are entered on a separate monthly personal account.

3. **A monthly summary of practice-related disbursements called an expense sheet**   The information needed for the specific types of expenditures can be taken directly from the checkbook and entered into this record when convenient.

4. **An annual summary of expenses**   The information for this report is obtained from the expense sheets. After totaling all columns on the expense sheets, the amounts are carried over to the summary.

5. **An annual summary of all income and expenses**   This report summarizes all information that is needed for the physician's tax returns.

Double-entry system   Double-entry bookkeeping is the method of keeping records used by most businesses, including medical practices. It is based on the fundamental accounting equation:

$$\text{Assets} \ = \ \text{Liabilities} \ + \ \text{Owner's Equity}$$

This means that the left side of the equation, assets (that which is owned), equals the right side of the equation, liabilities (that which is owed) plus owner's equity (the owner's residual interest).

In a double-entry system, the effects of a transaction are recorded in a general ledger. A general ledger is a book with a separate page for each account. Entries noted on the left side of the ledger are called *debits,* while entries entered on the right side are called *credits.* A bookkeeper posts (i.e., transfers information from one record to another) the totals from the daily log or journal to the general ledger, which is the basic reference for this bookkeeping system. The daily log or journal is a book of original entry.

At the end of a specified period of time, usually one month, a trial balance is taken to ensure that all accounts are in balance; that is, that the total of all debits equals the total of all credits. When the trial balance is balanced, a worksheet is completed that incorporates any adjustments or corrections that should be made to the accounts. From the worksheet, any desired financial statements can be produced.

The specified accounts used in the general ledger are listed on a chart of accounts. This chart is a list of accounts used by a specific medical practice or business and is normally one of the first items prepared in the development of a physician's bookkeeping system.

There are certain bookkeeping and accounting terms with which a medical assistant should be familiar. They are *current assets, fixed assets, current liabilities,* and *long-term liabilities. Current assets* are those resources that will be liquidated (turned into cash) or used in the operation of the practice within one business (operating) cycle or a twelve-month period—whichever is longer. *Fixed assets* are the physical assets that will be used in the operation of the business over a number

Patient's Ledger Card

DATE	SERVICE RENDERED	CHARGE	PAID	BALANCE
	NAME _Feathers, Mary (Mrs. John D.)_			
	ADDRESS _6 Melody Lane Jonesville, ST 12345_			
	TELEPHONE _536-1306_ INSURANCE _BCBS 6765325 hus_ REF BY _M. Korn, MD_			
3-7-78	NOB	500	100	400
4-7-78			200	200
5-7-78			200	—

FORM 5106 COLWELL CO., CHAMPAIGN, ILLINOIS

Reprinted by permission of The Colwell Company.

of business cycles. *Current liabilities* are obligations (debts) that will become due within the next business cycle. *Long-term liabilities* are obligations that will not mature within the next operating cycle.

An accountant designs the appropriate bookkeeping system for the physician and often does most of the actual bookkeeping. A medical assistant does not have the same financial knowledge as an accountant. Consequently, the assistant normally maintains only the daily log under a double-entry bookkeeping system. However, the more assistants understand about financial systems and problems, the more valuable they are to the doctors.

FACSIMILES OF BOOKKEEPING RECORDS
The next seven pages contain illustrations of typical bookkeeping records for a practice: the daily log, the business summary, the personal account, the expense sheet (including Expense Sheet One and Expense Sheet Two), the annual summary of expense, and the annual summary of all income and expenses.

Daily Log

HOUR	NAME OF PATIENT	SERVICE RENDERED	CHARGE		CASH		REC'D ON ACCOUNT		√
1	Arnold Wing	on acct					60	00	✓
2	Lester Remick	" "					10	00	✓
9:00	Mrs. Roger Curry (936 So. Elm)	emergency home visit			20	00			✓
9:30	Mrs. Mary Feathers	set fracture	100	00					✓
10:00	Charles Byrd	hospital	20	00					✓
10:15	Mrs. Cecil Dean	"	10	00					✓
10:30	Betty Witt	"	10	00					✓
11:30	John Nyberg	home - Rx	20	00					✓
11:45	M. C. Kabell	"	14	00					✓
1:30	Stan Hinton	office cons.			10	00			✓
1:50	Helen Shelby	" "	10	00			30	00	✓
2:00	Vern McBride	dressed arm	10	00					✓
2:30	Russell Steffy	change dressing	10	00					✓
2:50	Emma Finch	exam	10	00			18	00	✓
3:20	Gordon Bishop	exam - Rx			12	00			✓
3:50	Olive Smyth	office cons.	10	00					✓
4:00	Ella Loftis	treatment			10	00			✓
4:10	Luella Young	"	8	00					✓
4:25	Norm Fields	exam - Rx	14	00					✓
4:45	Marcia Austin	treatment	10	00					✓
5:00	M. V. Reynolds	"	10	00					✓
5:15	Fred Mattern	exam - inoc.	14	00					✓
7:15	Mrs. D. Steele	home - Rx	14	00					✓
26									
27									
28									
29									
30									
31									
32									
33									
34									
35									
36									
37									
38									
39									
40									
CARRY TOTALS FORWARD TO **BUSINESS SUMMARY**		TOTALS	294	00	52	00	118	00	

FORM 4201   COLWELL CO. CHAMPAIGN, ILL.

Reprinted by permission of The Colwell Company.

Business Summary

DAY OF MONTH	CHARGE BUSINESS		CASH BUSINESS		RECEIVED ON ACCOUNTS		TOTAL BUSINESS		TOTAL CASH RECEIVED	
1	166	00	20	00	10	00	186	00	30	00
2	186	00	18	00	204	00	204	00	222	00
3	124	00	8	00	234	00	132	00	242	00
4	168	00	44	00	196	00	212	00	240	00
5	154	00	40	00	210	00	194	00	250	00
6	—		—						—	
7	294	00	52	00	118	00	346	00	170	00
8	216	00	50	00	150	00	266	00	200	00
9	124	00	46	00	92	00	170	00	138	00
10	134	00	36	00	180	00	170	00	216	00
11	210	00	40	00	242	00	250	00	282	00
12	184	00	52	00	192	00	236	00	244	00
13	—		—		—		—		—	
14	174	00	36	00	184	00	210	00	220	00
15	164	00	30	00	198	00	194	00	228	00
16	142	00	32	00	272	00	174	00	304	00
17	176	00	40	00	174	00	216	00	214	00
18	166	00	48	00	210	00	214	00	258	00
19	158	00	40	00	122	00	198	00	162	00
20	10	00	—		—		10	00	—	
21	140	00	44	00	250	00	184	00	294	00
22	148	00	24	00	106	00	172	00	130	00
23	138	00	30	00	—		168	00	30	00
24	80	00	50	00	104	00	130	00	154	00
25	226	00	30	00	96	00	256	00	126	00
26	66	00	18	00	98	00	84	00	116	00
27	—		—		—		—		—	
28	150	00	14	00	170	00	164	00	184	00
29	166	00	10	00	184	00	176	00	194	00
30	84	00	8	00	96	00	92	00	104	00
31	120	00	—		136	00	120	00	136	00
TOTAL FOR THE MONTH	4,268	00	860	00	4,228	00	5,128	00	5,088	00
BROUGHT FORWARD	8,794	00	1,446	00	8,746	00	10,240	00	10,192	00
GRAND TOTAL	13,062	00	2,306	00	12,974	00	15,368	00	15,280	00

CARRY ALL **GRAND TOTALS** FORWARD TO **BUSINESS SUMMARY** OF FOLLOWING MONTH

FORM 4202A COLWELL CO. CHAMPAIGN, ILL.

Reprinted by permission of The Colwell Company.

Personal Account

Personal Account						
RECEIPTS (NON-PROFESSIONAL)			**DISBURSEMENTS** (NON-PROFESSIONAL)			
DAY	SOURCE	AMOUNT	DAY	ITEM	WITH-DRAWALS	INVEST-MENTS
2	Chet Holmes (sale of seed oats)	106 70	1	Cash – Household	130 00	
			4	W. Sangster Co.	49 70	
			4	General Ins. Co.		281 08
10	Bldg. & Loan-interest	35 00	4	Pure Milk Co.	13 40	
15	Ray Jonas (payment on note)	200 00	6	Model Laundry	15 40	
			8	Lyons Tailors	91 50	
			15	State Univ.		
21	Moore & Lovett (sale of bond)	1,005 00		– J's tuition	150 00	
			16	1st Nat'l Bank		
				– Bond		800 00
			20	Cash–Household	200 00	
			20	J's allowance	210 00	
			30	Cash	100 00	
	TOTAL FOR PRESENT MONTH	1,346 70		TOTAL FOR PRESENT MONTH	960 00	1,081 08
	FORWARDED (FROM PREVIOUS MONTH)	419 64		FORWARDED	2,722 44	530 00
	GRAND TOTAL	1,766 34		GRAND TOTAL	3,682 44	1,611 08

WITHDRAWALS AND DEPOSITS

BEGINNING CASH IN BANK . . . . $ _____

PLUS ALL DEPOSITS THIS MONTH . . . . _____

TOTAL TO BE ACCOUNTED FOR . . . . _____

LESS – OFFICE EXPENSES . . . $ _____

NON-DEDUCT. EQUIPMENT. . . _____

PERSONAL WITHDRAWALS. . . _____

END CASH IN BANK . . . . _____

ACCOUNTS RECEIVABLE

BEGINNING BALANCES, OPEN ACCOUNTS . . . . $ _____

PLUS CHARGES TO PATIENTS FOR MONTH . . _____

LESS RECEIPTS ON ACCOUNT. . $ _____

DISCOUNTS AND AMOUNTS JUDGED UNCOLLECTABLE. _____

END BALANCES, OPEN ACCOUNTS . . . . $ _____

FORM 42035 COLWELL CO., CHAMPAIGN, ILL.

Reprinted by permission of The Colwell Company.

Expense Sheet One

Expense Sheet One

DRUGS AND SUPPLIES			SALARIES			DUES, MEETINGS		
DAY	ITEM	AMOUNT	DAY	ITEM	AMOUNT	DAY	ITEM	AMOUNT
2	Lilly	27 36	2	Mary Wells	94 37	7	Washington	
3	Sargeant	15 80	9	" "	94 37		Co. Med. Soc.	50 00
4	Faulkners	37 74	16	" "	94 37			
10	Cunningham	8 44	23	" "	94 37			
23	Swandell	35 80	30	" "	94 37			
28	Abbotts	13 40						
							TOTAL	50 00
						OFFICE SUPPLIES, STAMPS ETC.		
						9	Petty Cash	47 00
						13	Colwell Co.	26 00
						15	Office Supply Co.	21 50
				TOTAL	471 85			
				OFFICE RENT, UPKEEP				
			3	Bldg. & Loan	300 00			
			6	H. Chin - painting	210 00			
	TOTAL	138 54						
	AUTOMOBILE UPKEEP							
3	Motor Club	30 00		TOTAL	510 00			
3	White Motors	15 70		LAUNDRY SERVICE				
5	Gas & Oil	25 66	3	Model Laundry	9 50			
10	" " "	66 14	16	" "	6 00		TOTAL	94 50
25	Tire	97 00	21	Acme Cleaners (draperies)	11 50		PROFESSIONAL INSURANCE	
						1	XYZ Ins. Co.	200 00
				TOTAL	27 00		TOTAL	200 00
				ELECTRICITY, GAS, WATER			BUSINESS TAXES	
			18	Power & Light	57 80		DO NOT INCLUDE WITHHOLDING TAX. INCLUDE ONLY ½ SOCIAL SECURITY TAX	
				TOTAL	57 80			
				TELEPHONES, TOLLS			TOTAL	
			13	State Bell	52 00		INTEREST PAID	
	TOTAL	234 50		TOTAL	52 00		TOTAL	

FORM 42028 COLWELL CO., CHAMPAIGN, ILL.

Expense Sheet Two

Expense Sheet Two

PROFESSIONAL INSURANCE			ENTERTAINMENT			MISCELLANEOUS		
DAY	ITEM	AMOUNT	DAY	ITEM	AMOUNT	DAY	ITEM	AMOUNT
15	Mutual Ins. Co.	127 20	4	Lunch		8	Med. Supply Co.	
				Dr. Ross	5 00		(ster. Repair)	20 00
			26	Flowers		17	Upholsterer	24 00
	TOTAL	127 20		Mrs. Gent	12 00	19	Med. Credit Bur.	16 00
	BUSINESS TAXES		26	Benefit	10 00	20	Time Mag.	12 00
8	County Collector	137 50				22	Picture Frame	6 62
	(pers. prop.)					25	Rep. Lamps	16 00
				TOTAL	27 00			
	TOTAL	137 50						
	INTEREST PAID							
	TOTAL			TOTAL			TOTAL	94 62

CARRY TOTALS FORWARD TO SUMMARY OF EXPENSE

SUMMARY OF EXPENSE	AMOUNT	MONTHLY BALANCES		
DRUGS AND SUPPLIES	138 54	FOR THE PRESENT MONTH		
AUTOMOBILE UPKEEP	234 50			
SALARIES	471 85	TOTAL CASH RECEIVED	5,088	00
OFFICE RENT, UPKEEP	510 00	TOTAL EXPENSE	2,022	51
LAUNDRY SERVICE	27 00	NET EARNINGS	3,065	49
ELECTRICITY, GAS, WATER	57 80	FOR THE YEAR TO DATE		
TELEPHONES, TOLLS	52 00			
DUES, MEETINGS	50 00	GRAND TOTAL CASH	15,280	00
OFFICE SUPPLIES, STAMPS, ETC.	94 50	GRAND TOTAL EXPENSE	5,331	99
PROFESSIONAL INSURANCE	127 20	NET EARNINGS	9,948	01
BUSINESS TAXES	137 50	EQUIPMENT (NONDEDUCTIBLE)		
INTEREST PAID				
ENTERTAINMENT	27 00	DAY	ITEM	AMOUNT
		9	Shay Furn. Co.	
			(red. room chair)	164 00
		10	Surg. Equip. Co.	196 90
MISCELLANEOUS	94 62			
TOTAL FOR PRESENT MONTH	2,022 51			
FORWARDED FROM PREVIOUS MONTH	3,309 48	* TOTAL	360	90
GRAND TOTAL	5,331 99	* ENTER THIS TOTAL DIRECT IN ANNUAL SUMMARY		

FORM 4203A COLWELL CO., CHAMPAIGN, ILL.

Reprinted by permission of The Colwell Company.

Annual Summary of Expense

Annual Summary of Expense

	DRUGS AND SUPPLIES		AUTO UPKEEP		SALARIES		OFFICE RENT UPKEEP		LAUNDRY SERVICE		ELEC GAS WATER		TELEPHONE TOLLS		DUES MEETINGS		OFFICE SUPPLIES		PROF INS	
							OFFICE OVERHEAD (DEDUCTIBLE FOR INCOME TAX)													
JAN	158	24	166	40	377	48	300	00	39	40	56	36	47	20	50	00	26	96	65	38
FEB	176	48	269	58	377	48	300	00	30	90	55	24	47	80	20	00	86	80	93	98
MAR	138	54	234	50	471	85	510	00	27	00	57	80	52	00	50	00	94	50	127	20
APR	154	88	197	62	377	48	300	00	30	24	51	90	52	80	—		68	50	—	
MAY	184	80	279	10	471	85	300	00	38	96	48	30	49	20	20	00	61	00	—	
JUN	182	46	189	20	377	48	300	00	38	70	57	90	43	80	620	00	44	44	—	
JUL	150	32	119	22	377	48	300	00	39	76	57	90	42	80	—		59	00	—	
AUG	103	64	172	46	471	85	300	00	37	44	58	70	51	78	—		50	00	—	
SEP	97	38	169	02	377	48	300	00	36	90	58	70	54	20	20	00	58	80	—	
OCT	106	52	163	80	377	48	300	00	39	70	61	90	52	80	—		41	00	110	24
NOV	117	80	284	80	471	85	300	00	40	58	61	24	56	50	410	00	50	00	—	
DEC	154	88	172	56	377	48	300	00	37	26	55	90	57	90	50	00	39	00	—	
TOT	1,725	94	2,418	26	4,907	24	3,810	00	436	84	681	84	608	78	1,240	00	680	00	396	80

	OFFICE OVERHEAD, CONTINUED								NONDEDUCTIBLE ITEMS							
	BUSINESS TAXES		INTEREST PAID		ENTERTAINMENT		MISCELLANEOUS		FEDERAL INCOME TAX		OFFICE FURN		INSTRUMENTS		BOOKS	
JAN					17	38	137	66	1,980	94	110	20				
FEB	66	00			13	60	144	52								
MAR	137	50			27	00	94	62			164	00	196	90		
APR	39	50			15	30	112	38	1,620	00						
MAY					13	44	98	84								
JUN					16	96	126	16			132	48				
JUL	39	50			13	84	92	24								
AUG					14	68	79	38					91	76		
SEP					11	20	124	08	1,620	00						
OCT	39	50			14	80	164	80								
NOV					19	20	148	22								
DEC	39	50			20	00	139	78	1,620	00						
TOT	361	50			197	40	1,460	68	6,840	94	406	68	288	66		

OTHER EXPENSE (NONDEDUCTIBLE)			OTHER EXPENSE (NONDEDUCTIBLE)			OTHER EXPENSE (NONDEDUCTIBLE)		
DATE	ITEM	AMOUNT	DATE	ITEM	AMOUNT	DATE	ITEM	AMOUNT

Reprinted by permission of The Colwell Company.

Annual Summary

					Annual Summary	
VOLUME (FROM DECEMBER GRAND TOTALS)		TOTAL CHARGE BUSINESS	56,544	00		
		TOTAL CASH BUSINESS	7,244	00		
		TOTAL BUSINESS			63,788	00
RECEIPTS (FROM DECEMBER GRAND TOTALS)		TOTAL REC'D ON ACCOUNTS	53,134	00		
		TOTAL CASH BUSINESS	7,266	00		
		TOTAL CASH FROM PROFESSION			60,400	00
DISBURSEMENTS (FROM OPPOSITE PAGE)		DRUGS AND SUPPLIES	1,725	94		
		AUTOMOBILE UPKEEP	2,418	26		
		SALARIES	4,907	24		
		OFFICE RENT UPKEEP	3,810	00		
		LAUNDRY SERVICE	436	84		
		ELECTRICITY GAS WATER	681	84		
		TELEPHONE TOLLS	608	78		
		DUES MEETINGS	1,240	00		
		OFFICE SUPPLIES STAMPS ETC.	680	00		
		PROFESSIONAL INSURANCE	396	80		
		BUSINESS TAXES	361	50		
		INTEREST PAID	—			
		ENTERTAINMENT ETC.	197	40		
		DEPRECIATION	1,526	96		
		MISCELLANEOUS	1,460	68		
		TOTAL PROFESSIONAL EXPENSE			20,452	24
		NET FROM PROFESSION			39,947	76
		DIVIDENDS, INTEREST			2,428	00
		NET FROM OTHER SOURCES			2,069	26
		TOTAL INCOME			44,445	02

OTHER EXPENSE (NONDEDUCTIBLE)		TOTALS		NON PROFESSIONAL DEDUCTIONS		TOTALS	
FEDERAL INCOME TAX (FROM OPPOSITE PAGE)		6,840	94	CONTRIBUTIONS (FROM NEXT PAGE)		1,490	00
OFFICE FURNISHINGS " "		406	68	REAL ESTATE TAX " " "		1,068	40
INSTRUMENTS " "		288	66	OTHER TAXES " " "			
BOOKS " "				*Sales Tax*		125	50
PERSONAL EXPENSE (FROM DECEMBER GRAND TOTAL)		22,601	72			420	00
INVESTMENTS " "		5,000	00	INTEREST EXPENSE " " "			
				BAD DEBTS " " "			
				LOSSES " " "			
	TOTAL	35,138	00		TOTAL	3,103	90

FORM 4230 COLWELL CO., CHAMPAIGN, ILLINOIS

Reprinted by permission of The Colwell Company.

PEGBOARD SYSTEM OF RECORD-KEEPING

Another method of maintaining records is the pegboard system, commonly referred to as the write-it-once bookkeeping system. This system is so called because, physically, it is a board with pegs down one side on which various financial forms are secured. With the help of carbon sheets, information need be written only once instead of a number of times to complete the forms.

A pegboard system features the daily log attached to the board. Shingled over the log are a series of imprinted, prenumbered, and carbonized receipt and charge slips. When a patient arrives, his or her financial ledger card is pulled. From this card, the previous balance and patient's name are entered on the charge slip. Simultaneously, the data are recorded on the daily log. The charge slip is then separated from the receipt and is given to the doctor. This procedure allows the doctor to know the patient's current financial status before the patient enters. After treatment has been rendered, the physician notes any fees on the charge slip, which is then returned to the assistant.

The patient's ledger card is then aligned under the receipt slip. The date, type of service rendered, charge, payment (if any), and new balance are posted with one writing to the receipt, the patient ledger, and the daily log. The receipt is then removed and given to the patient with a notation of the next appointment. The patient's ledger card is removed and the pegboard is ready for the next patient.

In summary, the pegboard system has some distinct advantages. It eliminates unnecessary clerical work and minimizes the possibility of errors. In addition, the patient is provided with a current statement of account, a receipt if payment is made, and a notation of the next appointment.

HANDLING PETTY CASH FUNDS

Since it is impractical to pay for small expenses by check, most practices maintain a petty cash fund for that purpose. Incidental expenses such as stamps, small quantities of office supplies, carfare, and coffee are normally paid for out of petty cash. Expenditures are made at the assistant's discretion and the physician usually gives the secretary responsibility for maintenance of the fund.

To start the fund, a check is drawn and made out to petty cash. It should be large enough to cover a specified period of time (a week or a month). The amount of the fund depends on the size of the practice and the frequency of small payments. When the check is presented at the bank, a separate sheet should indicate the breakdown of currency and coins desired. The cash is then kept in a locked box in a safe or in a drawer in the office.

Disbursements from the fund are recorded on petty cash receipts (written authorizations) or on a special expense book or sheet indicating the date, the amount, the purpose of the expenditure, and to whom the money was paid. Whenever possible, the assistant should obtain receipts or vouchers for expenditures. The receipts or book should be small enough to be kept in the box so that at all times the total of cash and expenditures equal the original amount of the fund. Cash register receipts should be attached to the petty cash receipts.

When the fund is low, the expenses are computed from the receipts or book and a check is written for this amount, restoring the cash in the fund to its starting amount. This is known as *replenishing the fund.*

KEEPING RECEIPT BOOKS

When a patient pays in cash, the assistant prepares a receipt in duplicate and gives the original to the patient. Carbon copies or stubs are used to corroborate cash entries in the daily log. The issuance of receipts assures the physician that cash is accounted for and also acts as protection for the assistant.

Reprinted by permission of The Colwell Company.

Pegboard System

Labels: Pegboard · Journal Page · Receipt & Charge Slip · Photocopy Ledger Card

DAILY LOG OF CHARGES AND RECEIPTS

DATE March 10, 1978   SHEET NO. 2 of 2

RECEIPT NUMBER	DATE	PROFESSIONAL SERVICE	A CHARGE	B PAID	C NEW BALANCE	D PREVIOUS BALANCE	NAME
						315 —	
						50 —	Mr. John Hardman
							Mrs. Pat Maple
						10 —	Carol Morrow
							Mr. Virginia Black
						35 —	Mr. Tom Granger
						15 —	Mrs. A.G. Temple
						35 —	Wm. Tarrant
							Mrs. Leo Lackey
							Roger Kaufman
1038	3/10	OC & Lab	15 00	15 00	—	—	Mrs. Patricia Maple

STATEMENT

LEONARD S. TAYLOR, M.D.
2100 WEST PARK AVENUE
CHAMPAIGN, ILLINOIS 61820

TELEPHONE 367-6671

Mrs. Patricia Maple
123 Horseshoe Lane
Wallington, ST 34567

RECEIPT NUMBER	DATE	PROFESSIONAL SERVICE	CHARGE	PAID	NEW BALANCE
1038	3/10	OC & Lab	15 00	15 00	—

YOU PAID THIS AMOUNT

LEONARD S. TAYLOR, M.D.
2100 WEST PARK AVENUE
CHAMPAIGN, ILLINOIS 61820

TELEPHONE 352-7658

OC - OFFICE CALL	INS. INSURANCE	PE PHYSICAL EXAMINATION
HC - HOUSE CALL	OB OBSTETRICAL CARE	EKG ELECTROCARDIOGRAM
HOSP - HOSPITAL CARE	PAP PAPANICOLAOU TEST	XR X-RAY
L - LABORATORY	OS OFFICE SURGERY	M MEDICATION
I - INJECTION	HS HOSPITAL SURGERY	NC NO CHARGE

NEXT APPOINTMENT 4/10/78   AT 9:30 a.m.

PROFESSIONAL SERVICE   OC & Lab
NO. 1038

	CHARGE
OFFICE CALL	10.00
LABORATORY	5.00
INJECTION	
OBSTETRICAL CARE	
OFFICE SURGERY	
PHYSICAL EXAMINATION	
ELECTROCARDIOGRAM	
X RAY	
MEDICATION	
PREVIOUS BALANCE	15.00

PAY LAST AMOUNT IN THIS COLUMN ◇

OC - OFFICE CALL	INS. INSURANCE	PE PHYSICAL EXAMINATION
HC - HOUSE CALL	OB OBSTETRICAL CARE	EKG ELECTROCARDIOGRAM
HOSP - HOSPITAL CARE	PAP PAPANICOLAOU TEST	XR X-RAY
L - LABORATORY	OS OFFICE SURGERY	M MEDICATION
I - INJECTION	HS HOSPITAL SURGERY	NC NO CHARGE

ACCOUNTS RECEIVABLE CONTROL

PREVIOUS ACCT. REC. BALANCE	4755.—
"PLUS" COLUMN A	453.—
SUB TOTAL	5308.—
"MINUS" COLUMN B	560.—
PRESENT ACCT. REC. BALANCE	4748.—

PROOF OF POSTING

COLUMN D TOTAL	988.—
"PLUS" COLUMN A TOTAL	453.—
SUB TOTAL	1441.—
"MINUS" COLUMN B TOTAL	560.—
EQUALS COLUMN C BALANCE	881.—

	Dr. W.	Dr. T.	Dr. O.
1	180 —	70 —	50 —
2	25 —		
3			
4			15 —
5			
6	15 —		
7			15 —
8			
9			
10			
11			
12	5 —		
13	10 —	125 —	
14	20 —		5 —
15			
16			10 —
...			
TOTALS	255 —	195 —	95 —

DAILY CASH SUMMARY

OPENING CASH ON HAND AT BEGINNING OF DAY	100.—
CASH RECEIVED DURING DAY	560.—
TOTAL	660.—
CASH PAID OUT	
BANK DEPOSITS	
CLOSING CASH ON HAND	

CASH PAID OUT $	560.—
BANK DEPOSITS $	100.—
CLOSING CASH ON HAND $	660.—
TOTAL $	
TOTAL $	
CASH LONG $	
CASH SHORT $	
TOTAL $	

FORM 7531 COLWELL CO., CHAMPAIGN, ILLINOIS

FORM 7512 COLWELL

Receipt

```
TELEPHONE 728-0153
                    TRUDY F. EISENMAN, M.D.
                    4640 NORTH MARINE DRIVE
                    CHICAGO, ILLINOIS  60640
                                                   16237
                              DATE   5-20-78
  RECEIVED OF   Jane M. Doe          $ 15.00
  ☐ CHECK      Fifteen  and no/100           DOLLARS
  ☒ CURRENCY
  ON ACCOUNT OF  $15.00
  ACCOUNT TOTAL  $ 15.00
  AMOUNT PAID    $ 15.00    PER   SMC
  BALANCE DUE    $   —
              Kindly retain this receipt for tax purposes
```

Reprinted by permission of The Colwell Company.

PHYSICIAN'S CASH DISBURSEMENT RECORDS
No matter which bookkeeping system is used, it must include a mechanism for recording cash disbursements. In many practices, a checkbook serves as the basic record of payment, with the checkbook stubs clearly reflecting the nature of expenditures. As in any business, receipts and invoices should be obtained whenever possible. These documents should be clearly marked *paid* with the check number and date recorded. They should then be filed in a systematic manner. The proper maintenance of receipts is vital to documentation of tax returns. An expense sheet is prepared from the checkbook. This summary can take whatever form deemed necessary in the circumstances. Combining the monthly summaries of disbursements results in the annual summary of expense which, with appropriate adjustments, can be used for the preparation of financial statements and tax returns.

ANNUAL FINANCIAL SUMMARY OF THE PRACTICE
The annual financial summary of a medical practice is the combination of the annual receipts and disbursement summaries mentioned previously. This combined summary can take any form, but it is usually similar to the annual summary. This report summarizes total business (both cash and charge) for the year, total cash receipts (cash received on account and actual cash business), and total cash disbursements. Most physicians practice on a cash basis. This means that the income is calculated only by cash actually received and that disbursements are determined by expenditures actually paid. Net income from the practice and income from other sources are computed from the annual summary.

In most medical offices a bookkeeper or an accountant prepares the annual summaries. However, it is important that the medical assistant be familiar with the reasoning behind keeping the summaries. This helps the assistant understand the need for accuracy in the records.

STAFF PAYROLL RECORDS
The federal Wages and Hours Law requires all employers to maintain an individual record for each employee. The employee earnings record contains the employee's name, address, Social Security number, number of exemptions claimed, date of birth, marital status, rate of pay, hours worked, earnings, deductions, net pay, check numbers, and year-to-date earnings.

An employee, especially in a practice where many people are employed, may be required to use time cards or time sheets. These forms are used to maintain records of employee arrival and departure times. The data on the cards are the basis for the hours worked in gross pay computations.

Employee Earnings Record

NAME Bart, Gwen   SOCIAL SECURITY NO. 046 12 1930

ADDRESS 14 Pawling Avenue   DATE OF BIRTH June 5, 19--

Troy, New York 12180   MARITAL STATUS Married

NO. OF EXEMPTIONS 2   HOURLY RATE $5.60

Line No.	Week Ended	Hours Wkd.	EARNINGS			DEDUCTIONS			Net Pay	Check No.	Year-to-date
			Reg.	Over-time	Total	FICA	FWT	Total			
1	1/7	41	229.60	2.80	232.40	13.60	41.00	54.60	177.80	22	232.40
2	1/14	40	224.00	—	224.00	13.10	40.00	53.10	170.90	65	456.40

Payroll Register

PAYROLL PERIOD   January 8-14, 19--

NAME	No. Exemp.	Hrly. Rate	Hours Wkd.	EARNINGS			TAXABLE EARNINGS		DEDUCTIONS			Net Pay	Chk. No.
				Reg.	Over-time	Total	FICA	Unemp. Ins.	FICA	FWT	Total		
Bart, Gwen	2	5.60	40	224.00	—	224.00	224.00	224.00	15.01	40.00	55.01	168.99	65
Evans, Sid	1	7.40	42	296.00	22.20	318.20	318.20	318.20	21.32	80.00	101.32	216.88	66
Murray, June	3	10.00	44	400.00	60.00	460.00	460.00	460.00	30.82	69.00	99.82	360.18	67
Sokol, Larry	2	8.00	36	288.00	—	288.00	288.00	288.00	19.16	24.00	43.16	244.84	68
				1208.00	82.20	1290.20	1290.20	1290.20	86.31	213.00	299.31	990.89	

A payroll register may also be kept. Information is entered from the time cards onto the payroll register, which also includes employees' names, the number of exemptions claimed, pay rates, gross pay, taxable earnings for FICA and unemployment insurance computations, deductions, net pay, and check numbers. This register includes all employees who work during a payroll period. If a register is used, the data from it can be copied onto the individual employee earnings records.

Employee earnings records and payroll registers can be typewritten by the assistant to meet the needs of the practice or they can be obtained from companies specializing in preprinted medical office documents.

THE PHYSICIAN'S SALARY

A doctor is not considered an employee in a medical practice unless the practice is a professional corporation. Not being an employee means that the physician is not really paid a salary; whatever funds the doctor takes are considered personal withdrawals. The practice, therefore, does not maintain an individual earnings record for the physician; neither income tax nor FICA is withheld from the amounts withdrawn by the doctor. The physician pays a tax as a self-employed person—a situation that provides benefits similar to those that the employees receive from FICA deductions.

WITHHOLDING FEDERAL AND STATE TAXES

Federal withholding taxes are the income taxes employers must withhold from their employees' gross salaries or wages as the money is earned. The withheld funds are sent periodically to the federal government and are determined from wage-bracket tables appearing in Circular E of the Employer's Tax Guide published by the Internal Revenue Service. It contains tables for weekly, biweekly, semimonthly, monthly, and daily or miscellaneous payroll periods.

The federal withholding tax deduction is based on the employee's gross pay for the payroll period and on the number of exemptions (dependents) claimed on the W–4 form (Employee's Withholding Allowance Certificate).

Some states have their own income tax programs that require employers to deduct these taxes from salaries and wages. The amounts deducted are determined by using withholding tables published by the respective states.

FICA

This term stands for the Federal Insurance Contributions Act and is used more frequently by accountants than the term *Social Security*. The FICA rate is set by Congress and has been increased several times over the years. FICA deductions support the old-age, survivors, and disability insurance programs (OASDI) and the Medicare program. The actual deduction for an employee can be determined from FICA tables supplied by the government, or by multiplying gross pay by the current FICA rate. Each year, the Congress sets a tax rate and the maximum amount of gross pay from which FICA taxes are deducted. The law also requires employers to match the taxes deducted from their employees' pay by remitting a like amount when the withheld FICA amounts are forwarded.

FEDERAL UNEMPLOYMENT TAX

This tax is used for the administration of unemployment insurance programs. Except in a few states, only employers are required to pay the tax. An *employer* is defined as one who in the previous calendar year either paid wages of $1,500 or more in any calendar quarter or had one or more employees at any time in each of twenty calendar weeks. The employer files an annual Federal Unemployment Tax Return (Form 940) by January 31 of the year following the taxable year and remits the tax with the form to the federal government.

STATE UNEMPLOYMENT TAX

The funds that are accumulated from this tax are used to pay unemployment insurance benefits. Merit-rating plans reduce the taxes for employers with stable payrolls. The form is filed quarterly and its contents vary with the state. Other data that are usually required on this form include employees' names, Social Security numbers, taxable wages, and tax computation. As with federal unemployment insurance, most states tax the employer only.

STATE DISABILITY INSURANCE

Many states impose a disability or sickness tax on employees that the employer must withhold from gross pay. The deductions are computed by applying the specified rates to taxable wages as determined by the respective state law. Along with contributions by employers, the taxes collected are used to pay benefits to employees who cannot work because of a disability (sickness).

SOURCES OF BOOKKEEPING INFORMATION

For a list of helpful books and articles regarding bookkeeping in a medical practice, see the Appendix of this book.

11.3

BANKING FOR THE PHYSICIAN

Bank services include checking accounts, collection of notes, loans, money orders, and many others. Business activities are so intertwined with banking that the assistants must be aware of how these services are used by their employers. Assistants are often called on to perform such duties as writing checks, depositing funds, paying bills, and arranging travel finances.

CHECKING ACCOUNTS

A checking account is opened at a commercial bank upon deposit of funds and the completion of bank forms listing the bank's rules and regulations. A signature card must be completed containing the signature(s) of anyone empowered to sign checks for the practice. The depositor is the *drawer,* the bank is the *drawee,* and the company or individual to whom a check is made out is the *payee.* A check made out to CASH can be cashed by anyone in possession of it.

Deposit slip   Funds deposited in the bank are accompanied by a deposit slip in duplicate containing the types and amounts of money being deposited. This money includes coins, bills, checks, and money orders. Interest coupons may be included, too. The duplicate is retained by the depositor.

The checkbook   A physician's checkbook usually contains three checks to a page, with prenumbered stubs attached by perforation to the prenumbered checks. Information about the check—date, payee, amount, and reason for the disbursement—is written on the stub prior to preparation of the check, thus assuring a permanent record of the payment.

Writing checks   Checks may be typed, printed, or written in ink. The signature should be written or printed in facsimile. Erasures and deletions are not permitted. If an error is made, the word VOID should be written on both the stub and the check. The symbols at the bottom of the check are printed in magnetic ink, and through the magnetic ink character recognition system, computers process large numbers of checks quickly and efficiently.

Overdrafts   Despite the best of intentions, or through an oversight, a physician's checks may occasionally be written for sums greater than the amount on deposit. As a customer service, the bank may honor the overdrawn check(s) and ask the doctor to deposit sufficient funds to cover the checks. On the other hand, it may refuse to honor the checks. Since the latter action can cause great embarrassment to the doctor, overdrafts should be treated seriously, and good relations with the bank should be cultivated. Dishonored checks may be returned to a depositor with a bank notice indicating the reason for its return. The term NSF (Not Sufficent Funds) is usually written on the notice.

Stop payments   Should a depositor want to stop payment on an issued check, the bank must be notified immediately. However, the bank cannot stop the check if it has already been cleared. Stop payments are usually requested on stolen or lost checks and on those that contain errors.

Checkwriters   These machines write check amounts so that they are difficult to change. They also reduce the time it takes to write checks.

Check endorsements In order to negotiate a check, the payee must endorse it on its reverse side. When endorsed in *blank*, only the payee's name appears as the endorsement. This may be done by a payee who is a private individual, but it is a dangerous practice because the bearer of the endorsed check can cash it or negotiate it further. A *full* or *special* endorsement contains the name of the company or person to whom the check is being given, followed by the payee's signature. Only the new payee can negotiate the check further. A *restrictive* endorsement indicates the condition of endorsement and limits the negotiability of the check. The words *For Deposit Only* followed by the payee's signature mean that the check is to be deposited in the payee's bank account. It cannot be negotiated again.

Types of Endorsements

Blank Endorsement	Full Endorsement	Restrictive Endorsement
Barbara Dee	*Pay to the order of George May Martin Lander*	*For Deposit Only Sue Foreman*

BANK STATEMENTS AND BANK RECONCILIATIONS

Depositors receive monthly statements from their banks which indicate the previous month's beginning balance, deposits made and checks paid during that month, other charges or additions, and the ending balance. Because it is likely that certain transactions have not been entered on both the bank's and the depositor's books by the last day of the month, their respective end-of-month balances will not coincide. A bank reconciliation statement must be prepared indicating the reasons for the disparity. The statement is prepared by the accountant or the assistant.

Canceled checks These are checks that have been paid by the bank and are returned in the envelope containing the bank statement. Banks are developing systems that eliminate the return of canceled checks, at no inconvenience to the depositor.

Outstanding checks If a depositor's check has not cleared the bank by the end of the previous month, it is considered outstanding.

Deposits-in-transit Depositors may enter receipt amounts in their records which do not reach the bank as deposits by the last day of the previous month and are therefore not included on the bank statement. Such deposits are said to be late or in transit.

Bank service charges Banks may charge depositors for services such as the collection of notes and stop payments. These charges are listed on the bank statements.

Bank memos Deductions and additions indicated on bank statements are sometimes explained in debit and credit memos sent along with the statement to the bank customer.

OTHER BANK SERVICES AND FEATURES

The assistant should be acquainted with the variety of services offered by banks. Such information is invaluable for use in assisting a busy physician.

Certified check   Should a payee require guaranteed payment, a bank will certify that a depositor's account contains sufficient funds to pay for the check. The amount is subtracted from the depositor's balance and the check is stamped "Certified."

Certificate of deposit   Banks pay interest on short-term deposits (a minimum of 30 days) to customers who do not want cash to lie idle. The bank issues a promissory note to the depositor which can be negotiated to other parties or cashed at the end of the time period.

Short-term checking account   A depositor can open a temporary checking account for a particular purpose. As soon as that purpose has been accomplished, the account is closed.

11.4

ACCOUNTING MACHINES

The term *data processing* covers much more than computers or punch cards. Many times our notion of data processing includes only computer programs, expensive equipment, and reports printed on special paper. The daily typewriting and routine arithmetic calculations performed in offices are also forms of data processing. This section describes the calculating machines used in typical offices to process data.

Most desk calculators perform only arithmetic operations; therefore, they are used for addition, subtraction, multiplication, or division problems. Other calculating machines may be quite complex: they perform arithmetic and logical operations, and they may have the ability to store and retrieve those data from machine-readable files. Although modern electronic data processing equipment may perform both arithmetic and logical operations, their arithmetic calculations utilize the same principles as their predecessors—the manual and electric adding machines.

ELECTRIC ADDING MACHINES

The electric adding machine is still available in some offices for basic arithmetic functions. However, this full-bank keyboard is becoming less popular than the newer 10-key model. The arithmetic function keys (the PLUS and the MINUS keys) are used as the data entry keys on the electric adding machine. The operator depresses the numeric keys that represent the number desired; that number is entered into the machine by next depressing either the plus (addition) or the minus (subtraction) keys. Multiplication on most electric adding machines is performed by depressing the addition key a repeated number of times. For example, to multiply the number 674 by 4, the operator would enter 674 and depress the addition key 4 times. Some electric adding machines require that a REPEAT key be held down while the addition key is depressed in order to perform multiplication. A paper tape is used on this machine. Each entry is shown on the tape. For example, with the depression of a TOTAL key, an accumulated total will print on paper tape. Usually, electric adding machines can perform only addition, subtraction, multiplication, and division.

ELECTRONIC CALCULATORS
Electronic calculators are much smaller and faster than electric adding machines; their operation is facilitated by a 10-key numeric keyboard. Electronic calculators perform all arithmetic functions rapidly as well as sequential operations, which are often stored in the calculator's memory. Some calculators print numbers and totals on paper tape, but other models display numbers and totals on a digital readout window.

Electronic printing calculators   These printing calculators are useful for accounting purposes when complex addition or multiplication problems must be verified for accuracy. Electronic printing calculators have a 10-key numeric keyboard for entering the values *zero* through *nine;* numbers and totals are printed on a paper tape. Some models may have a display (digital readout) window as well. (Dual-feature electronic printing calculators have both paper tape and digital readout windows.) On the keyboard a separate key is available for each of the basic arithmetic functions: addition, subtraction, multiplication, and division.

Many electronic printing calculators have additional function keys that allow such operations as the automatic calculation of percentages or of square roots. A separate key may facilitate chain arithmetic operations, such as repeated multiplications with different multiplicands. An additional key will allow a constant value to be stored in the machine's memory in order that the same value can be used in different, separate calculations. Most of the machines provide for a total to be accumulated in the machine's memory and that total can be increased as a result of separate additional calculations.

Electronic display calculators   The electronic display calculator is characterized by a digital readout window for displaying numbers and totals; there is no printing capability in this instance. Numbers are displayed as they are entered and totals are displayed as they are calculated. The keyboard is the typical 10-key numeric keyboard along with an assortment of function keys. The electronic display calculator is similar in most respects to the electronic printing calculator, except for the manner in which the data are displayed. The electronic printing calculator prints data on paper tape, while the electronic display model has only a digital readout window; however, some models offer both of these features. Since the electronic display calculator provides no audit tape or printed record of the numbers entered or the totals accumulated, the operator must verify these values by observing the display window. Although the lack of printed entries and totals may be a disadvantage, this model's purchase price is usually less than that of the electronic printing calculator.

There are few moving parts in this calculator; usually the result is fewer service calls and correspondingly lower maintenance costs. The relatively low cost of these machines often makes it more economical to discard a broken electronic display calculator rather than to have it repaired.

While the printing calculator usually draws its power from a standard electrical outlet, most display calculators are also equipped with a rechargeable battery.

PROGRAMMABLE ELECTRONIC CALCULATORS
A unique feature of the programmable electronic calculator is its ability to store a complex program in its memory. A programmable calculator can be directed by a

series of instructions to perform sequential calculations automatically. The operator merely (1) feeds the instructions into the calculator (2) enters any values required, and (3) starts the calculation series. These instructions are often called a *program*. Programs may be recorded on strips of magnetic tape which are inserted into the calculator whenever the program is required. The use of a program relieves the operator of the responsibility for making several repeated calculations in the proper, logical sequence.

Calculator vendors usually have libraries containing several routines or programs commonly used in business. In fact, many times the library accompanies the calculator without any additional payment. Additional programs are available with the calculator for a small additional fee. Customized programs designed especially for a particular office operation may also be acquired from most vendors. A common arrangement provides for a specific number of customized programs to be delivered with the calculator, and additional programs to be prepared at a later date for a specific programming fee. Some business offices have staff members who are able to write programs for these calculators.

Programmable display calculators vary in size and sophistication. Hand-held programmable calculators feature the typical 10-key numeric keyboard with additional function keys. These calculators usually perform the common arithmetic functions as well as additional calculations such as sine, cosine, square root, and percentage. These functions may be used by depressing the proper function key.

There are larger programmable calculators that may be called *minicomputers*. The desktop minicomputer usually has a typewriter keyboard and an additional cluster of 10 numeric keys together with special function keys. The desktop model is approximately the size of an electric typewriter. Programs for this calculator are often stored on a cassette tape similar to those used on dictating and transcribing machines. Many programs may be stored on one cassette tape. Some calculator keyboards may have as many as 10 function keys which are applicable to specific office calculations. These function keys initiate stored programs that automatically perform the arithmetic calculations and sequential processing steps that are frequently used in business offices. One example of such a program is the calculation of a repeated number of specified chain discounts. Such a program is helpful when there are as many as five chain discounts applied to any purchase, and when each discount is different. A long series of discounts can be recorded as a program, and the entire program can be used by merely depressing one function key. Another example of a program initiated by a function key is the calculation of payroll values. The payroll program can be stored on a cassette tape, and the individual function keys are used to calculate overtime pay, withholding tax, and social security tax. In each case, the calculation of payroll deductions requires several arithmetic steps. The program is the collection of these arithmetic steps in the proper sequence. The steps may be executed by depressing the proper function keys.

A calculator that is classified as a minicomputer obviously requires more memory than a hand-held calculator. A programmable desktop calculator usually has about 4,000 positions of memory storage, and the memory can be expanded by adding additional units of 4,000 storage positions.

COMMON FEATURES OF ELECTRONIC CALCULATORS

All electronic calculators have 10 number keys representing the values 0-9. These keys are used to enter numbers into the calculator's memory. Calculators also have separate function keys for each of the arithmetic functions—addition, subtraction, multiplication, and division. Another feature common to all electronic calculators is a key that will cause the total to be displayed or printed. This key—a TOTAL key—may be labeled TOTAL, T, =, or *.

Electronic calculators have a memory for storing numbers. The memory is divided into three separate parts: (1) keyboard memory, (2) operating memory, and (3) storage memory. The keyboard memory (sometimes called a *keyboard register*) contains the number entered from the keyboard. The operating memory handles addition, subtraction, multiplication, and division. The storage memory retains data that may be recalled in the future. The following calculator keys may be depressed in order to make changes in numbers stored in these three memory registers:

CLEAR ENTRY **CE**	This key will erase any number entered into the machine (keyboard register) if the CE key is depressed <u>before</u> striking the arithmetic function key. The CLEAR ENTRY key is used to erase a number entered in error. A typical error occurs when the operator accidentally depresses the wrong numeric key.
CLEAR **C**	The CLEAR key erases the keyboard register and the operating register, but not the storage memory. However, when a calculator does not have a CLEAR ALL key, this key will erase all three sections of memory.
CLEAR ALL **CA**	This key will erase the keyboard register, the operating register, and the storage memory. The CLEAR ALL key should be depressed before beginning each new calculation in order to clear all previous totals and numbers from the calculator.
MEMORY PLUS **M+**	This key will cause the number entered on the keyboard to be added to whatever value is in the storage memory.
MEMORY MINUS **M−**	This key will cause the number entered on the keyboard to be subtracted from the contents of the storage memory.
MEMORY RECALL **MR**	This function recalls the value in the storage memory in order that the recalled value may be displayed or used in an arithmetic calculation. The use of this key does not change or erase the value in the storage memory.

The following function keys are more commonly found on electronic calculators. These keys execute complete calculations:

ROUND OFF **R/O**	This key will cause all calculated answers to be rounded off to a selected decimal position. Some calculators have a ROUND OFF switch that may be set to round off all calculations. Other calculators have a key that may be depressed to round off only the answer stored in the storage memory—this answer is the last value calculated or the value displayed on the screen.
CONSTANT **K**	The CONSTANT key permits the calculator to retain a value and to use that same value in separate arithmetic operations. This function is usually used for repeated multiplication or division. An example of the use of the CONSTANT key is the calculation of a chain of discounts, when each discount is identical (5% − 5% − 5%).
PERCENT **%**	The PERCENT key converts the number entered into a decimal value (expressed in hundredths—.00), and it multiplies the accumulated total by that decimal value. The resulting answer is expressed as a percentage.
PERCENT OF CHANGE **%** **CHG**	Although this key is not found on small calculators, large calculators often provide this automatic function. The procedure for using this function is: (1) enter the base number (2) depress the PERCENT OF CHANGE key, and (3) enter the second number. The calculator will automatically show the amount of change and the % of change between the base number and the second number.

VERIFICATION OF ARITHMETIC

Since it is so easy to depress an incorrect key when entering numbers, all arithmetic should be verified. Because electronic calculators without a printed output tape display only the number entered and the accumulated total, there is no record of separate entries so that the accumulated total can be verified.

Verification with output tape The paper output tape produced by electronic printing calculators lists each entry as well as the accumulated total. Many calculators will also print a sign representing the arithmetic function applied to each entry, such as a *plus* (+) sign representing addition and a *minus* (−) sign representing subtraction. Verification of a calculator's paper tape simply involves a comparison of each entry number on the paper tape with the number that the operator had intended to enter. When the number on the paper tape is correct, the operator can place a check mark next to that number. The check mark helps the operator return to the proper checking location if interrupted. When all numbers on the paper tape have been verified by this procedure, the operator can be confident that the accumulated total is correct.

Verification with a display screen Electronic display calculators do not produce a printed record of the numbers entered. A number entered is shown on the display screen only until the arithmetic function key is depressed; then, the accumulated total is displayed. The procedure for calculating and verifying totals on an electronic display calculator is listed below:

1. Clear the machine's total.
2. Enter all numbers together with the desired arithmetic functions.
3. Write the *final* accumulated total on a sheet of paper.
4. Repeat Steps 1 and 2 by entering all numbers a second time.
5. Compare the second *final* accumulated total with the total already written on the sheet of paper (Step 2).
6. If the two totals are identical, the total is correct. In case the two totals are not identical, the operator should repeat Steps 1, 2, and 3 until at least two (2) consecutive *final* totals are identical.

HAND POSITIONS FOR THE CALCULATOR KEYBOARD

Since an operator often has many numbers to enter into a calculator, the operating speed is important. Practice will help anyone develop the skill necessary for touch operation of the keyboard. Calculators, like typewriters, have a home row for the index, middle, and ring fingers. The home row keys are the 4, 5, and 6 keys. Normally, the 5 key contains a bump or depression to assist the touch operator in locating the home row. The third of the following four illustrations shows the proper fingers placed on the home row keys. The second illustration shows the thumb reaching the zero key. Each of the fingers moves independently from its home row position immediately up to reach the top row of keys, and immediately down to reach the bottom row of keys. For example, the index finger moves up to reach the 7 key; the middle finger moves up to reach the 8 key; and the ring finger moves up to reach the 9 key, as shown in the fourth illustration. The first illustration shows the proper finger positions for the 1, 2, and 3 keys. Practice in keying numbers into a calculator will develop touch operation similar to touch typing.

ROUNDING NUMBERS

Electronic calculators contain electronic circuits that calculate answers; these answers are retained in the calculator's memory. The memory of an electronic calculator is sometimes called a *register*. Most calculators are designed so that any

Fingering Techniques

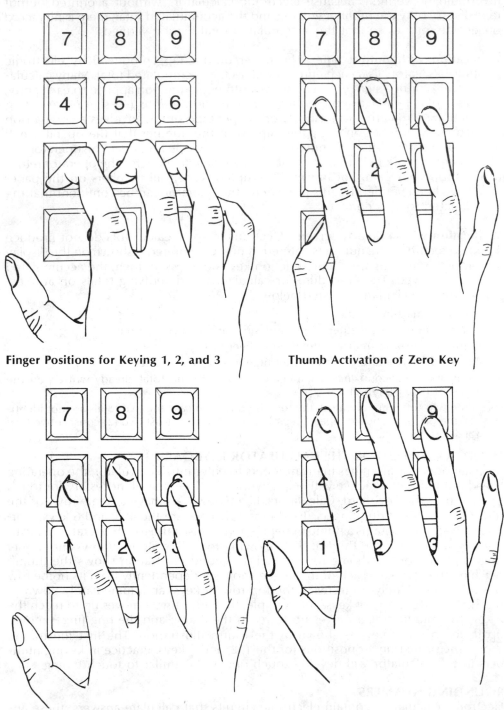

Finger Positions for Keying 1, 2, and 3

Thumb Activation of Zero Key

Proper Finger Position on Home Row Keys

Finger Positions for Keying 7, 8, and 9

calculated answer completely fills a memory register; therefore, a calculated answer may contain more numbers than are needed by the operator. For example, an 8-digit calculator will calculate answers containing 8 digits, regardless of the operator's need. Some calculators automatically suppress zeroes to the right of the desired answer, even though they are calculated and retained in the machine's memory. The following illustration shows the difference between an expected answer and the answer calculated and retained in the machine's memory.

Problem Multiply $2.42 by 11 (desired answer in dollars and cents)

Manual Calculation	Machine Calculation (8-digit Machine)	
2.42	2.42	enter
× 11	×	enter
2 42	11	enter
24 2	26.620000	machine register contents
26.62	26.62	right zeroes suppressed

While some calculators will automatically position the decimal point in the proper place, others depend on the operator to position the decimal point. The calculator in the example shown above retains an 8-digit answer in its register (26.620000) even though a 4-digit answer (26.62) is as accurate.

The operator is often required to *round* numbers to a desired length. Numbers that are to be rounded are calculated (or *carried*) two places beyond (to the right) of the rounding position. This rule is illustrated below:

When Rounding To	Number Desired	Carry To
Thousandths	.746	.74611
Hundredths	.57	.5724
Tenths	.6	.643

The procedure for rounding numbers is as follows:

1. Begin rounding with the right-most digit (this is called the *test digit*).
2. When the test digit is 5 or more, add 1 to the digit immediately to the left of the test digit.
3. Discard the test digit.
4. Repeat Steps 1, 2, and 3 until the number contains the digits required.

Problem Round 457.7561 to an accuracy of two places to the right of the decimal point (hundredths).

Solution	Step 1	457.7561	Test digit is 1.
	Step 2	1	is not equal to or more than 5.
	Step 3	457.756	Discard the test digit.
	Step 4	457.756	New test digit is 6.
	Step 5	6	is greater than 5.
	Step 6	457.76(6)	Add 1 to the digit left of the test digit.
	Step 7	457.76	Discard the test digit.

Example Problem Round $756.4227 to the nearest cent.

Solution	Step 1	756.4227	Test digit is 7.
	Step 2	7	is more than 5.
	Step 3	756.423(7)	Add 1 to the digit left of the test digit.
	Step 4	756.423	Discard the test digit.
	Step 5	3	is the new test digit.
	Step 6	3	is not equal to or more than 5.
	Step 7	756.42	Discard the test digit.

Table of Fractions with Decimal Equivalents

commonly used fractions	decimal equivalent	commonly used fractions	decimal equivalent
½	.5	1/9	.1111
		2/9	.2222
⅓	.3333	3/9	.3333
⅔	.6667	4/9	.4444
		5/9	.5556
¼	.25	6/9	.6667
¾	.75	7/9	.7778
		8/9	.8889
⅕	.2		
⅖	.4	1/12	.0833
⅗	.6	5/12	.4167
⅘	.8	7/12	.5833
		11/12	.9167
⅙	.1667		
⅚	.8333	1/16	.0625
		3/16	.1875
1/7	.1429	5/16	.3125
2/7	.2857	7/16	.4375
3/7	.4286	9/16	.5625
4/7	.5714	11/16	.6875
5/7	.7143	13/16	.8125
6/7	.8571	15/16	.9375
⅛	.125		
⅜	.375		
⅝	.625		
⅞	.875		

Table of Representative Decimal Equivalents With Complements

%	decimal equivalent	complement
.5 (½ of 1%)	.005	.995
1.0	.01	.99
2.0	.02	.98
2.5	.025	.975
3.0	.03	.97
4.0	.04	.96
5.0	.05	.95
7 ⅛		
7 ¼		
7 ½	.075	.925
7 ¾	.0775	.9225
10.0	.10	.90
12.0	.12	.88
12 ½	.125	.875
15.0	.15	.85
20.0	.20	.80
85.0	.85	.15
90.0	.90	.10

12

CHAPTER TWELVE

PROFESSIONAL FEES AND PATIENTS' CREDIT

CONTENTS
12.1   FEES
12.2   FEE ADJUSTMENTS AND CANCELLATIONS
12.3   CREDIT ARRANGEMENTS

12.1

FEES

DETERMINING FEES

When establishing a practice, a physician must determine a fee schedule. The following items are considered: the cost of maintaining the practice, the value of the doctor's education and experience, fairness to the patients, and prevailing community rates. A valuable step in setting fees is to check with the local medical association and other physicians to ascertain the prevailing community rates. This information should be used as a guide in setting fees, but it should not be considered as rigid criteria.

The concept of "usual, customary, and reasonable fees" is becoming more prevalent as a method of percentage payments by insurance companies. This concept is based on the usual fee that a physician would charge private patients for a certain procedure, the customary fee for that procedure performed by a physician with similar training and experience, and the reasonable fee that a patient might be expected to pay for similar services.

Despite the basis on which fees are established, setting fees remains a judgmental decision on the part of the physician. Only the doctor can estimate the value of the services rendered. Patients are willing to pay a fair fee for good service as long as they are aware of what is involved.

DISCUSSION OF FEES WITH PATIENTS

Patients do not usually shop around for inexpensive doctors. On the contrary, they will typically pay the customary fee if they are assured of the necessity and the quality of the services rendered. The best method of communicating the fairness of a physician's fees to a patient is for the doctor or the medical assistant to have an open, frank discussion with the patient prior to treatment. If necessary, additional discussions should take place as treatment continues. In this manner, the patient will be aware of what is expected and can make the necessary financial arrangements for payment. By encouraging financial discussions, the problems of collection of delinquent accounts are minimized.

FEE SCHEDULES

As the medical assistant is the one who usually discusses fees with patients, it is important that a typed fee schedule, approved by the doctor, be available for quick desk reference. With the schedule at hand, the assistant can quote accurate fees to the patients upon inquiry. In addition, a patient can be told the charges immediately after treatment. If so requested, the assistant should give the patient a written, itemized statement.

FEE SCHEDULE

Internal Medicine		Urology	
Office visit	25	Initial office visit	50
Initial office visit	50	Intravenous pyelogram	85
Chest X ray	35	KUB (flat X ray of abdomen)	35
EKG	50	Cystoscopy	85
Lab—			
CBC	15		
12–channel	25		
24–channel	35		
Sigmoidoscopy	75		
Urinalysis	10		
Urine culture	25		

PROFESSIONAL COURTESY

Professional courtesy is the traditional obligation of a physician to give free or reduced-cost treatment to certain members of the medical profession and their families. The medical assistant should know exactly which people are to receive free care, which groups are to be billed at a discounted amount, which ones are to be billed for insurance purposes only, and which people are to be billed as regular patients. The doctor—not the assistant—sets these guidelines for the practice. Recipients of professional courtesy include:

1. Physicians and their immediate families
2. Parents of physicians
3. Medical assistants and secretaries employed by colleagues
4. Nurses
5. Dentists
6. Pharmacists

"WE DO NOT BILL" POLICY

Many specialists such as orthodontists, podiatrists, oral surgeons, and veterinarians place conspicuous notices in their reception areas indicating in a tasteful fashion that "we do not bill." The notice explains that by not billing patients, office costs are reduced and fees are kept lower. This technique shifts the responsibility of immediate payment to the patient. If the patient cannot pay immediately, he or she must ask specifically to be billed. If patients know there is no billing policy, most of them will pay upon treatment if the charges are not exceptionally large. Normally, only those patients with financial difficulties or those with other extenuating circumstances will ask for special arrangements to be made.

However, it is important to know that the "we do not bill" technique works only in certain types of practices. Normally, this procedure is used in offices where the individual treatment charges are not overwhelming, the treatment period is of short duration, and it is an accepted custom in the community. If any of these factors is missing, a physician may decide wisely not to have a "no bill" policy, as the increase in cash payments may not compensate for the loss of patients. Although there are variations of this policy that can be adopted, careful consideration nevertheless must be given to it before implementation, especially if the physician has used a billing procedure in the past.

12.2

FEE ADJUSTMENTS AND CANCELLATIONS

MEDICAL CARE FOR THOSE UNABLE TO PAY

Medical care for the indigent is available in many practices. It is the medical assistant's responsibility to help both the doctor and patient(s) arrange for whatever free medical care is necessary. The assistant should be familiar with local organizations and/or agencies that provide related medical services for those who are medically indigent. Needed services such as hospitalization or therapy should be provided or arranged for by various organizations with which the assistant should be familiar. Records that are kept on a patient who is not charged are the same as those used for any other patient. The one difference is that the notation "N/C" (no charge), instead of a dollar amount, is entered in the debit column of the financial records.

REDUCTION OR CANCELLATION OF FEES

If the appropriate financial information has been obtained from the patient prior to the setting of a fee, there is usually no need for a fee reduction or fee cancellation. The reason for this is that any unusual circumstance would have already been taken into account. For example, it might be the doctor's policy to accept an insurance or a governmental payment as a fee if the patient falls below certain established levels. One such criterion might be an income level. If the proper information is obtained prior to setting the fee, it can be adjusted accordingly. Consequently, the necessity for recording a fee on the books and then reducing it is diminished. The following guidelines determine if fee reduction or cancellation is warranted:

1. Have an open and honest discussion with the patient about the patient's financial problems.
2. Recheck the initial information and the patient's credit rating to see if there have been any major changes.
3. Investigate the possibility of the patient's qualifying for a public assistance program.
4. Investigate whether the patient is covered by or is entitled to an insurance settlement.

Reduction of a fee can sometimes lead to malpractice suits, especially when the patient dies. Or, if a doctor has agreed to a fee reduction and the patient still doesn't pay, the doctor may be legally forced to accept the lower payment regardless of how much time has elapsed. Unless there is a written agreement that is witnessed, that contains the terminology "without prejudice," and that includes a specific time limit, the doctor forfeits his or her rights to the original fee if the patient doesn't pay the agreed-on reduced fee.

A fee should never be reduced just as a way to obtain quicker payment and to dispense with further collection efforts. In this case, the patient may feel that the doctor's original charges were inflated. However, there are two schools of thought on this subject. The first is that it is better to reduce a fee than to cancel it entirely. The rationale for this is that the patient's pride can be maintained; i.e., the patient is not a "charity case." The second school of thought is that a fee, if deemed necessary, should always be cancelled and not reduced since a doctor should not bargain with patients over fees. The medical assistant must follow whichever policy prevails in the practice. The following is an example of the way that a letter containing the reduction of a fee might be worded:

Dear _____:

Dr. Best has agreed to reduce his fee from $200 to $100 based on his discussion with you last week, provided that payment is received here before the end of the month.

Sincerely,

Secretary to Dr. Best

PROFESSIONAL COURTESY

As mentioned previously, doctors traditionally have given free medical treatment to other physicians and their families, to nurses, to dentists, and to others in related health care fields. The Principles of Medical Ethics, as currently interpreted by the American Medical Association, now permits doctors to accept insurance benefits in payment for professional courtesy services. As most doctors do subscribe to some type of health insurance plan, this practice is more widespread than in the past.

12.3

CREDIT ARRANGEMENTS

FEDERAL LAWS GOVERNING RETAIL CREDIT

There are several major federal laws affecting retail credit. These laws provide guidelines for the opening and collection of accounts including those of a medical practice. It is important that medical assistants know these laws because they affect relations with patients.

The credit law having the greatest impact on an assistant's responsibilities is the Truth in Lending Act, or, as it is commonly known, Regulation Z of the 1968 Consumer Protection Act. This provision calls for full written disclosure regarding payment of a fee in more than four installments. The disclosure must take place at the time the agreement is reached between the physician and patient. A standard-ized form can be used, disclosing: (1) the amount of total debt (2) the amount of down payment (3) the date of each payment (4) the date of final payment (5) the amount of each installment (6) the finance charges, and (7) the annual percentage rate. The physician retains one copy of the agreement and the patient receives the other. Regulation Z does not apply and disclosure is not required if the patient decides unilaterally to pay in installments or at other convenient times.

Other laws that deal with credit and collections are:

1. The Fair Credit Reporting Act (Title V of the Consumer Protection Act of 1968)
2. The Federal Trade Commission's Guides Against Debt Collection Deception
3. The Federal Communications Commission's Public Notice on Use of Telephone for Debt Collecting. This last act prohibits such behavior as calling at odd hours, making threatening calls, and other harassing tactics.

All of the above laws are important to a medical practice because of their impact on the establishment of collection procedures. In a tactful manner, medical assistants must inform patients that physicians are entitled to the same credit information as other businesses. The so-called "pay the doctor last" attitude should be discredited and the medical assistant is the person who has the opportunity and responsibility for doing so.

GUIDELINES TO EXTENDING CREDIT

It is imperative that detailed credit data be obtained from patients prior to their receiving treatment. When a new patient arrives, it is up to the medical assistant to obtain as much credit information as possible. Many practices have devised a form that new patients fill out before seeing the physicians. This eliminates resentment on the part of those patients who feel that the assistant is intrusive. It is advisable to have the practice's billing procedures written directly on the form to avoid misunderstandings. Once the credit data are obtained, they should be checked as soon as possible. More and more doctors are turning to credit bureaus for verification on patients' credit ratings. This is a perfectly acceptable method of checking out patients, and assistants should not feel embarrassed about doing so. An assistant would be remiss if credit data went unchecked and the account later became uncollectible.

THIRD-PARTY LIABILITY

It is important to ascertain from the patient who exactly is to be financially responsible for the medical care given. If it is another person, the correct name, address, employment data, and similar information on that person should be obtained. The third party should then be contacted for verification of the financial obligation. If the third party is not obligated by law, it is imperative that a signed statement of obligation be obtained, as verbal agreements are not binding. If the third party is an insurance carrier, it may be necessary to have the patient sign an order instructing the company to pay the physician directly. Forms for this purpose can be obtained from the insurance companies or from local medical associations.

RELEASE OF CREDIT DATA FOR HEALTH INSURANCE RECORDS

Credit data obtained about a patient is confidential and cannot be released without the patient's express permission. Many insurance carriers and government programs (e.g., Medicare) require information about a patient's advance payments, unpaid balances, and amounts to be financed. This information cannot be released without the patient's signature. A standard form obtainable from insurance carriers or local medical societies should be filled out, signed by the patient, and retained with the patient's medical records.

INSTALLMENT PAYING

All patients should be encouraged to pay immediately after treatment has been rendered. If there are extenuating circumstances, the physician should be prepared to help the patient make financial arrangements in a satisfactory manner. The use of credit cards has become an accepted way of life in the United States. They are even used to pay for college tuition. This trend may well spill over to the medical field. The Judicial Council and the Council on Medical Service of the American Medical Association have jointly agreed that it is not unethical per se for physicians to participate in credit card programs. They also concur that it is up to the individual physician to judge whether the use of such financing plans may result in unnecessary increases in the cost of medical care. Finally, they agree that the physician must decide whether the use of credit cards will be construed as advertising for patients and will provide profits from other than professional services.

Banks also offer plans to finance patients' medical bills. If a patient desires to finance a medical debt through a bank, the bank investigates the patient's credit reliability. If the credit is found to be acceptable, the bank usually agrees to finance the debt. The bank then pays the physician the total owed, less a small discount. The doctor may even decide to have the bank deduct the interest charges owed by the patient from the fee to encourage the patient to use the bank's financing. Some medical associations also make similar arrangements to help patients finance their medical care.

The physician may also recommend that an installment arrangement be initiated directly between the physician and the patient, usually with no financing charges. In accordance with Regulation Z, if the payments are to be made in more than four installments, a written disclosure statement must be signed. Before a budgeting or financing system is recommended to a patient, the physician should consider whether these methods are in the patient's best interest, and whether they are in line with medical professional ethics.

CREDIT BUREAUS

Credit bureaus are businesses that maintain credit data on individuals. Many companies have developed special departments that specialize in medical-dental collections. The various bureaus usually pool their information on borrowers and form an association such as the Associated Credit Bureaus of America. This organization has over 1200 affiliates and can supply such data as:

1. The patient's residence and moving habits
2. Verfication of employment
3. The patient's approximate salary
4. Other reports on how the patient pays his or her bills
5. Any other useful information including bankruptcy history, change of name, and so on.

Before using a credit bureau, the physician and/or the assistant should be sure that it is a reputable organization.

BUREAUS OF MEDICAL ECONOMICS

Bureaus of medical economics are credit bureaus operated by medical associations. These bureaus usually have their own credit information service or they have access to an ethical credit bureau. Physicians would be wise to consider the use of a bureau of medical economics, as they can rely on its ethical approach. These bureaus usually maintain specific information on all medical accounts assigned to them and can report ratings on individuals with poor medical credit records.

MEDICAL-DENTAL-HOSPITAL BUREAUS OF AMERICA

The Medical-Dental-Hospital Bureaus of America is an association of all agencies serving the medical profession and hospitals. It maintains high ethical standards among its affiliates and is committed to using collection procedures most acceptable to physicians. This group can give a physician information about a credit bureau or collection agency in relation to ethics and reliability.

13

BILLING AND COLLECTION

CONTENTS

13.1

BILLING PROCEDURES

In order to yield a high collection ratio, it is necessary to establish and maintain systematic billing habits. Whatever billing procedures are chosen, they should be decided on at the start of a doctor's practice. If a physician bills patients in a clear, professional, and systematic manner, the patients will be encouraged to remit payment promptly. If, on the other hand, a physician has an erratic and sloppy billing system, the patients may conclude that payments are unimportant to the doctor. Consequently, payments may be forgotten, or, at a minimum, delayed beyond a reasonable period of time. No matter what kind of system is used, this type of situation can be prevented by consistent implementation of the billing procedures.

STATEMENT FORMS
When to prepare them   It is most important that patients be given the opportunity to pay at the time the service is rendered. This means that a bill, or, at a minimum, a receipt, be made available immediately. Most patients are prepared to pay for routine visits at once. If patients prefer to be billed, it is vital that it be done promptly. A physician must have a regular billing schedule, e.g., at least once a month. Some doctors prefer to bill immediately after a visit; others choose to bill only once or twice a month; and still others prefer to use cycle billing.

If monthly billing is preferred, it is important that the statements be sent a few days before the end of the month. This ensures that patients will receive their bills by the first of the month, enabling them to include the bills in their monthly budgets. The preparation of statements need not be left to the end of the month. It can be done directly after treatment or sporadically; in either case, the statements are postdated and are mailed at the end of the month. The same type of system can be used for twice-a-month billing.

Cycle billing, which has been used quite effectively in business, is relatively new in medical practices. Under this system, accounts are divided alphabetically into equal groups. Each group is billed on a predetermined day each month, and each group is assigned a different day. This ensures that the burden of billing is spread rather evenly throughout the month. If an established practice opts for cycle billing, the patients must be told in advance of the change. The system should be explained to them so that ill will and confusion do not arise. New patients should be given complete information as to the billing procedures. A printed statement of the office billing policy can be handed to the patient at the time of the initial visit.

How to prepare statements   A statement can be prepared directly from the patient's ledger card. This card is an up-to-date record of all fees charged and collected. The statement can be prepared as a photocopy of the ledger card or as a carbonized copy of the ledger card. Still another alternative is to copy it onto a different bill form. Any method is acceptable as long as the bill is accurate and neat. The bill reflects the doctor's image: if it isn't correct, the patient may become concerned about other aspects of the practice and may also delay payment.

Determining to whom the statement is to be sent   In most cases, the person to whom the doctor renders treatment is the one to whom the bill is sent. This procedure is based on the law of contracts, as an implied contract exists between doctor and patient if there is no third-party involvement. It is sometimes difficult to determine third-party responsibility. A husband is legally responsible for debts incurred by his wife, so a bill may be sent to the husband at the wife's request. Parents are legally responsible for minor children who live at home and are not self-supporting, even if treatment is rendered without their knowledge.

   In other cases, it is much more difficult to establish third-party responsibility. In general, the physician should make an express contract with the third party in which the latter accepts responsibility over his or her signature. This will hold the third party responsible and will make it possible for the physician to avoid difficulties in collecting the fee. It is not enough to ask the patient to whom the bill should be sent, if the relationship of the named third party to the patient does not establish responsibility. When third-party responsibility has been established, the assistant makes sure that the correct name and address are recorded on the patient's ledger card for use in billing.

Coding and itemizing treatments   Although a great many doctors send statements to their patients containing the phrase "For Professional Services," and the amount, it is always desirable that the statements be itemized even if the fees have been explained in advance. Patients may forget the amount of the fee, or, if many visits and services are involved, they may lose track of the different fees. It is courteous and helpful to itemize statements for patients. By doing so, collection problems may be avoided since the patients will have a written record of dates, services rendered, and fees charged and collected.

   The simplest method of preparing itemized bills is to use a carbonized patient's ledger card that has frequently rendered treatments listed with corresponding key symbols. When a patient is treated, the appropriate date, the correct treatment symbol, and the fee are entered on the ledger card. If the form is not carbonized, it can be either photocopied or transcribed onto a similar billing form. This system provides the patient with information and keeps clerical work to a minimum.

PHYSICIANS' BILLING SERVICES

Various independent billing services are available to physicians. A major advantage of using such a service is that the people performing these functions are experts in the field of accounts receivable management. They remove the burden of time-consuming clerical tasks from the physician and the staff, thus leaving them free to

Codified Patient Ledger Card

STATEMENT

LEONARD S. TAYLOR, M.D.
2100 WEST PARK AVENUE
CHAMPAIGN, ILLINOIS 61820

TELEPHONE 367-6671

Mrs. Jonathan M. Wainright
4554 Newton Terrace
Champaign, IL 61820

RECEIPT NUMBER	DATE	PROFESSIONAL SERVICE	CHARGE		PAID		NEW BALANCE	
16240	9/29	OC	17	00	10	00	7	00
18000	10/22	PAP	10	00	17	00	0	00
21234	12/29	PE	15	00	10	00	5	00
							5	00

PAY LAST AMOUNT IN THIS COLUMN ⟶

1629

OC - OFFICE CALL	INS - INSURANCE	PE - PHYSICAL EXAMINATION
HC - HOUSE CALL	OB - OBSTETRICAL CARE	EKG - ELECTROCARDIOGRAM
HOSP - HOSPITAL CARE	PAP - PAPANICOLAOU TEST	XR - X-RAY
L - LABORATORY	OS - OFFICE SURGERY	M - MEDICATION
I - INJECTION	HS - HOSPITAL SURGERY	NC - NO CHARGE

THIS IS AN EXACT COPY OF YOUR ACCOUNT PREPARED ON 3M "JIFFMASTER" COPY PAPER

Reprinted by permission of The Colwell Company.

concentrate their efforts on the patients. There are, however, some disadvantages to the use of these services. The first drawback is cost. In most instances, it is impractical for a single practitioner or a small group practice to engage such services. In these circumstances, it would probably be better for the medical assistant to do all the billing. A larger practice, however, may find the investment in such services quite worthwhile. Another disadvantage of billing services is that patients' records may have to be removed from the doctor's premises, resulting in an inconvenience to the office routine. If some arrangement can be made for the removal of these records without interference with the practice (e.g., on weekends), the billing services can help the doctor significantly. However, removing records from the office is risky and may be an invasion of a patient's right to privacy.

COMPUTERIZED BILLING

The cost of computerized billing usually makes its use feasible only in large medical practices. Before a physician decides to institute a computerized billing system, it would be wise to consider the competency of the service firm. The following questions should be asked: Is the system capable of rejecting incorrect information?

Will the service firm give good service after the system has been adopted? And finally, is the doctor's present staff qualified to use the system? If the physician has major reservations about these problems, the use of a computerized system should be reconsidered.

When the decision has been made to use a computer, there are three types of systems that can be used. The first is the remote terminal system in which the information is taken from the doctor's office by hand and is delivered to the computer center for processing. The computer system services many businesses simultaneously, and there is usually a flat fee for each account plus an additional charge for each printout. The office computer is the second type of system available, and it can be purchased outright. Though it does not have the flexibility or the capacity of the large computers found in data processing centers, it is nevertheless available exclusively for the practice. The third type of computer system is the time-sharing system, wherein a telephone-linked terminal in the doctor's office relays input to the computer. This system is also employed simultaneously by many users, with costs and computer time being shared in an equitable manner. In effect, a computerized billing system can do everything a manual system can do. However, it does these things more efficiently, faster, and more accurately. It can produce statements, patient ledger cards, insurance forms, and many other documents required in a medical office.

13.2

COLLECTION PROCEDURES

With regard to nonpayment, patients can be categorized into four groups. First, they may be negligent about payment. If a patient falls into this group, the fault may lie in part with the medical office staff. If billing isn't done promptly or if there isn't timely follow-up on collections, the patient may feel that the bill is not important enough to be paid on time. There are also those patients who are unable to pay, although they would like to do so. Prompt collection efforts can establish the nature of the problems. Time-payment plans can then be arranged to fit the particular circumstances. Oddly enough, many honest people who cannot pay their medical bills promptly will, due to embarrassment, either do without needed medical care or will go to another physician. This situation can be avoided if prompt follow-up of bills is combined with understanding and planning. The third category includes those who are unwilling to pay. In most cases, the patient will have what he or she feels is a valid reason for nonpayment. Again, a prompt collection policy will help to ascertain what the reason is and will hasten the collection process. Frequently, payment is not forthcoming due to a misunderstanding about the fee. If this is the case, an honest open discussion of the fee should take place as soon as possible, preferably between the patient and the doctor. It is far better, of course, for discussions to take place prior to treatment. The fourth category includes the deadbeat, the patient who never had any intention of paying. The only way to detect a deadbeat prior to treatment is through a credit check. However, a discussion of the fee prior to treatment may help you to ascertain the patient's attitude and intentions.

AGING ACCOUNTS

All accounts receivable should be "aged." This means that the status of each account is analyzed on a monthly basis showing exactly what collection procedures have been followed to date. Aging is a systematic method of enabling one to see exactly what the next collection step should be.

It is best to use some type of coding system for aging accounts. Collection efforts lose their clout if an error is made in the order of procedures. For example, if a reminder letter is sent to a patient who has already received pointed requests for payment, the patient may conclude that the medical office is disorganized. That patient may also feel that the debt is of no importance, thereby leading to continued nonpayment. One coding system uses colored tabs to reflect the different ages (and therefore, different collection stages) of the accounts. These tabs are attached directly to the patients' ledger cards. Another popular coding system uses letters combined with numbers to represent the different collection procedures. For example, "L1" might mean that one collection letter had been sent; "L2," that a second collection letter had been sent, and so on. These codes would also be on tabs attached directly to the patients' ledger cards.

THE MEDICAL ASSISTANT'S ROLE IN OBTAINING PAYMENTS QUICKLY
A doctor does not usually discuss routine fees with patients, instead preferring that the medical assistant do so. Therefore, it is the assistant's job to obtain payment from patients as quickly and as tactfully as possible. The quicker the fees are obtained, the less collection effort is required. Tact is needed so that patients will maintain a high regard for the doctor and the staff. Medical office personnel are traditionally thought of as humanitarians; thus, hard, cold business-world approaches to collection do not work.

SAMPLE DELINQUENCY SITUATIONS
Situation 1   The patient has not paid the bill within a reasonable length of time (30 days after initial billing), and the patient is known to be a procrastinator. The best approach would be to remind the patient firmly of his or her obligation at short, regular intervals until payment has been received. On subsequent visits, an attempt should be made to collect all fees before the patient leaves the office.

Situation 2   The patient has not paid the fee within a reasonable length of time after initial billing and the patient is known to be a prompt payer. As the first collection effort, the assistant should determine the nature of the patient's problem. If the situation warrants it, the assistant may help the patient make other arrangements for payment, even to budgeting a specific sum every pay period for the physician's fees. In medical practices, interest or carrying charges are usually not added to bills.

Situation 3   The patient has not paid within a reasonable period after billing and the initial collection effort on the assistant's part indicates that the patient may have a valid complaint. The assistant should attempt to alleviate the situation by a frank discussion of the problem. If this does not help, the patient should be told that the matter will be discussed with the doctor and that the patient will be contacted again. After discussion, the physician may decide to discuss the matter with the patient. Whatever the outcome, the patient has been assured of a continued interest in his or her welfare, which is a big first step toward obtaining payment.

Situation 4   The patient neither pays nor responds to any type of collection effort. The assistant ascertains from the patient's attitude that he or she does not intend to pay. The best thing to do at this point is to stop the collection efforts and ask the doctor for guidance. The physician may decide that this type of account should be turned over to a collection agency or to an attorney.

COST OF USING COLLECTION AGENCIES

Collection agencies are usually employed as a last resort in the medical profession. The cost to the physician, both in dollars and in goodwill, is often more than he or she is willing to pay. (Collection agency charges are high in relation to the amounts owed by most patients.) The services of a collection agency should not be utilized until the doctor's staff has exhausted all other feasible collection methods. No matter what the situation is, patients resent the use of a collection agency. Most physicians understand this, and they believe that the loss of goodwill will be a definite result of using such an agency. Over the long term this could more than offset any immediate financial results the agency may have been able to achieve.

COLLECTION METHODS TO BE USED BEFORE RESORTING TO AGENCIES OR THE COURTS

There are many timetables usable for collection. Those that are used most commonly are as follows:

1. During the first month, an itemized statement is sent to the patient.
2. If no payment has been received by the end of the second month, another statement is sent with a reminder that it is a second statement.
3. If no payment is forthcoming by the end of the third month, a reminder letter is sent.
4. At this point, additional and progressively sterner letters are sent. Alternatively, a telephone contact with the patient can be made by the medical assistant. If a telephone interview is deemed desirable, the assistant must at all times be professional, tactful, to the point, and brief. The assistant also must try to obtain a definite commitment from the patient, preferably a specific amount by a specific date.
5. If this effort produces no results or if the patient does not fulfill his or her commitment, the physician may decide to telephone the patient. Having the physician call personally may prod the patient into paying or, at least, into discussing the problem. The physician may also decide that the situation warrants a meeting with the patient. In many cases, this procedure compels the patient to pay at least a portion of the bill and paves the way for a mutually satisfactory payment of the remainder.

It is generally thought that personal contact—either by letter or by telephone—produces far better results than the use of impersonal devices such as form letters, reminder stickers and stamped messages. The medical assistant, however, must always remember that it is the physician's practice and that delegated authority must not be exceeded. The doctor must decide how extensive the collection effort should be. The following examples illustrate the wording that might be used in various collection letters:

Example 1
You have always paid your account promptly in the past, so we assume that this unpaid balance must be an oversight.
Please accept our note as a friendly reminder that your account is due for $__.

Example 2
Since your last visit to this office on ____(date)____, we have not heard from you about your account due. If it is impossible for you to remit to us the full due amount (give the balance), please telephone this office within the next __ days so that we can work out satisfactory payment arrangements.

Example 3
As we agreed in our telephone conversation today, we are looking forward to receiving full payment on your account within the next __ days. Thank you very much for your cooperation.

Example 4
It has now been over __ months since your treatment was completed, and in spite of all the financial arrangements made with you before the treatment was administered, a balance still

remains on your account. As members of the local credit bureau, one of our responsibilities is to report the names of patients not meeting their financial obligations promptly. Although we are always reluctant to do this, for it damages such patients' credit ratings, we nevertheless must follow through if we do not receive payment within __ days. Please think of yourself and remit the balance due before we have to take further action.

Letter Ending Physician-Patient Relationship

MARTIN A. BROMLEY, MD
2100 PARK AVENUE
THOMPSONVILLE, ST 45678

TELEPHONE 123-9876

June 4, 19—

Mr. Donald D. Doe
34 Smith Lane
Thompsonville, ST 45678

Dear Mr. Doe:

This letter is to inform you that your overdue account has now been transferred to a collection agency for further action.

As of one month from June 4, 19—, no further appointments or services will be provided for you by my office. However, I am giving you a month's notice of this action so that you will be able to obtain the services of another physician.

Mr. Doe, I regret having to take this unpleasant action; however, you have continuously ignored my assistant's repeated requests for payment.

Very truly yours,

M.A. Bromley, MD

Martin A. Bromley, MD

FLAGGING OF OVERDUE ACCOUNTS

It is important that overdue accounts be flagged or marked to differentiate them from current accounts. Many practices have devised systems in which credit symbols representing the patients' status are entered directly on the patients' ledger cards. In this manner, a medical assistant can see at a glance which accounts are past due, as well as their exact status. It also alerts other staff members to delinquent patients. At the next appointment, the assistant can tactfully discuss the past due balance. It is hoped that at least partial payment can be obtained as a result of the discussion.

13.3

SPECIAL COLLECTION PROBLEMS AND PROCEDURES

TRACING "SKIPS"

When a patient still has an open account balance and moves without leaving a forwarding address, he or she is considered a "skip." Whether the patient's behavior is deliberate or inadvertent, it is still important to take steps quickly to find him or her. If the post office's forward order has expired, the insertion of the phrase "Address Correction Requested" on the statement's envelope may result in the statement being delivered. "Skips" can be traced in the following ways:

1. Recheck the patient's original registration form to ascertain that the correct address was used on the statement.
2. Call the telephone number that is on the form. It is possible that the number has been transferred to the person's new location or that a recording will inform you of the patient's new telephone number.
3. Call references given by the patient, but use the utmost discretion.
4. Check with the patient's employer without stating why you need to contact the person. If the employer is not willing to give you the information, he or she may be willing to give the patient a message.
5. Check with the state motor vehicle department for notification of a change of address.
6. Check the *City Directory* to locate the former landlord or neighbors of the patient; they may know the patient's location.
7. If the patient has children, check with the school nearest their former home. The school may have a forwarding address.
8. If the patient has an unusual name, check with the telephone company's information service to find out if there is a new listing.
9. Check with the patient's bank for a corrected address.

If none of the above methods locate the "skip," it is advisable to turn the account over to a collection agency with any information you have about the patient.

CLAIMS AGAINST ESTATES

When a patient dies, a bill should be submitted to the estate of the deceased. If the doctor chooses to cancel or reduce the fee, a registered letter to that effect with condolences should be sent to a member of the deceased's family. The letter is sent to dispel any belief on the part of the family that the cancellation or reduction is due to faulty action by the doctor. It is obvious that the consequence of such a family-held belief might result in a malpractice suit. Generally, there is a response to the doctor's correspondence. However, if the deceased's estate or next of kin cannot be located, the assistant can inquire of other physicians who treated the patient, the mortuary, or the hospital if the patient died there.

The bill should be itemized and sent in duplicate by certified or registered mail (return receipt requested), so that there will be proof of receipt. If no response is received within 10 days, or if the administrator of the estate rejects the claim, a claim against the estate should be filed with the county clerk in the county of probate. As the various states have different time limits, it is best to check with the physician's attorney for the exact procedure to be followed. If the claim is accepted by the administrator of the estate, the doctor will receive a written acknowledgment. Once a claim has been acknowledged, payment will be forthcoming, although this may take some time.

BANKRUPTCY
Bankruptcy laws are federal. A patient who files for bankruptcy becomes a ward of the court and is entitled to its protection. Therefore, when a physician is notified that a patient has declared bankruptcy, all collection efforts must cease. A creditor who continues to proceed against a bankrupt debtor can be fined for contempt of court. There are two types of bankruptcy: a straight petition in bankruptcy and a wage earner's bankruptcy. A person who declares a straight petition in bankruptcy simply indicates to whom money is owed and is not required to make payment. If a patient files this way, a claim for the doctor's fee has to be filed on a form that can be obtained by writing to the referee in bankruptcy. As the doctor's fee is not tied to collateral, it is usually one of the last debts to be paid. A patient in wage earner's bankruptcy, on the other hand, pays a fixed amount (i.e., an amount agreed to by the court) to the trustee in bankruptcy. These funds are then passed to the creditors. While a person is in wage earner's bankruptcy, creditors cannot garnish, attach, or in any way proceed against the bankrupt party.

STATUTES OF LIMITATIONS
Two aspects of Statutes of Limitations should be considered in the collection of medical fees. First, malpractice statutes of limitations exist, which set a specific time limit during which malpractice suits may be filed. It is usually advisable to wait until this time has elapsed before suing a patient. The second aspect involves collection limitations. These limitations refer to specific time limits during which a legal collection suit may be filed against a debtor. The statutes vary depending on which of three account categories are involved. If an account is considered an open-book account (an account that is open to charges made from time to time), the statute runs from the last date of an entry for a specific illness. Most physicians' accounts are open-book, and in cases where patients have chronic conditions, it is almost impossible to set a time limit. Accounts also can be written contracts (the statute runs from the date of the last installment or single due date) or single-entry accounts (usually for small amounts). The second type of account has only one entry so that the statute runs from that date. Many states have shorter statutes for single-entry accounts than for the other two categories.

SELECTION OF ACCOUNTS FOR COLLECTION AGENCIES
The only accounts that should be submitted to a collection agency are those that have already been subjected to the medical practice's routine collection efforts, with no patient response. If a patient has responded positively to collection efforts, it is advisable not to turn the account over to an agency unless the patient subsequently stops payments and does not respond to further efforts.

SELECTING A COLLECTION AGENCY
A physician may decide to use a collection agency after the staff has made an earnest effort to collect overdue accounts. The agency should be selected with care.

Different types of agencies are available. Most are privately owned and operated, with some specializing in the handling of medical and dental accounts. Other collection agencies are operated by medical associations. (Out-of-state or mail-order agencies usually are not suitable for the collection of medical accounts.) Certain guidelines should be followed in order to select a reliable, ethical collection agency. These are:

1. Check with the local medical association as to the reliability of the agency. It is also advisable to check with the Medical-Dental-Hospital Bureaus of America, the Associated Credit Bureau of America, or the National Retail Credit Association, all of whose members maintain high standards.

2. Check with the Better Business Bureau.

3. Investigate the ownership and financial responsibility of the agency and its promptness in settling accounts.

4. Investigate the agency's collection methods. Request copies of sample collection letters.

ECONOMICS OF USING AN AGENCY

As stated elsewhere in this chapter, a physician should not use the same collection tactics as a business because of the humanitarian aspects of medical practice. Before deciding to use a collection agency, a decision must be made as to the cost of using an agency—in both dollars and in the loss of goodwill. In many cases, it is better to write the account off than to use a collection agency. If an overdue account is for a small amount, the routine collection effort may cost more than the account is worth. If this occurs, it would be wise to write the account off after only superficial collection efforts have been made. Most physicians feel that it is inadvisable to resort to court action unless unusual circumstances warrant it. In many states, doctors can use small claims courts as a vehicle for collection after a nominal fee is paid for a summons to the patient. When deciding on the advisability of court action, several factors should be considered: the patient's ability to pay, justification of the fee by comparison with fees charged by other physicians, supporting documentation, legal liability of the patient or a third party, and the exhaustion of all other collection means. The threat of a lawsuit should not be used carelessly. However, once a patient is threatened with a suit, the matter should be pursued to a conclusion. Under no circumstances should the assistant threaten a suit unless the doctor has given permission for such action.

14

CHAPTER FOURTEEN

MEDICAL DICTATION AND TRANSCRIPTION SYSTEMS: An Overview

CONTENTS

14.1

GOALS AND STANDARDS

One of the primary transcription goals of the medical assistant/administrative is to commit the dictated word to paper in an accurate manner. An equally important goal is to transcribe all medical dictation on time. But before these goals can be accomplished effectively, the doctor must provide the assistant with standards and directions indicating how all transcription assignments are to be carried out. In this connection, job descriptions, task sheets, and written production standards are useful guides for medical assistants in single or group practices, for transcriptionists, and for supervisors in very large practices or institutions. The following paragraphs discuss each of these documents.

JOB DESCRIPTIONS

Job descriptions with concomitant task sheets are desirable in all offices where medical transcription is performed. (Each job description and task sheet should be written for the individual employment setting, of course.) While the job description gives a general outline of the responsibilities of the position, the task sheets list the specific daily, weekly, and monthly assignments that the assistant is expected to carry out. These documents are extremely helpful to the new employee, the seasoned employee, and the physician as well.

A typical job description for an assistant whose position requires much transcription contains most if not all of the boldface items in the following sample:

1. **Title of the position**   Medical Assistant/Administrative
2. **Immediate supervisor**   General Office Supervisor or the Physician
3. **Nature and purpose of work**   Medical assistants/administrative in this office transcribe complex confidential medical dictation from all clinical specialties [or, in the smaller offices, they transcribe all office dictation]. These materials may include medical histories, physical examinations, operative reports, laboratory data, drug reports, and clinical résumés. The medical assistant works directly for the physician or for the general office supervisor [in a very large office].
4. **Duties**   In accordance with individual office policies and procedures, the medical assistant
   a. Transcribes all medical dictation;
   b. Gives the completed transcription to the physician for signature;
   c. Prepares each report for photocopying and mailing;
   d. Files copies of completed reports;
   e. Performs other administrative duties that are assigned;
   f. Reports equipment malfunctions and breakdowns immediately;
   g. Keeps all equipment clean and the work area neat.
5. **Scope of work**   The medical assistant is required to have an exceptionally broad and thorough knowledge of medical terminology and is expected to transcribe dictation with rapidity and accuracy. (In addition to basic disease names and anatomical terms, the medical terminology includes the names of drugs, instruments, and therapeutic procedures.) The medical assistant must be knowledgeable in English grammar and composition. Good spelling is essential.
6. **Mental demand**   Transcription requires a high degree of concentration, and the employee must have the ability to work under pressure. Not only must the medical assistant be thoroughly familiar with the procedures for handling transcribed dictation, but the assistant must also be able to concentrate in the presence of extraneous noises (e.g., the sounds of electric typewriters and voices). The assistant is expected to recognize and correct obvious errors in dictation and to refer questionable items to the physician. The assistant must at all times protect the confidentiality of the dictated matter.
7. **Qualifications and skills**   General Education—high school graduate (minimum). Special Education—completion of an accredited medical assisting program that includes training in medical terminology, machine transcription, and typewriting. The assistant must have a copy typewriting speed of at least 55 words per minute. The assistant must understand thoroughly the operation of the equipment which is used and must be able to recognize any malfunction in it.

NOTE: The above job description is intended to identify a particular aspect of the profession and is not to be interpreted as a work schedule. Any employee assigned to this position may be required to perform other duties as requested by the physician.

TASK SHEETS

Task sheets, like the procedures manuals described in Chapters 6 and 7, generally serve as simple reminders of the assignments to be carried out on a regular basis. However, task sheets are usually more limited in scope than procedures manuals: the sheets are restricted in coverage to the duties of a particular staff member (such as a receptionist, a transcriptionist, a bookkeeper, or a file clerk). An administrative procedures manual, on the other hand, lists and explains all of the administrative office procedures of the practice.

The content of task sheets differs according to the size and nature of the office. For example, the number and diversity of duties performed by any individual generally depend on the number of nonphysician staff members. In the single-physician office, the sheets typically contain many more tasks than the ones in multi-physician offices do. Task sheets should never be used as standards, though: they merely specify what *shall* be done without addressing either quantity or quality of output. (Production standards delineate the latter.)

Thought should be given to the structure of the sheets so that a task can be easily added or deleted without the whole set of sheets having to be redone. An orderly way to do this is to begin with the first assignment of the day and to end with the last one. Weekly and/or monthly tasks may be listed on separate sheets. Because of their relative infrequency, the weekly and monthly tasks should be accompanied with special detailed instructions explaining how they are to be accomplished. (Inclusion of these details will refresh the employee's memory regarding procedures.) The sheets should state which tasks are to be performed each day, each week, and each month without exception. In this way, if the employee responsible for the fulfillment of a particular assignment is absent, another employee can easily determine what is to be done and how it is to be done.

Daily dictation and transcription tasks   The following examples typify the daily and weekly dictation and transcription tasks that might be performed in a two- or three-physician office where the patient load is heavy. (NOTE: Each office's routine will differ in detail according to the size of the practice, the nature of the patient population, and the preferences of the physician or physicians.)

Simulated task sheet   Beginning each day Monday through Friday the assistant whose job involves much transcription should:

MORNING
1. Check and replenish (if necessary) the secretarial supplies.
2. See that all equipment is functional.
3. Make the necessary pretranscription preparations (see section 14.3).
4. Transcribe priority or STAT dictation first. This is preadmission information required by a hospital on scheduled patient hospitalizations and referral correspondence. (If the letters do not contain the latest medical data, photocopies of the patient's most recent physical examination and/or lab tests need to be attached.)
5. Proofread the transcribed material.
6. Mail all reports and letters not requiring the physician's signature.

AFTERNOON
7. Complete the rest of the daily transcription and proofread it.
8. Make photocopies of all reports and test results as required and attach them to the completed transcription.
9. By a specified time in the afternoon (such as 4:00 p.m.), distribute all remaining transcribed reports and letters for signature and pick up all reports and letters that have already been signed.
10. Prepare the signed documents for mailing.
11. Turn off the equipment (e.g., the dictation/transcription unit, the electric typewriter, and the photocopying machine) at the end of the day.

WEEKLY DICTATION AND TRANSCRIPTION TASKS
1. One afternoon a week set up a portable dictation unit in the conference room for any required dictation by the doctors.
2. Each Thursday submit a weekly work time summary to the physicians or to the office manager.
3. Each Thursday submit supply purchase requests to the physicians or to the other staff member responsible for supplies.

4. Each Friday morning prepare a list of patients who are scheduled to be admitted to the hospital the following week, and give a copy to the physicians and to the receptionist.

PRODUCTION STANDARDS

Production standards are most often established simply to make the employee aware of what the employer expects. But in a very large group practice or in a hospital, such standards may be established to measure the production of the employees. Employees whose quantity and quality of output measure up to established standards may be rewarded by bonuses in some settings. The production level of a medical transcriptionist is determined by the total words, total lines, or total minute-units of transcription completed during a specified time period. An example based on the standards used by large facilities is as follows:

The minimum standard level of production is the accurate transcription of seventy (70) minute-units of dictation per day on a weekly average. The definition of a *minute-unit* of dictation is a minute recorded by the time device on the dictation equipment. A minute-unit may vary from 55 to 60 seconds, depending on the type of dictation equipment used. Some large institutions provide bonuses to those whose production exceeds seventy (70) minute-units per day.

The medical assistant/administrative ought to request some sort of quality and production standards from the physician regardless of the size of the office.

TRANSCRIPTION OUTPUT: Quantity Standards

Although the following information is relevant mainly to medical transcriptionists in large institutional settings, it also should be of interest to all medical assistants whose duties include lengthy transcription:

1. Copy typewriting skills for the good typist should be approximately 55 to 60 words per minute. Since the assistant who is transcribing must listen, type, listen, type, and so on, the assistant cannot be expected to transcribe at the same rate as that of copy typewriting. The average time to typewrite one minute of dictation is five minutes of actual "typewrite-listen" time.

2. The national averages for the lengths of the following kinds of medical reports are approximately:

history and physical examination	250 words
consultation	100 words
operative report	300 words
discharge summary	250 words
radiology report	75 words
pathology report	100 words
autopsy report	1600 words

3. The dictation volume measured in words could be approximated as follows:

Average Number of Reports per Day	Average Volume	Total Volume
20 Histories and physical examinations	250 words	5,000 words
4 Consultations	100 words	400 words
8 Operative reports	300 words	2,400 words
20 Discharge summaries	250 words	5,000 words

52 total reports/day   total words of dictation: 12,800 words/day

4. The average work day is eight (8) hours in length. Even though the employee is paid for the full 8 hours, lunch and other breaks occurring during the period reduce the 8 hours to approximately 6 ½ hours of actual productive time.

5. The average work week is five (5) days. To compute actual annual working time, start with 260 days or 2,080 hours work per year and subtract from this holidays and vacation time. The remainder is the actual time in days or hours to be used in computing actual output expected during the year.

6. The best typist using the best machine can transcribe approximately 25 words of verbal dictation per minute. The good typist using a good machine averages approximately 16 words per minute, and the slow typist using a poor machine averages only 8 words of dictated material. Average productive time is approximately 390 minutes per day based on calculations in #4.

Possible Productive Time 450 min/day	**Average Productive Time 390 min/day**
25 words/min = 11,250 words/day	25 words/min = 9,750 words/day
16 words/min = 7,200 words/day	16 words/min = 6,240 words/day
8 words/min = 3,600 words/day	8 words/min = 3,178 words/day

7. Another simple method of equating transcription production can be computed as 75 minutes of dictation per eight-hour day equals approximately 750 lines of typewritten material at 10 words per line, resulting in approximately 7,500 typewritten words per day

   80 minutes of dictation per 8-hour day
   800 lines of typewritten material at 10 words per line
   8,000 typewritten words per day.

You can compare these statistics with your own transcription rates to determine the areas in which your skills need improvement.

QUALITY STANDARDS

Production with emphasis solely on output is of little value if the product is unusable due to defects. Therefore, quantity standards must be accompanied by quality standards. Quality standards define the degree of accuracy and the minimal expected neatness of the completed transcription. These standards are set and defined by the employer. The specific work environment (e.g., a single-physician office or a large transcription pool) determines the standards. The following is a list of transcription quality standards useful in any medical office:

1. Type everything that is dictated. DO NOT assume the responsibility of changing, rewording, deleting, or adding to any dictated material.
2. All words must be spelled correctly.
3. No typographical errors should appear on the final copy.
4. There should be no strike-over characters.
5. Squeezed characters are allowable if they are neatly executed.
6. Corrections are allowable if they are undetectable.
7. Use only the formats for the various reports that the physician chooses.
8. Style all abbreviations according to the dictionary designated by the physician.
9. Never use abbreviations, signs, and symbols in recording the diagnosis, regardless of where the diagnosis appears in the report.
10. Always give the date on which the material was dictated and the date on which it was transcribed.
11. Always identify the transcribed material by using typist's initials.

You should strive to transcribe all dictated material in a way that will match the quality standards outlined above.

14.2

AN OVERVIEW OF DICTATION AND TRANSCRIPTION EQUIPMENT

No matter how sophisticated the dictation/transcription equipment in your office is, it will be worthless if you do not know how to use it properly. Therefore, you should be thoroughly familiar not only with the equipment in your own office but also with dictation/transcription equipment in general. You may be responsible for dictating responses to routine correspondence on a regular basis or during the times that the physician is away from the office for several days (see also Chapter 15 for sample letters composed by the medical assistant). In addition, you may be asked to evaluate new dictation/transcription systems and to recommend one for purchase by the office.

Modern dictation and transcription devices enable the medical assistant to reflect in correspondence and reports the physician's or the facility's image quickly, efficiently, and effectively. Attractive letters and medical reports can be swiftly returned to the dictator for signature and approval. Turnaround time—the time required to transcribe the dictated material and put the finished document on the dictator's desk—may be within minutes or an hour or two from the actual time of live dictation. Same-day service is standard in most physicians' offices and large institutions. In this connection, it is important to remember that priority or STAT situations often arise in which the dictated matter must be transcribed and ready for the dictator's signature within minutes of the original dictation. And finally, it must be emphasized that continuous use of machine dictation will expedite the office work flow and will reduce the backlog of medical reports and correspondence to be written by the physician.

Familiarization with the chosen dictation-transcription system   An alert medical assistant understands the basic mechanisms of the complete machine dictation-transcription system used in the physician's office. Therefore, you should read, become familiar with, and keep on file the operation manual for the dictation-transcription machine that you must use in your work. With the aid of the equipment sales representative, you should learn about a new device's idiosyncrasies (such as how much heat or how much cold the system can tolerate and still operate normally). You also should know if the presence of sophisticated medical equipment such as X-ray machines will interfere with the system's operation. Some systems are sensitive to heat and moisture. Also, special care must be taken by users to remove all surgical glove powder from their hands prior to beginning dictation because the powder can adversely affect the machine controls.

The basic operating instructions may be attached directly to the input device or to the dictation machine itself so as to aid the user. In some cases (and especially with desktop models), it may be prudent for you to preset the machine and then to tape the controls in place so that they cannot be altered.

You should write the telephone number of the dictation-transcription service firm in a prominent place for quick reference. But before making a call for service, check to see whether the equipment is receiving power and whether the input and output devices are properly connected. When you call for service, the firm may request a description of the disorder. You should describe the disorder briefly and ask the company when the office can expect a repair person.

THE NATURE OF DICTATION SYSTEMS
An overview of dictation systems should deepen your understanding of their use within the office. Also, knowledge of a system places one in a position to use it to good advantage as individual opportunities occur.

An analysis of office dictation system location and use reveals three general classes of equipment: portable machines, desktop models, and centralized units which interact with the mobile and the stationary units. Portable machines and desktop models are most often used in medical offices today, while centralized units are most often found in hospitals and large corporate organizations.

Portable machines The small comparatively lightweight (10–25 oz) portable dictation unit that fits easily into a pocket, handbag, or attaché case has won wide acceptance from busy physicians and other health care practitioners. It permits its user to dictate freely when telephones are not available. Portables are particularly useful in recording clinical facts immediately after the dictating physician has seen a series of hospital, office, or clinic patients. It is also useful during or after medical conventions and conferences. The recording time available on portable dictation machines ranges from 15 to 120 minutes depending on the recording medium (such as a standard cassette, a minicassette, a microcassette, a Mag card, or a visible belt). Special features of some portable dictation units include a wide range of useful controls, some of which are listed here:

The digital counter pinpoints the amount of tape available on the machine. It also helps to locate reports or letters quickly. Some units have an instant reset feature.

Side thumb-touch controls order the machine to stop, rewind, and play back.

Direct visual indication of document length and location eliminates the need for log pads and index strips.

A pause button permits the user to dictate at any desired pace.

Through the use of a recorder coupler, a dictator may prerecord the message in a remote area and immediately transmit it to the office by dialing the office. The information is transmitted from the portable's cassette to a cassette in the office for direct transcription.

NOTE: Not all of the features described above are available on all equipment models.

Desktop models Standard or desktop dictation machines are extremely useful in large offices having a heavy dictation flow. The skilled assistant can provide quick report or correspondence turnaround with the companion transcribing machine equipped with sophisticated and sensitive tone, speed, and volume controls.

Smaller offices may be equipped with a combination machine to be used for both dictation input and transcription output on a smaller scale. However, during times of peak work load, a combination dictation-transcription unit can present a problem, for it can perform only one operation at a time: it either records or plays back dictation. To prevent a backlog in the physician's work load, it is necessary to have additional compatible systems accessible by loan.

Centralized dictation systems Continuous service—24-hour service 7 days a week, with input from almost anywhere—is the most characteristic feature of centralized dictation systems in hospitals and in extremely large multi-physician offices. The components of the central recording system may vary widely from in-house operations/private-wire phone and recorder installations to PBX (private branch exchange) systems directing the dictation flow into banks of endless-loop tanks. As the job requirements of the facility change and as dictation needs vary, the system can be enlarged or modified.

The capabilities of some centralized dictation systems are illustrated just to show you their potential for adaptation within various facilities having special or limited dictation needs:

Sample System 1:   In-house Private-wire System
Ten remote microphone input stations are used.
Only one dictator may dictate at any given time.
Input stations are installed within 500 feet of
the central recorder or recorders.

Sample System 2:   Private-wire and PBX Systems
Recorder automatically loads and records.

Nine hours of recording time are available.
Filled cassettes drop out of the recorder.
Empty cassettes are automatically positioned.

Sample System 3:   Pushbutton Phone or Private-wire Systems
Private-wire input is achieved through special desk phones
which give access to a cassette recorder.

Sample System 4:   In-house, Private-wire, Pushbutton Phone Systems
Private-wire input is achieved through special desk phones which
give access to a bank of endless-loop tanks.
Several dictators may dictate at any given time.
There is a heat-moisure sensitive pushbutton input phone with
correction, fast forward, and reverse capabilities.

NOTE: Such systems are rarely if ever used in the smaller practices.

OUTPUT: Transcription Systems
The transcription output system parallels or is compatible with the dictation input:

1. Machine transcription by the medical assistant from belts, cassettes, discs, tapes, and other media results from the dictator's initial decision to use the media.
2. Conventional transcription from the stenographic notebook results from the dictator's decision to use this form of recording medical information. (This method is seldom used by practicing physicians.)

The production of accurate medical output documents (such as reports, letters, or abstracts) is the major goal of all medical assistants regardless of the transcription method used. In fact, work measurement of this output is a valid determinant of the worth of the person performing the transcription. An alert assistant can combine knowledge and skill to attain success in transcription production.

THE NATURE OF THE TRANSCRIPTION PROCESS
The product or output of the transcription process is the transcript. *Webster's New Collegiate Dictionary* defines *transcript* as " . . . a written, printed, or typed copy; *esp:* a usu. typewritten copy of dictated or recorded material." The actual transcription process involves three phases of responsibility for effective output:

1. Pretranscription preparations.
2. Transcription functions.
3. General post-transcription procedures.

PRETRANSCRIPTION PREPARATIONS
Organization and planning play a major part in the pretranscription preparations. First of all, the work module should be arranged efficiently. Especially in the smaller office where the person performing transcription shares space with other employees, the transcription work module can be more efficiently arranged by having the desk face a wall. In this way the activities of the other employees will be less disruptive because they are out of the transcriptionist's eye range. If the desk faces a wall, it is wise to place a picture or a wall hanging in front of the transcriptionist to help combat monotony and fatigue. In a large transcription pool, however, the medical transcribers should face the supervisor. This arrangement enables the supervisor to aid a transcriptionist without disturbing the other members of the pool.

If possible, the work module should contain sound absorbers (as carpets or an acoustic tile ceiling). The typewriter and transcription equipment should be checked regularly to see that it is in good working order.

Desk organization   Those items (such as the transcribing machine or the steno-graphic notebook) essential to transcription ought to be arranged on the desk for easy use. The following reference books also ought to be within easy reach: a general dictionary, a medical dictionary or dictionaries, a medical secretarial guide, and any other references designated by the physician. The basic kinds of stationery and report forms used regularly should be accessible in the stationery drawer. They include letterhead, plain bond continuation sheets, carbons, envelopes, preprinted forms, and other such materials. Correction tools (as tapes, liquids, or pencils) should be placed near the typewriter. The efficient assistant never has to look for these items but is able to locate them by touch. The right-handed person will usually place erasing tools at the right side of the typewriter; the left-handed person will, as a rule, choose the left side for convenience. However, the blind person may choose the lap instead. Of course, if the office has a self-correcting typewriter, there is little if any need for correction materials.

Chair adjustment   Chair adjustment so that the person performing the transcrip-tion can maintain a good, comfortable posture is important. A chair with an adjustable backrest should be made to fit the small of the back for maximum support. Correct chair and desk height definitely affect a typist's transcription production. For example, the typist's forearm slope should only equal that of the typewriter keyboard (i.e., there should be less slope for electric machines).

Typewriter condition   Careful attention to the condition of the typewriter before transcription will often save valuable time later. First of all, an inspection should be made to ensure a clean typeface. Daily brushing is vital to good typescript. Liquid cleaners may be used only on conventional manual or electric machines with type bars. One may use plastic cleaners and brushes on elements or fonts; however, liquid cleaners are definitely harmful to electric typewriter components.

A ribbon check before transcription will indicate whether or not a new fabric or film ribbon is needed; in this way, a uniform, dark typescript will be ensured. Having a spare spool or cartridge always at hand will ensure minimal interruption at the point when the ribbon change is needed.

Transcription machines   There are many manufacturers of transcribing machines. These companies provide helpful booklets with each new machine to assist the transcriber. If pertinent operating instructions are unavailable, the assistant need only telephone the company's local educational representative for information and assistance.

An Illustration of the Listen/Type Transcription Process

```
          TYPExxxxxxxx      TYPExxxxxxxx      TYPExxxxxxxx
LISTEN))))))))))))))))  LISTEN))))))))))))))  LISTEN))))))))))

The chest X ray shows   infiltration in the  left lower lobe.

TYPExxxxxxxxxxxxxxxxxx   TYPExxxxxxxxxxxxxxxx  TYPExxxxxxxxxxxxx
LISTEN))))))))))         LISTEN)))))))))))))))  LISTEN)))))))))))))))))))))))))

There has been          some clearing since   the previous examination.
```

A machine transcription simulation function   A simulation of the work flow of a machine transcriber is illustrated in the instructions below:

1. Place the recorded medium into the transcribing machine.
2. Put the earpiece or headset in place.

3. Position the foot control or the thumb control panel.

4. Check the machine controls (e.g., the start switch, the tone, the volume, and the speed).

5. Install an index strip (see the next illustration). There are 15 calibrations on a typical index strip. Each calibration represents one minute of dictation. One minute of dictation equals 10 typewritten lines. The diamond mark above the horizontal line indicates the end of a report. The triangle below the horizontal line represents an instruction or a correction. (ALWAYS LISTEN TO THESE SECTIONS *BEFORE* TRAN-SCRIBING.)

Index Strip

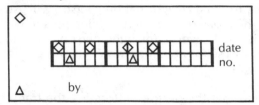

6. Move the index strip scanner (or pointer) to the first priority or STAT item.

7. Depress the foot control or the thumb control to activate the machine for listening. (Adjustments may be needed in tone, volume, or speed.)

8. Look at the index strip and determine the estimated line length of the first report or letter to be transcribed. The sample index strip provides the following information to the transcriber:
   Item 1, marked by the first diamond is five lines in length.
   Item 2, marked by the second diamond is 30 lines long.
   Item 3, marked by the third diamond is 35 lines long.
   Item 4, marked by the fourth diamond is 25 lines long.

9. Refer to the Letter Placement Table in this section to find the suggested marginal settings for the letter for either elite or pica spacing.

10. Set the typewriter margins, tabular stops, and correct vertical setting.

11. Find the triangle markings on the index strip, position the scanner at each triangle, and listen to the instructions and/or corrections of the dictator before transcribing. Doing so will avoid retyping because of changes.

12. Position the scanner at the beginning of the first item to be transcribed.

13. Use the Triple-Form Typewriting Copy Guide in Chapter 16 (the assistant can easily construct a copy) to insert the appropriate stationery into the typewriter.

14. Listen to the first transcription thought phrase.

15. Type only a portion of the first thought phrase.

16. Listen to the second thought phrase as typewriting of the first phrase is completed. Refer to the Listen-Type illustration.

17. Continue the transcription process toward the goal of continuous typewriting as listening continues in spurts by thought phrases.

POST-TRANSCRIPTION PROCEDURES

Regardless of the transcription method, the following procedures, if used by the assistant, will assure quality work:

1. Proofread the transcript and correct any previously undetected errors before removing the letter or report from the typewriter.

2. Compare the transcription of any data abstracted from another document with the original source.

3. If possible, enlist the aid of a proofreading assistant to help check statistical or technical data on transcript.

4. Make certain that any enclosures are attached to the letter or report.

5. Present the letter or report to the physician for signature.

Letter Placement Table
Three Sizes of Stationery

Lines in Letter Body	Words in Letter Body	Starting Line for Inside Address*	Typewriter Marginal Stops Elite/Pica	Length in Inches of Typing Line
Half-sheet Stationery: Assume Letterhead takes 7 vertical lines. (Baronial—center No. 36 for Elite; No. 30 for Pica)				
9–10	60–66	17**	15–60/10–50	4
11–12	67–73	16**	15–60/10–50	4
13–14	74–80	15**	15–60/10–50	4
15–16	81–87	14**	15–60/10–50	4
17–18	88–94	13**	15–60/10–50	4
19–20	95–100	12**	15–60/10–50	4
Executive-size Stationery: Assume Letterhead takes 8 lines. Monarch—center No. 44, Elite; No. 35, Pica)				
13–14	95–115	19**	15–75/10–60	5
15–16	116–135	18**	15–75/10–60	5
17–18	136–155	17**	15–75/10–60	5
19–20	156–175	16**	15–75/10–60	5
Full-size Stationery: Assume Letterhead takes 9 lines. (Standard—center No. 50, Elite; No. 42, Pica)				
11–14	175–200	20**	15–90/12–72	6
15–18	201–225	19**	15–90/12–72	6
19–22	226–250	18**	15–90/12–72	6
23–26	251–275	17**	15–90/12–72	6
27–30	276–300***	16**	15–90/12–72	6

*Begin to count at the very top edge of the stationery.
**The date should be typed three lines below the last line of the letterhead on all letters.
***Letters consisting of more than 300 words should be two-page letters.

14.3

THE USE OF MACHINE DICTATION SYSTEMS

Each dictation system is different, as are the dictation techniques used by each physician. However, the following paragraphs detail the most important steps that are followed by most dictators in the use of machine dictation systems.

ROUTINE INSTRUCTIONS
The assistant may be instructed by the doctor at the beginning of the dictation to follow routine instructions for a particular type of patient record. (You should have an indexed listing of instructions to follow.) For instance, the physician may dictate at the beginning of a medical report, "Medicare patient, routine." By giving this instruction, the doctor intends that you transcribe the report for the patient's medical record. From that dictated-transcribed medical report, the physician expects you to (1) fill out predetermined Medicare forms to be mailed to Medicare (2) write a letter to the patient telling the patient the results of any tests, and (3) tell

the patient that the Medicare reimbursement forms have been mailed. Thus, upon completion of this instruction, you will have created three documents for the physician's signature. Routine instructions vary with the office setting, however. Every doctor gives his or her own instructions to the assistant. A newly employed medical assistant must request the specific routines from the doctor right in the beginning: it is never wise to wait until the material is needed before asking for the routines.

STEPS IN PREPARATION FOR DICTATION

After completing a physical examination or a medical procedure, the physician will dictate the findings as soon as possible. The following guidelines in dictation techniques are included so as to assist not only medical assistants who might need to perform this task but also physician-employers who are interested in improving their dictating habits.

Get ready to dictate   Readiness to dictate involves *five* preparatory steps that will minimize time loss:

1. Plan ahead—dictate as soon as possible following each medical care intervention.
2. Alert the medical assistant for any upcoming STAT work.
3. Position the telephone or the microphone of the dictating machine: have extra input media (as cassettes or belts) available.
4. Review the examination findings, interventions, test results, or notes.
5. Organize your thoughts about any instructions that must be given.

Instruct the transcriber   It is important to remember that the transcriber needs special instructions from the dictator to produce acceptable transcripts. Following these instructions will produce better work:

1. Record the dictator's identification by name and title.
2. Indicate STAT work.
3. Identify the type of report (such as a history and a physical examination, an operation report, or a letter) and indicate whether the transcribed matter is to be a rough draft or final copy.
4. Give the patient's name and any other identification information.
5. Indicate routine instructions for particular types of patients.
6. Specify the number of copies needed.
7. Identify any extra reports (such as test results) that are to be attached.
8. Dictate numbers and complex medical words *slowly.*
9. Mention any subheadings in reports.
10. Give any special instructions.

Proceed to dictate   The art of effective dictation involves the correct tone of voice, naturalness of expression, sufficient volume to project the message, and clear enunciation. Special attention should be paid to the pronunciation of complex medical words since mistakes resulting from garbled dictation can have serious medicolegal implications. Try to pronounce such words slowly—syllable by syllable if necessary. The avoidance of distracting mannerisms is also essential for clean dictation. For example, the tapping of a pencil, the squeak of a chair, or a chance remark to the transcriber can later confuse the transcriber.

Since busy physicians rarely have the time to give detailed sentence punctuation instructions when dictating medical material, their assistants have to rely heavily on changes in pace or intonation to interpret the intended punctuation. The dictator should be aware of this and should try to modulate his or her voice accordingly.

A SIMULATION OF THE USE OF A MACHINE DICTATION SYSTEM

A simulation of dictation preparation, of instructions for the transcriber, and of actual dictation is given in this section following a few guidelines regarding the use of machine dictation systems.

Using the system   The dictation input phone is positioned on the desk. A light indicator tells the dictator which channel can be used. The tone, volume, and speed are automatically controlled by the system. The following information will be helpful to you in understanding the operation of the system and in using good dictation techniques.

1. Remove the dictating phone from the cradle in order to select a channel.
2. Select and depress the appropriate channel button to gain entrance into the system. It is important to remember not to put the phone back on the cradle until the entire dictation including instruction, additions, corrections, etc., have been completed. Once the phone is replaced, the system automatically locks out any access to the dictated material. The system is designed in this manner for security and confidentiality of dictated material. If you wish to pause, to review reports, or to stop dictating for a few minutes, simply lay the phone on the desk. This procedure retains the channel and yet allows you to resume dictation when ready or to reverse the tape to the first word of your dictation, if desired.
3. Press the dictate button (located on the input phone) with your thumb and speak directly into the instrument as if you were using a telephone. When not dictating (as when pausing for thought), simply release the dictate button. Upon resumption of dictation, again press the dictate button with your thumb and continue speaking.
4. Press the appropriate button (as correction, listen, reverse, or fast forward) for aid in making additions, deletions, and corrections.

How to instruct the transcriber   The dictator lifts the phone, depresses the channel selector, presses the dictate button, and dictates the needed secretarial transcription information (i.e., special instructions). (The assistant performing the transcription must have an indexed desk reference of the ROUTINES—the special instructions—for each specific task.)

A sample dictation and transcription   The following is a sample of centralized machine dictation and transcription. You will notice that in the sample the dictator has not given many instructions to the assistant. This is a fact of life. Very few busy dictators have the time to follow all of the helpful instructions listed earlier in this section. Consequently, the importance of the indexed desk ROUTINES cannot be overemphasized.

SIMULATION

Dictation A	This is doctor John Doe internal medicine clinical résumé on Thomas J Jones who was seen in the office today and whose birth date is March tenth nineteen twenty nine this patient was referred by doctor Rush W Smith ten Main Street Neighbortown US [ZIP Code given]
Routine instructions	The assistant will always refer to the ROUTINES desk reference for the specific task (clinical résumé, in this case) until this particular description has been memorized. The assistant will want to know the kind of paper to be used, the format (as for headings and for margin and line space alignment), and capitalization rules. The ROUTINES might state: 1. Plain bond paper, size 8½ × 11 inches.

2. Margins—five spaces right and left.
3. Title of report—six lines from top of page, centered and typewritten all in capitals.
4. Report style—entire report is to be typewritten in block style with two line spaces between each category heading.
5. Patient identification—two line spaces following the title of the report and flush with the left margin, single-space the patient's full name all in capitals with the last name first and the date of birth written as DOB: 01–01–29.
6. Category headings—flush with left margin and typewritten all in capitals and underlined followed by a colon.
7. Attending physician identification—typewrite it all in capitals on the same line with patient's name, ending at approximately the right margin.

   NOTE: *Doctor* is styled MD following the physician's name.
8. Medical specialties—on a line directly below the physician's name typewrite the medical specialty all in capital letters, and align the first letter of the specialty with the first letter of the physician's name.
9. Visit date—on a line directly below the medical specialty typewrite the visit date and align it with the first letter of medical specialty. The visit date is to be styled as:

   VISIT: 07–01–78 (Arabic numerals with hyphens, using two numbers for days, months, and years.) *Visit* is typewritten all in capitals followed by a colon.
10. Referring physician (if applicable) and referring physician's address—skip two line spaces and typewrite all in capitals flush left: REFERRING PHYSICIAN + a colon + two horizontal spaces on the same line + the referring physician's name. On a line directly under the first letter of the referring physician's name, typewrite the complete mailing address, using two single-spaced lines for the address. Refer to the ZIP Code reference book if the ZIP Code is not given.

CLINICAL RÉSUMÉ

Transcription A

JONES, THOMAS J.   JOHN DOE, MD
DOB: 03–10–29   INTERNAL MEDICINE
                                    VISIT: 07–01–78

REFERRING PHYSICIAN: Rush W. Smith, MD
                       10 Main Street
                       Neighbortown, US 00000

Dictation B

present illness this forty seven year old white male presents with a twenty four hour history of fever shaking chills and hemoptysis prior to his coming to the office his temperature reached a maximum of one hundred two degrees orally cough with hemoptysis is present with minimal sputum production there is no associated shortness of breath past history this patient has a long history of gastro-intestinal hemorrhages pancreatitis and other complications of alcoholic liver disease   the patient has a long extensive smoking history greater than sixty packs of cigarettes a month and a long standing moderately severe chronic pulmonary disease

Routine instructions

The ROUTINES desk reference identifies category headings (as *present illness, past history,* and *laboratory data*) and states:

1. Category headings—flush with the left margin, typewritten all in capitals and underlined followed by a colon.
2. The first word of the first sentence—two horizontal spaces following category heading.
3. Punctuation—punctuation to be added appropriately. (Refer to Chapter 17.)
4. Capital letters—capitalization to be used appropriately. (Refer to Chapter 17.)

Transcription B

PRESENT ILLNESS: This 47-year-old white male presents with a 24-hour history of fever, shaking chills, and hemoptysis. Prior to his coming to the office, his temperature reached a maximum of 102 degrees orally. Cough with hemoptysis is present with minimal sputum production. There is no associated shortness of breath.

PAST HISTORY: This patient has a long-standing history of gastrointestinal hemorrhages, pancreatitis, and other complications of alcoholic liver disease. The patient has a long, extensive smoking history, greater than 60 packs of cigarettes a month and a long-standing, moderately severe chronic pulmonary disease.

Dictation C

laboratory data hemoglobin eight point eight with a hematocrit of twenty five point eight wbc twelve thousand four hundred with eighty polys three bands thirteen lymphs and four monos prothrombin time is elevated with a control time of eleven and patient time is thirteen point three parenthesis sixty two percent activity parenthesis reticulocyte count is zero point eight percent with a platelet count of two hundred thirteen thousand creatinine zero point eight milligrams percent   sgpt is normal at fourteen iu urinalysis normal except three to five white cells with a negative culture chest x ray revealed a left lower lobe infiltrate

Routine instructions

For laboratory data, refer to the published office or facility laboratory manual for normal values of test results, abbreviations, etc. Arabic numbers are to be used in transcribing test results. At any time when there is uncertainty regarding a test or a result, leave blank spaces in the report. Attach a note to this effect to the right margin of the report. Ask the dictator to verify that particular item and to return the material for typewriting. (NOTE: Style all abbreviations according to the dictionary designated by the physician.)

Transcription C

LABORATORY DATA: Hgb. 8.8 with a hematocrit of 25.8, WBC 12,400 with 80 polys, 3 bands, 13 lymphs, and 4 monos.

Prothrombin time is elevated with a control time of 11, and patient time is 13.3 (62% activity). Reticulocyte count is 0.8% with a platelet count of 213,000. Creatinine is 0.8 mg%, SGPT is normal at 14 IU. Urinalysis normal except for 3–5 white cells with a negative culture. Chest X ray revealed a left lower lobe infiltrate.

Dictation D

final diagnoses number one left lower lobe pneumonia number two chronic alcohol abuse number three chronic obstructive pulmonary disease number four chronic pancreatitis number five history of gastrointestinal hemorrhages number six anemia

Routine instructions

The ROUTINES desk reference identifies *final diagnoses* as a category heading and states:

1. Category headings—typewrite all in capitals and underlined flush with left margin followed by a colon.
2. Enumeration of each diagnosis—*Number one* is on the same line with category heading, two horizontal spaces after the colon. Arabic numerals are followed by a period and two horizontal spaces.
3. Single-line space each enumerated diagnosis and align the numbers directly under one another.
4. Each transcribed diagnosis is followed by a period.

Transcription D

FINAL DIAGNOSES: 1.   Left lower lobe pneumonia.
2.   Chronic alcohol abuse.
3.   Chronic obstructive pulmonary disease.
4.   Chronic pancreatitis.
5.   History of gastrointestinal hemorrhages.
6.   Anemia.

Dictation E

end of report send one copy to the referring physician

Routine instructions

The ROUTINES desk reference states that upon completion of a report, the following tasks are to be carried out:

1. Dictating physician's name—six line spaces from the last item in the report, flush with the left margin, typewrite the dictating physician's name.
2. Identification initials—two line spaces below item #1 and flush with left margin, typewrite the transcriber's identifying initials.
3. Date of dictation and date of transcription—two horizontal spaces following the transcriber's initials, give the date of dictation and the date of transcription as in this example:
   ab   D: 07–01–78   T: 07–01–78
4. Copies of reports—one-line space below item #3 and flush with the left margin, typewrite CC followed by colon. Identify how many copies are to be sent and to whom.
5. All copies are to be photocopies.

6. Address all envelopes appropriately and attach them to the copies to be mailed.

7. Route the completed reports and copies to the appropriate sources for signature.

Transcription E

John Doe, MD
ab   D: 07–01–78   T: 07–01–78
CC: 1   Rush W. Smith, MD

14.4

THE USE OF LIVE DICTATION SYSTEMS

The term *stenographer* describes an individual who habitually uses shorthand or other live methods for recording material to be transcribed. While medical assistants use machine dictation/transcription much more often than stenography, it is nevertheless felt that live dictation should be discussed here for the benefit of those readers using stenographic techniques.

INPUT: Dictation for the Secretary/Stenographer
Dictation rates may vary from 80 to 140 words per minute. Even though average dictation normally ranges near the lower end of this scale—e.g., between 90 to 110 words per minute—the stenographer needs reserve speed for fast spurts of dictation.

Correspondence, medical reports, and staff conferences make up the major portion of medical dictation. In staff meetings and conferences, the medical assistant must be selective in note-taking. Only essential information and facts are recorded. Extraneous matter has to be carefully screened and deleted.

The assistant skilled in stenography may be trained in one of the various kinds of shorthand or in Speedwriting. However, as work experience accrues, the assistant will probably develop a unique and individual system of characters.

THE USE OF THE STENOGRAPHIC NOTEBOOK
Anyone using stenography needs to devise a system for handling the stenographic notebook. The system will be devised to meet individual circumstances; however, it is of prime importance to have the notebook, pens, and other items readily at hand so that you can respond immediately to the dictation call of the physician. Some basic procedures for handling the notebook are these:

Use several elastic bands around the top cover of the notebook in order to bind off transcribed notes.

Attach several paper clips at the side of the notebook cover for use in flagging STAT or important items to be transcribed first.

Assemble a work folder or binder consisting of a stationery pocket inside each cover. The stenographic notebook will fit easily in the right-hand pocket. The left-hand pocket will be useful for reference copies of correspondence, reports, agendas, or other items related to the day's dictation.

Place several pens, colored or black pencils, and a small ruler in the pocket of the folder beside the stenographic notebook.

Notebook identification systems   If you take dictation from several physicians, you should maintain a separate notebook for each one. Label each notebook cover with the name of the dictator and the date on which the notebook was last used.

Completed notebooks may then be filed chronologically under the name of each dictator. It is important to check with the physician concerning the retention policy for completed notebooks as well as how these notebooks may be destroyed. Paper clips, a triangularly folded notebook page corner, or colored pencil markings may be used to identify STAT items that must be transcribed first.

Space planning in the notebook Intelligent use of notebook space will enable you to add information with ease or to write in changes or instructions with care, either during or after dictation. Each item in a day's dictation series should bear an identification number or name. Allow several blank lines before and after each identified dictation item. This will normally provide enough space for changes and instructions.

Coding the stenographic notebook Changes in dictation are a part of the normal course of events in any stenographic recording session. You ought to be familiar with the symbols that are used to code changes. As time goes by, you will develop an individual coding system that you have found to be the most appropriate for your own work setting. Some examples of stenographic coding are shown in the following illustrations.

Delete or remove a word or phrase.

Add a word or a short phrase.

Use at the beginning and at the end of a change or an instruction.

Marks the first lengthy insert. (Each subsequent insert bears the letter b, c and so on.)

Indicates a STAT transcription item.

Strike out this section of notes.

Shows a transposition; invert the order of the words.

Move this sentence or section to the new position indicated by the arrow.

Examples of Speedwriting and Shorthand with Changes in the Stenographic Notebook

Correction
The regular monthly meeting of the Transfusion Committee will be held Tuesday, March 21, at 3 p.m., in my office. Please make every effort to attend.

Please change that to:
2-East Conference Room

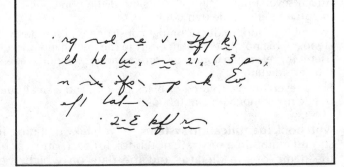

Deletion

At the moment, I am interested in researching some of the formats used to introduce obstetrical and newborn medical records into the computers.

Please omit:
At the moment

Insertion

Cardiac catheterization was done. No postoperative complications except for a mild fever spike without source of infection apparent.

Please insert this phrase after the word *done:*
showing excellent results

Addition

Item 1. Laboratory services—It may be possible to develop a computer program that gives an average ancillary cost per day.

Please add after the word *possible: and practical*

Correction

The Medical Staff Meeting was held on Tuesday, May 20th in the Ohio Room.

Please change day and date to: *Thursday, May 22nd*

Deletion

The Cancer Conference is tentatively scheduled every Friday at 2 o'clock with case presentations.

Please leave out: *tentatively*

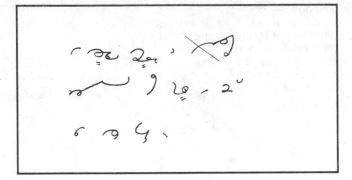

Insertion

The Chairman read the report from Mr. John J. Smith, Program Surveyor. The Committee discussed only the following points:

Please insert after the sentence nding with *Surveyor: For full details, see appended report.*

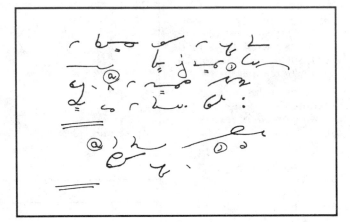

Restoration

The patient is a 12 year old white male who has a three day history of fever.

Correction, that should be: *two day;* let it stand as: *three day history*

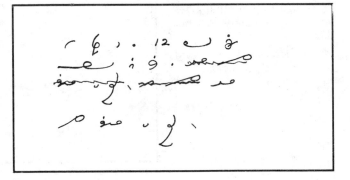

Stenographic transcription and copy typewriting   While the stenographic notebook transcription and copy typewriting processes differ in various ways from other forms of transcription, they also share similarities with them. A typical work-flow pattern for a secretary/stenographer is outlined below:

1. Elevate the stenographic notebook or the material to be typewritten in order to preclude eye fatigue. A copyholder may be used for this purpose.
2. Look for signaling devices (such as paper clips, folded corners of the notebook, or colored pencil notations) that are often used to flag STAT items for priority transcription.
3. Edit the shorthand or Speedwriting notes so that all changes, insertions, and special instructions are clearly understandable.

Referral Response: Transcription

(letterhead)

January 31, 1979

Henry Brown, MD
101 Elm Street
Hometown, OH 00000

Re: Adam M. Jones
DOB: 12-20-30

Dear Dr. Brown:

The above patient, Mr. Adam M. Jones, was seen on January 17, 1979. As you know, Adam desired a complete physical examination. He did not have any significant symptoms.

The examination was essentially normal. He does have a short ejection systolic murmur which has been noted previously of grade I/VI intensity heard best at the apex. No radiation. The murmur does not vary with various maneuvers. Blood pressure: 142/88. Chest X ray: Normal. CBC: Normal. Coagulation screen: Normal. BUN: Normal. Blood sugar: Normal. Sigmoidoscopy: Normal.

Resting electrocardiogram: The T waves are slightly flat in the V6 position. One PVC is noted.

He was exercised on a treadmill and his heart rate went to 160 per minute. Some junctional ST segment depression occurred, but no significant right angle ST segment depression. The monitored tracing after one minute of exercise reveals two premature beats.

Adam shows some minor changes. However, I do not feel they are significant. I again urged him to take a regular amount of exercise and maintain a normal body weight. I see no reason for any specific medications.

Thank you for allowing me to see him.

Sincerely,

John W. Doe, MD

Referral Response: Shorthand

4. Edit any special material (such as portions to be abstracted) so that all changes and extractions are clearly understood.

5. Determine the margin settings as required or as specified by the office setting or the type of report. (See the Letter Placement Table in section 14.2 for the margin settings for letters.)

6. Adjust the margin settings, the tab stops, and the spacing settings as necessary.

7. Place an envelope on the typewriter paper table. Insert the letterhead (and carbons) and the Triple-Form Typewriting Copy Guide (a sample of which appears in Chapter 16) into the space between the flap and the envelope. Spin the envelope into the machine to the date line. Remove the envelope.

8. If using a preattached multipart form, place the form on the typewriter paper table. Spin the form into the machine to the predetermined starting point.

9. Strive for smooth, continuous typewriting by reading a phrase ahead of the words that you are typewriting. (See the listen/type illustration in section 14.2; substitute the word *read* for the word *listen* when studying this illustration).

10. Refer to a dictionary for spelling. Use a medical secretarial handbook or an office manual and other references to verify data as the transcription progresses.

11. Compare the typescript with the shorthand notes or copy material to be certain that nothing has been inadvertently omitted.

12. Cancel the report or letter in the notebook by drawing a vertical line through it to show that it has been transcribed.

13. Code and date the original copy from which the copy typewriting was transcribed.

14.5

MEDICAL TRANSCRIPTION: Sources of Help with Special Problems

The medical assistant's most commonly encountered problem is that of poor enunciation on the part of the dictator. The assistant should <u>never</u> under any circumstances guess about unclear medical words or interpolate new words in an attempt to clarify them without first verifying the words used in the actual dictation. The following paragraphs give some sources of help that can be used in circumstances when the dictated matter is unclear.

In-house reference sources   In cases when you are unsure of a word or words, the patient's past and present medical records may be of assistance. Laboratory test data also may be of use. In addition, you can ask another staff member to listen to the machine dictation for help in interpreting what has been said. And finally, if all else fails, you can ask the physician who dictated the material in the first place to verify or clarify what has been said.

Outside reference sources   If you are unsure of a reporting procedure or a format for material being submitted to insurance companies or to local, state, and federal agencies, you can telephone the proper departments of these organizations for help. It is much better to find out how the materials should be handled in the beginning than to wait until the project has been completed, only to have to retype the data because of incorrect formats and/or transcription procedures.

Reference books   Essential reference books include the latest edition of at least one good unabridged medical dictionary. (See the Appendix for a list of titles.) Other important reference books include a good general dictionary, a medical secretarial handbook, a good grammar book, a medical spelling guide showing correct end-of-line divisions, and perhaps an abridged medical dictionary. (See the Appendix for a list of titles.) Some highly specialized titles that should be on your bookshelf are as follows: the *American Drug Index*, the *Guide to Surgical Terminology*, the *International Classification of Diseases, Adapted*, the *International Classification of Diseases for Oncology*, the *Merck Index*, *Modell's Current Drug Use*, the *National Formulary*, the *Physician's Desk Reference*, *A Syllabus for the Surgeon's Secretary*, and the *United States Pharmacopeia*. Locally published hospital, laboratory, X-ray, and physical therapy manuals also can be helpful in seeking answers to specialized questions.

14.6

SPECIAL TRANSCRIPTION PROCEDURES

Some medical reports require special transcription procedures that are unique to the field of health care. It is essential that the medical assistant understand the nature and the purpose of the documents that are commonly prepared and/or filed in the office. The following paragraphs discuss and illustrate the patient's problem list, a medical data base (including a medical history, a family history, a complete physical examination, a systems review, and laboratory data), and an example of an operation report. Typewriting guidelines are given beneath the illustrations of those documents that the medical assistant/administrative might have to type. Other illustrations in this section include an operating record and a discharge summary or clinical résumé. These documents often form an important part of a patient's total record, even though a medical assistant in private practice will not have to prepare them.

PATIENT'S PROBLEM LIST
As discussed in Chapter 9, the patient's problem list may be used in any setting (e.g., in a one-physician office, a multi-physician office, an ambulatory care clinic, or a hospital). A patient's problem list simply enumerates the patient's health problems with the approximate dates of onset and the dates on which the problems became inactive or were resolved. The ongoing problem list gives the physician a concise overview of the individual's health problems—both past and present. Durable heavy-duty paper should be used for this document. The problem list may be typewritten in a way similar to that used for the following illustration.

MEDICAL HISTORY AND PHYSICAL EXAMINATION
The primary purpose of the history and physical examination is to assist the physician in establishing a diagnosis on which to base the care and treatment of the patient. These are its main components:

Chief Complaint—a brief statement in the patient's own words of why the patient sought medical help.

Present Illness—a chronology of facts given by the patient concerning the symptoms, the onset, and the nature of the complaint as well as the events leading up to and including the current illness.

Past Medical History—a summary of all past illnesses, injuries, allergies, and childhood diseases (the physician may obtain the past history from the patient and from previous medical records).

Problem List with Fill-ins

MEDICAL RECORD			**PATIENT'S PROBLEM LIST**		
IMPORTANT — DO NOT USE ABBREVIATIONS WHEN LISTING PROBLEMS. This form may be used for inpatient/patient - members and outpatients. Upon DISCHARGE, place form in the Medical Records folder (Type II) - on the top of the right or left side, whichever is convenient. Upon READMISSION, remove form and place with current records on ward.					
Problem Number	Approx. Date of Onset	Date Problem Recorded	Active Problems	Inactive/Resolved Problems	Date Resolved
# 1	2-76	2-10-76	Left lower lobe pneumonia	Resolved	2-20-76
# 2	1977	4-22-77	Diabetes mellitus		
# 3	Years	1-20-78	Chronic obstructive pulmonary disease		
		1-20-78	A) Chronic bronchitis		
		1-20-78	B) Emphysema		
# 4	5-5-79	5-5-79	Acute appendicitis		
			with appendectomy	Resolved	5-15-79

Enter in space below: PATIENT IDENTIFICATION - TREATING FACILITY - WARD NO. - DATE

MEDICAL RECORD
PATIENT'S PROBLEM LIST

Guidelines
Align the form in the typewriter so that the typescript will be centered within the available line spaces.
Align all entries vertically.
Estimate the anticipated space required to include data in narrow-width columns before you start to type.
Do not use abbreviations when listing the patient's problems.

Family History—the health status of relatives (as mother, father, siblings, children, and spouse) in which heredity or contact may play a role. (If any family members are dead, the causes of death and the ages at the time of death are usually given.)

Review of Systems—a systematic review of all the body systems to reveal any subjective symptoms that the patient may have failed to mention.

Physical Examination—the result of a thorough examination of the patient by the physician with statements of his or her observations and significant findings, both normal and abnormal. A complete physical examination should cover the following:

1. **General inspection**   appearance, age, race, sex, nutrition, weight, height, temperature, pulse, respiration, blood pressure
2. **Skin**   color, texture, pigmentation, hair distribution, nail abnormalities, sweating
3. **Head**   size, shape, abnormalities
4. **Eyes**   conjunctiva, sclera, pupils, reflexes, fundi, vision
5. **Ears**   size, shape, position, canals, tympanic membranes, hearing
6. **Nose**   mucosa, septum, discharge
7. **Mouth**   breath, lips, teeth, gums, tongue, salivary ducts
8. **Throat**   tonsils, pharynx, postnasal drip, redness
9. **Neck**   stiffness, masses, thyroid
10. **Lymph nodes**   cervical, supraclavicular, axillary, inguinal
11. **Chest**   shape, respiration
12. **Breasts**   masses, discharge, tenderness
13. **Heart**   size, thrills, pulsation, rhythm, sounds, murmurs, gallop, friction rub
14. **Lungs**   breath sounds, adventitious sounds, friction rubs
15. **Blood vessels**   pulses, quality
16. **Abdomen**   contour, peristalsis, scars, rigidity, tenderness, masses, liver, kidney, spleen, hernia
17. **Genitalia, male**   scars, lesions, discharge
18. **Genitalia, female**   external, vagina, cervix, uterus, discharge
19. **Rectal**   fissure, hemorrhoids, masses, prostate, feces
20. **Bones, joints, muscles**   deformities, swelling, redness, tenderness, limitation of motion
21. **Extremities**   color, edema, tremor, clubbing, ulcers
22. **Neurological**   cranial nerves, peripheral nerves, coordination, reflexes, gait, sensory
23. **Impression or tentative diagnosis**   the physician's impression of the patient's illness before laboratory tests or diagnostic procedures have confirmed the final diagnosis.

Laboratory Data and X Rays—the results (normal and/or abnormal) of any ordered tests of any blood, urine, sputum, or stool samples; the interpretation of any ordered EKG; and the results and interpretation of any X rays ordered. (See also the Laboratory section of the Medical Data Base illustrated in this section.)

OPERATION REPORT
This is a report of the surgeon's findings during the course of an operation and of the procedures he or she used. It is a general requirement that the surgeon include the following items in the report regardless of the extent of the surgery:

1. **Preoperative diagnosis**—made before the operation and based on clinical findings
2. **Postoperative diagnosis**—based on findings at operation
3. **Name of operation or procedure**
4. **Findings**—a description of findings, both normal and abnormal, of tissues and organs.
5. **Procedure**—a detailed description of the techniques, equipment, and devices used.
6. **Specimens**—identification of any tissues or other specimens sent to the pathologist or to the laboratory.

Medical Data Base: History

Hometown Hospital   #090909

Smith, Mr. John James
10 Main Street
Hometown, US 00000

Birthdate: 03-20-29

HOMETOWN HOSPITAL
Hometown U. S.

MEDICAL DATA BASE
History and Physical

Person Recording: John Doe, MD
Time and Date: 12-30-79 10:30 p.m.

Age __50__ Sex __M__ Race __White__ Marital Status __Married__

Birth Place __Monroe County__ Residence __Hometown, US__

Education __High-school graduate__

Occupation __Transit Service__ Date Last Worked __Today__

Source of Information __Patient__ Reliability __Good__

CHIEF COMPLAINT: __"Chest pain"__

PRESENT PROBLEMS: Mr. Smith, a 50-year-old diabetic, notes that over the past two weeks he has had an increase in the number of hypoglycemic reactions. Once a day, always between 11:00 a.m. and 2:00 p.m., from 3 to 4 hours after breakfast prior to lunch. Also, he notes that he had had 2 to 5 episodes a day of pain that feels like someone "bursting a balloon" in the pit of his stomach, and that travels throughout his chest and both shoulders and into the left arm with a sensation like "bursting bubbles." This is not brought on by position, excitement, pressure, foods, etc. It is not affected by position, cough, breathing, etc. It lasts 5 to 15 seconds and is associated with shortness of breath but no diaphoresis, dyspnea, palpitations, nausea, or vomiting. Since these sensations began 10 to 12 days ago he has noted "soreness" in his chest, mainly anterior middle and both shoulders. This has been constant since then. No associated shortness of breath, cough, nausea, palpitations, or diaphoresis but the sensation is increased with deep breath and cough but not with swallowing or changes of position.

He has never had any pain like this before. He has a chronic cough which every morning is productive of whitish sputum - no change. He has had some nighttime sweats, and at

(Continue on next page if necessary)

times he feels like he has a fever.

In the past month, he has had two episodes like "the flu" associated with cough, fever, and myalgia lasting 24 to 48 hours.

He denies heart disease, murmurs, hypertension, edema, and claudication. He has been a 1,095 pack/year smoker with chronic bronchitis and emphysema. He had pneumonia once 20 years ago. No tuberculosis. No wheezing. Increased shortness of breath and cough for years.

Patient has a history of pancreatic insufficiency with diabetes. He is on a regular diet with 20 units of NPH insulin daily every morning. His urines are normal every day.

Guidelines

Type the patient's name and address and date of birth in the space provided. Align the data vertically.

Align the form in the machine so that no information will be obscured by the preprinted lines.

Skip two character spaces between sideheads and fill-ins.

In the Present Problems section, align the text flush left.

Medical Data Base: Family History

Hometown Hospital   # 090909

Smith, Mr. John James
10 Main Street
Hometown, US 00000

Birthdate: 03-20-29

FAMILY HISTORY:		Age	State of Health	Age at Death	Cause
Father				69	Heart disease
Mother				71	Hypertension
Siblings & Children					
No diabetes, cancer, thyroid disease or lung disorders.	Brother	51	Heart disease		
	Sister	47	Alive & well		
	Son	21	Alive & well		

Last chest x-ray, result —   1 year ago - emphysema

Transfusions —   None

Use of tobacco, alcohol —   20 years, three packs per day

Immunizations —   30 years ago

Long-term or current medications: Insulin 20 units NPH every day

Drug reactions: Penicillin - rash

PAST PROBLEMS: Hospitalizations, operations, injuries — date, place, result

Left hip - complete prosthesis January 1973

Cholecystectomy 1970

Pneumonia 20 years ago

Pancreatic insufficiency 1974

Rectal fistula repaired 1965

3

Guidelines
Align all inserts vertically as shown in the illustration.
Position all entries in the Past Problems section flush with the left margin.

Medical Data Base: Systems Review

SYSTEMS REVIEW: Circle positive responses, underline negative responses.

GENERAL
Weight change   Fever-chills   Weakness
Fatigue   Sweating-nightsweats

See present illness.

SKIN
Nail changes   Itching   Rash-eruptions

HEAD
Headache   Trauma

EYES
Vision-glasses   Blurring   Photophobia
Diplopia   Scotoma   Inflammation

Reading glasses

EARS/NOSE/MOUTH
Pain   Discharge   Vertigo
Deafness   Tinnitus

With hypoglycemia therapy - blurring vision

Sinusitis   Polyps   Postnasal drip
Epistaxis   Obstruction

Teeth   Gums   Breath
Taste   Pain   Dentures

Poor dental repair

RESPIRATORY
Wheezing   Dyspnea   Hemoptysis
Chest pain   Cough   Sputum

See present illness

BREASTS
Lumps   Pain   Discharge

CARDIOVASCULAR
Palpitation   Pain   Dyspnea
Orthopnea   Murmurs   Blood pressure
Cyanois   Edema   Claudication

GASTRO-INTESTINAL
Appetite   Pain   Hematemesis
Jaundice   Hernia   Melena
Constipation   Anal discomfort   Stool-shape, color
Dysphagia   Hemorrhoids   Diarrhea
Indegestion   Nausea-vomiting   Abdominal girth

GENITO-URINARY
Dysuria   Nocturia   Hematuria
Frequency   Urgency   Incontinence

Chronic one time per night nocturia

SEXUAL HISTORY
Syphilis, Gonorrhea, Sores   Other
Epididymitis, Pain   Discharge

Gradiva/Para/Abortions
Sterility   Impotence   Contraception

FEMALE-MENSES
Cycle/Duration/Amount/Menopause
Last Pelvic exam, PAP smear
Dysmenorrhea   Spotting   Irregularity

ENDOCRINE
Goiter   Glycosuria   Exophthalmos
Treatment with hormones (thyroid, steroids)

ALLERGIC
Sens. to allergens, drugs, vaccines
Eczema   Asthma   Hay Fever   Hives

BONES, JOINTS & MUSCLES
Trauma   Swelling   Pain-arthritis

BLOOD-LYMPATIC
Anemia   Bleeding tendency
Pain   Lymph node enlargement

NEUROLOGIC
Syncope   Convulsions   Sensation
Gait   Coordination   Paralysis-strength

PSYCHOLOGIC
Memory   Mood   Sleep pattern
Anxiety   Emotional disturbances
Drug, alcohol problems

Medical Data Base: Physical Examination

PHYSICAL EXAMINATION

Circle abnormal findings
and describe in detail.
Underline normal findings.
No mark means not examined.

Hometown Hospital   # 090909

Smith, Mr. John James
10 Main Street
Hometown, US 00000

Birthdate: 03-20-29

Temp. ____99____   Pulse ____72____   Reg/Irreg _____   Resp. ___12___

Blood pressure: Supine, right arm __130/75__   Left arm _____
              Sitting   _____
              Standing   _____
              Legs   _____

Weight __61 kg__   Height _____

General appearance: Pleasant appearing white male in no acute distress

SKIN
Color
Texture
(Pigmentation)   Multiple cherry angiomas and spider angiomas of full anterior chest
Cyanosis
Hair
Nails
Lesions (type, color, size, shape, distribution)

LYMPH NODES
Cervical
Post-auricular
Axillary
Epitrochlear
Inguinal
Remoral

HEAD
Trauma
Tenderness
Bruit

EYES
Lids
Conjuctivae
(Sclerae)
Pupils   Melanin pigment spot OD temporal sclera
Fundi
Exophthalmos

EARS/NOSE/THROAT
Pinna/Canals/Drum
Hearing
Septum/Mucosa

(Teeth)/Gums/Mucosa   Poor dental repair and hygiene
Lips/Breath
Tongue/Palate
Tonsils-pharynx

5

6

NECK
Mobility _____
Thyroid gland _____
Venous distension _____
Bruit _____
Tracheal shift _____

CHEST
Shape symmetry
Resonance   Increased anterior-posterior diameter with
Breath sounds
                   hyperresonance. Very slight diaphragm movement

                   on inspiration. Distant breath sounds with

                   prolonged expiration phase.

BREAST
Masses _____
Tenderness _____

CARDIOVASCULAR
Jugular vein distension ____0____ cm.
Hepatojular reflux (negative) positive _____ cm.
Point of maximum impulse ____xiphoid____ I.C.S. at _____

Auscultation S^1 S^2 S^1 S^2

S^1
S^2 S1 and S2 normal. No gallop, murmur, or rub.
Gallops
Ejection sounds
Systolic murmur
Diastolic murmur
Other

Peripheral pulses	R	L
Radial	2+	2+
Femoral	2+	2+
Popliteal	+	+
Dorsal pedis	2+	2+
Post tibial	+	+

R   L

0 = absent, 1 + weak, 2 + normal, 3 + hyperactive

Hometown Hospital   # 090909

Smith, Mr. John James
10 Main Street
Hometown, US 00000

Birthdate: 03-20-29

ABDOMEN
Contour
Tenderness
Masses
Organomegaly
Liver size_____8_____cm, total dullness

Increased bowel sounds. Slight

tenderness in midline just superior

to the umbilicus.

Hematest negative stool.

GENITALIA-RECTUM
Male
Penis
Scrotum
Testes
Prostate
Rectum

Atrophic left testicle.

Female
Perineum
Vagina
Cervix
Corpus
Adnexae

NERVOUS SYSTEM
Mental status
Speech
Memory
Intelligence
Cranial nerves
Coordination
Gait
Pathological reflexes
Sensory abnormalities

REFLEXES:	R	L
Biceps	2+	2+
Knee	2+	2+
Ankle	+	+

7

EXTREMITIES
Edema _____
(Varicosities)   Small distal bilateral lower extremity varicosities.
Temperature _____
Trophic changes _____

SKELETAL
Deformities _____
Tenderness _____

MUSCULAR
Bulk _____
Strength _____
Tenderness _____

JOINTS
Swelling _____
Tenderness _____
Redness _____
(Deformity)
(Loss of motion) Decreased length of left leg with loss of motion of the left hip post total
Instability _____ hip replacement.

LABORATORY

| Normal | | Abnormal | Normal | | Abnormal |

Data to be Obtained by Morning Report

( ) Hct __40.3__ Vol%
( ) WBC __13,200__ cells/mm^3
( ) Diff __58__ PFM __35__ L Plts __nl.__
( ) RBC Morph __nl.__
( ) Urine: Color __nl.__ Sp. gr. __1.015__ pH __6.0__
    Prot. __nl.__ Sugar __nl.__ Acet. __nl.__
    Micro __Bacteria 1+__
( ) BUN __15__ mgm%
( ) Bld. Sugar __55__ mgm%
( ) Na __143__ meq/L K __5.0__ meq/L
    Cl __106__ meq/L HCO$_3$ __27__ meq/L
( ) EKG: Rate __72__/min Rhythm __sinus__
    PR __0.14__ QRS __0.08__ QT __0.36__
    Interpretation __JD__

( ) Chest x-ray: (x)
Interpretation __Emphysema with very__
__large bullae. Bilateral fibrosis.__

            Date 12-31-79   Time 8:00 a.m.
Signatures: _Mary P. Martin_ _____ Student
James A. Longworth, MD _____ Intern
Martin Fisher, M.D. _____ Resident
John H. Doe, M.D. _____ Attending

Operating Record

MEDICAL UNIVERSITY HOSPITAL

OPERATING RECORD

Physicians in Attendance: Surgeon: John H. Doe, M. D.; Adam M. Smith, M. D.

Operation _____ Appendectomy _____ ☒ Major ☐ Minor

Anesthetist _____ Peter H. Jones, M. D. _____ Operation Started _____ 10:20 a.m.

Anesthetic _____ General _____ Operation Closed _____ 11:20 a.m.

Scrub Nurse _____ Jane Green, RN _____ Anesthesia Started _____ 9:55 a.m.

Circulating Nurse _____ Susan Brown, RN _____ Anesthesia Stopped _____ 11:35 a.m.

Clean contaminated Category _____ I ___ II ___ III ___ IV

Transfusions _____ None _____ Operating Room Number ___ # 8

Complications _____ None

Sponge Count: Peritoneal ___ Correct ___ Skin ___ Correct ___ Signature: *Ann Jones R.N.*

Date of Operation:

Preoperative Diagnosis:

Postoperative Diagnosis:

Findings:

Operations:

Operating Procedures:

Immediate Postoperative Condition

Signature of Surgeon

Form MUP-6

Operation Report

OPERATIVE REPORT

Preoperative diagnosis: Chronic tonsillitis.

Postoperative diagnosis: Chronic tonsillitis with tonsil and
                            adenoid hypertrophy.

Operations: Tonsillectomy and adenoidectomy.

Findings: Tonsils are scarred and retracted
                            bilaterally with crypts.
                            Hypertrophic lymphoid tissue.

Procedure: The patient was placed on the operating
                            table after general endotracheal anes-
thesia was obtained. The left posterior nasopharyngeal area was
palpated and was noted to have an enlarged adenoidal pad. An
adenotome was then used to excise adenoidal tissue. Packs were
placed in the posterior nasopharyngeal area. The left tonsil was
then grasped with a curved tonsil tenaculum. With the use of the
Nivert knife, the mucosa was incised and the tonsil freed from its
fossa. Attention was turned to the right side where the exact same
procedure was followed. Following this, the left fossa was then
visualized, bleeding points were identified, clamped, and ligated
with suture ties of 0 plain. The same procedure was carried out
on the right. The nasopharynx was again inspected. The patient
was then noted to be adequately hemostatic, was awakened from
general anesthesia, and was taken from the operating room to the
recovery room in good condition. Estimated blood loss 100cc.
Complications: None. The tonsillar tissue was sent to Pathology.

Guidelines

For long reports, use 1″ margins; for shorter reports (as shown above), use $1\frac{1}{2}$″ margins.
Align all fill-ins vertically with their introductory sideheads as illustrated here.
Double-space betwen major segments of the report.
Use single-spacing *within* major segments of the report.
Align all elements of the report flush left.

The first portion of the operation report (i.e., the operating record) is generally initiated in the operating room at the time of the operation and may look similar to the first of the previous two examples. The body of the operation report, which is dictated or written by the surgeon, may be similar to the second illustration.

DISCHARGE SUMMARY

A discharge summary or clinical résumé is required before a patient's medical record is considered complete in hospitals accredited by the Joint Commission on Accreditation of Hospitals. Most licensing agencies also have this requirement. A few exceptions are made for short-stay patients who have been hospitalized less than 48 hours for minor procedures such as tonsillectomies and adenoidectomies, minor accidents, or overnight observation. Then, a simple progress note is required in lieu of a discharge summary.

The discharge summary serves a variety of needs. It is quite often used in lieu of a letter to another physician or a facility involved in the patient's medical care at a later date. Copies are usually sent to the attending physician's office for inclusion in the office records and to the referring physician who had the primary encounter with the patient for the particular illness. These summaries also may be used with the patient's authorization to substantiate disability claims. The discharge summary may be written or dictated in the format most desirable to the author; however, the content requirement is generally consistent. The summary or the résumé should contain at least the following data:

1. **Reason for admission**   a summation of the present illness
2. **Positive findings**   a summary of the positive findings and significant negative findings from the history, physical examination, laboratory tests, X-ray examinations, and any other diagnostic procedures
3. **Hospital course**   a chronological account of the events that took place during the course of the patient's hospitalization including a record of any complications and/or infection and a record of any blood transfusions
4. **Disposition**   advice and arrangements for health care (such as instructions given to the patient in regard to diet, physical activity limitations, medications, and follow-up appointments) that are given to the patient upon discharge from the hospital
5. **Physician to whom the patient is referred for follow-up care**   name and address of the physician (NOTE: This item is not required in many institutions.)
6. **Final diagnoses and operative procedures**   a list of all diseases and/or conditions for which the patient has been treated or which the patient is known to have, as well as a list of operative procedures and the dates on which they were performed.

The following illustrations show a typical discharge summary and a clinical résumé. These are included for the benefit of medical assistants who should become familiar with the content of the documents and for the benefit of those readers of this book who are medical transcriptionists in hospitals.

NOTE: Several forms and formats for discharge summaries may be used in various settings to meet the needs of the medical community. When there are transcription delays or when there are incomplete test results, a brief summary may be handwritten instead of typewritten.

Discharge Summary

```
                        HOSPITAL DISCHARGE SUMMARY


     Glutz, Thelma Marie                      Admitted:  12-12-79
     DOB:  08-23-42                           Discharged: 12-12-79

     REASON FOR ADMISSION:  Right breast mass.

     PRESENT ILLNESS:  The patient is a 37-year-old white female with a history of
                       previous fibrocystic disease of the breast and biopsy of the
     right breast.  Approximately one month ago, she had a biopsy of a cystic mass
     in the left breast.  Histological examination revealed that this was an area
     of atypical ductal epithelial hyperplasia.  Because of the borderline nature
     of this lesion versus lobular in situ carcinoma, it was felt that a biopsy of
     the upper quadrant of the opposite breast was indicated.  There was no history
     of trauma or nipple discharge.

     PAST MEDICAL HISTORY:  Right breast biopsy in 1977 and left breast biopsy in
                            1979.

     REVIEW OF SYSTEMS:  Mild shortness of breath on exertion.  Allergy to tape.

     PHYSICAL EXAMINATION:  Physical examination revealed a well-developed, well-
                           nourished white female in no acute distress.  Breasts:
     Old scar in upper outer quadrant of the right breast.  Recent scar in the upper
     outer quadrant of the left breast.  No masses noted.  Lungs clear to percussion
     and auscultation.  Heart reveals no cardiomegaly, murmurs, or extra sounds.
     Normal sinus rhythm.  Abdomen is flat; no organomegaly or masses.  Normal bowel
     sounds.  No hernia.  Neurological examination is within normal limits.

     LABORATORY DATA:  Laboratory data revealed hemoglobin 16, hematocrit 48, WBC
                       7900.  Urinalysis negative.

     HOSPITAL COURSE:  The patient was taken to surgery on the day of admission for
                       a biopsy of the right breast, upper outer quadrant.  A 4 cm
     thin-walled cyst resting on the pectoralis fascia was located about 9 o'clock,
     and this was removed.  An additional biopsy of about 5 gm of breast tissue from
     the upper outer quadrant also was taken.  The biopsy was sent to Pathology.  The
     patient tolerated this procedure well and was discharged on the same day.

     DISPOSITION:  Appointment in my office 12-19-79 at 3:00 p.m.  No activity limi-
                   tations.  Patient discharged on no medications.

     FINAL DIAGNOSIS:  Fibrocystic disease of right breast with large apocrine cyst.

     OPERATIONS:  Biopsy of right breast, 12-12-79.


     James J. Brown, MD

     ab  D: 12-12-79  T:  12-13-79

     CC:  1 office file
```

Guidelines

For short summaries, use 1½" margins; for long ones, use 1" margins.
Center the heading on the first line.
Type the patient's name and date of birth on the left, and the admission and discharge dates on the right.
Single-space the text; double-space between segments of the summary.
Use capitalized sideheads.

Clinical Résumé

CLINICAL RÉSUMÉ

```
Smith, John James                              Admitted:   11-10-79
DOB:  03-20-09                                 Discharged: 11-14-79
```

REASON FOR ADMISSION: The patient is a 70-year-old white male who is admitted
                       for cataract extraction.

POSITIVE FINDINGS: Pearly white cataracts have developed over the past year
                    by his history. The patient denies systemic illness,
hypertension, diabetes mellitus, or cardiac symptoms. The past medical history
reveals no major illnesses and no history of surgical procedures. No medications. No allergies known. Family history and review of systems are unremarkable.

The physical examination is unremarkable with the exception of the ocular examination. Ocular examination: Visual acuity OD uncorrected, hand motion at 6
inches; OS hand motion at 6 inches. Examination of the anterior segment reveals
a moderately shallow anterior chamber with an applanation tension of 15 mm of
mercury in each eye. Pearly white cataracts are present in both eyes. Examination of the fundus was obscured; however, Beta scan of the left eye was within
normal limits.

LABORATORY DATA: On admission to the hospital, the CBC was within normal limits,
                  SMA-12 was within normal limits except for a borderline ele-
vated uric acid. The urinalysis revealed 11-20 white blood cells and a culture
was obtained which later grew multiple organisms, which are felt to be contami-
nants. An electrocardiogram was within normal limits. Chest X ray revealed
no abnormalities.

HOSPITAL COURSE: On the second hospital day, the patient was taken to the Oper-
                  ating Room where an intracapsular cataract extraction was per-
formed in the left eye without difficulty and a 19.5 diopter, Fetteroff-style
intraocular lens was inserted. The patient's hospital course subsequently was
unremarkable and he was discharged home on the fourth hospital day.

DISPOSITION: The patient was instructed how to use the eye drops and to limit
              his usual physical activity until he returns for his appointment
in my office in one week. Discharge medications are Garamycin Ophthalmic Solution, one drop OS q.i.d. and Inflammase Forte Ophthalmic Solution, one drop OS
q.i.d. Discharged in good condition.

FINAL DIAGNOSIS: Cataracts, both eyes.

OPERATIONS AND SPECIAL PROCEDURES: Cataract extraction, left eye and intraocu-
                                    lar lens implant, left eye. 11-12-79.

Mark S. Dean, MD

ab   D: 11-14-79 T: 11-15-79

CC: 1 file; 1 Rush W. Smith, MD

Guidelines

Follow the instructions given in the preceding illustration of a discharge summary format.
If a copy of the résumé is to be sent to a referring physician, indicate this in the
carbon-copy notation at the bottom of the résumé.

15

CHAPTER FIFTEEN

STYLE IN MEDICAL CORRESPONDENCE

CONTENTS

15.1

THE LETTER AS AN IMAGE-MAKER

The word *style* as applied to letter writing encompasses format, grammar, stylistics, and word usage. All of these elements conjoin in a letter to produce a tangible reflection on paper not only of the writer's ability and knowledge and the typist's competence, but also of an office's total image. For example, a physician may have spent considerable time and effort in building up the practice and in projecting a positive professional image; yet, this image may be seriously eroded or negated altogether by carelessly prepared letters especially when produced over a long time span. On a smaller scale, a few letters of that kind may create such negative impressions on their recipients that they will have second thoughts about pursuing professional relationships with the writer. The letter, then, is actually representative of the physician's professional stature, regardless of the size of the practice. And if there appears to be no pride in or concern for the quality of something as basic as one's correspondence, how then can there be concern for or pride in the quality of one's professional services?

Letters are still the most personal method of written business and professional communication. A physician may devote much less time to correspondence than do his or her counterparts in the business world; however, the fact that there is less letter-writing in the medical office does not diminish the importance of faultless correspondence. If both writer and typist keep in mind the following simple aids to good letter production, the time and money involved will have been well spent:

1. Stationery (usually Executive or Monarch) should be of high-quality paper having excellent correcting or erasing properties.
2. Typing should be neat and accurate with any corrections or erasures rendered invisible.
3. If the physician's stationery is Executive or Monarch, the typeface should be Elite.
4. The essential elements of a letter (such as the date line, inside address, message, and signature block) and any other included parts should conform in page placement and format with one of the generally acceptable, up-to-date business-letter stylings shown in section 15.7.
5. The language of the letter should be clear, concise, grammatically correct, and devoid of padding and clichés.
6. The ideas in the message should be logically oriented, with the writer always keeping in mind the reader's reaction.
7. All technical and statistical data should be accurate and complete.

Style in correspondence, like language itself, is not a static entity: it has changed over the years to meet the varying needs of its users, and it is continuing to change today. For example, the open punctuation pattern has gained wide currency. On the other hand, the closed punctuation pattern is now little used in the United States. Busy office schedules and increased communication in all media have rendered fast, clear, lean communication essential.

15.2

TOTAL-LETTER CONSIDERATIONS

It has often been said that an attractive letter should look like a symmetrically framed picture with even margins working as a frame for the typed lines that are balanced under the letterhead. But how many letters really do look like framed pictures? Planning ahead before starting to type is the real key to letter symmetry:

1. Estimate the approximate number of words in the letter or the general length of the message by looking over the writer's rough draft or one's shorthand notes, or by checking the length of a dictated source.
2. Make mental notes of any long quotations, tabular data, long lists or footnotes, or of the occurrence of scientific names and formulas that may require margin adjustments, a different typeface, or even handwork within the message.
3. Set the left and right margin stops according to the estimated letter length: about one inch for very long letters, about one and one-half inches for medium-length ones; and about two inches for very short ones.
4. Use a guide sheet.
5. Continuation-sheet margins should match those of the first sheet, and at least three lines of the message should be carried over to the continuation sheet.

A Quick Guide to Attractive Letter Placement on the Page

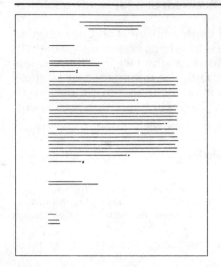

The Short Letter
100 words or less

side margins: about 2″

paragraphs may be double-spaced throughout

The Medium-length Letter
about 100–300 words

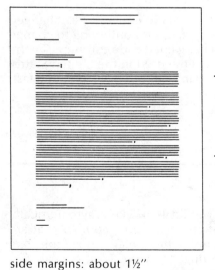

side margins: about 1½″

The Long Letter
300 words or more
(should comprise at least 2 pages)

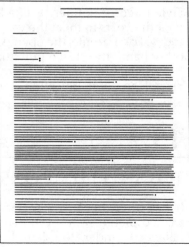

single-spacing
within
paragraph

double-spacing
between
paragraphs

side margins: about 1–1¼″

15.3

LETTERHEAD DESIGN AND LETTER BALANCE

Letterhead designs vary with one's office. For example, the letterhead used in a single- or a multi-physician practice will differ in size, layout, and design from that used in a clinic, a medical school, or a large health products company. Some letterheads are positioned dead-center at the top of the page, others are laid out across the top of the page from the left to the right margin, and still others are more heavily balanced right or left of center. Sometimes the doctor's name or the name of the practice appears at the top of the page, while the address and other data are printed at the bottom. Regardless of layout and design, a typical printed letterhead contains all or some of the following elements, with the asterisked items being essential:

*full legal name of the practice, clinic, institution, or group
*full street address
 suite, room, or building number, if needed—post office box number, if applicable
*city, state, and ZIP Code
 Area Code and telephone number(s)
 other data (as the names of individual physician-associates if not
 already shown as part of the legal name of a group practice

The names of particular services, groups, or divisions may be printed on the letterhead of extremely large or diversified institutions.

Personalized letterhead is used by physicians. Measuring 7¼ by 10½ inches ("Executive") or 7½ by 10 inches ("Monarch"), this stationery usually features a printed or sometimes engraved heading positioned at the top of the page. The heading includes the physician's full name, full street address, and geographical location (city, state, and ZIP Code). The office telephone number or numbers including the area code is often printed on the stationery. Envelopes ought to match the paper and must include the doctor's name and return address. The typestyle of the physician's printed appointment cards and prescription pads usually matches that of the office letterhead.

15.4

ALL ABOUT PAPER

Paper and envelope size, quality, and basis weight vary according to application. (The next table lists various paper and envelope sizes along with their uses.) Good-quality paper is an essential element in the production of attractive, effective letters. When one assesses paper quality, one should ask these questions:

1. Will the paper withstand corrections and erasures without pitting, buckling, or tearing?
2. Will the paper accept even and clear typed characters?
3. Will the paper permit smooth written signatures?
4. Will the paper perform well with carbons and in copying machines?
5. Will the paper withstand storage and repeated handling and will its color wear well over long time periods?
6. Is the color of the paper appropriate for a medical office?
7. Will the paper fold easily without cracking or rippling?
8. Will the paper hold typeset letterhead without bleed-through?

Stationery and Envelope Sizes and Applications

Stationery	Stationery Size	Application	Envelope	Envelope Size
Executive *or* Monarch	$7\frac{1}{4}'' \times 10\frac{1}{2}''$ *or* $7\frac{1}{2}'' \times 10''$	physicians' correspondence; usually used in single or group practices	*regular* Executive *or* Monarch	$3\frac{7}{8}'' \times 7\frac{1}{2}''$
			window Monarch	$3\frac{7}{8}'' \times 7\frac{1}{2}''$
Standard	$8\frac{1}{2}'' \times 11''$ *also* $8 \times 10\frac{1}{2}''$	general business or medical correspondence	*commercial* No. 6¾ No. 9 No. 10	$3\frac{5}{8}'' \times 6\frac{1}{2}''$ $3\frac{7}{8}'' \times 8\frac{7}{8}''$ $4\frac{1}{8}'' \times 9\frac{1}{2}''$
			window No. 6¾ No. 9 No. 10	$3\frac{5}{8}'' \times 6\frac{1}{2}''$ $3\frac{7}{8}'' \times 8\frac{7}{8}''$ $4\frac{1}{8}'' \times 9\frac{1}{2}''$
			airmail No. 6¾ No. 10	$3\frac{5}{8}'' \times 6\frac{1}{2}''$ $4\frac{1}{8}'' \times 9\frac{1}{2}''$

An important characteristic of paper is its fiber direction or grain. When selecting paper, one should ensure that the grain will be parallel to the direction of the typewritten lines, thus providing a smooth surface for clear and even characters, an easy erasing or correcting surface, and a smooth fit of paper against the typewriter platen. Every sheet of paper has what is called a felt side: this is the top side of the paper from which a watermark may be read, and it is from this side of the sheet that the letterhead should be printed or engraved. The table below illustrates various paper weights according to their specific uses.

Weights of Paper for Specific Business Correspondence Applications

Application: letter papers and envelopes	Basis Weight: letter papers and envelopes
Executive	24 *or* 20
Standard	24 *or* 20
Airmail	13
Form letters	20 *or* 24
Continuation sheets	match basis weight of first sheet

Continuation sheets, although blank, must match the letterhead sheet in color, basis weight, texture, size, and quality. Envelopes should match both the first and continuation sheets. Therefore, these materials should be ordered along with the letterhead to ensure a good match.

Letterhead and continuation sheets as well as envelopes should be stored in their boxes to prevent soiling. A smaller supply of these materials may be kept in the typist's stationery drawer but they should be arranged carefully so as not to become damaged over time.

15.5

GENERAL PUNCTUATION PATTERNS IN MEDICAL CORRESPONDENCE

As with letterhead designs, the choice of general punctuation patterns in correspondence is usually determined by the physician. However, it is important that specific punctuation patterns be selected for designated letter stylings, and that these patterns be adhered to for the sake of consistency and fast output. The two most common patterns are *open punctuation* and *mixed punctuation*. Their increased popularity in recent years is yet another reflection of the marked trend toward streamlining correspondence.

OPEN PUNCTUATION PATTERN

1. The end of the date line is unpunctuated, although the comma between day and year is retained.
2. The ends of the lines of the inside address are unpunctuated, unless an abbreviation such as *P.C.* terminates a line, in which case the period after the abbreviation is retained.
3. The salutation if used is unpunctuated.
4. The complimentary close if used is unpunctuated.
5. The ends of the signature block lines are unpunctuated.
6. This pattern is often used with the Block Letter.

MIXED PUNCTUATION PATTERN

1. The end of the date line is unpunctuated, although the comma between the day and year is retained.
2. The ends of the lines of the inside address are unpunctuated unless an abbreviation such as *P.C.* terminates a line, in which case the period after the abbreviation is retained.
3. The salutation is punctuated with a colon.
4. The complimentary close is punctuated with a comma.
5. The end(s) of the signature block line(s) are unpunctuated.
6. This pattern is used with either the Block, the Modified Block, or the Modified Semi-block Letters.

15.6

THE INDIVIDUAL PARTS OF A LETTER:
A Discussion of Each

The various elements of a letter are listed below in the order of their occurrence. While asterisked items are essential elements of any letter regardless of its general styling, those items that are unpunctuated may or may not be included, depending on the letter styling chosen and on the nature of the letter itself:

*date line	attention line	*signature block
reference line	salutation	identification initials
special mailing notations	subject line	enclosure notation
on-arrival notations	*message	carbon copy notation
*inside address	complimentary close	postscript

DATE LINE

The date line may be typed two to six lines below the last line of the printed letterhead; however, three-line spacing is recommended as a standard for most letters. Spacing may be expanded or contracted, depending on letter length, space available, letterhead design, and office policy. The date line consists of the month, the day, and the year. The use of an abbreviation or an Arabic numeral for the month is not permitted in date lines. The following page placements of date lines are all acceptable, and the choice depends on the general letter styling or the letterhead layout; however, the date line should never overrun either right or left margins:

1. The date can be blocked flush with the left margin. This style is essential with the Block Letter.
2. The date can be blocked flush with the right margin so that the last digit of the date is aligned exactly with the margin. This style may be used with the Modified Block and the Modified Semi-block Letters. In order to align the date at the right margin, the typist moves the carriage to the right margin stop and then backspaces once for each keystroke and each space that will be required in the typed date. The typist can then set the tab stops when typing the first of several letters that will bear the same date.
3. The date line can be centered directly under the letterhead. This style may be used with the Modified Block and the Modified Semi-block Letters.
4. The date can be positioned about five spaces to the right of dead center. This style may be used with the Modified Block and the Modified Semi-block Letters.

REFERENCE LINE

A reference line with file, correspondence, case, order, billing, or policy numbers is included in a letter when the addressee has specifically requested that correspondence on a subject contain a reference, or when it is needed for filing. It may be centered and typed one to four lines below the date, although some offices require that it be typed and single-spaced directly above or below the date. With the Block Letter, the reference line should be aligned flush left, regardless of its position either above or below the date. With the Modified Block and the Modified Semi-block Letters, the reference line may be centered on the page or blocked under or above the date line wherever it has been typed.

reference line blocked left	reference line blocked right
January 1, 19--	January 1, 19--
Case No. 12345	Case No.12345
or	*or*
Case No. 12345	Case No. 12345
January 1, 19--	January 1, 19--

Reference lines on the first sheet must be carried over to the heading of a continuation sheet or sheets. The styling of the date line and the reference line on a continuation sheet should match the one on the first page as closely as possible; for example, if the reference line appears on a line below the date on the first sheet, it should be so typed on the continuation sheet. The first setup below illustrates a continuation-sheet reference line as used with the Block Letter:

John B. Jones, MD
January 1, 19--
Case No. 12345
Page 2

The second example illustrates the positioning of a reference line on the continuation sheet of a Modified Block or a Modified Semi-block Letter:

John B. Jones, MD   January 1, 19--
                                                                 Case No. 12345

SPECIAL MAILING NOTATIONS

If a letter is to be sent by any method other than by regular mail, that fact is indicated on the letter itself and on the envelope. The all-capitalized special mailing notation (as REGISTERED MAIL or SPECIAL DELIVERY) is aligned flush left about four lines below the line on which the date appears, and about two lines above the first line of the inside address. While some physicians prefer that this notation appear on the original and on all copies, others prefer that the notation be typed only on the original.

Vertical spacing (as between the date line and the special mailing notation) may vary with letter length, i.e., more space may be left for short or medium letter lengths.

ON-ARRIVAL NOTATIONS

The on-arrival notations that may be included in the letter itself are PERSONAL and CONFIDENTIAL. The first indicates that the letter may be opened and read only by its addressee; the second, that the letter may be opened and read by its addressee and/or any other person or persons authorized to view such material. These all-capitalized notations are usually positioned four lines below the date line and usually two but not more than four lines above the first line of the inside address. They are blocked flush left in all letter stylings. If a special mailing notation has been used, the on-arrival notation is blocked one line beneath it. Spacing between the date line and the on-arrival notation may be increased to as much as six lines if the letter is extremely brief. If either PERSONAL or CONFIDENTIAL appears in the letter, it must also appear on the envelope.

On-arrival Notation

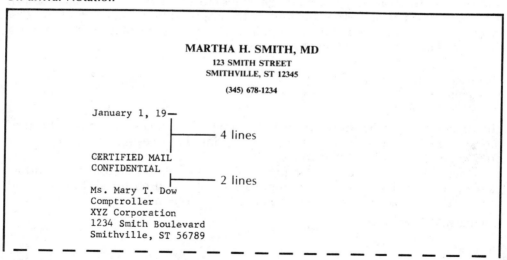

INSIDE ADDRESS

An inside address typically includes:

1. *if letter is directed to a particular individual*
    addressee's courtesy title + full name
    addressee's business or professional title if required
    full name of addressee's affiliation
    full geographical address
2. *if letter is addressed to an organization in general*
    full name of the practice, company, or institution
    individual department name if required
    full geographical address

The inside address is placed from about 3 to 8, but not more than 12 lines below the date. Inside-address page placement relative to the date may be expanded or contracted according to the length of the letter or the physician's preference. The inside address is always single-spaced internally. In all of the letters discussed in this book, the inside address is blocked flush with the left margin.

A courtesy title (as *Dr., Mr., Mrs., Miss, or Ms.*) should always be typed before the addressee's full name, even if a business or professional title (as *Treasurer* or *Chief of Staff*) is also included after the surname. Business and professional titles should not be abbreviated. Examples:

Dr. Jonathan T. Brown
Vice-president and Director
  of Research and Development

Ms. Ann B. Lowe, RRA
Director, Medical Records
City Hospital
Smithville, ZZ 11111

Arthur O. Smythe, MD
Chief Medical Director
XYZ Insurance Company
1234 Peters Street
Jonesville, XX 00000

Professor Ronald Peters
Chairman
Department of Biochemistry
State University Medical School
Statesville, UU 55555

Remember also that if *MD, PhD, DDS, DVM,* or a similar abbreviation for a doctorate degree appears after a person's surname, a courtesy title (as *Dr.* or *Professor*) is not used in the address block.

If an individual addressee's name is unknown or irrelevant and the writer wishes to direct a letter to an organization in general or to a unit within that organization, the organization name is typed on line 1 of the inside address, followed on line 2 by the name of a specific department if required. The full address of the organization is then typed on subsequent lines, as

XYZ Corporation
Pharmaceuticals Division
1234 Smith Boulevard
Smithville, ST 56789

The organization name should be styled exactly as it appears on the letterhead of previous correspondence, or as it appears in printed sources (as annual reports or business and professional directories).

Street addresses should be typed in full and not abbreviated unless window envelopes are being used. Arabic numerals should be used for all building and house numbers except *one*, which should be typed out in letters, as

One Bayside Drive
but
6 Link Road
1436 Freemont Avenue

and Arabic numerals should be used for all numbered street names above *twelve,* as

145 East 14th Street

but numbered street names from *one* through *twelve* should be spelled out:

167 West Second Avenue   One East Ninth Street

If a numbered street name over *twelve* follows a house number with no intervening word or words (as a compass direction), a spaced hyphen is inserted between the house number and the street-name number, as

2018 - 14th Street

An apartment, building, or suite number if required should follow the street address on the same line with two spaces or a comma separating the two:

62 Park Towers   Suite 9   62 Park Towers, Suite 9

Names of cities (except those following the pattern of *St. Louis* or *St. Paul*) should be typed out in full. The name of the city is followed by a comma and then by the name of the state and the ZIP Code. Names of states (except for the District of Columbia which is always styled *DC* or *D.C.*) may or may not be abbreviated: if a window envelope is being used, the all-capitalized, unpunctuated two-letter Postal Service abbreviation followed by <u>one space</u> and the ZIP Code must be used; on the other hand, if a regular envelope is being used, the name of the state may be typed out in full followed by one space and the ZIP Code, or the two-letter Postal Service abbreviation may be used. For the sake of fewer keystrokes and consistency, it is recommended that the Postal Service abbreviations be used throughout the material.

An inside address should comprise no more than five typed lines. No line should overrun the center of the page. Lengthy organizational names, however, like lengthy business or professional titles, may be carried over to a second line and indented two spaces from the left margin.

ATTENTION LINE

If the writer wishes to address a letter to an organization in general but also to bring it to the attention of a particular individual at the same time, an attention line may be typed two lines below the last line of the inside address and two lines above the salutation. The attention line is usually blocked flush with the left margin; it <u>must</u> be so blocked in the Block Letter. On the other hand, some writers prefer that the attention line be centered on the page: this placement is acceptable with all letters except the Block. However, for the sake of fast output, it is generally recommended that the attention line be aligned with the left margin. This line should be neither underlined nor entirely capitalized; only its main elements are capitalized. Placement of a colon after the word *Attention* is optional unless the open punctuation pattern is being followed throughout the letter, in which case the colon should be omitted:

Attention Mr. John P. Doe   *or*   Attention: Mr. John P. Doe

The salutation appearing beneath the attention line should be "Gentlemen" even though the attention line routes the letter to a particular person. Such a letter is actually written to the organization; hence, the collective-noun salutation.

SALUTATION

The salutation is typed flush with the left margin, usually two to four lines beneath the last line of the inside address or two lines below the attention line if there is one. Additional vertical lines of space may be added after the inside address of a short letter which is to be enclosed in a window envelope. The first letter of the first word of the salutation is capitalized, as are the first letters of the addressee's courtesy title and surname. If the mixed punctuation pattern is being followed in the letter, the salutation is followed by a colon; if open punctuation is being observed, the salutation is unpunctuated. The following are typical examples of salutations:

Gentlemen
Dear Mr. (*or* Mrs., Miss, Ms., Dr., etc.) Smith
Dear + *addressee's first name*

The salutation "Dear Sir" is rarely used today except in form letters and in letters to high-level personages.

With the advent of the Women's Rights Movement and the ensuing national interest in equal rights and equal opportunity, some writers—both male and female—have discarded the conventional salutation "Gentlemen" and have coined what they feel are more neutral, non-sexist replacements for letters addressed to organizations whose officers may be both male and female. Although a number of writers have used the following salutations, widespread general usage over a long time span has not yet been achieved and these expressions are therefore still not considered conventional:

Gentlepeople   Gentlepersons   Dear People   Dear Sir, Madam, or Ms.

The most conventional way of addressing a male-female group is to write

Ladies and Gentlemen   or   Dear Sir or Madam

although the latter expression has become less popular in recent years since the use of *Madam* in a letter to an unmarried woman may offend her.

Salutations for letters addressed to two or more persons having the same or different surnames may be found in the Multiple Addressees chart in section 15.7. See also section 15.8 for a discussion of the use of *Doctor/Dr.* with more than one addressee.

SUBJECT LINE

A subject line gives the gist of a letter. Its phrasing is necessarily succinct and to the point: it should not be so long as to require more than one line. The subject line serves as an immediate point of reference for the reader as well as a convenient filing tool for the secretaries at both ends of the correspondence. While subject lines are not frequently used in the medical correspondence of many practices, they are often used in letters relating to the business side of the practices and in letters referring to case numbers.

The subject line may be entirely capitalized and not underlined. As an alternative, the first letters of the key words in the subject line may be capitalized and every word underlined. If a subject line is included in a letter, it is positioned flush left, two lines beneath the salutation. Also, the word *subject* may be used to introduce the line as follows:

SUBJECT: CHANGE IN CLINIC HOURS
SUBJECT: Change in Clinic Hours

The first line of the message begins two lines below the subject line.

MESSAGE

The body of the letter—the message—should begin about two lines below the salutation or two lines below the subject line if there is one. Paragraphs are single-spaced internally. Double-spacing is used to separate paragraphs. If a letter is extremely brief, its paragraphs may be double-spaced throughout the letter. Paragraphs in extremely short letters should be indented so that they will be readily identifiable to the reader.

Equal margins measuring 1 inch for long letters, about 1½ inches for medium-length letters, and at least 2 inches for short letters should be kept (see Section 15.2 for a discussion of attractive letter page placement). The first lines of indented paragraphs (as in the Modified Semi-block Letter) should begin 5 to 10 spaces from the left margin; however, the 5-space pattern is the most common.

Long quotations (i.e., quotations comprising at least 4 typewritten lines or more) should be indented and blocked 5 to 10 spaces from the left and right margins with internal single-spacing and top-and-bottom double-spacing so that the material will be set off from the rest of the message. Long enumerations (i.e., enumerations of at least three or more elements) should also be indented: enumerations with items requiring more than one line apiece may require single-spacing within each item followed by double-spacing between items. Tabular data should be centered on the page. Individual elements or units in tabular data should be aligned vertically with double-spacing intervening between units or elements.

Page Placement of a Long Quotation   **Page Placement of an Enumeration**

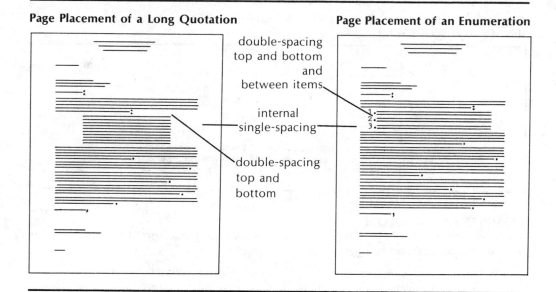

double-spacing
top and bottom
and
between items

internal
single-spacing

double-spacing
top and
bottom

If a letter is long enough to require a continuation sheet or sheets, at least three message lines must be carried over to the next page. The complimentary close and/or typed signature block should never stand alone on a continuation sheet. The last word on a page should not be divided. Continuation-sheet margins should match those of the first sheet. At least six blank lines equaling one inch should be maintained at the top of the continuation sheet.

Continuation-sheet Heading: the Block Letter

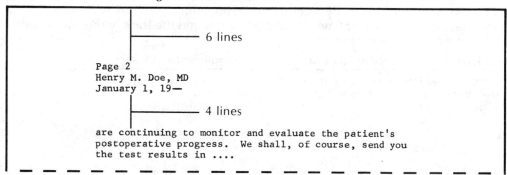

6 lines

Page 2
Henry M. Doe, MD
January 1, 19—

4 lines

are continuing to monitor and evaluate the patient's
postoperative progress. We shall, of course, send you
the test results in ....

The format shown above is used with the Block Letter. It features a flush-left heading beginning with the page number, followed on the next line by the addressee's courtesy title and full name, and ending with the date on the third line. Some physicians prefer that the page number appear as the last line of the continuation-sheet heading, especially if a reference number is included.

Another way to type the heading of a continuation sheet is to lay the material out across the page, six lines down from the top edge of the sheet. The addressee's name is typed flush with the left margin, the page number in Arabic numerals is centered on the same line and enclosed with unspaced hyphens, and the date is aligned flush with the right margin—all on the same line. This format is often used with the Modified Block and the Modified Semi-block Letters.

Continuation-sheet Heading: Used with the Modified Block and the Modified Semi-block Letters

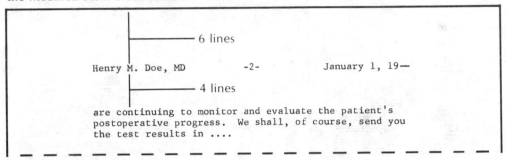

```
                    |——————— 6 lines
                    |
   Henry M. Doe, MD        -2-          January 1, 19—
                    |——————— 4 lines
                    |
   are continuing to monitor and evaluate the patient's
   postoperative progress.  We shall, of course, send you
   the test results in ....
```

COMPLIMENTARY CLOSE
The complimentary close is typed two lines below the last line of the message. Its alignment depends on the general letter styling being used:

1. With the Block Letter, the complimentary close is always aligned flush left.

2. With the Modified Block and the Modified Semi-block Letters, the complimentary close may be aligned directly under the date line (e.g., about five spaces to the right of dead center, or flush with the right margin) or under some particular part of the printed letterhead that the physician designates. It should never overrun the right margin.

Only the first word of the complimentary close is capitalized. If the open punctuation pattern is being used, the complimentary close is unpunctuated. If the mixed punctuation pattern is being followed, the complimentary close is punctuated with a comma. The typist should always use the complimentary close that has been dictated because the writer may have a special reason for the choice of phrasing. If the writer does not specify a particular closing, the typist may wish to select the one that best reflects the general tone of the letter and the state of the writer-reader relationship. See the next chart.

General Tone & Degree of Formality	Complimentary Close
highly formal—usually used to show respect and deference to a high-ranking addressee	Respectfully yours Respectfully Very respectfully
politely neutral—usually used in medical and general correspondence	Very truly yours Yours very truly Yours truly
friendly and less formal—usually used in medical and general correspondence	Most sincerely Very sincerely Very sincerely yours Sincerely yours Yours sincerely Sincerely

more friendly and informal—often used when writer and reader are on a first-name basis but also often used in general and medical correspondence	Most cordially Yours cordially Cordially yours Cordially
most friendly and informal—usually used when writer and reader are on a first-name basis	As ever Best wishes Best regards Kindest regards Kindest personal regards Regards

SIGNATURE BLOCK

Although the typist ought to style the signature block according to the doctor's wishes, a few general guidelines can be given here. The signature block typically includes the physician's name, followed by a comma and the abbreviation *MD*. However, it is not always necessary to include a typed signature block, especially if the doctor's name is the only one appearing in the printed letterhead. And, if the Official Letter styling is being followed, the typed signature block is always omitted. On the other hand, if the typist is employed by a group practice whose letterhead features the names of more than one doctor, the typist definitely should include the writer's name in the typed signature block. (Handwritten signatures are often illegible, thus causing the reader possible confusion.) Similarly, if the physician is part of a large organization (as an insurance company, a hospital, or an editorial board) whose printed letterhead features either a number of individuals' names or no personal names at all, the typist should include the physician-writer's name in the signature block.

With the Block Letter, the signature block is aligned flush left at least four lines below the complimentary close. Only the first letter of each element of the writer's name is capitalized, and only the first letter of each major element of the writer's professional title and/or department name is capitalized if included:

John D. Russell, MD Head Hematology Division	John D. Russell, MD Chief of Surgery	John D. Russell, MD, PhD Director, Research & Development

With the Modified Block and the Modified Semi-block Letters, the signature block may be centered on the page, aligned under the date line, positioned flush with the right margin, or aligned under a designated element in the printed letterhead. The signature block is typed four lines beneath the complimentary close. It is capitalized as shown in the examples above.

Regardless of page placement and letter styling, the name of the writer should be typed exactly as he or she signs it. Medical or academic degree abbreviations or professional rating abbreviations should be included after the writer's name so that the recipient of the letter will know the proper form of address to use in the reply. For example:

Typed Signature	**Salutation in Reply**
Francis E. Atlee, MD	Dear Dr. Atlee
Ellen Y. Langford, PhD Dean, Allied Health	Dear Dr. Langford *or* Dear Dean Langford
Carol I. Etheridge, RRA *or* (Mrs.) Carol I. Etheridge, RRA	Dear Ms. Etheridge *or* Dear Mrs. Etheridge

The only titles that may precede a typed signature are *Ms., Miss,* or *Mrs.,* even though they are not included in the writer's written signature. These courtesy titles are enclosed in parentheses as shown in the last example above.

The physician should always sign his or her letters and any letters composed by the medical assistant that will leave the office under the physician's name. Under no circumstances should the medical assistant sign the doctor's name followed by the assistant's initials. While acceptable in general business correspondence, this procedure is not appropriate for correspondence generated in a physician's office. If the doctor is away from the office for an extended period and routine correspondence must be answered without his or her signature, the assistant may sign the letters as shown below:

Sally T. Martin, CMA-A   *or*   Ann J. Jones
Office Manager   Secretary to Dr. Lee

IDENTIFICATION INITIALS

The initials of the typist and sometimes those of the writer are placed two lines below the last line of the signature block, and are aligned flush left in all letter stylings. There is a marked trend towards complete omission of the writer's initials if the name is already typed in the signature block or if it appears in the printed letterhead. Many offices indicate the typist's initials only on carbons for record-keeping purposes. These are common stylings:

FCM/HL   FCM:HL   Franklin C. Mason:HL
FM/hl   FCM:HOL
                             Franklin C. Mason
hol   FCM:hl   HL
hl   FCM:hol
               fcm:hol

ENCLOSURE NOTATION

If a letter is to be accompanied by an enclosure or enclosures, one of the following expressions should be aligned flush left and typed one or two lines beneath the identification initials, if there are any, or one or two lines beneath the last line of the signature block, if there is no identification line:

Enclosure   Enclosures (3)
enclosure   enclosures (3)
enc.   3 encs.
encl.   3 encls.

If the enclosures are of special importance, each of them should be numerically listed and briefly described with single-spacing between items:

Enclosures: 1. Preoperative test results
              2. Operation record
              3. Clinical résumé
              4. Pathology report

CARBON COPY NOTATION

A carbon copy notation showing the distribution of courtesy copies to other individuals should be aligned flush left and typed two lines below the signature block if there are no other notations or initials, or two lines below any other notations. If space is very tight, the carbon copy notation may be single-spaced below the above-mentioned items. The most common stylings are:

cc   cc: Copy to   Copies to

This notation may appear on the original and all copies or only on the copies.

Multiple recipients of copies should be listed alphabetically. Sometimes only their initials are shown, as

cc: WPB
TLC
CNR

or the individuals' names may be shown, especially if the writer feels that such information can be useful to the addressee:

cc: William L. Carton, Esq.   *or*   cc: Ms. Lee Jamieson
45 Park Towers, Suite 1   Copy to John K. Long, MD
Smithville, ST 56789   Copies to Dr. Houghton
                                                      Dr. Ott
Daniel I. Maginnis, MD   Dr. Smythe
1300 Dover Drive
Jonesville, ZZ 12345

If the recipient of the copy is to receive an enclosure or enclosures as well, that individual's full name and address as well as a description of each enclosure and the total number of enclosed items should be shown in the carbon copy notation:

cc: Ms. Barbra S. Lee, (2 copies, dental records)
123 Jones Street
Smithville, ST 56789
Ms. Sara T. Tufts
Ms. Laura E. Yowell

If the writer wishes that copies of the letter be distributed without this list being shown on the original, the blind carbon copy notation   bcc   *or*   bcc: followed by an alphabetical list of the recipients' initials or names may be typed on the carbons in the same page position as a regular carbon copy notation. The *bcc* notation may also appear in the upper left-hand corner of the carbon copies.

POSTSCRIPT
A postscript is aligned flush left and is typed two to four lines (depending on space available) below the last notation. If the letter's paragraphs are strict-block, the postscript reflects this format. If the paragraphs within the letter are indented, the first line of the postscript is also indented. All postscripts are single-spaced. Their margins conform with those maintained in the letters themselves. The writer should initial a postscript.

15.7

ESSENTIAL LETTER STYLES FOR MEDICAL CORRESPONDENCE

LETTER FACSIMILES
The following pages contain full-page facsimiles of the letter formats most often used by physicians in private practice or by physicians employed by large groups:

The Executive Letter: Block Style
The Executive Letter: Modified Block Style
The Official Letter
The Modified Block Letter with Continuation Sheet
The Modified Semi-block Letter with Continuation Sheet

Each facsimile contains a detailed description of letter format and styling.

The Executive Letter: Block Style

MARY A. MATTHEWS, MD
123 SMITHVILLE STREET   SUITE 100
SMITHVILLE, ST 12345

(345) 678-9090

June 1, 19—

Paul K. Lee, MD
Chief Medical Director
XYZ Insurance Company
45 Towers Square
Dowville, ST 56789

Dear Dr. Lee:

This is an example of the Block Letter typewritten on Executive stationery. The mixed punctuation pattern is being
used here. Margins are 1½ inches all around. In this facsimile, the date line is positioned flush left, three lines
beneath the letterhead. The inside address is typewritten
three lines below the date line and is positioned flush
left. Spacing may vary according to letter length. The
salutation appears two lines below the last line of the inside address.

All paragraphs are blocked flush with the left margin and
are single-spaced internally. Double-spacing is used between paragraphs. The complimentary close, also flush left,
is typewritten two lines below the last message line. The
signature block, containing the physician's name and degree
abbreviation, is positioned flush left and at least four
lines below the complimentary close.

Typist's initials, if included, are positioned two lines
below the signature block, and are aligned flush left. If
enclosure or carbon copy notations must be included, these
notations are blocked flush left and are placed two lines
below the signature block and/or the typists initials.

Very truly yours,

Mary A. Matthews, MD

Mary A. Matthews, MD

coc

Enclosures (2)

cc: Frederick L. Cooper, MD

The Executive Letter: Modified Block Style

DOWVILLE PEDIATRIC ASSOCIATES
456 LINDEN TOWERS   SUITE 4
DOWVILLE, ST 56789

PHILIP O. THOMPSON, MD
ANN T. THOMAS, MD
(456) 789-1000

January 23, 19—

Stephen D. Mills, MD
Chief of Surgery
Childrens Hospital
1246 Smith Avenue
Jones City, ST 34567

Dear Dr. Mills:

This is an example of the Modified Block Letter typewritten on Executive stationery with margins of 1¼ inches all around. The mixed punctuation pattern is being illustrated.

The Modified Block Letter differs from the Block Letter only in the page placement of the date line, the complimentary close, and the signature block, all of which are typewritten at the center, towards the right margin (as shown here), or flush with the right margin.

In this example, the date line is placed three lines below the last letterhead line, and five spaces to the right of the center of the page. The inside address begins three lines below the date line. The spacing of these two elements will vary from letter to letter, according to the length of each message.

The styling of the rest of the letter follows that of the Modified Block styling illustrated on full-size stationery further on in this section of the handbook.

Sincerely yours,

Ann T. Thomas, MD

coc

Enclosures (6)

cc: Paul K. Lee, MD

     Sarah Y. Zarrell, MD
     456 Downs Street Suite 1
     Martinsville, ST 55555

The Modified Block Letter

MORTON A. LANGLEY, MD
CERTIFIED, AMERICAN BOARD OF NEUROLOGICAL SURGERY

THE MEDICAL CENTER OF SMITHVILLE
1234 DOW PARK · SUITE 456 · SMITHVILLE, ST 12345 · (345) 456-7876

                                January 1, 19—

REGISTERED MAIL
PERSONAL

Mr. John Z. Taller
Treasurer
XYZ Corporation
1234 Smith Boulevard
Smithville, ST 56789

Dear Mr. Taller:

This is a facsimile of the Modified Block Letter. It differs from
the Block Letter chiefly in the page placement of its date line,
its complimentary close, and its signature block that are aligned
at center, toward the right margin, or at the right margin. Either
the open or the mixed punctuation pattern may be used: The mixed
pattern is illustrated here.

While the date line may be positioned from two to six lines below
the last line of the letterhead, its standard position is three
lines below the letterhead, as shown above. In this facsimile, the
date line is typed five spaces to the right of dead-center. If an
account or policy number is required, it is blocked and single-
spaced on a line above or below the date.

Special mailing notations and on-arrival notations such as the two
shown above are all-capitalized, aligned flush left, and blocked
together two lines above the first line of the inside address. If
used singly, either of these notations appears two lines above the
inside address.

The first line of the inside address is typed about four lines below the date line. This spacination can be expanded or contracted
according to the letter length. The inside address, the salutation,
and all paragraphs of the message are aligned flush left. The salutation, typed two to four lines below the last line of the inside
address, is worded as it would be in the Block Letter. A subject
line if used is typed two lines below the salutation in all-capital
letters and is either blocked flush left or centered on the page.
Underscoring the subject line is also acceptable, but in this case,
only the first letter of each word would be capitalized.

The message begins two lines below the salutation or the subject
line if there is one. Paragraphs are single-spaced internally and

Mr. Taller   - 2 -   January 1, 19—

double-spaced between each other; however, in very short letters,
the paragraphs may be double-spaced internally and triple-spaced
between each other.

Continuation sheets should contain at least three message lines.
The last word on a sheet should not be divided. The continuation-
sheet heading may be blocked flush left as in the Block Letter or
it may be laid out across the top of the page as shown above. This
heading begins six lines from the top edge of the page, and the
message is continued four lines beneath it.

The complimentary close is typed two lines below the last line of
the message. While the complimentary close may be aligned under
some portion of the letterhead, directly under the date line, or
even flush with but not overrunning the right margin, it is often
typed five spaces to the right of dead-center as shown here.

The signature line is typed in capitals and lowercase at least four
lines below the complimentary close. The writer's business title
and department name may be included if they do not already appear
in the printed letterhead. All elements of the signature block
must be aligned with each other and with the complimentary close.

Identification initials need include only those of the typist, providing that the writer and the signer are the same person. These
initials appear two lines below the last line of the signature
block. An enclosure notation is typed one line below the identification line, and the carbon copy notation if required appears
one or two lines below any other notations, depending on space
available.

                                   Very truly yours,

                                   Physician Signature

coc
Enclosures (5)

cc Dr. Doe
   Dr. Franklin
   Dr. Mason
   Dr. Watson

The Modified Semi-block Letter

NU

NORTHERN UNIVERSITY
SCHOOL OF MEDICINE
45 GRAHAM BOULEVARD
NORTHVILLE, ST 89101

January 1, 19—

Mr. Carroll D. Thompson
Sales Manager
XYZ Corporation
1234 Smith Boulevard
Smithville, ST 56789

Dear Mr. Thompson:

MODIFIED SEMI-BLOCK LETTER

This is a facsimile of the Modified Semi-block Letter. It features a date line aligned either slightly to
the right of dead center or flush right (as shown above).
Its inside address and salutation are aligned flush left,
while the paragraphs of the message are indented five to
ten spaces. Its complimentary close and signature block
are aligned under the date, either slightly to the right
of dead-center, or flush right. Identification initials,
enclosure notations, and carbon copy notations are aligned
flush left.

A special mailing notation or an on-arrival notation
if required would have been typed flush left and two lines
above the first line of the inside address. An account or
policy number if needed would have been blocked with the
date, one line above or below it. The page placement of
these elements parallels their positioning in the Modified
Block Letter. An attention line if required is aligned
flush left, two lines below the last line of the inside address. A subject line may be typed in all-capitals two
lines below the salutation and is typically centered on the
page.

The paragraphs are single-spaced internally and
double-spaced between each other unless the letter is extremely short, in which case the paragraphs may be double-
spaced internally and triple-spaced between each other.
Continuation sheets should contain at least three message
lines, and the last word on a sheet should never be divided. The heading for a continuation sheet begins at
least six lines from the top edge of the page, and follows the format shown in this letter.

Mr. Thompson   - 2 -   January 1, 19—

    The complimentary close is typed at two lines below
the last line of the message. The signature line, four
lines below the complimentary close, is aligned with it
if possible, or centered under it if the name and title
will be long. In this case, it is better to align both
date and complimentary close about five spaces to the
right of dead-center to ensure enough room for the signature block which should never overrun the right margin.
The writer's name, business title and department name (if
not already printed on the stationery), are typed in capitals and lowercase.

    Although open punctuation may be followed, the mixed
punctuation pattern is quite common with the Modified
Semi-block Letter, and it is the latter that is shown
here.

                        Sincerely yours,

                        Physician Signature

                        Physician Signature, MD
                        Professor of Radiology

coc

Enclosures: 2

cc: Bennett P. Oakley, MD
     Addison Orthopaedic Associates
     91011 Jones Street
     Smithville, ST 56789

    A postscript if needed is typically positioned two
to four lines below the last notation. In the Modified
Semi-block Letter, the postscript is indented five to ten
spaces to agree with message paragraphing. It is not
necessary to head the postscript with the abbreviation
P.S. The postscript should be initialed by the writer.

The Official Letter

XYZ INSURANCE COMPANY
45 TOWERS SQUARE
DOWVILLE, ST 56789

PAUL K. LEE, MD
CHIEF MEDICAL DIRECTOR

January 23, 19—

Dear Dr. Brighton:

    This is an example of the Official Letter typewritten on Monarch stationery. It is a letter style that is often used by high corporate executives.

    The Official Letter is characterized by the page placement of the inside address: It is typewritten flush with the left margin, two to five lines below the last line of the typewritten signature block or below the written signature. This spacing varies with the length of the message.

    It is not always necessary to include a typed signature, because the writer's name and title are usually printed in the corporate letterhead.

    The typist's initials if included are typed two lines below the last line of the inside address. An enclosure or carbon copy notation if needed appears two lines below the last line of the inside address or two lines below the typist's initials. These notations are flush with the left margin.

    Although the paragraphs may be indented as shown here, they also may be blocked flush left. The mixed punctuation pattern is shown in this illustration, but the typist may use the open punctuation pattern instead.

Sincerely yours,

Paul K. Lee

Nathaniel D. Brighton, MD
Dean, College of Medicine
Northville Medical University
890 Riverview Road
Centerville, ST 89012

Multiple Addressees

Inside Address Styling	Salutation Styling
two or more men with same surname	
Mr. Arthur W. Jones	Gentlemen
Mr. John H. Jones	
or	*or*
Messrs. A. W. and J. H. Jones	
or	Dear Messrs. Jones
The Messrs. Jones	
two or more men with different surnames	
Mr. Angus D. Langley	Gentlemen *or* Dear Mr. Langley and
Mr. Lionel P. Overton	Mr. Overton
or	
Messers. A. D. Langley and	Dear Messrs. Langley and Overton
L. P. Overton	
or	
Messrs. Langley and Overton	
two or more married women with same surname	
Mrs. Arthur W. Jones	Mesdames
Mrs. John H. Jones	
or	*or*
Mesdames A. W. and J. H. Jones	
or	Dear Mesdames Jones
The Mesdames Jones	
two or more unmarried women with same surname	
Miss Alice H. Danvers	Ladies
Miss Margaret T. Danvers	
or	*or*
Misses Alice and Margaret Danvers	
or	Dear Misses Danvers
The Misses Danvers	
two or more women with the same surname but whose marital status is unknown or irrelevant	
Ms. Alice H. Danvers	Dear Ms. Alice and Margaret Danvers
Ms. Margaret T. Danvers	
two or more married women with different surnames	
Mrs. Allen Y. Dow	Dear Mrs. Dow and Mrs. Frank
Mrs. Lawrence R. Frank	
or	*or*
Mesdames Dow and Frank	Mesdames *or* Dear Mesdames Dow and Frank
two or more unmarried women with different surnames	
Miss Elizabeth Dudley	Ladies *or* Dear Miss Dudley and
Miss Ann Raymond	Miss Raymond
or	*or*
Misses E. Dudley and A. Raymond	Dear Misses Dudley and Raymond
two or more women with different surnames but whose marital status is unknown or irrelevant	
Ms. Barbara Lee	Dear Ms. Lee and Ms. Key
Ms. Helen Key	

ENVELOPES

The following information may appear on any envelope regardless of its size. Asterisked items are essential and those that are unmarked are optional, depending on the requirements of the particular letter:

*1. The addressee's full name and full geographical address typed approximately in the vertical and horizontal center

2. Special mailing notation or notations typed below the stamp

3. On-arrival notation or notations typed about nine lines below the top left

*4. Sender's full name and geographical address printed or typed in the upper left corner.

The typeface should be block style. The Postal Service does not recommend unusual or italic typefaces. The typewriter keys should be clean.

The address block on a regular envelope should encompass no more than $1\frac{1}{2}'' \times 3\frac{3}{4}''$ of space. There should be $\frac{5}{8}''$ of space from the bottom line of the address block to the bottom edge of the envelope. The entire area from the right and left bottom margins of the address block to the right and left bottom edges of the envelope as well as the area under the center of the address block to the bottom center edge of the envelope should be free of print. With regular envelopes, most address blocks are begun about five spaces to the left of horizontal center to admit room for potentially long lines. The address block should be single-spaced. Block styling should be used throughout.

If a window envelope is being used, all address data must appear within the window space, and at least $\frac{1}{4}''$ margins must be maintained between the address and the right, left, top, and bottom edges of the window space.

Address-block data on a regular envelope should match the spelling and styling of the inside address. Address-block elements are positioned as follows:

first line

If the addressee is an individual, that person's courtesy title + full name are typed on the first line.

If the addressee is an organization, its full name is typed on the first line.

If an individual addressee's business title is included in the inside address, it may be typed either on the first line of the address block with a comma separating it from the addressee's name, or it may be typed alone on the next line, depending on the length of title and name.

If a particular department within an organization is specified, it is typed on a line under the name of the organization.

Examples:
Mr. Lee O. Idlewild, Administrator
or
Mr. Lee O. Idlewild
Administrator
or, addressed for automation
MR LEE O IDLEWILD
ADMIN
or
MR L O IDLEWILD
ADMIN
and
XYZ Pharmaceuticals
Sales Department
or, addressed for automation
XYZ PHARM
SALES DEPT

next line

The full street address should be typed out (although it is acceptable to abbreviate such designations as *Street, Avenue, Boulevard,* etc.). In mass mailings that will be presorted for automated handling, it is correct to capitalize all elements of the address block and to use the unpunctuated abbreviations for streets and street-designations that are recommended by the U.S. Postal Service. Room, suite, apartment, and building numbers are typed immediately following the last element of the street address and are positioned on the same line with it.

last line

The last line of the address block contains the city, state, and the ZIP Code number. Only <u>one space</u> intervenes between the last letter of the state abbreviation and the first digit of the ZIP Code. The all-capitalized, unpunctuated, two-letter Postal Service state abbreviations are mandatory, as is the ZIP Code.

Examples:

Dr. John P. Smith
4532 Kendall Place, Apt. 8B
Smithville, ST 56789

or

Dr. John P. Smith
4523 Kendall Pl. Apt. 8B
Smithville, ST 56789
or, addressed for automation
DR J P SMITH
4523 KENDALL PL APT 8B
SMITHVILLE ST 56789
or
CAMERON CORP
ATTN DR J P SMITH
765 BAY ST ROOM 100
SMITHVILLE ST 56789

When typing a foreign address, the typist should refer first to the return address on the envelope of previous correspondence to ascertain the correct ordering of the essential elements of the address block. Letterhead of previous correspondence may also be checked if an envelope is not available. If neither of these sources is available, the material should be typed as it appears in the inside address of the dictated letter. The following guidelines may be of assistance:

1. All foreign addresses should be typed in English or in English characters: if an address must be in foreign characters (as Russian), an English translation should be interlined in the address block.
2. Foreign courtesy titles <u>may</u> be substituted for the English; however, it is unnecessary.
3. The name of the country should be typed in all-capital letters. Canadian addresses always carry the name CANADA, even though the name of the province is also given.
4. When applicable, foreign postal district numbers should be included.

On-arrival notations Notations such as PERSONAL or CONFIDENTIAL must be typed all in capital letters about nine lines below the left top edge of the envelope. Any other on-arrival instructions such as <u>Hold for Arrival</u> or <u>Please Forward</u> may be typed in capitals and lowercase, underlined, and positioned about nine lines from the left top edge of the envelope.

If an attention line is used in the letter itself, it too must appear on the envelope. Attention lines are typed in capitals and lowercase for regular mailings using commercial envelopes, and they are typed entirely in capitals for mass mailings that will be presorted for automatic handling. The attention line may be placed anywhere in the address block so long as it is directly above the next-to-last-line, as:

XYZ Pharmaceuticals
Sales Department
Attention Mr. E. R. Lee
Smithville, ST 12345

XYZ PHARM
SALES DEPT
ATTN MR E R LEE
SMITHVILLE ST 12345

A special mailing notation (as CERTIFIED MAIL, REGISTERED MAIL, or SPECIAL DELIVERY) is typed entirely in capitals just below the stamp or about nine lines from the right top edge of the envelope. It should not overrun a ½″ margin.

Envelope

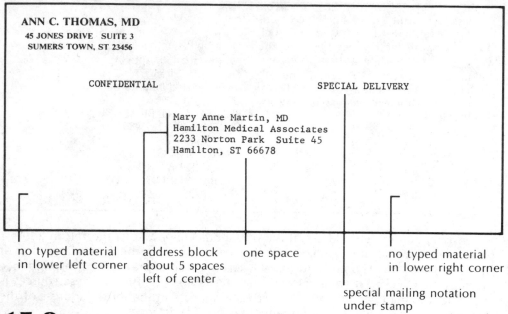

```
ANN C. THOMAS, MD
45 JONES DRIVE  SUITE 3
SUMERS TOWN, ST 23456


            CONFIDENTIAL                          SPECIAL DELIVERY


                        Mary Anne Martin, MD
                        Hamilton Medical Associates
                        2233 Norton Park  Suite 45
                        Hamilton, ST 66678
```

no typed material   address block   one space   no typed material
in lower left corner   about 5 spaces   in lower right corner
                          left of center

special mailing notation
under stamp

15.8

SPECIAL TITLES AND DESIGNATIONS

A GUIDE TO MEDICAL AND GENERAL USAGE

Doctor   If *Doctor* or *Dr.* is used before a person's name, academic or medical degree abbreviations are not used after the surname. The title *Doctor* may be typed out in full or abbreviated in the salutation, but if used in the address block it is abbreviated. When *Doctor* appears in a salutation, it must be used with the addressee's surname:

Dear Doctor Smith   *or*   Dear Dr. Smith   *not*   Dear Doctor

If a woman holds a doctorate, her title should be used in professional correspondence even if her husband's name is included in the letter too:

Dr. Ann R. Smith and
  Mr. James O. Smith
Dear Dr. Smith and Mr. Smith

If both husband and wife are doctors, one of the following patterns may be followed:

Ann R. Smith, MD	*more formal*
James O. Smith, MD	My dear Doctors Smith
or	*informal*
Dr. Ann R. Smith and	Dear Drs. Smith
Dr. James O. Smith	Dear Doctors Smith
or	
The Drs. Smith	
or	
The Doctors Smith	
or	
Drs. Ann R. and James O. Smith	

Address patterns for two or more doctors associated in a joint practice are:

Francis X. Sullivan, MD
Philip K. Ross, MD
or
Drs. Francis X. Sullivan and
   Philip K. Ross
more formal
My dear Drs. Sullivan and Ross
informal
Dear Drs. Sullivan and Ross
Dear Doctors Sullivan and Ross
Dear Dr. Sullivan and Dr. Ross
Dear Doctor Sullivan and Doctor Ross

Esquire The abbreviation *Esq.* for *Esquire* is used in the United States after the sur-names of professional persons such as architects, attorneys, and consuls, regardless of their sex. Under no circumstances should *Esq.* appear in a salutation. If a courtesy title such as *Dr., Hon., Miss, Mr., Mrs.,* or *Ms.* is used before the addressee's name, *Esq.* is omitted. The plural of *Esq.* is *Esqs.* and is used with the surnames of multiple addressees.

Examples:
Carolyn B. West, Esq.
Attorney-at-Law

Dear Ms. West

Samuel A. Sebert, Esq.
Norman D. Langfitt, Esq.
or
Sebert and Langfitt, Esqs.
or
Messrs. Sebert and Langfitt
Attorneys-at-Law

Gentlemen
Dear Mr. Sebert and Mr. Langfitt
Dear Messrs. Sebert and Langfitt

Simpson, Tyler, and Williams, Esqs.
or
Scott A. Simpson, Esq.
Annabelle W. Tyler, Esq.
David I. Williams, Esq.

Dear Ms. Tyler and Messrs. Simpson and Williams

Honorable In the United States, *The Honorable* or its abbreviated form *Hon.* is used as a title of distinction (but not rank) and is accorded elected or appointed (but not career) government officials. Neither the full form nor the abbreviation is ever used by its recipient either in written signatures, letterhead, business or visiting cards, or in typed signature blocks. While it may be used in an envelope address block and in an inside address of a letter addressed to him or her, it is <u>never</u> used in a salutation. *The Honorable* should never appear before a surname stand-ing alone: there must always be an intervening first name, an initial or initials, or a courtesy title:

The Honorable John R. Smith
The Honorable J. R. Smith
The Honorable J. Robert Smith
The Honorable Mr. Smith
The Honorable Dr. Smith

If *The Honorable* is used with a full name, a courtesy title should not be added. *The Honorable* may also precede a women's name:

The Honorable Jane R. Smith
The Honorable Mrs. Smith

However, if the woman's full name is given, a courtesy title should not be added. If a married woman holds the title and her husband does not, her name appears first on the business-related correspondence addressed to both persons:

The Honorable Harriet M. Johnson   Dear Mrs. (*or* Governor, etc.)
  and Mr. Johnson   Johnson and Mr. Johnson

if maiden name retained:

The Honorable Harriet A. Mathieson   Dear Ms. Mathieson
  and Mr. Robert Y. Johnson   and Mr. Johnson

Jr. and Sr. The designations *Jr.* and *Sr.* may or may not be preceded by a comma, depending on office policy or writer preference; however, one styling should be selected and adhered to for the sake of uniformity:

John K. Walker Jr.
or
John K. Walker, Jr.

Jr. and *Sr.* may be used in conjunction with courtesy titles, and with academic degree abbreviations or with professional rating abbreviations, as

Mr. John K. Walker[,] Jr.
Dr. John K. Walker[,] Jr.
General John K. Walker[,] Jr.
The Honorable John K. Walker[,] Jr.
Hon. John K. Walker[,] Jr.
John K. Walker[,] Jr., Esq.
John K. Walker[,] Jr., MD

Formation of the possessive with either *Jr.* or *Sr.* follows this pattern:

singular possessive
John K. Walker, Jr.'s new office is open.

plural possessive
The John K. Walker, Jrs.' daughter is my patient.

Plural patterns for *Jr.* and *Sr.* are:

The John K. Walkers Jr. are here.
The John K. Walkers, Jr. are here.
The John K. Walker Jrs. are here.
The John K. Walker, Jrs. are here.

Madam The title *Madam* is used only in salutations of a highly impersonal nature unless the writer is certain that the addressee is married. Avoid use of this term in medical correspondence.

Mesdames The plural form of *Madam, Madame,* or *Mrs.* is *Mesdames,* which may be used before the names of two or more married women associated together in a professional partnership or in a business. It may appear with their names on an envelope and in an inside address, and it may appear with their names or standing alone in a salutation:

Mesdames T. V. Meade and P. A. Tate
Mesdames Meade and Tate
Dear Mesdames Meade and Tate

Mesdames
Mesdames V. T. and A. P. Stevens
The Mesdames Stevens
Dear Mesdames Stevens
Mesdames

Messrs.   The plural abbreviation of *Mr.* is *Messrs.* It is used before the surnames of two or more men associated in a professional partnership or in a business. *Messrs.* may appear on an envelope, in an inside address, and in a salutation when used in conjunction with the surnames of the addressees; however, this abbreviation should never stand alone. Examples:

Messrs. Archlake, Smythe, and Dabney
Attorneys-at-Law
Dear Messrs. Archlake, Smythe, and Dabney
Gentlemen
Messrs. K. Y. and P. B. Overton
Architects
Dear Messrs. Overton
Gentlemen

Messrs. should never be used before a compound corporate name formed from two surnames:

McKesson & Robbins
SmithKline & French

Misses   The plural from of *Miss* is *Misses,* and it may be used before the names of two or more unmarried women who are being addressed together. It may appear on an envelope, in an inside address, and in a salutation. Like *Messrs., Misses* should never stand alone but must occur in conjunction with a name or names. Examples:

Misses Hay and Middleton
Misses D. L. Hay and H. K. Middleton
Dear Misses Hay and Middleton
Ladies
Misses Tara and Julia Smith
The Misses Smith
Dear Misses Smith
Ladies

Professor   If used with a surname, *Professor* should be typed out in full; however, if used with a given name and initial or a set of initials as well as a surname, it may be abbreviated to *Prof.* It is, therefore, usually abbreviated in envelope address blocks and in inside addresses, but typed out in salutations. *Professor* should not stand alone in a salutation. Examples:

Prof. Florence C. Marlowe, RRA
Department of Medical Record Administration
Dear Professor Marlowe
or
Dear Dr. Marlowe
or
Dear Miss Marlowe
     Mrs. Marlowe
     Ms. Marlowe
but not   Dear Professor

When addressing two or more professors—male or female, whether having the same or different surnames—type *Professors* and not "Profs.":

Professors A. L. Smith and C. L. Doe

Dear Professors Smith and Doe
Dear Drs. Smith and Doe
Dear Mr. Smith and Mr. Doe
Dear Messrs. Smith and Doe
Gentlemen

Professors B. K. Johns and S. T. Yarrell

Dear Professors Johns and Yarrell
Dear Drs. Johns and Yarrell
Dear Ms. Johns and Mr. Yarrell

Professors G. A. and F. K. Cornett
The Professors Cornett

Dear Professors Cornett   *acceptable for any combination*
Dear Drs. Cornett

Gentlemen   *if males*

Ladies *or* Mesdames   *if females*

Dear Mr. and Mrs. Cornett   *if married*
Dear Professors Cornett
Dear Drs. Cornett

Reverend   In formal or official writing, *The* should precede *Reverend;* however, *The Reverend* is often abbreviated to *The Rev.* or just *Rev.* especially in unofficial or informal writing, and particularly in correspondence where the problem of space on envelopes and in inside addresses is a factor. The typed-out full form *The Reverend* must be used in conjunction with the clergyman's full name:

The Reverend Philip D. Asquith
The Reverend Dr. Philip D. Asquith
The Reverend P. D. Asquith

The Reverend may appear with just a surname only if another courtesy title invervenes:

The Reverend Mr. Asquith
The Reverend Professor Asquith
The Reverend Dr. Asquith

The Reverend, The Rev., or *Rev.* should not be used in the salutation, although any one of these titles may be used on the envelope and in the inside address. In salutations, the following titles are acceptable for clergymen: *Mr.* (or *Ms., Miss, Mrs.*), *Father, Chaplain,* or *Dr.* The only exceptions to this rule are salutations in letters addressed to high prelates of a church (as bishops, monsignors, etc.).

Second, Third   These designations after surnames may be styled as Roman numerals:

II
III
IV

or as ordinals:

2nd/2d
3rd/3d
4th

Such a designation may or may not be separated from a surname by a comma, depending on office policy or writer preference:

Dr. J. L. Jones, III
Dr. J. L. Jones III

Possessive patterns are:

Samuel Z. Watson III's (*or* 3rd's *or* 3d's) office is open now.
The Samuel Z. Watson IIIs' (*or* 3rds' *or* 3ds') insurance policy covers it.

ABBREVIATIONS AND INITIALS

The following illustrates the proper order of occurrence of initials representing medical, academic, and allied health degrees and professional ratings appearing after surnames:

John D. Doe, MD, PhD, FACP
John D. Doe, MD, FAAP
John D. Doe, DVM, PhD
Joan M. Doe, RN, BSN
Joan M. Doe, RRA, MS

Note that most medical journals give precedence to the *MD* in by-lines. Thus, this degree would precede any other degrees held by the author. In most other instances, however, multiple degrees are listed in the order in which they were received.

List of abbreviations and initials   The following list of medical, allied health, and some general abbreviations and initials representing various degrees, fellowships, and professional ratings is a cross-section of the terms that the medical assistant may encounter in office communications (as in printed letterhead, signature blocks, and author by-lines). Since limited space precludes entry here of all such terms, the list below includes only the most common ones. More detailed information may be obtained by consulting the current edition of the *Allied Medical Education Directory,* published by the Council on Medical Education of the AMA, and the current edition of *Academic Degrees,* published by the Department of Health, Education and Welfare Office of Education. The entries are listed alphabetically, followed by their expansions:

AA   Associate in Arts
AB   Bachelor of Arts—also *BA*
AM   Master of Arts—also *MA*
ARRT   Registered Respiratory Therapist
ART   Accredited Record Technician
BA   Bachelor of Arts—also *AB*
BS   Bachelor of Science
BSN   Bachelor of Science in Nursing—also *BScN*
BScN   Bachelor of Science in Nursing—also *BSN*
BSNA   Bachelor of Science in Nursing Administration
BSNE   Bachelor of Science in Nursing Education
BSPh   Bachelor of Science in Pharmacy—also *BSPhar, PhmB*
BSPH   Bachelor of Science in Public Health
BSPhar   Bachelor of Science in Pharmacy—also *BSPh, PhmB*

BSPHN   Bachelor of Science in Public Health Nursing
BSPT   Bachelor of Science in Physical Therapy
ChB   Bachelor of Surgery (British)
CLA   Certified Laboratory Assistant
CMA-A   Certified Medical Assistant - Administrative
CMA-AC   Certified Medical Assistant - Administrative & Clinical
CMA-C   Certified Medical Assistant - Clinical
CMET   Certified Medical Electroencephalographic Technician; Certified Medical Electroencephalographic Technologist
CORT   Certified Operating Room Technician
COTA   Certified Occupational Therapy Assistant

CRTT   Certified Respiratory Therapy Technician
CT   Certified Technician
DC   Doctor of Chiropractic
DCM   Doctor of Comparative Medicine— also *MCD*
DDS   Doctor of Dental Science; Doctor of Dental Surgery
DHA *or* **DHAdm** Doctor of Hospital Administration
DMD   Doctor of Dental Medicine; Doctor of Medical Dentistry
DMJ   Doctor of Medical Jurisprudence
DMSc   Doctor of Medical Science—also *MedScD*
DO   Doctor of Osteopathic Medicine and Surgery; Doctor of Osteopathy
DOpth   Doctor of Ophthalmology—also *OphD*
DPH *or* **DrPH** Doctor of Public Health
DPM   Doctor of Podiatric Medicine
DSC   Doctor of Surgical Chiropody
DSc   Doctor of Science—also *ScD*
DVM   Doctor of Veterinary Medicine
DVS   Doctor of Veterinary Surgery
EdD   Doctor of Education
EMT   Emergency Medical Technician
FAAP   Fellow of the American Academy of Pediatrics
FACA   Fellow of the American College of Anesthesiologists; Fellow of the American College of Apothecaries
FACC   Fellow of the American College of Cardiology
FACD   Fellow of the American College of Dentists
FACOG   Fellow of the American College of Obstetricians and Gynecologists
FACP   Fellow of the American College of Physicians
FACR   Fellow of the American College of Radiology
FACS   Fellow of the American College of Surgeons
FAMA   Fellow of the American Medical Association
FAPA   Fellow of the American Psychological Association
FAPHA   Fellow of the American Public Health Association
FCAP   Fellow of the College of American Pathologists
FCCP   Fellow of the American College of Chest Physicians
FCGP   Fellow of the College of General Practitioners
FCPS   Fellow of the College of Physicians and Surgeons

FDS   Fellow of Dental Surgery
FICD   Fellow of the International College of Dentists
FICS   Fellow of the International College of Surgeons
FRCP   Fellow of the Royal College of Physicians (British)
FRCS   Fellow of the Royal College of Surgeons (British)
FRCSc   Fellow of the Royal College of Science (British)
FRS   Fellow of the Royal Society (British)
FRSC   Fellow of the Royal Society, Canada
IT   Inhalation Therapist
JD   Doctor of Laws—compare *LLD*
LLB   Bachelor of Laws
LLD   Doctor of Laws—compare *JD*
LLM   Master of Laws
LRCP   Licentiate of the Royal College of Physicians (British)
LPN   Licensed Practical Nurse
LRCS   Licentiate of the Royal College of Surgeons (British)
LVN   Licensed Vocational Nurse
MA   Master of Arts—also *AM*
MC *or* **MCh**   Master of Surgery (British)
MCD   Doctor of Comparative Medicine— also *DCM*
MD   Doctor of Medicine
MDS   Master of Dental Surgery (British)
ME   Medical Examiner
MedScD   Doctor of Medical Science—also *DMSc*
MHA   Master of Hospital Administration
ML   Licentiate in Medicine (British); Licentiate in Midwifery (British)
MLS   Master of Library Science
MLT   Medical Laboratory Technician
MN   Master of Nursing
MPH   Master of Public Health
MS   Master of Science
MSW   Master of Social Welfare; Master of Social Work
MT   Medical Technologist
MT (ASCP)   Medical Technologist Certified by the American Society of Clinical Pathologists
NP   Nurse Practitioner
OphD   Doctor of Ophthalmology—also *DOpth*
OptD   Doctor of Optometry
OT   Occupational Therapist
OTR   Registered Occupational Therapist
PA-C   Physician's Assistant - Certified
PC   Professional Corporation
PharD *or* **PharmD**   Doctor of Pharmacy
PhB   Bachelor of Philosophy
PhD   Doctor of Philosophy

PhG *or* **PhmG** Graduate in Pharmacy
PhM Master in Pharmacy
PhmB Bachelor of Pharmacy—also *BSPh,*
 BSPhar
PHN Public Health Nurse
PNP Pediatric Nurse Practitioner
RCPT Registered Cardio-Pulmonary Tech-
 nologist
RCVT Registered Cardio-Vascular Tech-
 nologist
RD Registered Dietician
REMT Radiological Emergency Medical
 Team

RLT Registered Laboratory Technician
RMT Registered Medical Technologist
RN Registered Nurse
RPh Registered Pharmacist
RPuT Registered Pulmonary Technologist
RRA Registered Record Administrator
RRL Registered Record Librarian
RT Radiological Technologist; Respiration
 Therapist
ScD Doctor of Science—also *DSc*
SF Senior Fellow
VN Visiting Nurse

15.9

SAMPLE LETTERS COMPOSED BY THE MEDICAL ASSISTANT

INTRODUCTION

Previous sections of this chapter have discussed the mechanical aspects of good letter production. Section 15.9 offers general pointers on the actual writing of letters. These pointers are supplemented at the end of the section with full-page facsimiles illustrating some of the most routine letters that the assistant might be asked to compose. (See also Chapter 2, section 2.2, for a sample letter of employment application; Chapter 12, section 12.2, for the wording of a fee adjustment letter; and Chapter 13, section 13.2, for sample fee payment reminder and collection letters and a facsimile of a letter ending the physician-patient relationship.)

While the correspondence flow in medical offices is markedly lighter than that encountered by secretaries in general business offices, the Medical Assistant/Administrative nevertheless should be able to compose some routine letters for the physician if he or she delegates this task to the assistant. Under no circumstances should the assistant attempt to answer any letters other than the types explicitly specified by the physician, regardless of how innocuous the letters may seem. After the assistant has learned which letters, if any, may be written for the doctor, the assistant may wish to examine the office correspondence to see how various types of routine letters have been treated in the past. A looseleaf binder consisting of appropriate letter models then can be set up for quick reference. Letter models should be arranged alphabetically according to their subject, as

Acknowledgment, in MD's absence
Fees, outline of
Reprint, request for

so that they will be easily retrievable when needed. The collection can be augmented from time to time as new kinds of letters answerable by the assistant accrue. Some offices already have letter models included in their procedures manuals. If this is the case in your own office, make sure that you are thoroughly familiar with the material—especially if you are a newcomer to the office staff.

At all times, the medical assistant should remember that every communication from the practice—be it by telephone, in person, or on paper—will be considered by its recipient as the voice of the doctor or the doctors. Thus, the wording of each letter should conform to the highest standards of English grammar. There should be no typographical errors or ugly strikeovers. Corrections, if any, ought to have been rendered absolutely invisible, preferably by use of correcting fluid or tape. Penned-in corrections are totally unacceptable. (Some doctors will not permit letters with corrections—no matter how neatly they have been made—to leave their offices.) The material ought to be politely yet succinctly worded. (Remember that the reader is apt to be as busy as the writer.) Finally, and most importantly, the medical assistant must keep in mind the legal implications inherent in every letter to every patient. For example, when composing a letter, the assistant should never make any statements that could later be construed as a diagnosis or a promise that the patient will be "cured" or "helped" by the doctor. In short, all of the precautions and ethical considerations that apply to face-to-face medical assistant-patient relationships also apply to written correspondence between the two. The medical assistant's letters are a tangible reflection of the role as an *agent* of the physician.

Kinds of letters that may be composed by the medical assistant   A physician may ask his or her assistant to compose letters that fall into two categories: those letters that will bear the signature of the medical assistant and those letters that will have the signature of the doctor. Letters written and signed by the medical assistant may include any or all of the following:

Letter of Acknowledgment During the Physician's Absence
Letter of Appointment Cancellation/Change
Letter of Cancellation (as of a subscription)
Letter of Correction (as of a previous clerical error)
Letter Ordering Supplies and Equipment
Letter Outlining Fees (as to an insurance company)
Letter Outlining Fees (as to a patient)
Letter Requesting Product Information
Letter of Reservation
Letter of Subscription

On the other hand, these letters may be written by the medical assistant but signed by the physician:

Letter of Acceptance (as of a speaking engagement)
Letter of Condolence (as to a recently deceased colleague's family)
Letter of Congratulation (as to a colleague)
Letter of Introduction/Recommendation
Letter Requesting a Reprint of a Colleague's Paper
Letter Thanking a Colleague for a Reprint
Letter of Transmittal (as of documents requested by another writer)

Models of the letters listed above are illustrated in that order at the end of section 15.9.

Appointment letters: special comments   If a letter about an appointment is being sent to a patient, the medical assistant usually writes and signs it. However, if a letter regarding an appointment is being sent to another doctor, the medical assistant may write it (if so directed by the doctor), but the doctor generating the correspondence usually signs it.

Referral letters and their responses: special pointers   Patient referrals are made by one physician to another physican, the latter of whom is often a specialist. A referral is usually made by telephone, followed by a confirmation note or a confirmation letter. Letters are used mostly when the two doctors are not located in the same geographic area. During the initial telephone conversation, the referring physician gives the patient's full name, address, and telephone number, followed by a description of the complaint for which the patient is being referred. And, most importantly, the physician describes the nature of the treatment (if any) that he or she has so far prescribed for the patient. The referral letter confirms the above data, and, at the physician's discretion, may amplify the details already conveyed to the specialist in a previous conversation. Referral letters are usually dictated to the typist by the physician. However, this book gives an example of a strictly routine referral letter.

A physician receiving a referred patient will usually telephone his or her opinions, findings, diagnosis, and recommendations for treatment to the referring

Referral Letter

```
                        ROBERT M. YOUNGBLOOD, MD
                            678 MEDICAL TOWERS
                                 SUITE 10
                            BEDFORD, ST 76543

                            TEL.: (545) 890-2345


                                        January 1, 19--


        Thomas Y. Lynch, MD
        Evans Orthopaedic Associates
        56 Swarthmore Building  Suite 3
        Evans City, ST 65433

        Dear Dr. Lynch:

            This letter confirms my December 30 telephone referral of
        Mrs. Sarah D. Johnson to you.  Mrs. Johnson's address and tele-
        phone number are:

                        543 Sandy Lane
                        Bedford, ST 76543
                        (555) 891-4567

            I am referring this patient to you because (give reason).
        On December 30, 19--, during a routine office check-up, the
        patient complained of (state the chief complaint and other per-
        tinent data).  The following tests and examinations were per-
        formed:  (list them).  Test results were as follows:  (give the
        results).  I have prescribed the following medication for Mrs.
        Johnson:  (give the medication/dose).

            My assistant tells me that your secretary has set up an
        appointment for you to see Mrs. Johnson at 10:15 a.m. on Monday,
        January 5.  I appreciate your taking the time to examine her,
        and I look forward to hearing your opinion.

                                    Very truly yours,

                                    Robert M. Youngblood, MD
                                    Robert M. Youngblood, MD

        RMY:as
```

doctor. This conversation will often be followed up by a written report on the patient's condition, a statement of opinion regarding the nature of the complaint, and/or a progress report. Medications either prescribed or recommended will also be described in detail. This letter will be dictated by the doctor. A model response to a referral is illustrated below. (Another example of a referral response, together with its counterpart in shorthand, is found in chapter 14.)

THE WRITING OF ROUTINE LETTERS: General Pointers
Planning ahead before starting to write   Before your fingers touch the keyboard,

Response to a Referral

EVANS ORTHOPAEDIC ASSOCIATES

56 SWARTHMORE BUILDING   SUITE 3
EVANS CITY, ST 65433

THOMAS Y. LYNCH, MD
THORNTON P. BROWN, MD
SAMUEL I. KENNEDY, MD

TELEPHONE (678) 432-9876 • 432-9875 • 432-9874

January 10, 19--

Robert M. Youngblood, MD
678 Medical Towers Suite 10
Bedford, ST 76543

Dear Dr. Youngblood:

    Today I saw your patient, Mrs. Sarah D. Johnson, whom you referred to me on January 1, 19--, and whose chief complaint is (give the complaint). The patient is suffering from (state the diagnosis). I have recommended (state complete recommendations: further treatment, medication/dosages, surgery, or whatever).

    I will keep you informed of her progress, of course. Thanks very much for referring this interesting patient to me.

                    Very truly yours,

                    Thomas Y. Lynch, MD

                    Thomas Y. Lynch, MD

TYL:al

---

you should have already planned what you are going to say, and you ought to have before you a written-out draft of how you are going to say it. When you are planning to answer an incoming letter, you can make marginal notes on the letter itself as a first step in organizing your thoughts prior to the actual writing process. A rough draft can then be made on scratch paper. This draft is really essential: you can make any number of corrections, deletions, and additions on it without wasting typing time and expensive office stationery. When you are thoroughly satisfied with the organization, the wording, and the content of the draft, you can then type the letter in final form. Or, if the letter requires the physician's review, approval, and/or signature, you can show the physician the draft prior to final typing.

If your are writing a letter for the physician (i.e., a letter that will bear the doctor's signature), try to use in it those expressions that you know are popular with the physician. In some cases, a busy doctor will merely outline what is to be said in the letter and leave the final writing to the assistant, if the assistant has shown sufficient writing ability. See the letters of congratulation, condolence, and introduction/recommendation given at the end of 15.9.

Creating the opening Since the writer's image can be enhanced or tarnished through his or her choice of words, the writer must be certain that just the right words are used. This statement is especially applicable to the opening paragraph of a communication. Always keep the reader's point of view in mind, especially when you are beginning a letter. The following is an example of a good opening paragraph:

How lucky we are that you said "Yes" to our invitation to appear before a group of new medical assistants at our annual "Get-Acquainted Day" on Thursday, December 2! After hearing you speak at the AAMA national meeting in October, I am convinced that we couldn't have found a better speaker.

Cues to the reader You should regard every potential reader of your letters as a critic of your letter production. Thus, each communication to a patient or to any other correspondent provides an opportunity to epitomize the very best in service, goodwill, and helpfulness. Here are some ways to create a positive impression on the reader:

1. Use tactful, easy-to-understand language. Short words, clear-cut and direct, are easier to read and to understand than lengthy words. Write as you speak, using natural everyday expressions. Example:

It is a real pleasure to know that you will lead our Health Insurance Seminar on May 14.

2. Organize your language carefully and concisely. Time is a precious commodity, and the busy reader wants to get the gist of the message on the first reading. Interesting messages contain sequences that vary in length and in internal structure. Coherence and continuity are other prime requisites of modern communications. (See also Chapter 17, section 17.8, for sentence and paragraph strategy.)

3. Construct sentences correctly. Technical correctness in writing is a worthy goal for any assistant. In order to attain it, one should proofread the material and make sure that none of the following infelicities is present: misplaced commas, misspelled words, incorrect word division, numbers written incorrectly, hackneyed and stilted expressions, a lack of agreement between subjects and verbs, and other such grammatical and stylistic pitfalls.

4. Give accurate, precise information. The omission of one important detail can spell the difference between order and confusion in the reader's mind. This is an example of a letter written by a medical assistant for a physician accepting a

speaking engagement (note the questions):

Thank you for your gracious invitation to participate in your pediatrics conference on October 19 at Sanford Hall. It is thoughtful of you to include me in your program. Would you please send along a map showing the best driving route to your campus, and also mention the amount of time allotted for my message?

If the writer of the original letter had checked the outgoing letter carefully for details, it would not have been necessary for the respondent to request information on the length of the speech and on conference location.

5. Write clearly to avoid any hint of double meaning. It has often been said that if a statement can be misunderstood, it will be! By scanning all written messages for unintended hidden meanings, the writer can avoid many problems. For example, which way will the following statement be interpreted?

I am writing to you about the report on Mr. John Doe's osteotomy which was mailed to you on January 12.

reader's reaction
Surely Mr. Doe's osteotomy was not mailed to the reader on January 12!
A careful rewording of the original statement will prevent any misunderstanding:

I am writing to you about the report (mailed to you on January 12) regarding Mr. John Doe's osteotomy.

6. Respond to questions raised. It is a serious omission when you neglect to answer a question that has been raised in previous correspondence. Here is another safeguard that will ensure good writing: double-check to see that no such omissions have been made, by rereading relevant previous correspondence and then comparing it with your response.

7. Introduce an unfavorable comment with a favorable one. It is helpful to present all the positive aspects of a situation first and then to lead into any negative or unfavorable comments. Find points of agreement with the reader and mention them before talking about an unfavorable fact. Example:

Dr. Jones has asked me to assure you that he values you very much as his patient. However, he has also requested that we devise a new appointment reminder system for you. You see, when you repeatedly cancel appointments without giving us advance notice, it does create great inconvenience for the doctor, for the staff, and for our other patients. Won't you help us?

Devising a friendly way to close a letter   Give the reader a pleasant closing thought in the final paragraph of the letter, as in this example:

Again, Dr. Warren asks that I thank you for giving her permission to reprint the article on your company's research in the field of nonsteroidal anti-arthritics. This information will be a valuable asset to her forthcoming textbook.

One should avoid thanking someone for something in advance. It is really rather impertinent to assume beforehand that one's request will be honored. Wait until the service is rendered; then, make an appropriate acknowledgment of it.

The signature block   If you are writing a letter in your own name on the printed letterhead of the practice, follow the guidelines that have been set down and illustrated on pages 343–344 of this chapter.

LETTER MODELS
The following pages illustrate in facsimile form seventeen of the more routine letters that may be written by a Medical Assistant/Administrative.

Letter of Acknowledgment During the Physician's Absence

MARIANNE E. DALTON, MD
2-A MEDICAL BUILDING
DOWVILLE, ST 56789

TELEPHONE (123) 456-7890

January 2, 19—

John P. Stafford, MD
President
State Medical Society
44 Tarleton Towers Suite 3
Statesville, ST 77777

Dear Dr. Stafford:

In the absence of Dr. Dalton, I would like to let you know that the office has received your gracious invitation for Dr. Dalton to be the speaker at the May 1 meeting of the State Medical Society at the Willoughby Hotel in Samson City.

Dr. Dalton will return two weeks from today, after a trip to Western Europe. As soon as she is back, I am sure that she will give your letter her prompt attention.

Sincerely yours,

Alice A. Simms

Alice A. Simms, CMA-A
Office Manager

Letter-writing Guides:
Acknowledge the request.
Explain the reason for the delay.
Use a courteous close.

Letter of Appointment Cancellation/Change

MARTHA D. SIMPSON, MD
123 DOW STREET ROOM 1
BARR CITY, XX 88888

TELEPHONE (456) 789-1234
789-1243

January 2, 19—

Mr. Adam R. Lawson
4400 Dover Street
Barr City, XX 88888

Dear Mr. Lawson:

At Dr. Simpson's request, I have tried several times (but, alas—unsuccessfully!) to reach you by telephone this week. Our problem is that Dr. Simpson, who has found that she must be out of town next week, will not be able to see you on Friday, January 12 at 9:30 a.m., as previously scheduled.

Dr. Simpson regrets that this change may inconvenience you; however, she has asked me to tell you that she will be in the office on Monday, January 15. Open hours in her schedule on that day are from 9:30 a.m. to 10:30 a.m., and from 4:40 p.m. to 5:30 p.m.

Would you please give us a call as soon as you can, regarding which time would be best for you? If none of these times are convenient, I'm sure that we can work out another appointment on another day.

Sincerely yours,

Sara T. Kingley

Sara T. Kingley, CMA-A
Assistant to Dr. Simpson

Letter-writing Guides:
Mention any previous efforts to contact the patient.
Explain the reason for the cancellation or change.
Offer the patient an alternative appointment.
Politely ask the patient to respond as soon as possible.

Letter of Cancellation (as of a subscription)

HARRISONBURG PEDIATRIC ASSOCIATES

MEDICAL BUILDING   SUITE 1-A
HARRISONBURG, XY 43210

BARBARA K. LEE, MD
SARAH T. JONES, MD
DANIEL T. WILLIAMS, MD

(345) 678-9101 • 678-9102 • 678-9103

January 2, 19—

The Jenkins Publishing Co., Inc.
Pediatrics Monthly
145 69th Street
Yorktown, ST 33445

Attention: Subscription Department

Gentlemen:

Dr. Williams has asked me to let you know that he would like to
cancel his subscription to Pediatrics Monthly, effective after
he receives the March 19— issue. I am enclosing his mailing
label and account number for your convenience.

Thank you.

Sincerely,

Annabel T. Barton

Annabel T. Barton, CMA-A
Office Manager

enclosure

Letter-writing Guides:

Use an attention line directing the letter to the appropriate office.
Cancel the subscription.
Mention when the cancellation should become effective.
Include the appropriate account data to expedite cancellation.

Letter of Correction (as of a previous error)

JOHN K. LYONS, MD
45 SMITH ROAD
SHORTVIEW, LL 12345

TELEPHONE: (301) 692-4800

January 2, 19—

James T. Alcott, MD
Medical Building Suite 4-A
Smithville, ST 56789

Dear Dr. Alcott:

   As I mentioned to your secretary this morning on the telephone, I have discovered that I inadvertently omitted page 3 of
the report regarding Mr. Kenneth H. Lee's osteotomy. I mailed
the report to you on December 30.

   Enclosed is the missing page. I regret very much this inexcusable oversight, and I hope that you have not been unduly
inconvenienced by it.

                    Sincerely,

                    Nancy A. Graham

                    Nancy A. Graham

enclosure

Letter-writing Guides:
Explain the nature of the error.
If it's your fault, take the blame.
Be polite but don't fawn.

Letter Ordering Supplies and Equipment

FRANK K. PETERSEN, MD
68 PULLER STREET SUITE 1
CANTONVILLE, XX 11111

TELEPHONE (999) 111-2345
111-3456

January 2, 19—

STA-VER Office Supplies, Inc.
6912 Main Street
Statesville, ST 99887

Gentlemen:

Please accept this order for immediate shipment to Dr. Petersen
of the following office equipment:

Catalog No.	Quantity	Description	Unit Price	Total
XZ-4289	1	6-drawer white filing cabinet	$85.00	$85.00
XY-9281-A	2	10-drawer white vertical card file	$100.00	$200.00
			total	$285.00
			handling	9.00
				$294.00

A check for $294.00 is enclosed. We would appreciate your
prompt attention to this order, since we are planning to reorganize our filing system shortly, and your equipment will be
essential to the new system.

Very truly yours,

Ellen C. Parker

Ellen C. Parker, CMA-A
Office Manager

enclosure

Letter-writing Guides:
Place the order, including all data needed for fulfillment.
Include a check if prepayment is required.
If the order is urgent, say so politely.

Letter Outlining Fees (as to an insurance company)

L. ROBERT SWANSON, MD
980 RIVERDALE MEDICAL CENTER
SUITE 12-J
RIVERDALE, VV 77777

TELEPHONE: (984) 654-3210
654-2310

January 2, 19—

XYZ Insurance Corporation
Office of the Medical Director
98 Tarrytown Tower Square
Tarrytown, ST 78910

Gentlemen:

Dr. Swanson has asked me to write to you concerning your prospective client, Mr. Thomas Y. Dowe of 4545 Creekside Lane,
Riverdale, VV 77777 (birth date: August 1, 19—). Mr. Dowe was
referred to Dr. Swanson on December 28, 19— by your company's
local agent, Mr. David R. Smith, for a complete physical examination to be completed prior to Mr. Dowe's receiving life insurance.

Our office has copies of all the required forms. Dr. Swanson
has read your physical examination form PE 1-223 and has asked
me to tell you that it is his policy to request prepayment of
his usual fee of $25.00 for an examination of this type.

Upon his receipt of your check, Dr. Swanson will perform the
necessary examination of the patient and will immediately forward the findings to you.

Very truly yours,

Frances E. Rogers

Frances E. Rogers, CMA-AC

Letter-writing Guides:
Mention the client/patient's full name, address, and any other identifying data.
Give the name of the insurance company's agent.
Mention the referral date and the type of examination required.
Politely explain the doctor's fee for the examination or procedure.
Explain the doctor's fee policy.
End the letter on a friendly note.

Letter Outlining Fees (as to a patient)

NANCY F. WHITMAN, MD
ANN A. YOWELL, MD
468 STACEY BUILDING
ROOM 8
BELTSVILLE, ST 34567

TELEPHONE (301) 456-7890
456-7891

January 2, 19—

Ms. Kathleen A. Smith
66 Maple Street
Longwood, ST 34566

Dear Ms. Smith:

 At your request, Dr. Whitman has asked me to send you a
written outline of her usual fee for the following office
procedure: (give a complete description of the type of procedure along with the fee).

 I do hope that this information is sufficient for your
purposes. If we can be of further assistance to you, please
call.

Sincerely yours,

Grace A. Ullander

Grace A. Ullander, CMA-A

Letter-writing Guides:
Describe each examination, procedure, or operation.
Give the applicable fee or fees.
Include any other statements desired by the doctor.
End the letter pleasantly.

Letter Requesting Product Information

HELEN D. THOMPSON, MD
55 SINGER STREET
MARTINSVILLE, ST 76543

January 2, 19—

SCI-FIB Corporation
Hospital Products Division
Industrial Park Drive #6
Smithville, ST 56789

Attention: Product Information Department

Gentlemen:

    Would you please send Dr. Thompson complete information on
your newly developed disposable drape pack trademarked (<u>give the
capitalized trademark of the product</u>)?

    Your consideration of this request will be appreciated.

                  Sincerely yours,

                  Sally Ann Roberts

                  Sally Ann Roberts
                  Office Manager

Letter-writing Guides:
Address the letter to the proper department.
Politely request the product information.
Use the trade name as well as the generic name of the product.
End the letter politely.

Letter of Subscription

AIMEE P. RAWLINGS, MD
MEDICAL BUILDING
SUITE 45
NORTONVILLE, ST 34342

(987) 654-3210
654-3211

January 2, 19—

XYZ Publications, Inc.
Medical News
123 87th Street NW
Witherstown, ST 12345

Attention: Subscription Department

Gentlemen:

    Please enter a subscription to Medical News in Dr. Rawlings'
name, effective immediately. A check for a one-year subscription
@ $12.00 is enclosed.

    Thank you.

Sincerely yours,

Kate Y. Carson

Kate Y. Carson, CMA-A

enclosure

Letter-writing Guides:
Request the subscription.
Give the date on which it should become effective.
Enclose complete prepayment, if necessary.
End the letter politely.

Letter of Reservation

STATE MEDICAL SOCIETY
44 TARLETON TOWERS   SUITE 3
STATESVILLE, ST 77777

JOHN P. STAFFORD, MD
PRESIDENT

TELEPHONE (321) 123-4567

January 2, 19—

Reservations Manager
Willoughby Hotel
674 Dennis Boulevard
Samson City, ST 88888

Gentlemen:

Dr. Stafford has asked me to set up reservations at the
Willoughby Hotel for the May 1, 19— meeting of the State Medical
Society. The meeting hours will be from 5:30 p.m. to 11:30 p.m.
on that date. The Society will require a room seating approximately 75 persons. We would prefer the "U" formation of tables
and chairs, and a movie screen as well as a slide projector.

Dr. Stafford would like to arrange cocktails and dinner prior to
the business part of the meeting. As soon as the membership
reservations have been firmed up, he will let you know exactly
how many people will attend, at what hours the cocktails and the
dinner will be served, and at what hour the business meeting will
begin.

In the meantime, would you please consider this a definite reservation? Also, we would like you to send us a copy of your menu
for group functions.

An early confirmation of this reservation will be appreciated.

Cordially,

Ann F. Hall
Secretary to Dr. Stafford

Letter-writing Guides:
Give the name and dates of the event.
List the details of required room arrangements.
Tactfully request an early written confirmation.

Letter of Acceptance (as of a speaking engagement)

HERBERT C. SIMON, MD, PhD
42 NORTH STREET
ABBOTVILLE, ST 66554

TELEPHONE (333) 222-1111
222-1112

January 2, 19—

John C. Thomas, MD
Associate Professor of Psychology
Department of Psychology
State University
Statesville, ST 12345

Dear Dr. Thomas:

Thank you very much for the kind invitation to lead your
senior seminar on Friday, March 23, 19—, in Milton Hall, Room
1289, from 2:30 p.m. to 5:30 p.m. The topic—as we discussed
earlier—will be "Empathy in Learning-disabled Children."
Enclosed is a reference list which your students will probably
want to delve into before the seminar, so that they will be as
familiar as possible with the subject matter.

I appreciate your thinking of me, and I'm looking forward
to working with your students.

Best regards,

Herbert C. Simon, MD, PhD

Enclosure

Letter-writing Guides:
Acknowledge the request.
Mention again the date, location, and time.
Mention any enclosed materials.
Express appreciation for the invitation.
Present the letter to the physician for signature.

Letter of Condolence

HENRY T. TAGGERT, MD
42 LAWTON STREET
HIGHTSTOWN, FF 12345

January 2, 19—

Dear Mr. Lee:

My staff and I wish to extend our deepest sympathy to you and your wife at this very distressing time. I considered your son to be a fine colleague, and he was greatly respected by my staff as well. He will be missed by all of us.

If there is anything that we can do to help you and Mrs. Lee especially now or in the future, please do not hesitate to call on us.

Although there is really nothing that can be said or written that will alleviate the pain that you feel, I hope that you will understand that my thoughts are with you.

Sincerely,

Henry T. Taggert, M.D.

Mr. David R. Lee
4328 Manson Boulevard
Hightstown, FF 12346

Letter-writing Guides:
Extend *sincere* sympathy.
Avoid emotional statements.
Offer assistance if possible.
Try to end on a note of comfort and friendship.
Present the letter to the physician for signature.

Letter of Congratulation

CHARLES B. WATSON, MD
FOREST VIEW MEDICAL BUILDING
SUITE 4-A
FOREST VIEW, ST 66666

January 2, 19—

Dear Norm:

Yesterday's Forest View <u>Recorder</u> carried the splendid news of your selection as a Fellow of the American College of Anesthesiologists. Congratulations! It's an honor well-deserved.

Had you been in town at this time, I'd have called instead, of course. But since our schedules seem to leave us no free time at all to visit even when we're both in town, I thought I'd write.

I am very proud that you have received this—the highest honor that can be bestowed on one in our specialty. May you have many years of continued success!

As always, give my warmest wishes to Molly and the kids.

Best regards,

Charlie

Norman A. Langley, MD
Fairview Hospital
Forest View, ST 66666

Letter-writing Guides:
Commend the recipient of the honor or the promotion.
Make additional comments on the nature of the achievement.
Close the letter with personal good wishes.
Present the letter to the physician for signature.

Letter of Introduction/Recommendation

DIANAH T. ROSSMANN, MD
99 SWARTHMORE BUILDING
ADAMSVILLE, ST 44444

TELEPHONE (659) 596-9990
596-9991

January 2, 19—

Martin A. Otto, MD
David T. Roth, MD
4268 Watkins Road
Smithville, ST 56789

Dear Drs. Otto and Roth:

This is a letter of introduction and recommendation for Ms.
Anita A. Brandt who has ably served as one of my office assistants for the past three years. Ms. Brandt received her CMA-A
rating from the AAMA during her second year of employment with
me.

Ms. Brandt's main duties have been bookkeeping, stenography,
and filing. She is well-versed in the business side of a rather
busy OB/GYN practice, so I don't think that moving from a one-
physician office to a joint practice will overwhelm her. She
has been quick to learn routines, to improvise when necessary
and under pressure, and to accept responsibility. When asked to
work overtime, she has always been willing to do so.

In short, I'm glad that Anita is getting married, but I'm sorry
that she is leaving Adamsville in the process. If you'd like
further comments regarding her, please give me a call.

Very truly yours,

Dianah T. Rossmann, M.D.

Dianah T. Rossmann, MD

DTR:coc

Letter-writing Guides:
Make the introduction.
Present relevant professional data.
Give an evaluation and a recommendation.
Offer more data upon request.
Present the letter to the physician for signature.

Letter Requesting a Reprint of a Colleague's Paper

JASON A. LONGMANN, MD
HILLVILLE MEDICAL COMPLEX
SUITE 34
HILLVILLE, ST 99999

(432) 461-4444
461-4445

January 2, 19—

Samuel P. Danner, MD, PhD
Professor of Clinical Psychiatry
Department of Psychiatry
State University College of Medicine
State City, US 55555

Dear Dr. Danner:

I have read with interest on page 301 of the December 19— issue
of Psychology Times an abstract of your paper entitled "An
Evaluation of Biofeedback Training Effects for Tension Headache
Patients" that was published in Therapy Review (62:44-54, 19—).

Would you be kind enough to send me a reprint of the entire
article? This particular topic is of great interest to me, and
I would very much appreciate your consideration of my request.

Very truly yours,

Jason A. Longmann, MD

Letter-writing Guides:
Address the letter to the person responsible for reprints.
Politely request a reprint.
Give the title and all pertinent publication data.
Conclude the letter politely.
Present the letter to the physician for signature.

Letter Thanking a Colleague for a Reprint

JASON A. LONGMANN, MD
HILLVILLE MEDICAL COMPLEX
SUITE 34
HILLVILLE, ST 99999

(432) 461-4444
461-4445

February 1, 19—

Samuel P. Danner, MD, PhD
Professor of Clinical Psychiatry
Department of Psychiatry
State University College of Medicine
State City, US 55555

Dear Dr. Danner:

 Thank you very much for sending me the reprint of your article entitled "An Evaluation of Biofeedback Training Effects for Tension Headache Patients" that appeared in Therapy Review (62:44-54, 19—). It arrived in the office on Friday, January 28.

 Your evaluation of the current literature is most thorough and informative.

Sincerely yours,

Jason A. Longmann, MD

Letter-writing Guides:
Send the letter immediately upon receipt of the reprint.
Thank the colleague for sending the reprint.
Mention the title of the article and the publication.
Close the letter with a nice comment about the article.
Present the letter to the physician for signature.

Letter of Transmittal

GEORGE A. ROMAN, MD
77 MANSON STREET
KEYSTONE, ST 33333

January 2, 19—

Roberta S. Downs, MD
Editorial Director
Radiologic Review
11 Towers Building Suite 12
Middleborough, ST 33447

Dear Dr. Downs:

Enclosed are the revised galleys of my article "Skin Response to
X-irradiation in the White Rat" which is intended for publication
in the May issue of Radiologic Review. Corrections (all of them
minor, by the way) have been made on pages 7, 9, and 11a.

Thank you for sending me an extra set of galleys; I'll keep them
here.

Sincerely yours,

George A. Roman, M.D.
George A. Roman, MD

Enclosures: 15

Letter-writing Guides:
Mention the nature of the enclosed material.
If specific page numbers are important, mention them.
Be sure to add an enclosure notation.
Present the letter to the physician for signature.

15.10

OFFICE NEWSLETTERS TO PATIENTS

Physicians often write open letters (typically termed *newsletters*) to their patients. These letters may contain special information detailing changes in office hours, new billing procedures, emergency call-in hours, medical problems currently prevalent in a particular locale, warnings about certain contagious diseases, and the like. Depending on the circumstances and the nature of the practice, an open letter may deal only with one important topic (such as a measles epidemic due to a lack of public interest in immunization). Newsletters may be issued regularly or sporadically, depending on the doctor's wishes. They are duplicated and are usually placed conspicuously in the reception area or in the treatment rooms. Photocopying is the easiest method. (See also Chapter 18.)

The physician will dictate the material that is to appear in the letter. The typist's responsibility is to read through the shorthand notes or to listen to the entire tape or cassette before typing the document. Any material that is not clearly understandable to the typist should be clarified by the physician before the final typing begins.

Depending on the length of the letter, the typist may choose 1-inch or 1½-inch margins all around. The printed letterhead of the practice is appropriate for newsletters. If the physician has printed 8½ × 11-inch stationery, use it: the larger size paper affords more page space than Executive or Monarch paper. If 8½ × 11-inch printed letterhead is unavailable, use plain bond paper of the same measurements. Typewrite the name of the practice and all other pertinent letterhead data at the top of the page. Center the material, and type it all in capital letters.

The Block Letter styling is the simplest for such a project. Insert a date line (month and year will suffice). Use the salutation (if any) that is dictated by the doctor ("Dear Parents" or "Dear Parent" is typical for letters written by pediatricians, and "Dear Patients" or "Dear Patient" is typical for those dictated by other physicians). Position the date line, the salutation, and all paragraphs flush with the left margin. Single-space the paragraphs. Use double spacing between paragraphs. Set off main topics with all-capitalized sideheads. The sideheads—also positioned flush left—should stand alone on separate lines. Double-space between the sidehead and the first line of the following paragraph. Terminate the letter with the complimentary close (if any) that is dictated by the physician. "Sincerely" and "Sincerely yours" are typical closings. The doctor's full name and degree abbreviation should be typed below the complimentary close. If the letter represents the views of a joint practice, type the name of the practice under the complimentary close. See the facsimile.

Office Newsletter

R. M. ABRAMS, M.D.
H. BURKHARDT, M.D.
H. GOLD, M.D.

D. R. SIGELMAN, M.D.
R. STEBBINS, M.D.

HOLYOKE PEDIATRIC ASSOCIATES
1787 NORTHAMPTON STREET
HOLYOKE, MASSACHUSETTS 01040
(413) 536-2393

August 1977

Dear Parent:

CHILDHOOD SAFETY

We would like to remind you of some of the more common serious
accidents that you can prevent. Automobile and bicycle accidents
continue to be the most grave. Infants should <u>always</u> be secured
in a car seat (as discussed in our previous newsletter), and all
other passengers should wear seat belts. Proper use of a bicycle
should be insisted upon before a child is allowed to ride one.
In addition, this year there has been a dramatic increase in the
number of debilitating skateboard injuries. Skateboards may
appear to be harmless enough, but the injuries that occur from
falling from skateboards are surprisingly destructive.

ROUTINE PHYSICAL EXAMS

If your child is scheduled for a routine checkup, preschool exam,
or a summer camp exam, please bring in a urine sample in a clean
bottle or jar when you come for your child's appointment. This
will save all of us much time and effort.

UNLISTED OR CHANGED TELEPHONE NUMBERS

Recently we have tried to contact a number of our patients' families for a variety of reasons, but have been unable to do so because the telephone numbers were not listed or had been changed.
Please notify us of your phone number changes and be assured that
your number will be kept in the same confidence that information
on your medical records is kept.

SWIMMERS EAR

Infections of the ear canal, known as swimmers ear, are very common in children who swim in pools. An effective preventive
measure is to place 2 or 3 drops of alcohol in each ear immediately
after swimming. This will dry the ear canal and help kill bacteria
that can cause the infection.

Sincerely,

Holyoke Pediatric Associates

16

CHAPTER SIXTEEN

SPECIAL EDITORIAL AND TYPING PROJECTS

CONTENTS

16.1

THE PHYSICIAN'S LIBRARY

INTRODUCTION

Physicians whose practices are near hospital or medical school libraries will usually not keep extensive private collections of books and periodicals in their offices. Rather, most doctors will use the resources of the large institutions, because it is easier and less expensive for them. However, physicians who are not conveniently located near such facilities will usually maintain libraries in their offices. In any event, almost all physicians want at least small libraries of books and periodicals in their offices.

The time spent by the medical assistant in taking care of the physician's library depends on the individual doctor's personal preferences. Another influencing factor is the size and the type of collection. Furthermore, the nature of the practice itself affects the library tasks assigned to an assistant: if the practice is a large one whose associates are specialists in different fields, the libraries of each of the doctors may be combined into a single collection that will be used by all of them. On the other hand, the doctors in a joint practice may prefer to maintain separate collections. In the first instance, the assistant may be asked to catalog and arrange the entire collection in a central location, maintain and update the catalog system, and inventory the library once a year. In the latter instance, however, the assistant may be expected merely to help each doctor keep his or her books in order and dust-free. Extensive collections include all or most of the following types of publications:

books
monographs
published proceedings of medical society and association meetings
medical journals—bound and unbound
reprints of articles published by colleagues

reprints of the physician's own articles
pamphlets
various instruction sheets, descriptions of diseases and conditions, and/or outlines of
  procedures commonly used by the practice

CATALOGING THE COLLECTION
Library of Congress cards   For extremely large and varied collections, a card catalog system is really essential. One way of cataloging the collection is to use the preprinted Library of Congress (LC) cards that can be obtained by writing to the Card Division of the Library of Congress, Washington, DC 20541. LC cards—containing author name(s), title(s) and subtitle(s), publishing data, table(s) of contents, and subject categories—are available for the author and/or coauthor name(s), the title, and the subject category or categories of each book. The Library of Congress will send instructions regarding the proper use of the cards and the appropriate ways of classifying the books. One advantage of the LC system is that the assistant typewrites a minimum amount of data, since the cards themselves are preprinted. Also, the assistant does not have to select subject categories for each book, since this has already been done by the Library of Congress subject catalogers. (Subject categories are printed at the bottom of each card.) The disadvantages of the LC system are the cost of the cards and the waiting period before they arrive.

Making one's own cards   A more informal and less expensive way of cataloging a collection is to typewrite the needed data on blank 3 × 5-inch white cards. Make up the following cards for each book:

an author card or coauthor cards (i.e., one card for a single author and an additional card for each coauthor); if the book has an editor or editors but no author(s), make up a card or cards for the editor(s).
a title card
a subject card or cards (i.e., one card for each subject)

Note that multiple subject cards may also be useful. Example: the phrase "diabetes in cystic fibrosis" could be typed on one card, with separate cards headed "diabetes" and "cystic fibrosis" also prepared for each condition. The data to be included on each card are:

1. author name(s), surname(s) first
2. title and subtitle (if there is a subtitle)
3. edition number if other than the first
4. publishing data: city of publication, name of publisher, publication date
5. total number of volumes if part of a multivolume series
6. a penciled notation of the specific volumes currently held in the office if the set is still incomplete: these data can be updated as new volumes are acquired
7. a notation of the current or customary location of the book if not kept in the library stacks but in the physician's private office or in another room

The assistant can typewrite each card individually; however, a convenient shortcut is to type up the author card, including all needed information. Then, the author card is photocopied once for each coauthor if the work is the product of more than one writer, once for the title, and once for each appropriate subject category. (The material on the original author card should be typed three or four vertical line spaces below the top edge of the card so as to leave enough space for later insertion of the coauthor names, the title, and the subject categories.) The assistant types the needed headings on the photocopies and then files the cards according to whichever system is being used in the library. See page 390 for an illustration of sample cards prepared for a book on medical writing.

Library Index Cards Made Up by the Assistant
Author Card

```
Fishbein, Morris

Medical writing:  the technic and the art
Ed 4

Springfield, IL:  Charles C Thomas, 1972


1.  Writing  2.  Style  3.  Manuscript
preparation
```

Title Card

```
Medical Writing:  The Technic and the Art

Fishbein, Morris

Medical writing:  the technic and the art
Ed 4

Springfield, IL:  Charles C Thomas, 1972


1.  Writing  2.  Style  3.  Manuscript
preparation
```

Subject Card

```
Writing

Fishbein, Morris

Medical writing:  the technic and the art
Ed 4

Springfield, IL:  Charles C Thomas, 1972


1.  Writing  2.  Style  3.  Manuscript
preparation
```

Selecting subject categories for made-up cards   Recently published books contain Library of Congress subject categories on their copyright pages. For instance, the copyright page of *Webster's Medical Speller* has these data:

Library of Congress Cataloging in Publication Data
Main entry under title:
Webster's medical speller   1. Medicine—Terminology. 2. Spellers.

The numbered items shown above are the two subject categories selected for this book: one file card for each category would have to be made up.

   In books that do not contain LC data, the assistant can check the table of contents for ideas on subject selection. With highly technical books, the assistant will have to consult the physician for suggestions as to the correct subjects.

Filing LC and/or made-up cards   The easiest way to file the cards is to arrange the author cards, the coauthor cards, the title cards, and the subject cards in one alphabetized sequence. Another procedure is to file all author and coauthor cards alphabetically in one box, all title cards alphabetically in another box, and all subject cards alphabetically in a third box. A third alternative is to follow one of the decimal classification/filing systems used by large medical libraries. This, however, is a specialized task that may demand the guidance of a professional librarian. The decimal system also requires that the appropriate classification numbers be appended to the cards and to the books themselves.

The selection of a filing system will depend on the physician's preferences and on the type of library. A helpful book for the assistant is the third edition of *A Handbook of Medical Library Practice,* edited by Gertrude L. Annan and Jacqueline W. Felter. It can be purchased in paperback from the Medical Library Association.

SERIAL PUBLICATIONS
Medical journals and the so-called controlled-circulation professional magazines are serial publications. They may be published on a weekly, monthly, bimonthly, quarterly, or even a yearly basis. Supplements to the journals also may be published. Obviously, it is necessary to control all journals and their supplements so that if an issue is lost or is never received, it may be found or reordered as soon as possible. It is extremely irritating for a physician to discover that a particular journal needed on the spot has been lost or never arrived in the first place.

If the physician subscribes to only a few journals, a control chart can be typewritten and photocopied. The chart can then be used for each of the incoming journals. If there are many journals in the office, it is simpler and easier to purchase preprinted serial control cards that can be filed vertically or in horizontal cabinets. If the assistant makes up a serial control chart, it should have columns and rows for these data:

top lines of the chart
journal name
number of subscription copies
publisher's name, address, and telephone number

body of the chart
year(s) in left column
volume number in middle column
month(s)—one column apiece for each month
NOTE: For dailies (such as newspapers used in the reception area), a chart can be made showing the months and the days of each month.

bottom of the chart
number of volumes per year to be bound
title page and index for bound volumes

Each number or issue is then checked off when it is received. Each journal should be stamped with the date received. See the example of a made-up chart.

If the physician subscribes to a large number of journals, the preprinted control cards mentioned earlier should be used. The horizontal filing system is preferable with these cards, since the system allows the assistant to see at a glance exactly what has been received and what is missing. Also, the cards can be flagged with colored stickers or tape to indicate subscription renewal times. Typical preprinted cards contain these data:

name of journal
number of copies in subscription
subscription expiration date
subscription rate

date of payment
period paid for
years—to be filled in for each volume
months—to be checked off as each number or issue arrives
days—to be checked off as each issue arrives

See the facsimiles of preprinted serial control cards.

Subscription renewals   Regardless of the type of control system being used, the assistant should flag each serial card in some way to indicate when the subscription is renewable. Colored stickers, tape, or metal clips can be used for this. In busy offices where daily, weekly, monthly, bimonthly, and perhaps yearly periodicals are arriving at different times, it is unwise to trust one's unaided memory to keep up-to-date with every subscription; a reminder system should be followed. The physician should not have to remind the assistant about such a routine task. However, before renewing a periodical, the assistant should obtain the doctor's approval.

Binding volumes of journals   It is standard practice to bind complete volumes of journals so that the issues will be well protected and sequentially organized. Medical journals are usually paginated consecutively throughout a volume with the index to that volume appearing in the last issue of the volume. When preparing material for binding, be sure that all issues of the volume are in the proper sequence, and that the index issue is accounted for. Never send journals to the bindery without being sure that the index issue is included in the package. Sometimes only two or three months' worth of journal issues can be bound together, especially if the journal is published on a weekly or a biweekly basis. The number of bound books within one volume will thus depend on the total number of issues comprising that volume. Supplements to volumes are usually bound in with the regular issues of the volumes if the pagination is consecutive throughout the volumes and the supplements. Supplements not consecutively paginated within journal issues or volumes are usually bound separately, and are labeled by the binder.

Serial Control Card Made Up by the Assistant

journal J Name _____   no. subscription copies 12 _____

published by Smith Publishers   address 12 Doe St, Statesville St, 12345

telephone (456) 789-1234 _____

year	volume	Jan	Feb	Mar	Apr	May	Jun	Jul	Aug	Sept	Oct	Nov	Dec	Supplements
1975	30	✓	✓	✓	✓	✓	✓	✓	✓	✓	✓	✓	✓	
1976	31	✓	✓	✓	✓	✓	✓	✓	✓	✓	✓	✓	✓	
1977	32	✓	✓	✓	✓	✓	✓	✓	✓	✓	✓	✓	✓	
1978	33	✓	✓	✓	✓									

no. volumes/year to be bound _____   title page & index for bound volumes _____

In many medical journals, pertinent and useful information is included on pages whose reverse sides contain advertising matter. Sometimes, there is even a different pagination system for the advertising. The physician should be asked if this kind of information should be included in the bound volume. After the assistant has found out from the doctor whether or not the ads are to be retained, the assistant should instruct the bindery accordingly.

Doctors often receive printed newsletters (such as *The Regan Report on Medical Law*) which may appear on weekly, monthly, or sporadic schedules, depending on the individual publication. Most of these publications feature

Preprinted Serial Control Cards

Card for a Monthly Journal

(Name of Magazine)											(Due)		
Year	Vol.	Jan.	Feb.	Mar.	Apr.	May	June	July	Aug.	Sept.	Oct.	Nov.	Dec.	T.P.&I.

No. Copies   Depts.   Indexed in

(OVER)

Card for a Daily Publication

Name																No. Copies						Expires							
	1	2	3	4	5	6	7	8	9	10	11	12	13	14	15	16	17	18	19	20	21	22	23	24	25	26	27	28	29	30	31
Jan.																															
Feb.																															
Mar.																															
Apr.																															
May																															
June																															
July																															
Aug.																															
Sept.																															
Oct.																															
Nov.																															
Dec.																															
	1	2	3	4	5	6	7	8	9	10	11	12	13	14	15	16	17	18	19	20	21	22	23	24	25	26	27	28	29	30	31

numbered issues within numbered volumes. If the newsletter subscription does not include a looseleaf or other binder for complete volumes, it is wise to purchase a binder to protect the documents and to keep them in order. Current issues should be arranged so that the newest issue appears first.

SHELVING THE MATERIAL

The system used to arrange books and periodicals on the shelves will be suggested by the physician in most instances. After all, it is the physician who will use the material. Some individuals prefer to arrange all books together, alphabetically by author names. Others prefer that the books be grouped according to subject and then alphabetized according to author names. Still others desire that the books and periodicals be arranged according to one of the decimal systems used by medical libraries. The assistant should follow the physician's preferences in this matter. Periodicals—whether they be bound or unbound—are usually shelved separately from the books; they are most often arranged alphabetically by title. Bound volumes should be kept together and should be arranged sequentially by volume number and year.

Inventorying the collection   At least once a year, the assistant should check to see that all the books and periodicals listed in the card catalog are indeed on the shelves in their proper locations or are otherwise accounted for. Books needing repair can be found and mended. Volumes of periodicals that are to be bound can be checked and sent to the bindery. The shelves can be cleaned thoroughly and the books and periodicals dusted.

CHARGEOUT PROCEDURES IN AN OFFICE LIBRARY

Unless the library is very large and a number of physicians use it on a regular basis, there is no need to use a preprinted library charge card system. A simple, easy, and effective chargeout system is to place boxes of 3×5-inch slips and pencils at intervals among the stacks. When checking out material, the user merely notes on a slip the publication title; the author, if the publication is a book; the volume and issue, if the publication is a journal; the chargeout date; and his or her initials. The slip is then filed in a chargeout box that is located in a place easily accessible to all. When the material is returned, it is properly shelved and the chargeout slip is destroyed.

REPRINTS

The physician's own reprints   A vertical file of reprints of articles written by the physician should be carefully maintained. The assistant ought to keep copies of each article appropriately labeled in separate file folders. Label the folders by article title and file them alphabetically. Make sure that the reprints have been neatly inserted into their folders so that they will not become dirty or crumpled. Keep a separate filing cabinet available for the reprints belonging to each physician in a joint practice, especially if all of the associates are prolific writers. If this is not in fact the case, keep one filing cabinet available for all of the associates' reprints, with one or two drawers assigned to each doctor. The space allotted to each writer can be adjusted when necessary. The assistant should tell the physician when the supply of reprints is getting low so that replacements can be ordered from the publisher.

Reprints received by the physician from colleagues   Maintain a separate vertical file for reprints coming into the office from other physicians. Stamp each reprint with the date received, and make sure that a thank-you letter or telephone call goes out to the author immediately. (See Chapter 15 for a sample thank-you letter.)

Keep each reprint in a separate file folder. Arrange the folders alphabetically by author surname or by the surname of the first coauthor, by the title, or by the subject. The doctor will suggest the most desirable method. An index file of 3 × 5-inch cards can then be placed near the reprint file. The index file should contain a card for each reprint. The cards are alphabetized by the author or the first coauthor surname, by the title, or by the subject. The physician should choose the system, since it is he or she who will use the material. A more elaborate system for an extensive reprint collection is: three cards for each reprint—an author or coauthor card, a title card, and a subject card. However, this method is necessary only in very large practices which receive hundreds of reprints every year.

16.2

TYPEWRITING MANUSCRIPTS

INTRODUCTION
The Medical Assistant/Administrative may be asked to help the physician prepare material that will be submitted for publication. The amount of time spent on manuscript preparation will vary from employer to employer: some doctors are very active researchers and prolific writers, while others are not. In addition, the prepublication tasks that may be assigned to the medical assistant will differ according to the physician-writer's own preference. Some of the tasks that might be given to the assistant are: helping the doctor locate and assemble materials, typewriting drafts, double-checking the accuracy and completeness of references, typewriting the final manuscript, counting the total number of words in the manuscript, proofreading the manuscript, and checking carefully the printed proofs of the material prior to publication. The manuscript may be a medical journal article or it may be an entire book. The guidelines given in this section apply to both, but the material has been slanted to the former.

Section 16.2 has been written so as to offer the reader an inclusive illustrated reference to all major aspects of manuscript typewriting. The reader will rarely need to refer to the entire section all at one time; however, during the course of manuscript development, the physician-writer and/or the typist will undoubtedly need to consult individual units within the section. These units appear in the following order:

Medical Journals: General Comments on Style
  Kinds of medical journal manuscripts
  Materials needed and general procedures to be followed
Drafts
The Manuscript Itself: A Description of its Parts
  Articles: the title page
  Title of the article
  Author by-line
  Author affiliation and/or professional title
  Abstract
  The text of an article
  Drug names used in a text
  Acknowledgments
  Permissions
  References
  Special reference problems
  Checking references

Tables
Graphics
Copyrights
Conclusion: comments from journal editors
Books
Proofreading What Has Been Typed
Handling Corrections Made by Editors

MEDICAL JOURNALS: General Comments on Style

If the physician is a contributor to the *Journal of the American Medical Association* (*JAMA*) or to any other of the AMA Scientific Publications Division journals (such as *Archives of Internal Medicine, American Journal of Diseases of Children, Archives of Otolaryngology, Archives of Dermatology, Archives of Neurology, Archives of General Psychiatry, Archives of Surgery, Archives of Ophthalmology,* or *Archives of Pathology & Laboratory Medicine*), the office should have at least one copy of the current edition of the AMA *Stylebook/Editorial Manual.* This paperback publication is available from the Association. The *Stylebook*'s detailed illustrated guidelines to manuscript development are definitive for *JAMA* and the other journals just mentioned. While the *Stylebook* does contain much information of interest strictly to editors, it nevertheless pinpoints and illustrates details of style that typists and writers ought to be familiar with.

An examination of 15 medical journals other than those published by the AMA indicates the presence of a number of stylistic differences, especially with regard to the typewriting and the formatting of reference lists. Therefore, it cannot be overstressed that both writer and typist should familiarize themselves with an individual journal's own Instructions to Authors. These instructions can usually be found either at the beginning or at the end of each issue. However, some journals print their Instructions to Authors in only one issue per year; in such a case, consult the cumulative index of the journal in order to find the appropriate issue. If, during the preparation of a manuscript, questions arise that have not already been answered in the Instructions to Authors, the physician can contact the journal editor for clarification.

The assistant's role in manuscript preparation is very important: if the material itself is medically and scientifically sound but its physical format is untidy and does not conform to publication guidelines, the manuscript may be returned to the writer unread. The importance of careful manuscript preparation is further emphasized by the late Morris Fishbein, MD, on page *viii* of the Introduction to his book *Medical Writing: The Technic and the Art,* ed 4 (Springfield, IL: Charles C Thomas, 1972):

Competition is certainly as great in medical writing as in medical practice. The leading medical publications are overwhelmed with offers of material. Many of the periodicals devoted to medical specialties find it necessary to hold manuscripts from six months to a year or more before space can be found for their publication. Therefore, the physician who launches a literary venture poorly clad, unsound in its constitution, limping in some of its sections and bruised by bad grammar may expect to have his manuscript returned with the statement, "The editor regrets. . . ."

It is therefore the responsibility of the assistant to see that the manuscript is at least *mechanically* perfect.

One way of becoming familiar with the format of a particular journal is to spend a few spare moments reading through several of its articles. Check the positioning of the titles of the articles, the style used in the by-lines, and the format of the abstracts. Look at the page placement of the sideheads and the subheads. Notice where the Arabic numerals indicating references are positioned within the running text (are they typed inside or outside other punctuation?). Find out where the acknowledgments are placed, and read the material in several acknowledgments footnotes (do acknowledgments of financial assistance precede or follow those indicating professional assistance?). Read carefully the numbered reference lists in <u>several</u> articles. How, for example, does one type a reference to a book? a reference to an article? a volume in a series? a supplement to a journal volume? an address given at a medical meeting but yet unpublished? One can make a card file listing various types of style examples for later use during manuscript preparation.

Sample Note Card Showing Journal Style

```
   references, JAMA

   authors, more than 3

   use et al
   no period & no ital with it
```

Kinds of medical journal manuscripts   The physician may ask the medical assistant to typewrite the following kinds of manuscripts that will be submitted for publication: a major article (as a research report or a complete, detailed consideration of a disease or syndrome), a review of the literature (as in a particular specialty or subspecialty and dealing with a specified topic), a case report, an editorial, a clinical note or suggestion, or a letter to the editor.

Major articles vary in length due to the topic chosen by the writer and the restrictions imposed by the journal. Articles may vary from about 3,800 words to 6,000 words (or from about 15 to 30 manuscript pages), excluding abstracts, tables, graphics, footnotes, and references. Reviews average from 2,500 words (about 10 manuscript pages) to 5,000 words (about 20–25 manuscript pages). Case reports average about 1,000 words (or about 5–8 manuscript pages) and are limited by some journals to not more than 3 pages with a reference list not exceeding 10 entries. Editorials, devoted to pertinent and timely subjects, usually comprise 2–2½ manuscript pages and ought not to exceed 3 manuscript pages. They do not contain graphics, but they do sometimes contain one or two listed references. Letters to the editor (often devoid of graphics but often having references) generally average 1–1½ manuscript pages and should not exceed 2 pages.

The medical assistant may be asked to make a word count when the manuscript of a major article, a review, or a case study has been finished. (Some journals, such as the *American Journal of Psychiatry,* currently require that the word count be noted on the title page of the manuscript.) When requested to make a word count, the assistant should count only the running text: all abstract material, legends, titles, tables, footnotes, and references should be <u>excluded</u>.

Materials needed and general procedures to be followed   The typewriter must be in excellent mechanical condition and it must be clean. Broken or fuzzy type is unacceptable. Avoid using typewriters with exotic fonts: Pica and Elite are the conventional typestyles for manuscripts. Ink should be black. Corrections ought to be rendered invisible by use of correcting fluid or tape. If the typewriter has self-correcting features, use them when it is necessary to correct errors. Virtually all journals require that the manuscripts submitted to them be typewritten on 8½ × 11-inch white unlined paper. Most journals prefer heavy <u>bond</u>. Erasable bond should <u>not</u> be used since it smudges easily in being handled by several reviewers and editors. While one or two journals require margins of at least 1 inch, the majority specify 1½-inch margins all around. (In the absence of explicit recommendations from the publisher, the typist should routinely use 1½-inch margins.) Manuscripts should be double- or triple-spaced in capitals and lowercase *throughout:* this includes the by-line, the abstract, any footnotes or acknowledgments, any case reports included within a larger text, tabular data, legends and titles for tables and graphics, lists of drug names referred to in the article, and listed references, as well as the body of the text itself. These spacing requirements apply not only to articles but also to letters to the editor. <u>Single-spacing is absolutely unacceptable.</u> Material should be typed on only one side of the paper.

The title itself—also double- or triple-spaced—may be typed all in capital letters, in capitals and lowercase, or with an initial capital only. Since title style differs with the publication, the typist ought to check the style of the journal.

Most journals require the writer to submit the original manuscript plus one complete duplicate. "Complete" means that the duplicate manuscript contains all tables, graphics, and references in addition to the entire text. (Other journals, however, require that manuscripts be submitted in triplicate.) In addition, the writer should keep a reference copy of the entire manuscript. Thus, the typist should find out in advance from the physician exactly how many copies will be needed for a particular project. If the typewriter performs poorly with multiple carbons, it would be wise to plan on photocopying all duplicates (see Chapter 18 for an overview of office copying systems and equipment). In any case, all copies—regardless of how they have been produced—should be razor-sharp black-on-white reproductions of the original. Smudged, black-on-gray copies with text lines runing off the pages or copies that have been reproduced askew are not acceptable.

Finally, the writer and the typist should have adequate reference books at hand that can be used in resolving spelling, compounding, end-of-line division, and capitalization dilemmas. Three excellent medical dictionaries are: *Dorland's Illustrated Medical Dictionary, Stedman's Medical Dictionary,* and *Blakiston's Gould Medical Dictionary. Webster's Medical Speller* can be used specifically for solving word division problems. Use the *Index Medicus* to determine the abbreviation styling of journal names in listed and in parenthetic textual references. The AMA's *Current Procedural Terminology,* the *International Classification of Diseases, Adapted,* and the *AMA Drug Evaluations* are also essential reference sources, especially for the writer.

DRAFTS

Typewrite the draft or drafts of a manuscript on one side of the paper with wide (1½- to 2-inch) margins. Triple-space the material so that the writer will have ample room for making corrections and/or additions. It is also helpful to use colored paper for drafts: use one color for the first draft, another for the second, and so on. This practice will enable the writer to distinguish each draft later on. Be sure to proofread every draft as carefully as if it were the final form of the manuscript. A busy physician does not have time to correct typographical errors and misspellings that are the typist's responsibility.

THE MANUSCRIPT ITSELF: A Description of its Parts
Articles: the title page   Although some details of format and punctuation vary among journals not published by the AMA, all journals do require a title page for

major articles and case studies. These are the basic elements included on a typical title page:

full title (including subtitle, if there is one)

full name(s) of the author(s), followed by appropriate abbreviation(s) of the highest medical and/or academic degree(s) of the author(s)

author affiliation(s) and sometimes professional title(s)

name, full address, and telephone number of the author responsible for editorial questions regarding the manuscript and for fulfilling later reprint requests

Some journals request that a word count be included on the title page—typically in the upper right corner. Also included in the upper right corner may be a notation indicating the total number of tables and figures in the article; be sure to check individual Instructions to Authors. Some journals ask their authors to supply a shortened version of the full title that will later serve as a running head or running title on each printed page. The shortened title, if included, should be typed two lines above the name and address of the author who is responsible for the manuscript. Do not paginate the title page.

Title of the article   The title is typically centered on the page about one-quarter of the way from the top edge of the sheet. If longer than one line, it is double- or triple-spaced. It can be typed all in capitals, in capitals and lowercase, or in lowercase with an initial capital only, depending on individual journal style. (Note that proper names always begin with a capital.) Be sure to check a current issue of the journal in question before proceeding to type the material. Greek letters, formulas, trade names, and italicized words may be used in titles if necessary (see Chapter 17, section 17.9 for further discussion.) A subtitle (if used) is usually set off from the main title by a colon. The initial word in a subtitle is usually capitalized unless it is a formula requiring lowercase letters or numerals.

The title should be a clear, succinct, informative statement of the main topic of the article. Some journals limit title length from about 35 character spaces to about 70 character spaces. If this type of limitation applies to a manuscript that the medical assistant is typing, the assistant should count all of the spaces in the title including spaces between words and spaces filled by punctuation marks. Alert the writer tactfully if a title overruns a particular limitation.

Author by-line   The author by-line, typed in capitals and lowercase and double- or triple-spaced below the title, should be attractively aligned with or centered under the title. The use of "by" as in "by John R. Doe, MD" is not necessary in author by-lines for manuscripts being submitted to AMA publications. However, most non-AMA journals currently use "by." Check individual journals for style.

The by-line should include the author's full name followed by a comma and the abbrevation of the highest medical/academic degree held by the author. If the author is a fellow of a medical college or society, the fellowship abbreviation may follow the degree abbreviation. The two abbreviations are separated by commas. The following is an example of a single-author by-line:

Sarah G. Goodman, MD, FAPA

Two authors' names are typically separated by commas (although some journals prefer semicolons):

Martin A. Lee, MD, Theresa W. Lindley, MD, PhD

However, a semicolon often separates the authors' names in multiauthor by-lines containing more than two names:

R. Lewis Armstrong, MD; Annabel T. Lyons, MD, PhD; Peter A. Royce, MD, FAPA

Check individual journals for style before typing the material.

Do not abbreviate first names (i.e., "Chas." for *Charles* is unacceptable), and do not divide names or degree abbreviations at the ends of lines. If there is not enough space to include all of the names on a single line, begin a new line. Some journals (as shown in the illustration on page 401) do not print medical and academic degree abbreviations in by-lines.

The average number of names in a multiauthor by-line is six. In AMA publications, the conjunction *and* is currently omitted in a series of names. However, a number of non-AMA publications do use *and* in multiauthor by-lines. Be sure to check the style of the individual journal beforehand.

Author affiliation and/or professional title In manuscripts destined for AMA publications, the author affiliation is indicated in an unnumbered footnote. This note may be double-spaced under the by-line on the title page or it may be typed on a separate sheet following the title page. Examples:

From the College of Medicine, Statesville
University, Statesville.

From the Department of Pediatrics (Dr. Smith) and Internal
Medicine (Dr. Lang), College of Medicine, Statesville
University, Statesville.

Dr. Jones is in private practice.

Or, if the doctor has relocated since doing the research and completing the paper, the affiliation note should read:

From the College of Medicine, Statesville
University, Statesville. Dr. Long is now with
the Department of Ophthalmology, Medical
University of Smithville, Smithville.

Notice that all of the footnotes are terminated by periods.

Give the name, address, and telephone number of the author responsible for the manuscript and for the fulfillment of later reprint requests. The journal editor will position this material in a footnote on the first printed page of the article.

Some journals not affiliated with the AMA include author titles either as part of the by-line or as part of the affiliation. If the journal specifies that titles should be given, make sure that the writer has included the necessary data where it is called for. Many journals limit the number of usable titles to *two*, and require that the title or titles be directly relevant to the context of the article.

Abstract The second manuscript page typically contains an abstract of the article. An abstract is a terse, clear digest of a particular problem central to the article, the methods of investigation used in examining or studying the problem, the results of the investigation or study, and the conclusions derived from it. In some instances, the abstract may also include a very brief explanation of the significance of the findings.

The length of an abstract generally depends on the type and length of the article itself. For example, an average abstract of a single case report might not be longer than 60 words. On the other hand, abstracts of major articles may average from 100 to 250 words, depending on the length and complexity of the article, the space problems of the publishing journal, and the general limitations that a journal may impose on all of its abstracts. Be sure to count the words in the abstract. Make sure that the count conforms to the publisher's specifications. If the word count overruns these specifications, tactfully bring the matter to the author's attention. These are typical elements in a very brief abstract:

Title Page of a Manuscript

REGULATION OF MEGAKARYOPOIESIS IN LONG-TERM

MURINE BONE MARROW CULTURES

By Neil Williams, Heather Jackson, A. P. C. Sheridan

Martin J. Murphy, Jr., A. Elste and Malcolm A. S. Moore

From the Department of Developmental Hematopoiesis, Sloan-Kettering

Institute for Cancer Research, 145 Boston Post Road, Rye, New York 10580

This work was supported in part by American Cancer Society grant ACS-CH3,

National Cancer Institute grant CA-17085 and the Gar Reichman Foundation.

Running Title: _In Vitro_ Megakaryopoiesis

Correspondence to: Neil Williams, Ph.D.

Sloan-Kettering Institute for Cancer Research

145 Boston Post Road

Rye, New York 10580

Reproduced by permission of BLOOD The Journal of the American Society of Hematology, Volume 51, pp. 245–255, and by Neil Williams, PhD. (Dr. Williams acknowledges the special assistance of Ms. Patricia Higgins and her typing staff.)

text of the abstract
source of the article abbreviated and enclosed
   in parentheses on a separate line at the end
   of the abstract text (these data to be supplied
   by the journal editor)
key words (if required by the journal)

And these are typical elements in a more elaborate abstract:

heading
   author name(s)
   abbreviated journal title
   publishing data (volume number, issue,
   pagination, and date) to be supplied by journal editor
text of abstract
   problem
   methods
   results
   conclusions
key words (if required by the journal)

See the illustration of a typical abstract.

Abstracts contain neither footnotes nor references. Tabular data and graphics are also excluded from them. Some journals request the authors to include at the ends of their abstracts a list of four or five key words that can be later used for indexing and/or for computer information storage and retrieval systems. If key words are required, make sure that they have already been used in the abstract and in the article itself. If they have not been so used, it would be wise to alert the author politely.

A brief but very helpful article on abstract writing can be found in the *Journal of the American Medical Association* (222:1307, 1972).

Abstract

Bernad, Peter, Synder, David A., and Levey, Michael: A civilian case of fatal meningococcemia due to Neisseria meningitidis, group Y. Am J Clin Pathol 68: 296-298, 1977. The present report is that of a civilian episode of fatal, fulminant group Y meningococcemia in a previously healthy adolescent, who denied prior vaccination against group C meningococcus. The patient suffered abrupt onset of purpura, hypotension and cardiopulmonary arrest. A detailed clinical and pathologic report is included.

(Key words: Group Y meningococcal disease; Neisseria meningitidis.)

The text of an article Follow the spacing and margin guidelines given at the beginning of this section. Number the first text page *1*. Page numbers can be typed (1) at the top center of the page and positioned according to the margin specifications being followed (2) in the top right corner of the page but not overrunning the right margin setting, or (3) at the bottom center of the page and positioned according to the margin specifications being followed. Unspaced hyphens can be used to enclose *centered* page numbers. Recheck all pagination twice after the manuscript has been typed in final form.

A typewriting margin guide can be constructed on heavy colored paper and then inserted behind the sheet being typed. A guide set up for 8½ × 11-inch paper will contain 66 single-spaced lines. The typist can mark the guide at the appropriate numbers to indicate top and bottom margin settings, page number position, and first and last text lines. The first text line should begin four vertical line spaces from the line on which the page number has been typed at the top of the sheet. If the page number has been typed at the bottom of the page, the first text line should conform to the margin setting designated. A Triple-Form Typewriting Copy Guide, useful for correspondence as well as for manuscripts, is illustrated in this section.

A few journals require that the surname of the author (or the surname of the first coauthor in multiauthor manuscripts) be typed in the upper right corner of each manuscript page. If the specifications call for this technique, be sure to do it and then check each page accordingly.

When typewriting the text, do not include tabular data or graphics. Do not leave gaps in the text for later inclusion of this material. All tables and figures should be prepared separately and should be placed after the references. However, light penciled indications of the desired placement of tabular data and figures can be made by the author in the right margins. These notations ought to be circled.

If the writer wishes to include sideheads or subheads within the text, insert them exactly as the writer indicates. (Some journals prefer to insert their own text dividers, while others request that their contributors place them at "sensible" intervals within the text.) If the journal has definite policies regarding the styling of text dividers, follow them exactly. For example, if italics are desired, underscore the head or use an italic type ball if the typewriter has this feature. If boldface (i.e., heavy) type is called for, indicate it by placing a wavy underline beneath the head. Avoid dividing words at the ends of the last lines of pages. Do not insert footnotes at the bottoms of pages; instead, use parenthetic comments or citations.

While there is no set and unchanging formula for the textual organization of a major article, the following are typical main elements:

introduction
methods (as of research or testing)
results
discussion
conclusions/findings
summary

Case reports—shorter than main articles—usually contain these elements:

introduction
report of a case
methods (as of treatment)
results
comment

It is not the responsibility of the assistant to change the wording or the order of an article.

See the illustration on page 405.

Triple-Form Typewriting Copy Guide

Baronial (half-sheet) stationery
Monarch (executive) stationery
Standard (full-sized) stationery

Baronial (half-sheet)	Monarch (executive)	Standard (full-sized sheet)
1	1	1
2	2	2
3	3	3
4	4	4
5	5	5
6	6	6
7	7	7
8	8	8
9	9	9
10	10	10
11	11	11
12	12	12
13	13	13
14	14	14
15	15	15
16	16	16
17	17	17
18	18	18
19	19	19
20	20	20
21	21	21
22	22	22
23	23	23
24	24	24
25	25	25
26	26	26
27	27	27
28	28	28
29	29	29
30	30	30
31	31	31
32	32	32
33	33	33
34	34	34
35	35	35
36	36	36
37	37	37
38	38	38
39	39	39
40	40	40
41	41	41
42	42	42
43	43	43
44	44	44
45	45	45
46	46	46
47	47	47
48	48	48
49	49	49
50	50	50
51	51	51
52	52	52
53	53	53
54	54	54
55	55	55
56	56	56
	57	57
	58	58
	59	59
	60	60
	61	61
	62	62
	63	63
		64
		65
		66

Suggestions for Copy Guide Use: A triple-form typewriting copy guide may easily be constructed on colored paper for ready identification. This vertical placement device can then be positioned behind the page or behind the carbon pack on which typewriting is to be done. The numbers on the copy guide should be exposed at the right-hand side. In this way, the typist may be guided as to the remaining lines on a page. A red pencil may be advantageously used to mark the copy guide at significant points such as the starting point of a date line, the place where the bottom margin is to begin, the length of an executive or half-page letter, and so on.

Manuscript Page

3

Of interest is the low incidence of prescriptions for the
drugs' antidepressant effect—1% of all uses for general practitioners, internists, osteopaths, and "all others"; 5% for obste-
trician-gynecologists; and none for all other specialty groups
(including psychiatrists). It thus appears that patients for
whom these drugs are prescribed and who are categorized as depressed are being treated with benzodiazepines for the anxiety
that so often accompanies melancholia of all types.

Although they are used both in and out of hospitals, the
benzodiazepines are more often prescribed in office practice, by
a factor of 2.5 to 1. The patients who receive these drugs are
more often women than men (by a factor of 1.8 to 1). The age
group 40-59 accounts for about 40% of the use, and the 20-39 and
65-and-over age groups account for 28% and 21%, respectively.

USES IN OTHER DISORDERS

Is there reason to suspect that the benefits derived from
benzodiazepines go beyond sedation, antianxiety effects, and muscular relaxation? Are there additional benefits in terms of concomitant gastrointestinal or cardiovascular dysfunction, for
instance?

As Greenblatt and Shader (2) pointed out, "The benzodiazepines are frequently used to treat organic or functional gastrointestinal disorders in which anxiety is judged to have a precipi-
tating or exacerbating role." Both the gut and the cardiovascular
system are well known to be affected by "stress," "anxiety," and
autonomic activity. Although the benzodiazepines are essentially

Drug names used in a text   Nonproprietary drug names may be used in the text of an article: trade names should be avoided in the title, the abstract, and the text unless the article is an adverse action report or a comparison/evaluation of one drug developed by two or more companies.

AMA publications and a few non-AMA journals request that their authors include a separate list of the nonproprietary names and trade names of all drugs referred to in the article. This list should be positioned flush with the left margin on the last text page—a few lines below the last line of the article, or on a separate sheet appearing immediately after the last text page. The heading of the list should be: Nonproprietary Name(s) and Trademark(s) of Drug(s). Beneath the heading is the double-spaced list, set up according to the following formula:

nonproprietary name in Roman type and styled
   with an initial capital letter
unspaced em dash
trade name in italics or underscored and typewritten in capitals and lowercase
terminal period

If there are several trade names for one nonproprietary name, the typist should list the trade names in alphabetical order. Examples:

Nonproprietary Name and Trademark of Drug
Chlordiazepoxide—*Librium.*

Nonproprietary Names and Trademarks of Drugs
Gentamicin sulfate—*Garamycin.*

Ampicillin sodium—*Alpen-N, Amcill-S, Omnipen,*
   Penbritin S, Polycillin-N.

Acknowledgments   An acknowledgment of assistance—either financial or professional—is usually given in an unnumbered footnote typed at the bottom of the last text page a few lines below the list of drug names, if there is one. An alternative procedure is to typewrite the acknowledgment note on a separate sheet. A third method is to type the footnote near the bottom of the title page. Check the journal's Instructions to Authors for the appropriate style. Acknowledgment footnotes are very brief and to the point:

   This study was supported in part by
Veterans Administration Grant (give number).
   Sarah Smith gave technical assistance;
John D. Jones and Lynn T. Prescott assisted
in the preparation of the manuscript.

   Statistical analysis was provided by
Kenneth Y. Lee of the Division of Biometrics,
Department of Preventive Medicine. Sally
Young and Linda Doe assisted in performing the
chemical analyses.

Notice that in the first example above, the financial assistance is credited first, followed by mention of personal assistance.

Permission   It is the writer's responsibility to obtain written permission to use material that has already been published elsewhere. Examples of permission footnotes that may appear at the end of the article or beneath specific drawings or tables are as follows:

Figures 1, 3, and 4 are reproduced by
permission of the *Journal of the
American Medical Association*
(238:603–604, 1977).

Martin A. Reiser, MD, gave permission to
report case 6.

Table 1 is reproduced by permission
of Reiser.[2]

In the last example above, *Reiser*[2] refers the reader to the reference numbered 2 that appears at the end of the article. It is in that source that the original data for Table 1 has been already published. When mailing the completed manuscript to the publisher, be sure that the physician has included copies of all permissions. The physician should keep the original correspondence.

References Writers give credit to other authors' published work by the use of textual citations and numbered references listed at the ends of articles. All published matter and material accepted for publication that have been cited in a text are usually listed at the end of the piece (in some cases, however, they may be parenthetically mentioned in the running text itself). Depending on individual journal style, textual indicators of material being cited may be Arabic numerals enclosed in parentheses, or they may be unspaced superscript Arabic numerals typed after the surnames of authors being referred to or after specific nouns (as "study," "examination," "investigation," and the like) indicating the published work. Examples:

Doe and Smith (16) and Jones (4) have shown that . . . .

Studies by Doe et al (1) and our own evaluations (3) raise the
possibility that . . . .

. . . glucose administration by Langley et al (9) in two patients . . . .

. . . in six famous studies (1–6).

and

Doe and Smith[16] and Jones[4] have shown that . . . .

Studies by Doe et al[1] and our own evaluations[3] raise the
possibility that . . . .

. . .glucose administration by Langley et al[9] in two patients . . . .

. . . in six famous studies.[1-6]

In all of the above examples, the numerals refer the reader to references 16, 4, 1, 3, 9, and 1–6, respectively.

Parenthetic reference numerals are typewritten <u>inside</u> periods, commas, colons, and semicolons. Examples:

. . . studied by Smythe (2), Frank (3), and Jones (4).

. . . is indicated in these data from Kingsley (6): . . . .

. . . was identified by Graham (7) and Stanley (8); however, other studies have also shown that . . . .

Superscript numerals, on the other hand, are typewritten <u>outside</u> periods and commas but <u>inside</u> colons and semicolons:

. . . were indicated in earlier studies.[1-3,5,19]

. . . as reported earlier,[12]

but

. . . revealed these data[6-9]:

. . . felt that it had been proved in those studies[1,7-9]; however . . . .

When more than one reference in a closed series (such as a citation indicating references 1 through 6) is listed at one point in the text, it is standard practice to join the superscript series with a hyphen, as

. . . in previously examined patients.[1-6]

Unspaced commas separate single elements in a multipart superscript citation:

. . . these investigations.[1-6,10,19]

If the physician desires to cite different page numbers from a single published source at different points in the text, the appropriate pagination is enclosed in parentheses and is included in the superscript citation, as

. . . these studies.[2(p 345),10]
. . . these studies.[2(pp 345-346,349),10]

Notice that all of the elements in the above citations are <u>unspaced</u>. Never use *op. cit., loc. cit.,* or *ibid.* in medical/scientific references.

In the text, the writer may wish to make parenthetic references to other published sources. If this is done, the name of the cited author may or may not be given, and the title of the article itself is usually omitted. However, the journal name, the volume of the journal (if there is a volume number), the appropriate pagination, and the date <u>are</u> given. Journal names are written out in full unless they appear in parentheses with inclusive pagination, in which case they are abbreviated according to the *Index Medicus* styling. Examples:

The test data were reported last year by Jones in the
British Medical Journal (2:771-775, 19-).

but

The test data were reported last year by Jones
(*Br Med J* 2:771-775, 19-).

Other parenthetic data included in the text may be citations of material not yet officially accepted for publication, personal correspondence with other physicians or with scientists, and general publications. These citations must be noted only in the text. It is standard practice not to include them in lists of numbered references. Examples:

The test results have been substantiated (J. R. Doe, MD, unpublished data, June 2, 19-).
According to a letter from J. R. Smith, MD (June 2, 19-) . . . .
Similar investigations were carried out by J. R. Doe, MD (written communication, January 2, 19-).
An article on HMOs appeared recently in a national business magazine (*Business Week* 30 May 1977, p 20), in which . . . .

Although the style for listed references varies from one journal to another (excluding AMA publications), there are, nevertheless, some general features common to all or most of them:

1. References are double-spaced on a sheet or sheets separate from the text.
2. References are usually listed in the order of their first occurrence in the text, although some journals require alphabetization by author surname.
3. Each reference is introduced by an Arabic numeral to which the textual citations referring to it are keyed.
4. The author surname appears first, followed by first and middle initials and a colon.
5. If there is no author, the title of the published matter begins the reference.
6. In multiauthor references whose coauthors number more than three, the first three coauthors' names are given followed by "et al".

7. Titles of books follow their authors' names: book titles are often italicized and are capitalized and lowercased as they appear in their original form.

8. Titles of articles follow their authors' names: only the first word of the title is given an initial capital, and the title is not enclosed in quotation marks.

9. Numbered subtitles are introduced in references by Roman numerals (for example, Doe JR: Title of the article: I. Numbered subtitle. *J Name* 123:45–46, 19–.).

10. A period terminates the titles of articles and books (exception: a comma terminates a book title followed by an edition number or other closely related appendage).

11. The title of a book is followed by pertinent publishing data: the place of publication + a comma + the name of the publisher + a comma + the date of publication.

12. The title of an article is followed by the abbreviated name of the journal, which is styled according to the *Index Medicus*.

13. The name of a journal is followed by pertinent publishing data: an Arabic numeral or numerals indicating the volume number + a colon + pagination + a comma + the year.

The following are major style variations occurring among non-AMA journals as opposed to AMA publications:

1. The AMA uses minimal punctuation; other journals, however, use punctuation in degrees varying from heavy to medium.

2. AMA publications currently indent the first reference line three spaces: some other journals set their references flush left, run their references in with each other, or set the first lines flush left with the runovers being hanging-indented.

3. AMA publications italicize journal names and book titles, while a large number of non-AMA journals currently set journal names and book titles in Roman.

4. AMA publications terminate references with a period, but usage among non-AMA journals is evenly divided as to the inclusion or the omission of the terminal period.

5. There are numerous differences among the non-AMA publications as to the styling of editions, translations, edited volumes, books in series, and supplements to journals.

6. Some journals expect the writer to list the references in alphabetical order according to author or coauthor names rather than to list them in the order of their first citation in the text.

The medical assistant should be familiar with some of the basic types of references often encountered in medical manuscript typewriting. These are given in the list below:

a single-author article
a multiauthor article
an authored book
an edition of a book if other than the first
an edited book
a part of a book
a volume in a series of books
a monograph or a report in a series
a federal or a state government publication
a legal reference: a citation of a case
material accepted for publication but still in press
a paper delivered at a meeting
other unpublished material or correspondence

The next paragraphs illustrate and then discuss briefly the types of references listed above. The style generally reflects AMA preferences for the sake of consistency. Where there are major stylistic variations among non-AMA publications, warning notes are included.

a single-author article
　　1. Doe JR: Title of the article: Subtitle if there is one.
J Name 12:345−348, 19−.

Indent the first line three spaces, give the appropriate numeral, and terminate it with a period. (Style among non-AMA journals varies considerably as to first-line indention; consult the publication in question to ascertain the proper style.) Typewrite the auther surname first followed by the initials. AMA style currently excludes punctuation within author names; however, usage is divided among other journals on this point. Insert a colon after the last element of the author name, skip two spaces, and type the title of the article in Roman with an initial capital followed by lowercase. If there is a subtitle, style it as if it were the title, with the initial capital after the colon dividing the title from the subtitle. If there are proper names in the title or subtitle, capitalize them. If the title appears in a foreign language with capitalized words, style the title exactly as shown in the original. Terminate the title with a period unless it has been phrased as a question. (Never use quotation marks around the title.) Abbreviate journal names according to the *Index Medicus*. Italicize all journal names if the manuscript is intended for an AMA publication; if not, check the house style of the particular journal to which the material is being sent. Enter the volume number followed by an unspaced colon and the appropriate pagination. Do not use the abbreviation *vol*. Use *p* and/or *pp* before the pagination of journals not having volume numbers or journals not consecutively numbered throughout a single volume (see also pages 412−413). Follow the pagination with a comma, a space, and the year of publication. End the reference with a period.

a multiauthor article
　　2. Doe JR, Roe SM, Smith TT, et al: Title of the article. *J Name*
12:345−348, 19−.

Separate the coauthor names with commas in references for material being submitted to AMA publications. Do not join the series of names with *and*. With references intended for non-AMA journals among which usage is greatly divided on these points, check the individual journal in question to ascertain proper house style. When there are four or more coauthors, give only the first three names followed by a comma and "et al" (typed in Roman and unpunctuated).

an authored book
　　3. Doe JR: *Title of the Book*. City, Publisher,
19−, p 123.

Style the author name or names as if for an article. Capitalize, lowercase, and italicize the book title. (Since some non-AMA publications style book titles in Roman, be sure to check the individual house style.) A period is placed after the title and is followed by appropriate publication data: the geographic location (city) of the publisher, the name of the publisher, and the date followed by the cited page or pages introduced by *p* or *pp*. Tie these units together with commas and end the reference with a period.

an edition of a book if other than the first
　　4. Doe JR: *Title of the Book*, ed 2. City, Publisher, 19−,
pp 34−35.

Style the author, title, and publication data as shown above and in note 3. It is standard to indicate an edition if other than the first by use of the lowercase unpunctuated abbreviation *ed* + the appropriate Arabic numeral. This information immediately follows the title and is separated from it by a comma. A few journals have distinctive house styles for editions: be sure to double-check the Instructions to Authors.

an edited book
   5. Doe JR, Roe SM, Smith TT, et al (eds):   *Title of the Book.*
City, Publisher, 19—, pp 45–67.
   6. Doe JR: *Title of the Book,* Roe SM (trans-ed). City, Publisher,
19—, pp 90–98.

Typewrite the name (or names) of the editor(s), following standard style for authors as shown above and in previous notes. Indicate editorship by placing the lowercase parenthetic abbreviation (ed) or (eds) after the name(s); see note 5 above. Give the book title and publication data as shown above and in previous notes. If the book is authored, edited, and translated (see note 6 above), begin the reference with the author's name followed by the title, a comma, and the inverted name of the translator-editor, indicated by the lowercase parenthetic abbreviation (trans-ed). Place a period after this abbreviated designation. Proceed to type the publication data and the pagination as would be done for other books. NOTE: Since usage among non-AMA publications is greatly divided as to the style for editorial and translation designations, be sure to check the journal in question before typing this sort of material.

a part of a book
   7. Doe JR: Title of the part of the book being cited, in Roe SM
(ed):   *Title of the Book.* City, Publisher, 19—, vol 4, pp 123–133.

Begin the reference with the name(s) of the author(s) responsible for the part being cited. Give the title of the part, section, chapter, or subsection cited, and style the material as if it were a journal title—i.e., with an initial capital only (see note 1). Place a comma after the cited part, insert the lowercase Roman word *in*, and then give the inverted name of the editor of the book, the editorial abbreviation (ed) followed by a colon, and the book title. Style the title and the publication data as shown in previous references. If the physician has given inclusive pagination for the part being cited as shown above, there is no need to give chapter or section or part numbers. However, if the physician omits the inclusive pagination, the number of the cited part or chapter or section should be given. Example:

   8. Doe JR: Title of the chapter in the book being cited, in Roe
SM (ed):   *Title of the Book.* City, Publisher, 19—, vol 1, chap 4.

Typical abbreviations used in this case are *pt* for *part,* *sect* for *section,* and *chap* for *chapter.* Note that they are unpunctuated and lowercased.

a volume in a series of books
   9. Doe JR: *Title of the Book.* City, Publisher, 19—,
vol 4, p 123.

Typewrite the author, title, and publication data as shown for books. Insert the lowercase unpunctuated abbreviation *vol* + the appropriate Arabic numeral right after the publication date and just before the pagination. Tie all publication data together with commas. NOTE: If the volume number comprises part of the book title, include it as part of the title and style it exactly as it appears in the original.

a monograph or a report in a series
   10. Doe JR: *Title of the Monograph or the Report,* publication 123,
Name of the Series, City, Publisher, 19—.

Style the author's name as for a journal article or a book. Give the monograph or the report title in italicized capital and lowercase letters followed by a comma, the publication number, another comma, the capitalized and lowercased name of the series in which the material appears, another comma, and the rest of the publication data styled as for books.

a federal or a state government publication
    11. Doe JR: *Title of the Publication,* publication identification
number FDA 1234. Publishing Government Agency, 19—.
    12. *Title of the Publication,* publication identification number
CDC 4567. City, Publishing Government Agency, 19—.

If the author is known, give the author's name followed by a colon and the italicized, capitalized, and lowercased publication title styled as for a book. Follow the title by a comma and the publication identification number: in reference 11, the sample number is shown as if it were for an FDA publication; in reference 12, as if it were for a CDC publication. If the publishing agency is located in Washington, DC, omit the city designation (see reference 11), and follow the publication number with a period. The name of the publishing agency is followed by a comma and the publication date. If the publishing agency is located in a city other than Washington, DC (see reference 12), give the city where the agency is located followed by a comma, the agency name followed by a comma, and the publication date.

a legal reference: a citation of a case
    13. *Doe vs Roe Community Hospital,* 200 App Div 400, 50 NYS 3d 200,
19—.

For legal references, give (1) the name of the case typewritten in italicized capitals and lowercase letters followed by a comma (2) the volume number (3) the abbreviated and unpunctuated identification of the record (4) the pagination, and (5) the year. Some designations may include a supplement (Suppl) or perhaps a series number (as 3d). Since legal citation styling is highly specialized, it is suggested that the physician make sure that the material is formatted according to the style guidelines of the publisher to which the manuscript is being sent. The AMA *Stylebook* offers detailed treatment of the topic, as does *A Uniform System of Citation* (Cambridge, MA: The Harvard Law Review Association).

material accepted for publication but still in press
    14. Doe JR: Title of the article. *J Name,* to be published.

Style the material as if it were a published journal article (see note 1). However, instead of inserting publication data and pagination, typewrite the phrase *to be published* after the abbreviated journal name.

a paper delivered at a meeting
    15. Doe JR, Roe, SM, Smith TT, et al: Title of the paper: Subtitle
if there is one. Read before Name of the Organization, City, ST,
January 31–February 1, 19—.

Give the author or authors' name(s) and the title of the paper styled as for a journal article (see note 1). Insert the phrase *Read before* or *Presented at* after the title and just before the full official name of the organization. Follow the organization name with a comma and the geographic location of the meeting (city + two-letter state abbreviation or the name of the country if the meeting took place outside the United States), followed by another comma and the inclusive dates of the meeting (months, days, and year).

other unpublished material and correspondence
Personal correspondence and other unpublished material should not be included in listed references. This type of information should be inserted within the running text in parenthetic citational form.

Special reference problems   Occasionally, the physician will refer to a thesis. The generally accepted format for this type of reference is:

1. Doe JR: *Thesis Title,* thesis. Name of the Graduate School, City, 19—.

Typewrite the author name as for a book or an article. Italicize the capitalized and lowercased thesis title and the subtitle, if there is one. Be sure to capitalize the first word after the colon in the subtitle. Terminate the title and/or the subtitle with a comma followed by the word *thesis* and a period. Give the full official name of the graduate school followed by a comma, its geographical location (city), another comma, and the date.

As mentioned earlier, the abbreviations *p* and *pp* generally are not used to introduce journal pagination, although they are so used in references to books. However, *p* and *pp* are used in references to journals not having volume numbers. Examples:

1. Doe JR: Title of the article. *J Name,* 19—, pp 13–14.
2. Smith TT: Title of the article. *J Name,* April 19—, pp 22–24.

Notice that the date of publication (whether just the year or the month and the year) is given <u>before</u> the pagination.

If a volume of a particular journal has two or more parts and only one part is cited, the following style is used:

1. Doe JR: Title of the article. *J Name* 20(pt 1):244–245, 19—.

In the above reference, 20 is the volume, pt 1 is the first part of volume 20, and 244–245 is the inclusive pagination of the part cited. Notice that the material from 20 through 245 is unspaced.

Special supplements are sometimes published by journals. If the physician wishes to refer to a supplement, the following style may be used:

1. Doe JR: Title of the article. *J Name* 20(suppl):80–89, 19—.

In the above example, 20 is the volume, (suppl) indicates that a supplement to volume 20 is being cited, and 80–89 is the inclusive pagination. Note that the material from 20 through 89 is unspaced.

If the pagination of a particular supplement is not consecutive with that of the volume being supplemented, the following style is used:

1. Smith TT: Title of the article. *J Name* 20(June suppl):120–125, 19—.

In the above reference, the June supplement to volume 20 is being cited. Its pagination is not consecutive with that of volume 20. The pagination being cited is included after the parenthetic designation of the supplement. Note that the material from 20 throught 125 is unspaced. The same style is used for numbered supplements published separately from regular issues or volumes:

1. Roe SM: Title of the article. *J Name* 23(suppl 4):200–203, 19—.

Checking references   The physician may ask the medical assistant to verify reference data before typing the material. In this case, the assistant can check the original books or articles or can refer to the *Index Medicus.* Every unit within every reference should be verified: author names, titles, publication names, and all publishing data. Be sure that in multiauthor references all coauthor names are in the correct sequence—i.e., they should appear in the references just as written in the original by-lines.

Listed References

References

1. Bhaskar SN: Oral tumors of infancy and childhood: A survey of 293 cases. J Pediat 63:195-210, 1963.

2. Andrews AD, Yoder FW, Barrett SF, et al: Cockayne's syndrome fibroblasts have decreased colony-forming ability but normal rates of unscheduled DNA synthesis after ultraviolet irradiation. Clin Res 24:624A, 1976.

3. Spector WS: Handbook of Toxicity. Philadelphia, WB Saunders Co, 1956, vol 1, p 240.

4. Bohler L: The Treatment of Fractures. ed 5, New York, Grune and Stratton, 1956, vol 1.

5. Wilk SP (trans-ed): Skeletal Roentgenology, ed 3. New York, Grune and Stratton, 1968, p 76.

6. Wintrobe MW, Thorn GW, Adams RD, et al (eds): Harrison's Principles of Internal Medicine, New York, McGraw-Hill, 1974, pp 785-788.

7. Leek BF: Abdominal visceral receptors, in Neil E (ed): Handbook of Sensory Physiology. Berlin, Springer-Verlag, 1972, vol 1, pp 113-160.

8. De Bakey M (ed): Transplantation and artificial organs, in The Year Book of General Surgery 1967-1968, Year Book Series, Chicago, Year Book Medical Publishers, pp 31-75.

9. Stout AP, Latles R: Tumors of the soft tissues, in Atlas of Tumor Pathology, Armed Forces Institute of Pathology, 1967, series 2, fasc 1.

10. Persky H, O'Brien CP, Smith KD, et al: Differences in the testosterone-aggression relationship between men and women. Read before the first annual meeting of the American Society of Andrology, Worcester, MA, March 31-April 12, 1976.

11. VD Fact Sheet, publication (CDC) 76-8195. US Department of Health, Education and Welfare, Public Health Service, Center for Disease Control, 1975.

12. Tennessee Morbidity Report. Nashville, Tennessee Department of Public Health, 1975.

13. AEtna Life Insurance Company vs Davey, 8 S Ct 331, 332, 123 US 739, 31 L Ed 315.

Tables   The suggestions regarding tabular data that are given below are based on an examination of both AMA publications and non-AMA publications:

1. Before typewriting the material, read carefully the journal's instructions to authors regarding the setup of tabular data. Then check a current issue of the journal to verify those instructions. Notice where the titles of the tables are placed, how the tables are numbered, how the titles and internal data are capitalized, and so forth.
2. Do not insert tables in the running text.
3. Typewrite each table on a separate sheet.
4. Typewrite the author's surname (or the surname of the coauther responsible for the manuscript) in the top right corner of each sheet.
5. Do not paginate the sheets, but do number the tables consecutively.
6. The majority of journals use Arabic numerals to number the tables; however, one or two still use Roman numerals for this purpose. Be sure to find out which system is to be followed.
7. Make sure that all textual references to tables have the correct numbers in them.
8. Make sure that each table has a title: these titles should be brief and must be written by the physician, of course.
9. Check totals and percentages for accuracy.
10. Tabular data should read down and not across the sheet.
11. Do not insert vertical or horizontal rules.
12. Make sure that footnotes have been inserted to explain any unusual symbols, signs, or abbreviations in the tables.
13. Ensure that permission footnotes have been included below tables taken from other published sources.

Graphics   Graphics include line drawings, photographs, photomicrographs, and graphs. They are commonly designated as "Figure" + the appropriate Arabic numeral(s). Although instructions regarding graphics vary from journal to journal, the following general rules apply to all:

1. Do not insert figures within running text.
2. The physician should not submit original artwork: all drawings should be *professionally* rendered in black india ink on white boards. Do not submit photocopies of drawings. If the drawings are to be mounted, use rubber cement.
3. Do not write on the faces of photographs.
4. Photographs should be *professionally* shot and unretouched. Do not crop or mount them unless instructed otherwise by the journal.
5. Black and white glossy prints are generally acceptable; however, policies regarding color photographs vary from journal to journal.
6. Duplicates of photomicrographs are usually acceptable.
7. The physician should indicate the following on the *back* side of each figure:
   the top of the figure by lightly penciling "top"
   the surname of the author or of the first coauthor
   the number of the figure
8. Legends and keylines must be typed on a separate sheet. Double-space the material. Make sure that each legend and any required keylines are introduced by the appropriate figure numbers. Arabic numerals are used to indicate figures.
9. Since blueprints will not reproduce, don't submit them.
10. Do not attach staples or paper clips to any of the figures. Do not paste labels to the backs of photographs.
11. Put all figures into a separate envelope that has been stiffened with protective cardboard. Label the envelope "Figures." It is also wise to indicate on the envelope how many figures are enclosed.

Copyrights   The Congress passed a new copyright law—The Copyright Revision Act of 1976—an act that became effective on January 1, 1978. This law has affected AMA procedures for manuscript review, with the result that covering letters accompanying manuscripts submitted for publication by the AMA must contain a sentence in which the writer (or the writers) transfers and assigns copyright ownership of the piece to the AMA if the work is published by the AMA. This rule applies not only to articles but also to questions submitted for publication. The proper wording for copyright ownership transferral of articles in AMA publications may be found in *JAMA* (238:2188, 1977) and that of questions in the same volume of *JAMA* (p 2200). For non-AMA publications, the writer should examine a current issue of the journal in question to ascertain the proper copyright transferral procedure.

Conclusion: comments from journal editors   Editors of several medical journals have expressed concern about the following points of mechanical style:

1. Be sure that you and the writer have adhered to the textual line spacing requirements of the journal. The one and one-half vertical line setting is <u>not</u> an acceptable substitute for double-spacing when double-spacing has been called for by the journal. Incorrect spacing will not slip by an editor. In fact, one managing editor of a prestigious journal has said that incorrectly spaced manuscripts are routinely returned to their writers unread.

2. If key words are required, make sure that the writer has included the correct number of them.

3. Some journals request that the writer submit a short running head (a truncated title) for use as page leaders in the printed article. Ensure that the writer has included the running head and that it does not exceed the word count stipulated by the journal. Running heads are usually appended to the title pages of articles.

4. Many editors complain that illustrations are routinely submitted with nary a legend in sight. The careful assistant will double-check to see that all legends have been included in the envelope with the complete manuscript and the figures.

5. Do not fold the manuscript when preparing it for the mail. Rather, mail it in a large manila envelope stiffened with cardboard. All illustrative material should have been placed in an inner envelope also stiffened with cardboard for extra protection.

6. Double-check the numerical textual citations referring to listed references: when they do not coincide with the reference sources, the editors are forced to return the material to the writers for correction.

7. Reference lists not styled according to journal specifications are eventually returned to the writer for reworking (*and* retyping).

8. Some writers insist on submitting manuscripts typed on legal-sized paper. All American medical journals request that $8\frac{1}{2} \times 11$-inch paper be used.

9. Most editors request that the writer and typist consult the *Index Medicus,* a reputable medical dictionary, the AMA *Stylebook,* or the *CBE Style Manual,* ed 3 (Council of Biology Editors Committee on Form & Style, 1972) for the appropriate styling of abbreviations.

BOOKS

The typewriting guides given at the beginning of this section also apply to book manuscript production. However, most publishers furnish their authors with style booklets outlining the procedures they wish to be followed. The typist should become familiar with these stylistic guidelines.

The author ought to include a table of contents, as well as any other necessary front matter (as a preface or an introduction). The table of contents should be double-spaced; however, it is not necessary to paginate it. Each chapter should open on a new sheet. Chapter openers and titles should be styled according to the publisher's guidelines. Text pages should be numbered consecutively.

Numbered footnotes may be used in books; however, footnote style should conform to the publishing house's guidelines. It is wise to typewrite all footnotes and listed references on separate sheets, since they will undoubtedly be set in a typesize smaller than that of the text. If footnotes and listed references are to appear at the ends of individual chapters, make sure that they have been positioned correctly within the manuscript. For listed reference styling, consult the publisher's style guide.

Tabular data in book manuscripts should be handled as follows:

1. Typewrite each table separately (i.e., on a separate sheet) and ask the physician to indicate in the margin of the text the desired placement of the table when the material is printed.
2. Number the tables according to the style of the publisher: note that tables are usually numbered consecutively *within* chapters.
3. Do not draw rules around or within tables.
4. Double-space and align all tabular data.
5. Recheck all sums and percentages in tables to ensure accuracy.

Drawings are usually produced by the publisher's art department. The writer should, however, include sketches of exactly what is desired (if line drawings are to be used), along with appropriate legends, keylines, and labels. Photographs submitted by the writer should conform to the general specifications listed earlier.

Permissions ought to be handled as described earlier in this section; it is very important to include all permission correspondence with the manuscript. The assistant should ensure that the correspondence is ordered in the sequence in which the permission footnotes and/or credit lines appear in the text. Otherwise, it can be confusing to the editor.

Since indexing is usually done by the publisher, the typist need not plan on setting up and typing an index to the book.

PROOFREADING WHAT HAS BEEN TYPED

Regardless of whether the material is a draft or the final copy of a manuscript, it should be carefully proofread before it is presented to the physician for final review. Do not assume that the doctor will have either the time or the inclination to pick up and correct the typist's mistakes. It is best to read the entire manuscript through for errors—all at one time. During this reading, the typist should make light pencil corrections in the margins when necessary. After the first reading has been done, the errors can be corrected. Then, the manuscript should be reread to pick up any stray typos that may have escaped the first reading, to locate misspellings not already caught, to recheck overall style, and to find and correct any areas of imperfect typescript.

The following table, reprinted from *Webster's New Collegiate Dictionary*, illustrates proofreaders' marks which can be used in correcting manuscripts as well as galleys or page proofs.

HANDLING CORRECTIONS MADE BY EDITORS

Of course, it is the physician-writer's responsibility to check and approve all suggestions and corrections made by editors. Sometimes the changes will be minor and will involve handwritten author alterations or comments on the copy. But in other instances (such as those in which an editor requests a writer to reorder and restyle the listed references or to rework several text pages), the manuscript or parts thereof will have to be retyped. The editor will usually inform the writer if retypes are needed; however, if the writer is uncertain as to what is actually desired by the

PROOFREADERS' MARKS

ℰ or ୪ or ⟋	delete; take it out
⌒	close up; print as one word
ℬ	delete and close up
∧ or ⟩ or ⋏	caret; insert here (something)
#	insert a space
eq#	space evenly where indicated
stet	let marked text stand as set
tr	transpose; change order the
/	used to separate two or more marks and often as a concluding stroke at the end of an insertion
[L	set farther to the left
] set ⌐	farther to the right
⌒	set ae or fl as ligatures æ or fl
=	straighten alignment
‖ ‖	straighten or align
x	imperfect or broken character
☐	indent or insert em quad space
¶	begin a new paragraph
(SP)	spell out ⟨set (5 lbs.) as five pounds⟩
cap	set in capitals ⟨CAPITALS⟩
sm cap or s.c.	set in small capitals ⟨SMALL CAPITALS⟩

lc	set in lowercase ⟨lowercase⟩
ital	set in italic ⟨italic⟩
rom	set in roman ⟨roman⟩
bf	set in boldface ⟨**boldface**⟩
= or -/ or ⌢ or /H/	hyphen
$\frac{1}{N}$ or en or /N/	en dash ⟨1965–72⟩
$\frac{1}{M}$ or em or /M/	em — or long — dash
∨	superscript or superior ⟨∨ as in πr^2⟩
∧	subscript or inferior ⟨∧ as in H_2O⟩
⌄ or ⋏	centered ⟨⌀ for a centered dot in $p \cdot q$⟩
⌂	comma
⌄	apostrophe
⊙	period
; or ;/	semicolon
: or ⊙	colon
⌄⌄ or ⌄⌄	quotation marks
(/)	parentheses
[/]	brackets
OK/?	query to author: has this been set as intended?
⊥ or ⊥[1]	push down a work-up
⊙[1]	turn over an inverted letter
wf[1]	wrong font; a character of the wrong size or esp. style

[1] The last three symbols are unlikely to be needed in marking proofs of photocomposed matter.

editor, he or she may ask the assistant to telephone the editor for further instructions. A good general rule to remember is this: retype any parts of the manuscript that are so heavily edited as to be difficult to read. Clean manuscript copy saves time in composition and avoids costly author alterations later on in galleys and page proofs. When the retypes have been completed, be sure that the doctor checks them and that you make photocopies of them for the office files.

16.3

TYPEWRITING SPEECHES

Physicians are often called on to deliver papers at medical society meetings, at medical conventions, and at other gatherings. It is desirable to typewrite the material so that it will be readable even if the lighting is poor or if the speaker's eyesight is not absolutely perfect (some individuals prefer not to wear reading glasses when addressing audiences). The typist can typewrite the paper or the speech in magnatype—a large-print typestyle. Machines having this typestyle can be rented for short periods. On the other hand, if the office typewriter is an IBM Selectric®, an Orator® ball can be used in typing speeches (see the facsimile on page 420). A third alternative is to use the office typewriter, but to type the material all in capital letters with triple-spacing between lines and three character spaces between sentences (see the facsimile on this page).

A few general guidelines apply to the formatting of all speeches, regardless of the typestyle chosen. These are:

1. The margins of the plain white paper should be at least 1½ inches but preferably 2 inches in width.
2. Ink must be black to afford the best readability.
3. The typeface ought to be razor-sharp, with no breaks or fuzzy spots in the type.
4. Double- or triple-space the speech.
5. End-of-line hyphenation should be avoided altogether: presumably, no one other than the speaker will see the speaker's copy, so right-margin justification is unimportant. Hyphened words can often cause a speaker to hesitate or to misread a word.
6. The last sentence on a page should not be carried over to another sheet. In addition, the assistant ought to type in the lower right corner of each page the first two or three words that will appear at the beginning of the next page. This procedure will facilitate the speaker's delivery, and will assist the speaker in avoiding awkward page shufflings and hesitations.

A Speech Typewritten with the IBM Orator ® Ball

```
        I WOULD LIKE TO TALK WITH YOU TODAY ABOUT THE

        EXPANDING ROLE OF ALLIED HEALTH PROFESSIONALS.

        THIS SUBJECT IS TOPICAL, FOR . . . . . . . . .
```

A Speech Typewritten all in Capitals with Pica Type

```
        I WOULD LIKE TO TALK WITH YOU TODAY ABOUT THE

        EXPANDING ROLE OF ALLIED HEALTH PROFESSIONALS.

        THIS SUBJECT IS TOPICAL, FOR IT IS AN


            .   .   .   .   .   .   .   .   .   .
```

7. Ellipsis points may be used to indicate slow or measured speech; dashes may be inserted to indicate quick, sharp delivery for special effects.
8. Short, very tightly connected phrases (as clusters of points or concepts) within sentences or paragraphs can be indented and blocked together in the center of the page to facilitate the speaker's delivery.
9. Number each page consecutively.
10. Make two copies of the speech—one for the office and an extra one for the physician in case the original is lost.

If the organization to which a speech has been delivered requests a copy for later publication, the typist will then type the material as if it were the running text of an article. The general guidelines given in section 16.2 apply also to speeches prepared for publication in proceedings.

16.4

THE PHYSICIAN'S CURRICULUM VITAE, BIBLIOGRAPY, AND LIST OF PRESENTATIONS

The office ought to have on hand at all times updated copies of the physician's professional profile. This profile is called a *curriculum vitae*. In addition to the vita, there ought to be updated copies of the doctor's bibliography listing the published material that he or she has authored or coauthored. Physicians who have addressed various groups but whose speeches are not to be published in proceedings also may wish to keep lists of these presentations. Such lists are often called "invited presentations." Since it is very important to keep the vita, the bibliography, and the list of presentations up-to-date, the medical assistant should recheck these documents every two or three months to make sure that they are complete and current.

THE CURRICULUM VITAE
The curriculum vitae—a terse yet objective and complete synopsis of the physician's education, experience, and professional activities—should be typewritten on 8½ × 11-inch white bond paper with 1½-inch margins all around. Use a conventional typestyle: avoid italic or script. Pica and Elite are the most common choices. The typewriter typeface should be clean so that there will not be any occurrences of smudged or fuzzy type. All elements of the document have to be evenly spaced and correctly aligned and balanced. While it is possible to achieve acceptable copies of an original document by photocopying, it is nevertheless strongly recommended that the vita and other related documents be offset. Offset printing produces truly professional-looking reproductions of the highest quality. (For a discussion of this copying process, see Chapter 18.) In short, the vita—just like a letter, a report, or a manuscript—is a tangible reflection of the physician's professional stature. Thus, great care should be taken in the production of the material.

The heading   A vita typically comprises one or two pages. The data on the first page are introduced by the all-capitalized heading CURRICULUM VITAE centered and typed 1½ inches from the top edge of the sheet. The doctor's name and appropriate degree abbreviation(s) are centered and typed two line spaces beneath the heading. Capital and lowercase letters are used: Kenneth D. Langley, MD, PhD

The subheads   Major subheads are usually typed flush with the left margin, since this layout is the easiest and the cleanest-looking. Single-space each cluster of data beneath each subhead. Skip two lines between the subhead and the first line of the data to be typed beneath it. Double- or triple-space between subheads. The choice of line spacing will depend on the amount of page space available for the data to be typed. (It is wise to type a draft of the vita first so that all space and alignment problems can be solved before the final copy is produced.) Subheads may be styled in one of these ways:

1. all in capital letters and underscored
2. all in capital letters with no underscoring
3. in capital and lowercase letters and underscored

Do not mix the stylings within one vita: select a style and retain it throughout the document.

Continuation sheets   Continuation-sheet styling conforms to that of the first page. Number each sheet consecutively (the second sheet is numbered 2, but the first sheet is unnumbered). Use Arabic numerals. Position the numerals in the upper right of each page. Typewrite the physician's surname all in capital letters before the numeral, as: JOHNSTONE 2

Content of a curriculum vitae   Commonly used subheads are: (1) PERSONAL DATA (2) EDUCATION (3) EXPERIENCE, and (4) PROFESSIONAL ACTIVITIES. Very prominent physicians having especially lengthy vitae often use more subheads, with the following being typical: (1) PERSONAL DATA (2) EDUCATION (3) FELLOW-SHIPS (4) EXPERIENCE (5) BOARDS (6) HONORS (7) EDITORIAL POSITIONS [or EDITORSHIPS] (8) SOCIETIES, and (9) ADVISORY CAPACITY. This section illustrates the first and most basic group of subheads. Lengthy vitae may be styled just as shown for the shorter version.

The physician may choose to include under PERSONAL DATA any of the following: age or birth date, marital status, office and/or home address, and a telephone number.

The EDUCATION category comprises a list of all medical and academic degrees held by the physician, usually starting with the MD or with an additional doctorate in another discipline that has been received more recently than the MD. For instance, if the physician holds both an MD and a PhD, the one most recently received is entered first in the education summary. (However, the MD is shown first after the physician's surname in the first-page vita heading.) Include the full names and the geographical locations of the institutions where studies were carried on and from which degrees were received. Include all pertinent attendance and graduation dates. If the physician has undertaken special postdoctoral studies, include a brief description of them with pertinent attendance dates and the names of the institutions where the studies were carried out. Names and numerical designations of grants or fellowships should be included. This material may be appended to the end of the education category. A typical sub-subheading for it might be Postdoctoral Study.

The EXPERIENCE section lists all positions held by the physician, starting with the present one (or ones) listed in the order of their importance, and working back in time to residency and internship. Service (if any) in the armed forces or the U.S. Public Health Service ought not to be omitted. Geographic locations and inclusive dates are shown with each entry. If the physician is or has been in private practice, it should be so stated. If the doctor has left the practice of medicine to engage in teaching, the academic position ought to be listed along with the name and location of the college or university. If the physician holds or has held professorships—even if they are part-time—these titles should be noted. Any active directorships (as with corporations) or trusteeships (as with universities or hospitals) should be included.

The doctor then lists his or her fellowships, memberships in medical societies and associations, and memberships in honorary medical or academic societies in the section entitled PROFESSIONAL ACTIVITIES. The states in which the doctor is licensed to practice medicine may also be included here. If the physician serves on an examining board or on a licensing board, a notation of it should be made in this section. It is standard to omit from a medical vita all general activities and honors. A typical curriculum vitae is illustrated below.

A Curriculum Vitae

```
                          CURRICULUM VITAE

                        Jonathan T. Preston, MD


     Personal Data

     Age:  42

     Office address:  Doctors' University Hospital
                      4400 Jefferson Street
                      Smithville, ST 56789


     Education

     MD  Medical College of State                         1957
           Location, ST

     BA  University of State                              1953
           Location, ST


     Experience

     Chief of Surgery, Doctors' University Hospital       1975-
     Professor of Surgery, Doctors' University            1975-
     Associate Professor of Surgery, Doctors' University  1974-1975
     Assistant Professor of Surgery, Doctors' University  1971-1974
     Instructor in Surgery, Doctors' University           1967-1971
     Surgeon, Doctors' University Hospital                1967-1975
     Surgeon, Beltsville General Hospital                 1965-1967
     Resident in General Surgery, West State Medical Center 1962-1965
     Intern, State University General Hospital            1961-1962


     Professional Activities

     Diplomate, American Board of Surgery
     Fellow, American College of Surgery
     Member, American Medical Association

     President, Smith County Medical Society             1977-1978
     Editor in Chief, Surgery Review                     1976-1977
     Associate Editor, The General Surgeon               1973-1974
     Vice-president, Smith County Unit, American Cancer Society  1972-1973
```

BIBLIOGRAPHY
Published material authored or coauthored by the physician is listed on a separate sheet or on several sheets, if there are many titles.

Format The material may be introduced by the all-capitalized headings BIBLIOG-RAPHY or PUBLICATIONS. Typewrite the physician's full name and degree abbreviation(s) two lines below the heading unless the bibliography is attached to the vita, in which case repetition of the doctor's name is unnecessary. Single-space each bibliographic entry but double- or triple-space between entries, depending on the page space available. Use the hanging-indented bibliographic style:

1. Typewrite the first line of each entry flush with the left margin. Do not introduce the entry with an Arabic numeral.
2. Indent runover lines 5 character spaces and begin typing on space 6.

See the facsimile of a typewritten bibliography found at the end of this section on page 426.

Order of entries If all titles are to be included together (i.e., single-author entries are to be listed together with joint-author titles in the same bibliography), the entries should be alphabetized by author surname(s). When listing in one bibliography all of the articles or books that the physician has written as the sole author, the typist should arrange them according to publication dates, with the earliest coming first in the list, as

Doe JR: Title of the article. *J Name* 12:34–36, 1971.
Doe JR: *Title of the Book*. City, Publisher,
       1972.
Doe JR: Title of the article. *J Name* 14:56–60, 1973.

Titles published by the physician in the same year are ordered alphabetically by the title of the book or article (excluding the words *a*, *an*, and *the*).

Single-author entries precede multiauthor entries beginning with the same surname:

Doe JR: . . . .
Doe JR, Roe SM, Smith, TT, et al: . . . .

Entries with the same first author but with different second or third coauthors are alphabetically ordered according to the surname of the second coauthor:

Doe JR, Roe SM, Smith TT, et al: . . . .
Doe JR, Swarthmore RA, Smith TT, et al: . . . .

Do not change the coauthor order from that of the original article or book: in other words, if the physician whose bibliography is being prepared is the second coauthor of a work, do not type his or her name first in the entry for that work.

On the other hand, the physician may choose to list all of his or her own single-author titles on one sheet or in one group, followed on another sheet or in another group by the joint authorships. If this is the case, the first sheet or grouping of entries should be headed PUBLICATIONS OF JOHN R. SMITH, MD and the second sheet or grouping of entries should be headed JOINT PUBLICATIONS OF JOHN R. SMITH, MD. Entries in the single-author group are introduced by title. (There is no need to repeat the physician-author's name at each entry, because the name heads the list.) Entries are conventionally ordered by publication date, with the earliest coming first. The hanging-indented format explained earlier in this section is acceptable for entries having runover lines. Examples of the single-author list are as follows:

Title of the journal article. *J Name*
12:34–36, 1971.
Title of the Book, City, Publisher,
1972.
Title of the journal article. *J Name*
14:56–60, 1973.

Entries in the joint-author list should be introduced by the coauthors' surnames, as already discussed. Include in the joint-author list any chapters, sections, or parts of larger works that were written by the physician. Begin the entry with the physician's surname and initials, and then follow the AMA pattern currently recommended for edited works, as

Doe JR: Title of the section or the chapter or the part
of the book, in Smith TT (ed): *Title of the Book*.
City, Publisher, vol 2, 19–, pp 42–46.

LIST OF PRESENTATIONS
Speeches (but not papers delivered at meetings whose proceedings have been or definitely will be published) and other formal oral presentations and lectures may be listed separately from the bibliography. The page is often headed INVITED PRESENTATIONS or LIST OF PRESENTATIONS with the heading typed all in capital letters and centered in the same way as those of the vita and the bibliography.

Each entry is single-spaced internally, and double-spacing is generally used between subunits of entries. Entries are usually separated by double- or triple-spacing. Margins should conform to those chosen for the vita and the bibliography if at all possible. List each presentation in chronological order beginning with the earliest. This practice will allow the later addition of new entries as they accrue. Give the date (month and year) of each presentation. Position the date flush with the left margin. Skip from about 8 to 16 horizontal character spaces and then type (on the same line as that of the date) the title of the presentation enclosed in quotation marks. Skip two vertical line spaces and typewrite the name of the group to which the presentation was made.

A Bibliography

BIBLIOGRAPHY

Carolyn A. Stephenson, MD

Stephenson CA: Title of the article. J Name 18:94-96, 1977.

Stephenson CA, Martin PA, Aaron AA, et al: Title of the article.
     J Name 17:64-69, 1976.

Stephenson CA, Zimmer AE: Title of the article. J Name 16:50-55,
     1975.

Thompson HT, Stephenson CA: Title of the article. J Name 15:44-46
     1974.

Watson CBW, Preston JT, Stephenson CA, et al: Title of the article.
     J Name 13:45-47, 1973.

Wilkins GN, Stephenson CA: Title of the article. J Name 12:22-25,
     1972.

Yazinsky MI, Watson CBW, Stephenson CA, et al: Title of the article.
     J Name 12:45-48, 1972.

Zolotov AN, Stephenson CA: Title of the section or the chapter or
     the part of the book, in Smith TT (ed): Title of the Book.
     City, Publisher, vol 5, 19—, pp 567-569.

Invited Presentations

INVITED PRESENTATIONS

A. Samuel Levi, MD, PhD

March 1973	"An Examination and an Evaluation of the Effect of Modeling on Drinking Rates" Medical College of State Lecture in Behavioral Psychology Department
September 1974	"Smoking Control: An Evaluation" Smith County Unit American Cancer Society
January 1976	"An Overview of Toxicomania in American Adolescents" Smith County Medical Society
March 1978	"A Study of the Influence of Life Change in Alcohol Addiction" Read before the State Psychiatric Association Thirtieth Annual Meeting
November 1978	"A Comparative-Contrastive Analysis of the Rehabilitation Needs of Male and Female Alcoholics" State Medical University Lecture to Senior Residents in Clinical Psychiatry
February 1979	"Abuse of (Nonproprietary Drug Name) by 10 Chronic Drug Addicts" State Medical College Department of Pharmacology and Toxicology Lecture to Senior Pharmacy Students

17

CHAPTER SEVENTEEN

A CONCISE GUIDE TO ENGLISH AND MEDICAL WRITING

CONTENTS

17.1

INTRODUCTION

The importance of cleanly typed correspondence is discussed in Chapter 15, and special typing projects (as manuscripts and abstracts) are treated in Chapter 16. However, the mechanics of typing attractive-looking material is only one factor contributing to effective written communication. Other equally important elements are standard grammar, correct spelling, felicitous style, and sound presentation of ideas within logically constructed sentences and paragraphs. While the physical appearance and mechanical setup of the material will impress a reader at first glance, these other factors will create even more lasting impressions as a reader studies the material carefully and reflects on its content.

Thus, all of the interrelated elements illustrated in the diagram are vital to effective communication: If the grammar is substandard, if the spelling is incorrect, if the sentence structure is contorted, if the paragraph orientation is cloudy or irrational, and if the text is riddled with padding and clichés, one can reasonably anticipate negative reader reaction. Although the writer or dictator does bear the prime respon-

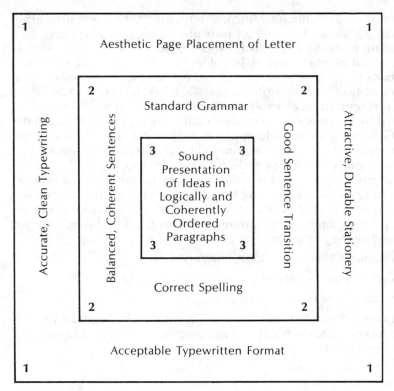

1. Physical appearance of the material creates a first-glance impression on the reader

2. Grammatical elements are noticed as the material is being read

3. Validity of ideas and logical organization of content are noticed as the reader studies the material carefully

sibility for his or her own grammar, diction, and usage, the assistant still should be competent enough in these areas to recognize basic grammatical and stylistic infelicities. Before typing questionable material, the assistant should research any doubtful points and tactfully query the physician. The following sections have been prepared as a quick reference tool for just this sort of situation. Highly specialized questions may be answered by consulting a current book on English grammar (see the Appendix for a list of titles).

17.2

ABBREVIATIONS

The occurrence of abbreviations in typed or printed material is directly related to the nature of the material itself. For example, technical literature (as in the fields of aerospace, engineering, data processing, and medicine) abounds in abbreviations, but formal literary writing features relatively few such terms. By the same token, the presence or absence of abbreviations in business writing depends on the nature of the office. A secretary in a university English department and one in a medical school each will encounter widely different abbreviations.

Abbreviation styling is, unfortunately, inconsistent and at the same time arbitrary. No rules can be set down to cover all possible variations, exceptions, and peculiarities. Abbreviation styling depends most often on the writer's preference or on a particular medical journal's own style guidelines. It can be said, however, that some abbreviations (as *a.k.a., e.g., etc., f.o.b., i.e., No.,* and *viz.*) are backed by a strong punctuation tradition, and that others (as *SGOT, WHO, ECG, EEG, DNA, RNA,* and *CAT scanner*) tend to be all capitalized and unpunctuated. Styling problems can be alleviated by (1) consulting a general dictionary especially for capitalization guidance (2) following the guidelines of the American Medical Association *Stylebook,* and (3) consulting one of the major medical dictionaries for answers to highly specialized questions (see the Appendix for a list of titles).

Abbreviations are used (1) to avoid repetition of long words and phrases that may distract the reader (2) to save space and time (3) to reduce keystrokes and increase output, and (4) to reflect statistical data in limited space. When using an abbreviation that may be unfamiliar or confusing to the reader, one should give the full form first, followed by the abbreviation in parentheses, as

Hamsters can carry and transmit lymphocytic choriomeningitis (LCM) . . . .

followed in subsequent references by just the abbreviation, as

Eleven cases of hamster-associated LCM occurred . . . .

The following chart offers illustrated abbreviation guidelines. These guidelines are listed alphabetically by key words in boldface type. See also 17.9 for additional data on abbreviations in manuscripts.

ABBREVIATIONS

1. **a** or **an** before an abbreviation; *see* page 473.

2. **A.D.** and **B.C.** are usually styled in printed matter as small punctuated unspaced capitals, but in typed material as punctuated unspaced capitals.

   [41 B.C.] [41 B.C.]
   [A.D. 185 *also* 185 A.D.]
   [A.D. 185 *also* 185 A.D.]
   [fourth century A.D.]
   [fourth century A.D.]

3. **Beginning a sentence with an abbreviation** should be avoided unless the abbreviation represents a courtesy title.

   [Page 22 contains . . . .]
   but not
   [P. 22 contains . . . .]
   however
   [Dr. Smith is here.] *or*
   [Doctor Smith is here.]

4. **Capitalization** of abbreviations; *see* CAPITALIZATION, RULE 2.

5. **Compass points** are abbreviated when occurring after street names, and they can be unpunctuated;
   however
   compass points are usually typed out in full when they form essential internal elements of street names.

   [2122 Fourteenth Street, NW]

   [192 East 49th Street]

6. **Dates** (as days and months) should not be abbreviated in running texts, and months should not be abbreviated in general business-letter date lines.

[I expect to meet with you in Chicago on Monday, June 1, 19--.]
general business-letter date line
[June 1, 19--]

---

7. **Division of an abbreviation** either at the end of a line or between pages should be avoided.

[received the MD degree . . . .]
but not
[received the M-
D degree . . . .]

---

8. **Company names** are not abbreviated unless abbreviations comprise their official names;
and
the words *Airlines, Associates, Consultants, Corporation, Fabricators, Manufacturing,* and *Railroad* should not be abbreviated when part of proper names.

[Stuart Pharmaceuticals]
[USV Pharmaceutical Corporation]
but
[SmithKline Instruments, Inc.]
[Applied Fiberoptics & Scientific Specialties, Inc.]
[Unifab Corporation]
[Eastern Airlines]

---

9. **Geographical and topographical names.** U.S. Postal Service abbreviations for states are all-capitalized and unpunctuated, as are the Postal Service abbreviations for streets and localities when used on envelopes addressed for automated mass handling,
and
ordinals are abbreviated in some street addresses
also
names of countries are typically abbreviated in tabular data, but are typed in full in running texts (exception: *U.S.S.R.*)
and
United States is often abbreviated when it modifies names of federal agencies, policies, or programs; when it is used as a noun, it is usually typed in full.

[Smithville, ST 56789]
addressed for automated handling
[1234 SMITH BLVD
SMITHVILLE, ST 56789]
regular address styling
[1234 Smith Blvd. (*or* Boulevard)
Smithville, ST 56789]

[147 East 31st Street]
[147 East 3d Avenue]
[147 East 3rd Avenue]

in a table [U.A.R. *or* UAR]
in a text [The United Arab Republic and the U.S.S.R. announced the research exchange.]

[U.S. Public Health Service]
[U.S. Department of Health, Education and Welfare]
[U.S. foreign policy]
but
[The United States has offered to. . . .]

---

10. **Latin words and phrases** commonly used in general writing and prescriptions are often abbreviated.

general:
[etc.] [i.e.] [e.g.] [viz.]
apothecary:
[a.c.] [b.i.d.] [p.r.n.] [q.i.d.]

---

11. **Latitude and longitude** are abbreviated in tabular data, but are typed in full in running texts.

in a table
[lat. 10°20'N *or* lat. 10-20N]
in a text
[from 10°20' north latitude to 10°30' south latitude. . . .]

12. **Laws and bylaws** when first quoted are typed in full; however, subsequent references to them in a text may be abbreviated.

first reference
[Article I, Section 1]
subsequent references
[Art. I, Sec. 1]

---

13. **Measures and weights** may be abbreviated in figure + unit combinations; however, if the numeral is written out, the unit must also be written out.

[15 mg]
but
[fifteen milligrams]

---

14. **Number** when part of a set unit (as a policy number), when used in tabular data, or when used in references may be abbreviated to *No.* (sing.) or *Nos.* (plural).

[Policy No. 123-5-X]
[Publ. Nos. 12 and 13]

---

15. **Period** with abbreviations; *see* PERIOD, RULE 3.

---

16. **Personal names** should not be abbreviated; however, initials of famous persons are sometimes used in place of their full names.

[George S. Patterson]
not
[Geo. S. Patterson]
but
[J.F.K. *or* JFK]

---

17. **Plurals** of abbreviations may be formed by addition of -s
or

[MLDs] [MDs] [LPNs]

by the addition of -'s especially if the abbreviation is internally punctuated, except for a few such terms that are punctuated only with terminal periods, in which case the apostrophe is omitted
or

[f.o.b.'s] [CMA-A's]
but
[Nos. 3 and 4] [Figs. A and B]

by repeating a letter of the abbreviation
or

[p. → pp.] [f. → ff.]

by no suffixation.

[1 sec → 30 sec]   [1 ml → 24 ml]

---

18. **Possessives** of abbreviations are formed in the same way as those of nouns: the singular possessive is signaled by addition of -'s
and

[our MD's diagnosis]

the plural possessive, by addition of -s'.

[our MDs' diagnoses]

---

19. **Saint** may be abbreviated when used before the name of a saint; however, it may or may not be abbreviated when it forms part of a surname or the name of a disease.

[St. Peter] *or* [Saint Peter]
but
[Ruth St. Denis] [Augustus Saint-Gaudens]
[Saint Vitus' dance]

---

20. **Scientific terms** In binomial nomenclature a genus name may be abbreviated after the first reference to it is typed out.

[(first reference) *Escherichia coli*]
[(subsequent references) *E. coli*]

21. **Time** When time is expressed in figures, the abbreviations that follow may be set in unspaced punctuated lowercase letters; if capitals or small capitals are used, one space should separate the letters (the writer's preference will dictate the style)
and
measurements of time (as in tables) are expressed in figures and typically unpunctuated abbreviations.

[8:30 a.m. *or* 8:30 A. M. *or* 8:30 A. M.]

[10 sec] [18 min] [24 hr]
[17 yr] [52 wk] [19 mo]

---

22. **Titles** The only courtesy titles that are invariably abbreviated are *Mr., Ms., Mrs.,* and *Messrs.* Other titles (except for *Doctor* which may be written out or abbreviated) are given in full form in business-letter salutations;

[Ms. Lee A. Downs]
[Messrs. Lake, Mason, and Nambeth]
[Dear Doctor Howe] *or*
[Dear Dr. Howe]
but
[Dear Professor Howe]
[Dear General Howe]

but
titles may be abbreviated in envelope address blocks and in inside addresses;

[Dr. John P. Howe]
[COL John P. Howe, USA]
[GEN John P. Howe, USA]

also
Honorable and *Reverend* when used with *The* are typed out, but if used without *The,* they may be abbreviated.

[The Reverend Samuel I. O'Leary]
[The Honorable Samuel I. O'Leary]
but
[Rev. Samuel I. O'Leary]
[Hon. Samuel I. O'Leary]

---

23. **Titles of journals** are abbreviated in references.

[Doe JR: Title of article.
JAMA 12:441–442, 19–.]

---

24. **Versus** is abbreviated as the lowercase Roman letter *v.* in legal contexts; it is either typed in full or abbreviated as lowercase Roman letters *vs.* in general contexts.

in a legal context
[*Smith* v. *Vermont*]
in a general context
[positive versus negative]
or
[positive vs. negative]

17.3

CAPITALIZATION

Capitals are used for two broad purposes in English: They mark a beginning (as of a sentence) and they signal a proper noun or adjective. The next seventy-seven principles, each with a bracketed example or examples, describe the most common uses of capital letters. These principles are alphabetically ordered under the following headings:

Abbreviations
Beginnings
Proper Nouns, Pronouns, and Adjectives
    armed forces

awards
eponyms
geographical and topographical references
governmental, judicial, and political bodies
names of organizations
names of persons
numerical designations
particles and prefixes
personifications
pronouns
scientific terms
time periods, zones, and divisions
titles of persons
titles of printed matter
trademarks
transport

When uncertain about the capitalization of a term not shown below, the assistant should consult a dictionary such as *Webster's New Collegiate Dictionary*.

CAPITALIZATION

Abbreviations

1. Abbreviations are capitalized if the words they represent are proper nouns or adjectives; most medical abbreviations are capitalized when they represent single letters of words.	[98 F for *Fahrenheit*] [Nov. for *November*] [AMA for *American Medical Association*] [CBC for complete blood count] *but* [fsd for *focus-to-skin distance*]
2. Most acronyms are capitalized unless they have been assimilated into the language as parts of speech, and as such are lowercased.	[SCID] [MEND] [DIC] *but* [quasar] [laser] [radar] [sonar] [tepa] [chlormerodrin]
3. Abbreviations of government agencies, military units, and other organization names are capitalized.	[FDA] [DEA] [HEW] [WHO] [USAF] [NIH] [DUMC] [ITT]
4. Abbreviations of air force, army, coast guard, and navy ranks are all-capitalized; those of the marine corps are capitalized and lowercased.	[BG John T. Dow, USA] [LCDR Mary I. Lee, USN] [Col. S. J. Smith, USMC]
5. Abbreviations of compass points are capitalized; punctuation styling depends on the writer's or organization's preference.	[lat. 10°20′N] [2233 Fourteenth Street, N.W. 2233 Fourteenth Street, NW. 2233 Fourteenth Street, NW]
6. Abbreviations of degrees, ratings, and fellowships may be all-capitalized or capitalized and lowercased, depending on the word; consult a dictionary when in doubt of styling. See also pages 361–363.	[DDS] [MPH] [RRA] [FACP] [PharmD] [PhD]

Beginnings

7. The first word of a sentence, of a sentence fragment, or of a complete sentence enclosed in parentheses is capitalized;

    however
    the first word of a parenthetical phrase or sentence enclosed by parentheses and occurring within another sentence is lowercased.

    [The meeting was postponed.]
    [No! I cannot.] [Will you go?]
    [A suspicious and hostile attitude. The patient cannot believe anyone has good intentions.
    —*Medicine Today*]
    [The meeting ended. (The results were not revealed.)]
    but
    [She studied medicine with Dr. Heller (he wrote this text, you know) at the university.]

8. The first word of a direct quotation is capitalized
    but
    a split direct quotation tightly bound to the rest of a sentence may be lowercased at the beginning of its continued segment or segments.

    [He said, "We must consider the health problems."]
    ["The Administration has denied the story," the paper reports, and goes on to say that "the President feels the media are irresponsible."]

9. The first word of a direct question within a sentence or of a series of questions within a sentence may be capitalized.

    [The question is this: Exactly what is the function of the medical assistant?]
    [How often should the vital signs be recorded postop? For how long?
    —*Supervisor Nurse*]

10. The first word following a colon may be lowercased or capitalized if it introduces a complete sentence; while the former is the more usual styling, the latter is common especially when the sentence introduced by the colon is fairly lengthy and distinctly separate from the preceding clause.

    [The advantage of this particular system is clear: it's inexpensive.]
    [The situation is critical: This hospital cannot hope to recoup the fourth-quarter losses that were sustained this fiscal year.]

11. The first words of run-in or blocked enumerations that form complete sentences are capitalized as are the first words of phrasal lists and enumerations blocked beneath running texts;

    [The advantages of the task inventories are . . . as follows: 1. The technique is economical. 2. The information . . . is quantifiable.
    —*Business Education World*]
    [. . . representation should include personnel from
        1. Auditing staff
        2. Nursing
        3. Health care
        4. Medical records
        —*Supervisor Nurse*]
    but
    [The scales have a six-point continuum as follows: (1) strongly agree, (2) agree, (3) not sure but probably agree . . . .
    —*J of Psychiatric Nursing and Mental Health Services*]

    however
    phrasal enumerations run-in with the introductory text are lowercased.

12. The words *Whereas* and *Resolved* are capitalized in minutes and legislation, as is the word *That* or an alternative word or expression which immediately follows either.

[Resolved, That. . . .]
[Whereas, Substantial benefits. . . .]
[Whereas, The Executive Committee. . . .]
[Resolved by the ----, the ---- concurring, That. . . .]

---

13. The first letter of the first word in an outline heading is capitalized.

[I. Clinical tasks
 II. Administrative responsibilities
      A. Office management
      B. Correspondence]

---

14. The first letter of the first word in a salutation and a complimentary close is capitalized as is the first letter of each noun following SUBJECT and TO headings (as in memorandums).

[Dear Bob] [Gentlemen] [My dear Dr. Smith] [Very truly yours]
[Yours very truly] [SUBJECT: Pension Plan]
[TO: All Department Heads]

Proper Nouns, Pronouns, and Adjectives

Armed Forces
15. Branches and units of the armed forces are capitalized as are short forms of full branch and unit designations.

[United States Army Medical Corps]
and
[a hospital run by the Medical Corps]

Awards
16. Awards and prizes are capitalized.

[the Nobel Prize for Medicine]
[Nobel Peace Prize] [Nobel Prize winners]
[Academy Award] [Oscar] [Emmy]

Eponyms
17. Eponyms are capitalized; see also RULES 44, 58.

[Gillmore needles] [Ishihara test]
[Madura foot] [Mules operation]
[Aschoff body] [Rouget cell]
[Drinker respirator]
[Duffy antigen] [Schneider index] [Thomas splint] [Lippes loop] [Romberg sign] [van den Bergh test] [Huygens eyepiece] [Cerenkov radiation] [Maddox rod]
[Romanowsky stain] [Zinn's ligament] [Purkinje cell] [Luer syringe]
[Pacchionian body] [Louis' angle] *or* [angle of Louis] [Nissl substance] [Sylvian fissure]

Geographical and Topographical References
18. Divisions of the earth's surface and names of distinct areas, regions, places, or districts are capitalized, as are adjectives and some derivative nouns and verbs; consult a dictionary when in doubt.

[the Middle East] [the Middle Eastern situation] [Eastern Hemisphere]
[the Great Divide] [Tropic of Cancer]
[Geneva] [Texas]
[Vietnam] [Vietnamization]
[Vietnamize] *but* [sovietism *often* Sovietism] [sovietize *often* Sovietize]

19. Compass points are capitalized when they refer to a geographical region or when they are part of a street name, but are lowercased when they refer to simple direction.

[out West] [back East] [down South] [up North] [the South] [the Middle West] [the West Coast] [157 East 92nd Street] *but* [west of the Rockies] [traveling east on I-84] [the west coast of Florida]

20. Adjectives derived from compass points and nouns designating the inhabitants of some geographical regions are capitalized; when in doubt of the proper styling, consult a dictionary.

[a Southern accent] [a Western drawl] [members of the Eastern Establishment] [Northerners]

21. Popular names of localities are capitalized.

[the Corn and Wheat Belts] [the Gold Coast] [the Loop] [the Eastern Shore] [City of Brotherly Love] [Foggy Bottom] [the Village]

22. Topographical names are capitalized, as are generic terms (as *channel, lake, mountain*) that are essential elements of total names.

[the English Channel] [Lake Como] [the Blue Ridge Mountains] [Atlantic Ocean] [Great Barrier Reef] [Mississippi River] [Black Sea] [Bering Strait] [Strait of Gibraltar] [Ohio Valley]

23. Generic terms occurring before topographical names are capitalized except when *the* precedes them, in which case the generic term is lowercased.

[Lakes Michigan and Superior] [Mounts Whitney and Rainier] *but* [the rivers Don and Volga] [the river Thames]

24. Plural generic terms occurring after multiple topographical names are lowercased, as are singular or plural generic terms that are used descriptively or alone.

[the Himalaya and Andes mountains] [the Don and Volga rivers] [the valley of the Ohio] [the Ohio River valley] [the river valley] [the valley]

25. Words designating global, national, regional, or local political divisions are capitalized when they are essential elements of specific names; however, they are usually lowercased when they precede a proper name or stand alone.

[the British Empire] *but* [the empire] [Oregon State] *but* [the state of Oregon] [Bedford County] *but* [the county of Bedford] [New York City] *but* [the city of New York] [Ward 1] *but* [fires in three wards]

26. Terms designating public places are capitalized when they are essential elements of specific names; however, they are lowercased when they occur after multiple names or stand alone.

[Fifth Avenue] [Brooklyn Bridge] [Empire State Building] [St. John's Church] [the Dorset Hotel] [Central Park] [Washington Square] [Bleecker Street] [Ford Theater] *but* [on the bridge] [Fifth and Park avenues] [the Dorset and the Drake hotels] [St. John's and St. Mark's churches]

27. Well-known short forms of place names are capitalized.

[Fifth Avenue → the Avenue] [Wall Street → the Street] [New York Stock Exchange → the Exchange]

Governmental, Judicial, and Political Bodies

28. The terms *administration* and *government* are capitalized when they are applicable to a particular government in power.

[The Administration announced a new oil and gas program.] [the Ford Administration] *but* [White House parties vary from one administration to another.]

29. The names of international courts are capitalized.

[the International Court of Arbitration]

30. The U.S. Supreme Court and the short forms *Supreme Court* and *Court* referring to it are capitalized.

[the Supreme Court of the United States] [the United States Supreme Court] [the U.S. Supreme Court] [the Supreme Court] [the Court]

31. Official and full names of higher courts are capitalized; however, the single designation *court* is usually lowercased when referring to them.

[the United States Court of Appeals for the Second Circuit] [the Michigan Court of Appeals] [the Virginia Supreme Court] [the Court of Queen's Bench] *but* [the federal courts] [the court of appeals ruled that . . . .] [the state supreme court] [the court]

32. Names of city and county courts are usually lowercased.

[the Lawton municipal court] [the Owensville night court] [police court] [the county court] [juvenile court]

33. The single designation *court* when specifically applicable to a judge or a presiding officer is capitalized.

[It is the opinion of this Court that. . . .] [The Court found that. . . .]

34. The term *federal* is capitalized only when it is an essential element of a name or title, when it identifies a specific government, or often when it refers to a particular principle of government.

[the Federal Bureau of Investigation] [. . . efforts made by the Federal Government. . . .] [the Federal principle of government] *but* [federal court] [federal district court] [federal agents] [federal troops]

35. Full names of legislative, deliberative, executive, and administrative bodies are capitalized as are the easily recognizable short forms of these names; however, nonspecific noun and adjective references to them are usually lowercased.

[United Nations Security Council] *and* [the Security Council] *but* [the council] [United States Congress] *and* [the Congress] *but* [congressional elections] [the Maryland Senate] *but* [the state senate] [Department of State] *and* [the State Department] *and* [State] *but* [the department]

36. The term *national* is capitalized when it precedes a capitalized word or when it forms a part of a specific name or title; however, it is lowercased when used as a descriptive word or as a noun.

[National Socialist Party] *but* [in the interests of national security] [the screening of foreign nationals]

37. The names of political parties and their adherents are capitalized, but the word *party* may or may not be capitalized, depending on the writer's or organization's preference.

[Democrats] [Republicans] [Liberals] [Tories] [the Democratic party] *or* [the Democratic Party]

Names of Organizations

38. Names of firms, corporations, organizations, and other such groups are capitalized.

[McKesson & Robbins Drug Company] [USV Pharmaceutical Corporation] [American Medical Association]

39. Common nouns used descriptively and occurring after two or more organization names are lowercased.

[Bellevue and Doctors hospitals] [the ITT and IBM corporations]

40. The words *company* and *corporation* are capitalized when they refer to one's own organization even when the full organization name is omitted; however, they are lowercased when they refer to another organization.

[It is contrary to the policies of our Company to. . . .] *but* [He works for a company in Delaware.] [Give me the name of your company.]

41. Words such as *group, division, department, office,* or *agency* that designate corporate units are capitalized when used with a specific name.

[The Pharmaceuticals Research Division is developing that medication.] *but* [The memorandum was sent to all operating divisions.]

Names of Persons

42. The names of persons are capitalized.

[John W. Jones, Jr.]

43. Words designating peoples and their languages are capitalized.

[Canadians] [Turks] [Swedish] [Welsh] [Iroquois] [Ibo] [Vietnamese]

44. Derivatives of proper names are capitalized when used in their primary sense; consult a dictionary when in doubt of styling. See also RULE 58.

[German measles epidemic] [Morganian cyst] [Wolffian duct] [Wormian bones] *but* [fallopian tubes] [pasteurize] [cesarean section]

Numerical Designations

45. Monetary units typed in full (as in legal documents and on checks) are capitalized.

[Your fee is Two Thousand Dollars ($2,000.00), payable upon receipt of. . . .]

46. Nouns introducing a set number (as on a policy) are usually capitalized.

[Order 123] [Policy 123-4-X] [Flight 409] [Regulation 15] [Stock Certificate X12345] [Exhibit A] [Form 2E] [Catalog No. 65432]

47. Nouns used with numbers or letters to designate major reference headings (as in a literary work) are capitalized; however, minor reference headings and subheads are typically lowercased.

[Book 2] [Volume 5] [Division 4] [Section 3] [Article IV] [Table 5] [Figure 8] [Appendix III] [Plate 16] [Part 1] *but* [experiment 1] [page 101] [line 8] [note 10] [paragraph 6.1] [case 123] [question 21]

Particles and Prefixes

48. Particles forming initial elements of surnames may or may not be capitalized, depending on the styling of the individual name; however, if a name with a lowercase initial particle begins a sentence, the particle is capitalized.

[Du Pont] [Da Costa's syndrome]
[De Bakey] [von Kossa stain]
[Von Meyenburg's disease]

[The writings of de Chauliac are. . . .]
but
[De Chauliac's writings are. . . .]

49. Elements of hyphened compounds are capitalized in running texts if they are proper nouns or adjectives; consult a dictionary when in doubt of styling.

[Jarish-Herxheimer reaction]
[Hand-Schüller-Christian disease]
[Schultz-Dale reaction] [Tay-Sachs disease] [Watson-Crick model]
[Guillain-Barré syndrome]
but
[a nineteenth-century physician]
[para-Wernicke's encephalopathy]
[sickle-cell anemia]

50. Prefixes occurring with proper nouns or adjectives are capitalized if they are essential elements of the compounds or if they begin headings or sentences; they are lowercased in other instances. NOTE: If a second element in a two-word compound modifies the first element or if both elements constitute a single word, the second element is lowercased.

[Anglo-American medical research]
[Anti-Rh serums contain. . . .]
but
[. . . containing anti-Rh serums.]

[French-speaking patients]
[T-lymphocytes] [X-irradiation]
[T-group] [X-disease]

Personifications

51. Personifications are capitalized.

[The Chair recognized the delegate.]

Pronouns

52. The pronoun *I* is capitalized.

[. . . said that he and I would go.]

Scientific Terms

53. Names of geological eras, periods, epochs, and strata and of prehistoric ages are capitalized, but the generic nouns which they modify are lowercased except when those generic nouns appear <u>before</u> the names of eras, periods, epochs, strata, or divisions, in which case they are capitalized.

[Silurian period] [Pleistocene epoch]
[Neolithic age]
but
[Age of Reptiles]

54. Names of planets, constellations, asteroids, stars, and groups of stars are capitalized, but *sun, earth,* and *moon* are lowercased unless they are listed with other astronomical names.

[Venus] [Big Dipper] [Sirius] [Pleiades]
but
[sun] [earth] [moon]
[unmanned space probes to the Moon and to Mars]
[a lengthy study comparing the gravitational effects on monkeys in Earth conditions as opposed to conditions on the Moon and simulated conditions on Mars]

55. Meterological phenomena are lowercased.

[northern lights]
[aurora borealis]

56. Genera in binomial nomenclature in zoology and botany are capitalized; however, species names are lowercased.

[the rhesus monkey (*Macaca mulatta*)]
[opium poppy (*Papaver somniferum*)]
[the brown rat (*Rattus norvegicus*)]
[a bacterium (*Clostridium botulinum*) causing botulism]

57. New Latin names of classes, families, and all groups above genera are capitalized, but their derivative nouns and adjectives are lowercased.

[Gastropoda] *but* [gastropod]
[Thallophyta] *but* [thallophyte]
[Nematoda] *but* [nematodes]

58. Proper names forming essential elements of terms designating diseases, syndromes, signs, tests, and symptoms are capitalized.

[Parkinson's disease] [Down's syndrome]
[syndrome of Weber] [Duchenne-Erb paralysis] [German measles] [Rorschach test]
but
[mumps] [measles] [herpes simplex]

59. Proprietary (i.e., brand and trade) names of drugs are capitalized, but generic names of drugs are lowercased.

[. . . was tranquilized with Thorazine.]
but
[. . . recommended chlorpromazine—a generic name for. . . .]

60. Proper names forming essential elements of scientific laws, theorems, and principles are capitalized; however, the descriptive nouns *law, theorem, theory,* and the like are lowercased.

[Weber-Fechner law]
[the Pythagorean theorem]
[Planck's constant]
[Einstein's theory of relativity]
[Dulong and Petit's law]
[Du Bois-Reymond's law]

Time Periods, Zones, and Divisions

61. Names of the seasons are not capitalized unless personified.

[The book will be published in the fall.]

62. Days of the week, months of the year, holidays, and holy days are capitalized.

[Tuesday] [July] [Independence Day]
[Good Friday] [Easter]

63. Historic periods are capitalized, but latter-day periods are often lowercased.

[Christian Era] [Golden Age of Greece]
[Roaring Twenties] [Augustan Age]
often
[nuclear age] [the atomic age]
[space age]

64. Numerical designations of historic time periods are capitalized when they are essential elements of proper names; otherwise, they are lowercased.

[the Roaring Twenties]
but
[the seventeenth century] [the twenties]

65. Historical events and appellations referring to particular time periods or events in time are capitalized.

[the Reign of Terror] [the Cultural Revolution] [Prohibition] [the Great Depression] [the New Frontier] [the Third Reich] [the Fourth Republic]

66. Time zones are capitalized when abbreviated, but lowercased when written out.

[EST] *but* [eastern standard time]

Titles of Persons

67. Corporate and professional titles are capitalized when referring to specific individuals; when used in general or plural contexts, they are lowercased.

[Mr. John M. Jones, Vice-president]
and
[Mr. Carl T. Yowell, Administrator]
but
[The hospital administrator called me.]
[All of the administrators will be here.]

68. Specific organizational and governmental titles may be capitalized when they stand alone or when they are used in place of particular individuals' names.

[The Board of Trustees approved the Treasurer's report.]
[The Secretary of HEW gave a news conference. The Secretary said . . . .]
[The Chief of Surgery will respond to your request when he returns.]

69. All titles preceding names are capitalized.

[President Doe] [Queen Elizabeth]
[Dr. Doe] [Professor Doe] [The Honorable John M. Doe] [The Reverend John M. Doe]

Titles of Printed Matter

70. Words in the titles of printed matter are capitalized except for internal conjunctions, prepositions (especially those having less than four letters), and articles.
NOTE: Only the first word of the title of an article is capitalized in medical/scientific reference lists. See also pages 407–410.

[*Writing and Communicating in Medicine*] [*The Professional Medical Assistant*] ["A Logical Basis for Medical Mythology"]

[Solomon F: Binding sites for calcium on tubulin. *Biochem* 16(3):358–363, 1977.]

71. Major sections (as a preface, an introduction, or an index) of books, long articles, or reports are capitalized when they are specifically referred to within the same material.

[The Introduction explains the scope of the book.]

72. The first word following a colon in a title is capitalized.
NOTE: In medical/scientific references, the first word after a colon in an article title is capitalized.

[*Medicine Today: A Report on a Decade of Progress*]
[Lown B, Matta RJ, Besser HW: Programmed "trendscription": A new approach to electrocardiographic monitoring. *JAMA* 232:39, 1975.]

73. The *the* before a title of a newspaper, magazine, or journal is capitalized if considered an essential element of the title; otherwise, it is lowercased,
and
descriptive nouns following publication titles are also lowercased.

[*The Wall Street Journal*]
but
[the New York *Times*]

[*Medical Economics* magazine]

74. Constitutional amendments are capitalized only when referred to by title or number.

[I took the Fifth Amendment]
but
[states ratifying constitutional amendments]

75. Formal titles of accords, acts, pacts, plans, policies, treaties, constitutions, and similar documents are capitalized.	[the Geneva Accords] [the Controlled Substance Act of 1970] [Kellogg-Briand Pact] [the Five Year Plan] [New Economic Policy] [Treaty of Paris] [the U.S. Constitution] [the Utah Constitution] *but* [narcotics legislation] [the state constitution]

Trademarks

76. Brand names, trademarks, and service marks are capitalized. For drug names, see RULE 59.	[the IBM Selectric] [Xerox] [Wite-Out correction fluid] [Air Express] [Laundromat]

Transport

77. The names of ships, airplanes, and often spacecraft are capitalized.	[M. V. *West Star*] [Lindbergh's *Spirit of St. Louis*] [*Apollo 13*]

17.4

ITALICIZATION

The following are usually italicized in print and underlined in typescript or manuscript:

1. foreign words and phrases that have not been naturalized in English	[*quater in die*] [*oculus dexter*] [*modo prescripto*] [*ad manus medici*] *but* [in vitro] [in vivo]
2. legal citations, both in full and shortened form, except when the person involved rather than the case itself is being discussed, in which instance the reference is typed in Roman	[*Jones v. Massachussetts*] [the *Jones* case] [*Jones*] *but* [the Jones trial and conviction]
3. letters when used as run-in enumerations (as in printed matter)	[Side effects were: (a) drowsiness (b) dizziness, and (c) gastrointestinal distress.]
4. names of ships and airplanes and often spacecraft	[M. V. *West Star*][Lindbergh's *Spirit of St. Louis*] [*Apollo 13*]
5. New Latin scientific names of genera, species, subspecies, and varieties (but not higher taxa as phyla, orders, or families, derivatives of these, or vernacular equivalents of genera)	[the spirochete *Treponema pallidum*] [the bacterium *Clostridium botulinum*] [*E. coli*] [Anoplura] [felid] [a streptococcus]
6. sideheads dividing sections of an article	[*CNS effects.*—Caution should be used . . . .]

7. **titles** of books, journals, published theses, magazines, newspapers, organizational policy papers (as bylaws), and government bulletins when used in running texts

[Fishbein's *Medical Writing*] [the magazine *Drug Topics*] [a thesis entitled *Recent Trends in Lung Cancer Mortality among Coal Miners*] [*The Wall Street Journal*] [our medical society's *Bylaws*] [PHS bulletin (CDC)76–8195 *VD Fact Sheet*] *but* [In his article "Binding Sites for Calcium on Tubulin," he . . . .] [the unpublished paper "Using Calculators in the Medical Office"]

NOTE 1: Titles of articles and unpublished works are not italicized but are enclosed by quotation marks when they are used in running texts or in *general* bibliographies.

NOTE 2: Titles of published articles are set off neither by italics nor by quotation marks in medical references. Book titles are italicized.

[Solomon F: Binding sites for calcium on tubulin. *Biochem* 16(3):358–363, 1977.] [Fishbein M: *Medical Writing*, ed 4. Springfield, IL, Charles C Thomas, 1972.]

8. **words, letters, and figures** when referred to as words, letters, or figures

[The word *liter* is not abbreviated.]

17.5

NUMERALS

In medical writing, most numerals—and especially those above *ten*—are expressed in figures. There are, however, exceptions to this rule. If material is being prepared for publication in a medical journal, the writer and the typist should familiarize themselves with the style guidelines of the publication to which the manuscript will be submitted. The guidelines given below are generally based on those of the American Medical Association *Stylebook,* which the reader can consult for answers to highly specialized style problems with numerals. See also 17.9 for more data on the styling of numerals in manuscripts.

NUMERALS

1. **Ages** are expressed in figures.

[her 6-month-old son] [the 11-day-old infant] [a man 65 years old]

2. **Beginning of a sentence** Numbers that begin a sentence are written out.

[Thirty-two physicians attended the meeting.] [Thirty-two physicians examined 100 patients, 11 of whom were outpatients.]

3. **Compounds** When two numbers comprise one item or unit, one of the numbers (usually the first) should be expressed in words, and the other (usually the second) should be expressed in figures; if, however, the second number is the shorter, it may be expressed in words.

[two 7-drawer files] *but* [20 ten-drawer files]

4. **Compounds adjacent to other figures** Two sets of figures (except for those in monetary units) should not be typed in direct succession in a text unless they comprise a series.

[By 1978, one hundred hospitals will have closed.]
but not
[By 1978, 100 hospitals will have closed.]

---

5. **Date lines** Figures are used to express days and years in business-letter date lines; do not use ordinals.

[January 1, 19–]
not
[January 1st, 19–]

---

6. **Decimals** Place a zero in front of a decimal if the amount is less than *one*.

[0.2 gm] [received 0.1 mg/kg diazepam i.v.]

---

7. **Dosages** are expressed with metric values. Although *teaspoonful, ounces, drams, grains* and other apothecary measurements should be avoided, *drops* is acceptable.

[required an increase in dosage from 200 to 500 mg]
[. . . at a rate of 20 drops per minute.]

---

8. **Enumerations** Run-in and vertical enumerations are often numbered.

[felt that she should (1) increase her clinical skills (2) upgrade her administrative skills, and (3) increase her production.]
[. . . tasks include:
  1. Making appointments
  2. Processing health insurance claims
  3. Billing and collection
  4. Typewriting reports]

---

9. **Figures** Figures are usually used to indicate policy, page, and section numbers; street, room, apartment, or suite numbers; and sizes, mixed amounts, shares, percentages, case numbers, and mixed fractions.

[Policy No. 123-X] [page 3] [p 3] [section 10] [123 Smith Blvd.] [Room 7] [Apt. 2] [Suite 4] [size 7] [9′ × 12′] [14,000 shares] [56.890] [90%] [case 14] [17½]

---

10. **Four-digit numbers** A number of four or more digits has each set of three digits separated by a comma except in set combinations such as policy, contract, check, street, room, suite, or page numbers, which are unpunctuated.

[15,000 units] [a fee of $12,500] [a population of 1,500,000]
but
[check 34567] [page 4589] [the year 1979] [Room 6000] [Policy No. 3344]

---

11. **Fractions** Common fractions are written out in words; mixed fractions are expressed in figures.

[one half of the control group . . .]
but
[waited 3½ hours for the appointment]

---

12. Inclusive numbers (as of dates or pages) should be expressed in full and in figures.

[1977–1978] *not* [1977–78]
[pp. 140–149] *not* [pp. 140–49]

---

13. **Measures** may be styled as figure + abbreviated unit combinations (as in tables); however, if the unit of measure is typed in full, the number is expressed in words.

[reported that 40 mg of propranolol had been administered . . .]
[dosage: 40 mg]
but
[Forty milligrams of propranolol were administered . . .]

14. **Monetary units** when containing both mixed and even-dollar amounts and typed in series should each contain: decimal point + 2 ciphers for the even-dollar amounts; also, the $ should be repeated before each unit. Units of less than one dollar are usually typed in running texts as: figure + *cents* (or ¢). Monetary units of one dollar or more or of less than one dollar are usually typed in vertical tabulations as: $ + decimal + figures on the first line, followed by decimals and figures only.

[The price of the book rose from $7.95 in 1970 to $8.00 in 1971 and to $8.50 in 1972.]
but
[The bids were $80, $100, and $300.]
[$10–$20]
[The pencil costs 15 cents.]
or
[The pencil costs 15¢.]
[$16.95
  .06
$17.01]

15. **Ordinals** less than *tenth* are written out; those greater than *tenth* are expressed in figure + abbreviation combinations unless they begin a sentence, in which case they are written out.

[the tenth patient today]
[the 11th patient today]
but
[Eleventh grade students were immunized.]

16. **Percentages** are styled as: figure + *percent* symbol (%); if a percentage begins a sentence, the number is written out, followed by *percent*.

[The death rate was halved to 9.5%.]
but
[Nine percent of the subjects were . . .]

17. **Roman numerals** are used in formal medical writing only when they are part of fixed combinations (as designations for blood-clotting factors). They are rarely used to specify volume numbers in references. See also 17.9.
NOTE: Roman numerals are used in references to cite numbered subtitles.

[blood-clotting factor VII]
but
[Vol. 1] [vol 1] [vol. 1]

[Eppig JJ, Leiter EH: Exocrine pancreatic insufficiency (EPI) syndrome in CBA/J mice. I. Ultrastructural study. *Am J Path* 86:17–30, 1977.]

18. **Round numbers in millions and above** are expressed as figures + words.

[1 million] [5.55 million]
[a $10 million building program]

19. **Series** Figures are used to express a series of numbers in one sentence if one of the numbers is greater than *ten,* is a mixed fraction, or contains a decimal fraction.

[examined 3 new patients, 12 returning patients, and 1 referral.]
[waited 3, 12, and 1½ hours, respectively.]
[The percentage of deaths increased from 3.5% in 1970 to 5% in 1976.]

20. **Temperatures** are expressed in figures + C (Celsius) and are followed by the Fahrenheit equivalent in parentheses.

[The temperature was 37.8 C (100 F).]

21. **Time of day** is expressed in figures + *a.m.* or *p.m.*

[The patient was admitted at 9:15 a.m.]
[The patient was discharged at 2:30 p.m.]

22. **Titles and subtitles** Numerals less than *ten* are written out unless they are part of a chemical compound or a formula; those over *ten* are expressed in figures.

[*Drug Addiction in Pregnancy: A Study of Nine Patients*] but [*Influence of Aromatic Compounds on the Interaction of Activated C4 and EAC1*]
[*A Follow-up Study of 19 Methadone Maintenance Program Participants*]

23. **Weight and height** Body weight and height are commonly expressed in metric values, especially in material submitted for publication.

[The patient weighed 63.50 kg.]
[The patient's height was 190.50 cm.]
[The infant's length was 53.34 cm.]

17.6

PUNCTUATION

The English writing system uses punctuation marks to separate groups of words for meaning and emphasis; to convey an idea of the variations of pitch, volume, pauses, and intonation of speech; and to help avoid contextual ambiguity. Punctuation marks should be used sparingly: overpunctuating often needlessly complicates a passage and also increases keystrokes. English punctuation marks, together with general rules and bracketed examples of their use, follow in alphabetical order. At the end of the section, a Punctuation-Spacination Chart will be found.

' APOSTROPHE

1. indicates the possessive case of singular and plural nouns and indefinite pronouns, as well as of surname and terminal title combinations

[Dr. Wilson's office] [Senator Ceccacci's office] [the boy's mother] [the boys' mothers] [anyone's guess] [everyone's questions] [his father-in-law's car] [their father-in-laws' cars] [John Burns' *or* Burns's insurance policy] [the Burnses' insurance policy] [Jay Adams' *or* Adams's boat] [the Adamses' boat] [a witness' *or* witness's testimony] [John K. Walker Jr.'s house] [the John K. Walker Jrs.' house]

NOTE: The use of an apostrophe + *s* with words ending in /s/ or /z/ sounds usually depends on the pronounceability of the final syllable: if the syllable is pronounced, the apostrophe + *s* is usually used; if the syllable is silent, the apostrophe is retained but an *s* is usually not appended to the word.

[Dr. Gomez's office]
[Knox's products]
[the class's opinion]
[Wilms's tumor]
[Treitz's muscle]
[Willis's artery]
[Vaquez's disease]
but
[Keats' poetry]
[Moses' laws]
[for righteousness' sake]
[Vleminckx' solution]
[Chagas' disease]

2. indicates joint possession when appended to the last noun in a sequence

[Appleton and Delaney's report]
[McKesson & Robbins' advertisement]
[Merck Sharp & Dohme's products]
[Smith Kline & French's executives]
[Martin, Doe, and Rowe's findings]

3.	indicates individual possession when appended to each noun in a sequence	[Appleton's and Delaney's report] [John's, Bill's, and Tim's boats] [Merck's and McKesson & Robbins' advertisements]
4.	indicates possession when appended to the final element of a compound	[Norfolk, Virginia's newest hospital] [XYZ Corporation's clinic]
5.	indicates understood possession	[The pills are at your druggist's.]
6.	marks omissions in contractions	[isn't] [you're] [aren't] [o'clock]
7.	often forms plurals of letters, figures, or words especially when they are referred to as letters, figures, or words; however, in formal medical writing, the apostrophe is usually omitted in plurals of capitalized abbreviations	[His *1*'s and *7*'s looked alike.] [She has trouble pronouncing her *the*'s.] [EEGs] [his late 60s] [the 1970s]
8.	is often used with *s* in expressions of time, measurement, and money *but* is not used with a plural noun used as a modifier	[a dollar's worth] [a year's subscription] [ten cents' worth] [six weeks' vacation] *but* [earnings statement]

[ ] BRACKETS

1.	set off extraneous data (as editorial comments in quoted material)	He wrote, "Only one of the samples were [sic] sent to the lab."
2.	function as parentheses within parentheses in running texts	A tranquilizer (as chlorpromazine [Thorazine]) should be prescribed.
3.	Sometimes separate units in chemical/math formulas	Pregn–4–ene 3, 20–dione, 17–[(1–oxohexyl)oxy] $\sqrt{[(x + y - z)/(a - b + c)]}$

● COLON

1.	introduces a clause or phrase that explains, illustrates, amplifies, or restates what has gone before	[The sentence was poorly constructed: it lacked both unity and coherence.]
2.	directs attention to an appositive	[He had only one pleasure: eating.]
3.	introduces a series	[Three countries were represented: England, France, and Belgium.]
4.	introduces lengthy quoted matter set off from a running text by blocked indentation but not by quotation marks	[I quote from Part I of the study:]

5. is used in medical/scientific references between an author's name and a title, between a title and a subtitle, and in periodical references between volume and page numbers

[Lown B, Matta RJ, Besser HW: Programmed "trendscription": A new approach to electrocardiographic monitoring. *JAMA* 232:39, 1975.]

6. punctuates the salutation in a letter featuring the mixed punctuation pattern

[Gentlemen:] [Dear Bob:] [Dear Mr. Smith:]

7. punctuates some correspondence headings

[TO:] [THROUGH:] [VIA:] [SUBJECT:] [REFERENCE:]

8. separates writer/dictator/typist initials in the identification lines of business letters

[WAL:coc]
[WAL:WEB:coc]

9. separates carbon copy or blind carbon copy abbreviations from the initials or names of copy recipients in business letters

[cc: RWP
        JES]

[bcc: MWK
        FCM]

, COMMA

1. separates main clauses joined by coordinating conjunctions (such as *and, but, for, nor, or,* and sometimes *so* and *yet*) and very short clauses not so joined
NOTE: Two very brief and tightly connected clauses joined by a coordinating conjunction and two predicates also so joined may be unpunctuated.

[Seven out of eight patients claimed that the drug improved their symptoms, and three said that it completely relieved them.]
but
[We have tested the computer and we are pleased.] [He discussed several important contraindications in great detail and followed them with an appraisal of the drug.]

2. sets off an adverbial clause that precedes a main clause

[When she found that the tests were positive, she called the doctor.]
[Although the test results were uncertain, I was still able to draw some preliminary conclusions.]

3. sets off an introductory phrase (as a participial, infinitive, or prepositional phrase) that precedes a main clause

NOTE: If a phrase or a noun clause is the subject of the sentence, it is unpunctuated.

[Having made that decision, he turned to other matters.] [To understand this situation fully, you have to be familiar with the background.] [On Monday, he left early.]
but
[To have believed your statement would have been wrong.] [Whatever is worth doing is worth doing well.]

4. sets off from the rest of a sentence interrupting transitional words and expressions (such as *on the contrary, on the other hand*), conjunctive adverbs (such as *consequently, furthermore, however*), and expressions that introduce an illustration or example (such as *namely, for example*)	[Your second question, on the other hand, is unanswerable.] [The diagnosis, however, is correct.] [He expects to evaluate two drugs, namely, chlorpromazine and prazepam.] [He believes in responsibility, i.e., professional responsibility.]
5. often sets off contrasting and opposing expressions within sentences NOTE: When *and, or, either . . . or*, or *neither . . . nor* join items in a pair or in a series, the series is internally unpunctuated.	[I note that he has changed his style, not his ethics.] [The fee is not $65.00, but $56.65.] [A holiday, but not a vacation day, is still open.] *but* [The fee is either $65.00 or $56.65.] [A holiday and a vacation day are still open.] [He has changed neither his style nor his ethics nor his attitude.]
6. separates words, phrases, or clauses in series joined at the end by a coordinating conjunction NOTE: The final comma before the conjunction in a series is optional; its purpose is to clarify meaning.	[Men, women, and children crowded into the office.] [On the morning of of the scan, the patient should eat only eggnog, fruit jelly, juice, and hot tea with four tablespoons of sugar.] [The lesions were green, black, and blue.] *but meaning could be different* [The lesions were green, black and blue.]
7. separates coordinate adjectives and phrases modifying the same word. NOTE: Two or more tightly connected adjectives in series each of which modifies the same word or a whole phrase may not require punctuation.	[It was a bright, beautiful, sunny day.] [This study is as thorough, though not as organized as his others.] *but* [The clinic rented office space in a new 90-story concrete and glass building.] [six ill-defined nodules]
8. sets off from the rest of a sentence parenthetic elements (as nonrestrictive modifiers and nonrestrictive appositives) NOTE: The comma does not set off restrictive or essential modifiers or appositives required to give a sentence or a phrase meaning.	[These programs, which should be under a physician's supervision, are not recommended for patients with high blood pressure.] [The Nursing Supervisor, Mary Dowd, attended the meeting.] *but* [the late astronaut Gus Grissom]
9. introduces a direct quotation, terminates a direct quotation that is neither a question nor an exclamation, and encloses segments of a split quotation	[Jim said, "I am leaving."] ["I am leaving," Jim said.] ["I am leaving," Jim said with determination, "even if you want me to stay."]
10. sets off words in direct address, absolute phrases, and mild interjections	[We would like to discuss your account, Mr. Baker.] [I fear the encounter, his temper being what it is.] [Ah, that's my idea of a sensible man.]

11. separates a tag question from the rest of a sentence	[It's been a fine convention, hasn't it?]
12. indicates the omission of a word or words, and especially a word or words used earlier in a sentence	[Some medical assistants work for single-physician practices; others, for joint practices.]
13. is used to avoid ambiguity and also to emphasize a particular phrase; *compare* COMMA, RULE 6, NOTE	[To Mary, Jane was someone special.] [The more difficult the operation, the higher the risks.]
14. groups numerals into units of three in separating thousands, millions, etc.; it is generally not used with numbers of four or more digits in set combinations; *see also* NUMERALS, RULE 10	[Smithville, pop. 100,000] [3,600 rpm] *but* [the year 1980] [page 1411] [1127 Smith Street] [Room 3000]
15. punctuates the date line of a business letter, an informal letter, and the expression of dates in running texts	[January 1, 19--] [On January 1, 19--, this hospital reported assets of. . . .]
16. follows a personal-letter salutation	[Dear Bob,]
17. follows the complimentary close of a business letter or of an informal letter featuring the mixed punctuation pattern	[Very truly yours,] [Sincerely,]
18. sometimes separates names from corporate titles in envelope address blocks, inside addresses, and signature blocks	[Mr. John P. Dow, Administrator SWC Hospital Smithville, ST 56789] [Very truly yours, Lee H. Cobb, MD Chief of Surgery]
19. may separate elements within some official corporate names	[Riker Laboratories, Inc.] [Manville Rubber Products, Inc.]
20. often punctuates an inverted name	[Smith, John W.]
21. separates a surname from a following academic, honorary, religious, governmental, or military title	[John W. Smith, MD] [John W. Smith, Esq.] [The Reverend John W. Smith, SJ] [General John W. Smith, USA]
22. Sets off geographical names (as that of a state or county from that of a city), items in dates, and addresses from the rest of a running text	[Houston, Texas, is the site of a large Air Force medical center.] [On June 1, 1977, the patient was examined.] [Mail your check to: XYZ Hospital, 1234 Smith Boulevard, Smithville, ST 56789.]

▬▬▬▬ DASH

1. usually marks an abrupt change or break in the continuity of a sentence	[The concern for any symptom—a headache, or a fear, or anxiety—is a part of total patient care.]
2. is used after numerical indicators in sideheads and in table titles (as in reports or medical journal articles)	[CASE 1.—A nine-year-old boy was seen on July 20, 1977.] [TABLE 6.—Clinical Uses of Radioisotopes.]
3. introduces a summary statement that follows a series of words or phrases	[Oil, steel, and wheat—these are the sinews of industrialization.]
4. is often used in formal medical writing after sideheads	[*Dose.*—The initial daily dosage for middle-aged patients is 250 mg. Caution should be exercised. . . .]
5. separates nonproprietary and trade names of drugs especially in lists	[Proproxyphene hydrochloride—*Darvon*] [Chlorpromazine hydrochloride—*Thorazine*]
6. may be used with the exclamation point or the question mark	[The faces of the crash victims—how bloody!—were shown on TV.] [Your question—was it on our test results?—just can't be answered.]

● ● ● ELLIPSIS *or* SUSPENSION POINTS ● ● ● ●

1. indicates by three periods the omission of one or more words within a quoted passage	[The use of methadone maintenance therapy alone . . . may not be in his best interests. —*United States Dispensatory*]

2. indicates by four periods (the last of which represents a period) the omission of one or more sentences within a quoted passage or the omission of a word or words at the end of a sentence	[Historically, powders represent one of the oldest dosage forms. They are the natural outgrowth of man's attempt to prepare crude drugs and other natural products . . . . However, with the declining use of crude drugs . . . powders as a dosage form have been replaced largely by capsules and tablets.
	    —*Remington's Pharmaceutical Sciences*]
	
	[Fifty patients 70 years of age underwent coronary artery bypass surgery . . . .
	    —*JAMA*]

3. is used as a stylistic device especially in advertising copy to catch and hold the reader's attention	[Backed by manpower and print promotion to physicians . . . to build prescription flow! —*Drug Topics*]
4. indicates halting speech or an unfinished sentence in dialogue	["I'd like to . . . that is . . . if you don't mind. . . ." He faltered and then stopped speaking.]

5. may be used as leaders (as in tables of contents) when spaced and extended for some length across a page
NOTE: leaders should be in perfect alignment vertically and should end precisely at the same point.

EXCLAMATION POINT

1. ends an emphatic phrase or sentence   [Do this—now!]

2. terminates an emphatic interjection   [Stat!]

HYPHEN

1. marks division at the end of a line concluding with a syllable of a word that is to be carried over to the next line

[tick-
borne]

[trans-
sect]

2. is used between some prefix and root combinations, such as
prefix + proper name;

some prefixes ending with
vowels + root;

sometimes prefix + word
beginning often with the same vowel;

stressed prefix + root word, especially when this combination is similar to a different word

[pseudo-Graefe phenomenon]

[re-ink] *but* [reissue]

[co-opted] *but* [cooperate]
[intra-abdominal] *but* [intraarterial]
[re-treat a patient]
but
[retreat from an argument]

3. is used in some compounds, especially those containing prepositions; consult a dictionary when in doubt of styling

[a double-blind study] [attorney-at-law]
[read the X rays]
but
[X-ray readings]

4. may be used between elements of a compound modifier in attributive position in order to avoid ambiguity; however, most clinical designations styled as open compounds are not hyphened when used as attributives

[a large-bowel constriction]
i.e., a constriction of the large bowel
[a large bowel constriction]
i.e., a large constriction of the bowel
but
[a myocardial infarction]
[Myocardial infarction invalidism is . . . .]
[were studied in vivo.]
[a constant in vivo response.]

5. suspends the first part of a *hyphened* compound when joined with another hyphened compound in attributive position

[a 4- to 8-mg dose]
but
[a dose of 4 to 8 mg]

6. is used in expressing written-out numbers between 21 and 99	[Forty-one patients were seen.]
7. is used between the numerator and the denominator in writing out fractions especially when they are used as modifiers; however, fractions used as nouns are usually styled open	[a two-thirds majority of the staff] *but* [used two thirds of the stationery]
8. serves as an arbitrary equivalent of the phrase "(up) to and including" when used between numbers and dates	[pages 40-98] [the years 1960-1970]
9. is used in the compounding of two or more capitalized names *but* is not used when a single capitalized name is in attributive position	[Tay-Sachs disease] [U.S.-U.S.S.R research] *but* [a New York hospital] [Middle East exports]

( )   PARENTHESES

1. set off supplementary, parenthetic, or explanatory material when the interruption is more marked than that usually indicated by commas and when the inclusion of such material does not essentially alter the meaning of the sentence; *see also* CAPITALIZATION, RULE 7	[A large number of patients (44.8%) required 2 calls before follow-up could be obtained.] [. . . as shown in the graph (Fig. 1).] [We appreciate your nice remarks (especially your reference to our new assistant).]
2. enclose Arabic numerals confirming a typed-out number	[Delivery will be made in thirty (30) days.]
3. enclose a reference given in a running text	[A similar response was noted by Doe and Jones (*J Med Soc NJ* 64:609, 1967).]
4. may enclose numbers or letters separating and heading individual elements or items in a series	[We must set forth (1) our long-term goals, (2) our immediate objectives, and (3) the means at our disposal.]
5. enclose abbreviations synonymous with typed-out forms and occurring after those forms	[. . . these patients had acute respiratory failure, requiring treatment with positive-end expiratory pressure (PEEP) in excess of 20 mmHg . . . . —*Biological Abstracts*]
6. enclose proprietary names of drugs when they follow generic names in running texts	[administration of cholestyramine (Questran) . . .]
7. are used as follows with other marks: **a.** If the parenthetic expression is an independent sentence standing alone at the end of another sentence, its first word is capitalized and a period is typed <u>inside</u> the last parenthesis.	[The discussion was held in the boardroom. (The results are still confidential.)]

b. Parenthetic material within a sentence may be internally punctuated by a question mark, a period after an abbreviation only, an exclamation point, or a set of quotation marks.

[Years ago, someone (who?) told me. . . .] [The conference was held in Vancouver (that's in B.C.).] [Our schedule has been light (knock on wood!), but. . . .] [The patient was depressed ("I want to die") and refused to cooperate.]

c. No punctuation mark should be placed directly before parenthetic material in a sentence; if a break is required, the punctuation should be placed <u>after</u> the final parenthesis.

[I'll get back to you tomorrow (Monday), when I have more details.]

● **PERIOD**

---

1. terminates sentences or sentence fragments that are neither interrogative nor exclamatory

[Take dictation.] [She took dictation.] [She asked whether he wanted her to take dictation.]

---

2. often terminates polite requests especially in business correspondence

[Will you please return these forms as soon as possible.]

---

3. punctuates some abbreviations and some contractions, as

[f.o.b] [a.k.a] [sec'y.] [min.]

  a. courtesy titles and honorifics backed by a strong tradition of punctuation

[Mr.] [Mrs.] [Ms.] [Dr.] [Prof.] [Rev.] [Hon.] [Esq.] [Jr.] [Sr.]

  b. some abbreviations (as of measure) especially when absence of punctuation could cause misreading

[p. 20] [Paper, 521 ff.] [18 in.] [No. 2 pencils] [fig. 15]

  c. abbreviations of Latin words and phrases commonly used in texts

[etc.] [i.e.] [e.g.] [a.c.] [b.i.d.] [q.i.d] [p.r.n.]

  d. compass points
NOTE: Punctuation styling varies.

[1400 Sixteenth Street, N.W.]
or
[1400 Sixteenth Street, NW.]
or
[1400 Sixteenth Street, NW]

  e. some geographical-name abbreviations
NOTE: Punctuation styling varies.

[U.S.-U.S.S.R. research]
or
[US-USSR research]
but not
[U.S.-USSR research]
and not
[US-U.S.S.R. research]

  f. abbreviated elements of some official corporate names

[A. H. Robins Company]

---

4. is used with an individual's initials

[Mr. W. A. Morton]
[Dr. J. H. R. Smythe]
[Professor Ann A. Dow]

5. is used after Roman numerals in general outlines but not with Roman numerals used as part of a title	[I. Objectives] *but* [John D. Jones, III]
6. is often used after Arabic numerals in enumerations whose numbers stand alone	[Required skills are: 1. Shorthand 2. Typing 3. Transcription]

? QUESTION MARK

1. terminates a direct question	[Who signed the memo?] ["Who signed the memo?" he asked.]
2. punctuates each element of an interrogative series that is neither numbered nor lettered; however, only one such mark punctuates a numbered or lettered interrogative series	[Has the patient completed the needed insurance forms? Checked the data? Signed the forms where indicated?] *but* [Has the patient (1) completed the needed insurance forms (2) checked the data (3) signed the forms where indicated?]
3. indicates the writer's ignorance or uncertainty	[John Jones, the President (?) of that company said. . . .]

66   99 QUOTATION MARKS, DOUBLE

1. enclose direct quotations in conventional usage	[He said, "I am leaving."] *but* [He said that he was leaving.]
2. enclose fragments of quoted matter when reproduced exactly as originally stated	[. . . investigators say there is evidence "that a viral gene which causes cancer may have originated from normal cells." —*JAMA*]
3. enclose words or phrases borrowed from others, words used in a special way, and often a word of marked informality when it is introduced into formal writing	[To acknowledge this difference, we denoted the cellular element as "sarc." —*JAMA*] [. . . some 58,000 cancer patients . . . die each year of "local disease." —*JAMA*]
4. enclose titles of reports, catalogs, short poems, short stories, articles, lectures, chapters of books, songs, short musical compositions, and radio and TV programs; *compare* ITALICIZATION, RULE 7	[the report "College Graduates and Their Employers"] [the catalog "Surgical Supplies and Equipment"] [Robert Frost's "Dust of Snow"] [Pushkin's "Queen of Spades"] [The third chapter of *Treasure Island* is entitled "The Black Spot."] ["America the Beautiful"] [Ravel's "Bolero"] [NBC's "Today Show"]

5. are used with other punctuation marks in the following ways:

the period and the comma fall <u>within</u> the quotation marks

[Methamphetamine is sometimes called "speed."] ["I am leaving," he said.] [The bandage was described as "waterproof," but "moisture-resistant" would have been a better description.]

the semicolon and the colon fall <u>outside</u> the quotation marks

[He spoke of his "little cottage in the country"; he might have called it a mansion.]

the dash, question mark, and the exclamation point fall <u>within</u> the quotation marks when they refer to the quoted matter only; they fall <u>outside</u> when they refer to the whole sentence

[He asked, "When did you leave?"] [What is the meaning of "clipboard supervisor"?] [He shouted, "Halt!"] [Save us from his "mercy"!]

6. are <u>not</u> used with quoted material comprising more than three typed lines and only one paragraph: such material is blocked and single-spaced internally but double-spaced top and bottom to set it off from the rest of the text

[An article entitled "Containing the Cost of Employer Health Plans" on page 75 of the May 30, 1977, issue of *Business Week* makes this point:

> Today the Health, Education & Welfare Dept. has certified only 30 of the nation's 180 HMOs, but additional ones are seeking certification and employers, consumer groups, and even traditional health insurers are announcing plans for new groups.

This, then, summarizes the current development of HMOs.]

NOTE: The illustration is reprinted from the May 30, 1977, issue of BusinessWeek © 1977 by McGraw-Hill, Inc., 1221 Avenue of the Americas, NY, NY 10020. All rights reserved.

7. are used with long quoted matter comprising more than three typed lines and having two or more paragraphs: double quotation marks are typed at the beginning of each paragraph and at the end of the final paragraph

[*Psychology Today* has this to say about pain:

> "Until recently, nobody really understood how the mind exacerbated or relieved pain. It was believed simply that in times of acute danger, the body would suppress the sensation of pain to survive . . . .
>
> "We know now that chronic pain feeds on itself, creating a self-reinforcing cycle that must be broken and then reversed to bring relief."

This material is from Julie Wang's article "Breaking out of the Pain Trap" found on page 78 of the July 1977 issue of the magazine.]

NOTE: The illustration is reprinted from PSYCHOLOGY TODAY MAGAZINE. Copyright © 1977 Ziff-Davis Publishing Company.

❝ ❞ QUOTATION MARKS, SINGLE

1. enclose a quotation within a quotation in conventional English

[The witness said, "I distinctly heard him say, 'Don't be late,' and then I heard the door close."]

2. are sometimes used in place of double quotation marks in British usage

NOTE: When both single and double quotation marks occur at the end of a sentence, the period typically falls <u>within</u> both sets of marks.

[The witness said, 'I distinctly heard him say, "Don't be late," and then I heard the door close.']
[The witness said, "I distinctly heard him say, 'Don't be late.'"]

•

⁊ SEMICOLON

1. links main clauses not joined by coordinating conjunctions

[So do a rapid neurologic exam; document any deficits as you go since all of this information must accompany the patient when he is sent on.
—*Emergency Medicine*]

---

2. links main clauses joined by conjunctive adverbs (as *consequently, furthermore, however*)

[Drug abuse is illegal and dangerous; furthermore, it is uneconomical.]

---

3. links phrases or clauses which themselves contain commas even when such clauses are linked by coordinating conjunctions

[Laboratory studies have disclosed the following values: hemoglobin, 12.5 g/dl; hematocrit, 37%; platelet count, 120,000/cu mm; WBC count, 5,100/cu mm, with 56% neutrophils . . . .
—*JAMA*]

---

4. often occurs before phrases or abbreviations (as *for example, for instance, that is, that is to say, namely, e.g.,* or *i.e.*) that introduce expansions or series

[A crisis is a peak from which there is no turning back; that is, a parent can no longer think of himself or herself as a single individual.
—*Contemporary OB/GYN*]

/ VIRGULE

1. separates alternatives

[The medication dose schedule can be made simpler by using calendar packs or by developing daily schedules and/or written reminders of times to take medications.
—Ann M. Gray, CMA-AC
*The Professional
Medical Assistant*]

---

2. often represents *per* in specific numeral + abbreviation combinations expressing measure; see also 17.9

[5.1 beats/min] [100 mg/kg body weight]
[a high concentration (0.60 mg/0.1 ml) of the drug] [hemoglobin level: 14 gm/100 cc]

---

3. often is an arbitrary punctuation mark within an abbreviation

[A/G ratio] [W/V]

PUNCTUATION-SPACINATION SUMMARY

Position	Example
Degree of Spacination No Space	
1. between any word and the punctuation immediately following it	[Here is the car.] [Is the·car here?] [Here is the car!] [The car is here; however, I don't need it now.] [The car is here: now, do I get in, or not?] [The car is here. . . .]
2. between quotation marks and the quoted matter	["I am leaving," he said.] [He said, "I am leaving."]
3. between parentheses and the items they enclose	[He is (should I say it?) just a bit peculiar.]
4. between brackets and the words or figures they enclose	[had recieved [sic] the gift]
5. between initials comprising punctuated or unpunctuated abbreviations	[q.i.d.] [b.i.d.] [i.e.] [p.m.] [MEND] [ACTH] [WHO] [PhD *or* Ph.D.]
6. between elements in figure + abbreviation or other word combinations when they are in attributive position	[a 200-hp engine] [a $15-million project]
7. between periods in leaders except for initial and terminal periods which are preceded & followed by one space; *compare* ONE SPACE, RULE 12	[Item 1 .... page 1]
8. between elements of hyphened compounds	[gram-negative] [$10-$20] [diphtheria-pertussis-tetanus]
9. on both sides of a colon separating volume and pagination in references; *compare* TWO SPACES, RULES 3, 4, 5	[*Behav Res Ther* 5:357–365]
10. on either side of a dash	[If she understands the contract—and I'm sure she does—we'll have no trouble.]
11. between words, letters, or figures separated by a virgule	[1976/77] [and/or] [A/G ratio]
12. between figures and symbols	[$12.95] [75%] [90F] [7.654] [8¢] [$.08]
13. within units expressing time of day	[9:30 a.m.] [9:30 p.m.]
14. in identification lines, and in carbon copy notations indicating only one recipient designated by initials	[FCM:hol] [MWK:FCM:hol] [cc:FCM] [bcc:MWK]
15. between referenced textual material and the reference number(s)	[. . . is a prime factor in successful hospital management"[1]] *or* [. . . is a prime factor in successful hospital management."[1,4–6]]
Degree of Spacination One Space	
1. after a comma	[The car is here, isn't it?] [Scarsdale, New York] [January 1, 19--]

Position	Example
Degree of Spacination One Space	
2. after a semicolon	[The car is here; however, I don't need it now.]
3. after a period following an initial	[Mr. H. C. Matthews]
4. before and after *x* meaning "by" or "times"	[a 3 x 5 card] [3 x 5 = 15]
5. after a suspended hyphen	[the long- and short-term results]
6. on each side of a hyphen in some street addresses	[2135 - 71st Street, NW]
7. between a question mark and the first letter of the next word in a series question	[Are you coming today? tomorrow? the day after?]
8. between Postal Service state abbreviations and ZIP Codes	[Smithville, ST 56789]

9. after the heading cc that is unpunctuated in letters following the open punctuation pattern and that introduces a list of names	[cc Mr. Slaughter
	    Mr. Tate
	    Mr. Watson]

10. between a final quotation mark and the rest of a sentence	["I am leaving," he said.]
11. between numerals and abbreviations of units of measure	[400 cc] [2000 R] [7 mm] [280 nm] [132 kgN] [56 sec] [150 mmHg] [3 ng/min]
12. between ellipses in leaders except for initial and terminal ellipsis points which are preceded and followed by at least two spaces, respectively (this styling is optional); *compare* NO SPACE, RULE 7	[Item 1 . . . . . page 1]
Degree of Spacination Two Spaces	
1. after a period ending a sentence	[Here is the car. Do you want to get in?]
2. after a question mark or an exclamation point ending a sentence	[Get out of here! Well, what are you waiting for? I've said enough.]
3. after a colon in running texts, in bibliographic references, in publication titles, and in letter or memorandum headings	[The car is here: Now, do I get in?] [*Medicine Today: A Report on a Decade of Progress*] [SUBJECT: Project X]
4. in references, after a colon separating an author from a title	[Stuart RB: Behavior control of overeating. *Behav Res Ther* 5:357–365, 1967.]
5. after a carbon copy notation punctuated with a colon + a full name	[cc: Mr. Johnson]

6. after a figure + a period that introduces an item in an enumeration	[The following skills are essential:
	    1. typing
	    2. shorthand]

17.7

WORD DIVISION

In the United States more time and energy have been spent worrying about the division of words at the end of a printed or typed line than the subject merits. The very fact that widely used and respected dictionaries published by different houses indicate different points at which to divide many words is evidence enough that there is no absolute right or wrong, and that for numerous words there are acceptable end-of-line division alternatives. The best policy to follow in individual instances is to consult an adequate dictionary whose main entries indicate points of division. End-of-line division is not based solely upon pronunciation, and in any case there is great variety in pronunciation throughout the English-speaking world. The question of end-of-line division occurs only in written contexts, and it is perhaps unreasonable to expect the spoken form of the language to dictate a consistent set of principles for an essentially mechanical problem.

Common sense suggests some guidelines which will help to minimize the time spent consulting a dictionary. For instance, the division of a single letter at the beginning or end of a word should be avoided. On the one hand, in typed material a single letter hanging onto the end of a line with a hyphen may be dropped to the next line without leaving unsightly right-hand margins, and in printed material the space required for two characters (the letter and the hyphen) is, in most circumstances, easily filled. On the other hand, if there is room for a hyphen at the end of a line, there is room for the last letter of a word in its place. Thus, *abort* and *obex* should not be divided, for such divisions as

a-	*o-*	*obe-*
bort	*bex*	*x*

would detract from rather than add to the appearance of the page.

Compounds containing one or more hyphens will cause a reader less trouble if divided after the hyphen. For the words *diphtheria-pertussis-tetanus, Voges-Proskauer reaction,* and *growth-inhibiting* the divisions

diphtheria-	*diphtheria-pertussis-*	*Voges-*	*growth-*
pertussis-tetanus	*tetanus*	*Proskauer reaction*	*inhibiting*

are less obtrusive than such divisions as

diph-	*diphtheria-per-*	*Vo-*	*growth-in-*
theria-pertussis-tetanus	*tussis-tetanus*	*ges-Proskauer reaction*	*hibiting*

although there are no "rules" against the latter set of examples, and such divisions may occasionally prove necessary especially in narrow columns.

Similarly, closed compounds are best divided between component elements; thus, the divisions

every-	*post-*	*blood-*
one	*humous*	*mobile*

appear more natural and will cause the reader less trouble than

ev-	*posthu-*	*bloodmo-*
eryone	*mous*	*bile*

though divisions such as the ones above may be required in exceptional circumstances.

For words that are not compound, it is best to consult a dictionary or a guide to word division, and in order to maintain greatest consistency it is preferable always to consult the same source (such as *Webster's New Collegiate Dictionary* or *Webster's Medical Speller*).

There are, in addition, some specific instances in which one should avoid end-of-line division if at all possible. These are as follows:

1. The last word in a paragraph should not be divided.

2. The last word on a page (as of a business letter or a memorandum) should not be divided.

3. Items joined by *and/or* and the coordinating conjunction *and/or* itself should not be divided.

4. Proper names, courtesy titles, and following titles (as *Esq.*) should not be divided either on envelopes, in inside addresses, or in running texts:

correct	*incorrect*
. . . to	. . . to Mr.
Mr. J. R. Smith.	J. R. Smith.

The one exception to this rule is the separation of long honorary titles from names especially in envelope address blocks and in inside addresses where space is often limited:

correct	*incorrect*
The Honorable	The Honorable John
John R. Smith	R. Smith

5. If dates must be divided (as in running texts), the division should occur only between the day and the year:

correct	*incorrect*
. . . arrived on	. . . arrived on Jan-
January 1, 19--.	uary 1, 19--.
. . . arrived on January 1,	. . . arrived on January
19--.	1, 19--.

6. Set units (as of time and measure) as well as single monetary units should not be divided:

correct	*incorrect*
. . . at 10:00 a.m.	. . . at 10:00
	a.m.

correct	*incorrect*
. . . had a temperature of 98.6 F	. . . had a temperature of 98.6
	F.

correct	*incorrect*
. . . a fee of $4,900.50.	. . . a fee of $4,900.-
	50.

7. Abbreviations should not be divided:

correct	*incorrect*
. . . received the MD	. . . received the M-
from Harvard.	D from Harvard.

8. Compound geographic designations (as city + state combinations) should not be divided:

correct	*incorrect*
. . . to St. Paul, Minnesota.	. . . to St.
	Paul, Minnesota.

17.8

COMPONENTS OF DISCOURSE

The word *discourse* is defined in *Webster's New Collegiate Dictionary* as "formal and orderly and usually extended expression of thought.·. . ." Thus, no guide to effective communication can ignore the fundamental components of discourse: the word, the phrase, the clause, the sentence, and the paragraph. Each of these increasingly complex units contributes to the expression of a writer's points, ideas, and concepts.

The word, of course, is the simplest component of discourse. Words have been traditionally classified into eight parts of speech. This classification system is determined chiefly by a word's inflectional features, its general grammatical functions, and its positioning within a sentence. On the following pages, the parts of speech—the adjective, adverb, conjunction, interjection, noun, preposition, pronoun, and verb—are alphabetically listed and briefly discussed. Each part of speech is introduced by an applicable definition from *Webster's New Collegiate Dictionary*. The phrase, the clause, the sentence, and the paragraph are discussed later in this section.

PARTS OF SPEECH

Adjective

²**adjective** *n* : a word belonging to one of the major form classes in any of numerous languages and typically serving as a modifier of a noun to denote a quality of the thing named, to indicate its quantity or extent, or to specify a thing as distinct from something else

The main structural feature of an adjective is its ability to indicate degrees of comparison (positive, comparative, superlative) by addition of the suffixal endings *-er/-est* to the base word (*clean, cleaner, cleanest*), by addition of *more/most* or *less/least* before the base word (*meaningful, more meaningful, most meaningful; less meaningful, least meaningful*), or by use of irregular forms (*bad, worse, worst*). Some adjectives are compared in two ways (as *smoother, smoothest/more smooth, most smooth*), while still others (as *prior, optimum,* or *maximum*), called "absolute adjectives," are ordinarily not compared since they are felt to represent ultimate or highest conditions.

Adjectives may occur in the following positions within sentences:

1. preceding the nouns they modify, as
   the *black* hat
   a *dark brown* coat
2. following the nouns they modify, as
   an executive *par excellence*
   I painted my room *blue.*
3. following the verb *to be* in predicate-adjective position, as
   The hat is *black.*
   and following other linking (or "sense") verbs in predicate-adjective position, as
   He seems *intelligent.*
   The food tastes *stale.*
   I feel *queasy.*
4. following some transitive verbs used in the passive voice, as
   The room was painted *blue.*
   The passengers were found *dead* at the crash site.

Adjectives may describe something or represent a quality, kind, or condition (a *sick* man); they may point out or indicate something (*these* men); or they may convey the force of questions (*Whose* office is this?). Some adjectives (as *Galenic, Wolffian, Hippocratic,* and others) are called "proper adjectives." They are derived from proper nouns, take their meanings from what characterizes the nouns, and are capitalized.

The following are general points of adjective usage:

Absolute adjectives   Some adjectives (as *prior, maximum, optimum, minimum, first,* and the like) ordinarily admit no comparison because they represent ultimate conditions. However, printed usage indicates that many writers do compare and qualify some of these words in order to show connotations and shades of meaning that they feel are less than absolute. The word *unique* is a case in point:

. . . required a fairly *unique* mode of viewing things.
　　　　　—*Change*

. . . psychology strives toward a rather *unique* concept of "understanding."
　　　　　—*The Social Sciences*

The appearance of gas gangrene at the sites of parenteral injections is truly *unique*.
　　　　　—*JAMA*

. . . children each so *unique* . . . .
　　　　　—*Education Digest*

. . . the most *unique* human faculty, that of speech . . . .
　　　　　—*Hartford Studies*
　　　　　　in Literature

While many examples may be found of qualification and/or comparison of *unique,* it is difficult to find printed evidence showing comparison of a word like *optimum.* When one is in doubt about the inflection of such an adjective, one should consult a dictionary.

Coordinate adjectives   Adjectives that share equal relationships to the nouns they modify are called coordinate adjectives and are separated from each other by commas:

a concise, coherent, intelligent article

However, in the following locution containing the set phrase *short story*

a concise, coherent short story

the adjectives *concise* and *coherent* are neither parallel nor equal in function or relationship with *short* which is an essential element of the total compound *short story.* The test to use before inserting commas is to insert *and* between questionable adjectives, and then to decide whether the sentence still makes sense. Whereas *and* could fit between *coherent* and *intelligent* in the first example, it could not work between *coherent* and *short* in the second example.

Adjective/noun agreement   The number (singular or plural) of a demonstrative adjective (*this, that, these, those*) should agree with that of the noun it modifies:

these kinds of typewriters	*not*	these kind of typewriters
those sorts of jobs	*not*	those sort of jobs
this type of person	*not*	these type of people

Double comparisons   Double comparisons should be avoided since they are considered nonstandard:

the easiest
or
the most easy solution   *not*   the most easiest solution

an easier
or
a more easy method   *not*   a more easier method

Incomplete or understood comparisons   Some comparisons are left incomplete because the context clearly implies the comparison; hence, the expressions

Get *better* buys here!
We have *lower* prices.

These are commonly used especially in advertising. It should be understood, however, that the use of incomplete comparisons is often considered careless or illogical especially in formal writing.

Adverb	¹**ad·verb.** . . . *n* . . . : a word belonging to one of the major form classes in any of numerous languages, typically serving as a modifier of a verb, an adjective, another adverb, a preposition, a phrase, a clause, or a sentence, and expressing some relation of manner or quality, place, time, degree, number, cause, opposition, affirmation, or denial

An adverb admits three degrees of comparison (positive, comparative, superlative) ordinarily by addition of *more/most* or *less/least* before the base word (*quickly, more quickly, most quickly*). However, a few adverbs (such as *fast, slow, loud, soft, early, late,* and *quick*) may be compared in two ways: by the method described above, or by the addition of the suffixal endings *-er/-est* to the base word (*quick, quicker, quickest*).

Adverbs may occur in the following positions within sentences:

1. before the subject, as
   Then he announced his resignation.
2. after the subject, as
   He *then* announced his resignation.
3. before the predicate, as
   He praised the committee's work and *then* announced his resignation.
4. at the end of the predicate, as
   He announced his resignation *then.*
5. in various other positions (as before adjectives or other adverbs), as
   He also made an *equally* important announcement—that of his resignation.
   He adjourned the meeting *very* abruptly.

Adverbs answer the following questions: "when?" (Please reply *at once*), "how long?" (She wants to live here *forever*), "where?" (I work *there*), "in what direction?" (Move the lever *upward*), "how?" (The staff moved *expeditiously* on the project), and "how much?" or "to what degree?" (It is *rather* hot).

Adverbs modify verbs, adjectives, or other adverbs, as

He studied the operative report *carefully.*
He gave the operative report *very* careful study.
He studied the operative report *very* carefully.

and may also serve as clause joiners or sentence connectors, as

clause joiner
You may share our car pool; *however,* please be ready at 7:30 a.m.
sentence connector
He thoroughly enjoyed the symposium. *Indeed,* he was fascinated by the presentations.

In addition, adverbs may be essential elements of two-word verb collocations commonly having separate entry in dictionaries, such as

He looked *over* the figures.
He looked the figures *over*.
The attendant took the tray *away*.
The attendant took *away* the tray.

See also page 467 for a discussion of conjunctive adverbs, words like *however* in the example on page 465 that are adverbs functioning as conjunctions in sentences. The following are general points of adverb usage:

Placement within a sentence   Adverbs are generally positioned as close as possible to the words they modify if such a position will not result in misinterpretation by the reader:

unclear
The project that he hoped his staff would support completely disappointed him.

Does the writer mean "complete staff support" or "complete disappointment"? Thus, the adverb may be moved to another position or the sentence may be recast, depending on intended meaning:

clear
The project that he hoped his staff would completely support had disappointed him.
or
He was completely disappointed in the project that he had hoped his staff would support.

Emphasis   Adverbs (such as *just* and *only*) are often used to emphasize certain other words, Thus, a writer should be aware of the various reader reactions that may result from the positioning of an adverb in a sentence:

strong connotation of curtness
He just nodded to me as he passed.
but
emphasis on timing of the action
He nodded to me *just* as he passed.

In some positions and contexts these adverbs can be ambiguous:

I will only tell it to you.

Does the writer mean that he will only tell it, not put it in writing, or does he mean that he will tell no one else? If the latter interpretation is intended, a slight shift of position would remove the uncertainty, as

I will tell it only to you.

Adverbs vs. adjectives: examples of misuse
a. Adverbs but not adjectives modify action verbs:
not   He answered very harsh.
but   He answered very harshly.

b. Complements referring to the subject of a sentence and occurring after linking verbs conventionally take adjectives but not adverbs:
questionable   I feel badly.
                        The letter sounded strongly.
acceptable   I feel bad.
                        The letter sounded strong.
but
acceptable   He looks good these days.
                        He looks well these days.

In the last two examples, either *good* or *well* is acceptable, because both words may be adjectives or adverbs, and here they are functioning as adjectives in the sense of "being healthy."

c. Adverbs but not adjectives modify adjectives and other adverbs:

not   She seemed dreadful tired.
but   She seemed dreadfully tired.

Double negatives   A combination of two negative adverbs (as *not* + *hardly, never, scarcely,* and the like) used to express a single negative idea is considered substandard:

not   We cannot see scarcely any reason why we should try this drug.
but   We can see scarcely any reason why we should try this drug.

We can't⎫
cannot ⎬ see any reason why we should try this drug.

Conjunction

con·junc·tion . . . *n* . . . **4** : an uninflected linguistic form that joins together sentences, clauses, phrases, or words : CONNECTIVE

Conjunctions exhibit no characteristic inflectional or suffixal features. They may occur in numerous positions within sentences; however, they ordinarily do not appear in final position unless the sentence is elliptical. Three major types of conjunctions are listed and illustrated according to their functions in the table on page 468.

A comma is traditionally used <u>before</u> a coordinating conjunction linking coordinate clauses especially when these clauses are lengthy or when the writer desires to emphasize their distinctness from one another:

The patient is in serious condition, and he shows few signs of improvement.
Shall we consider this person's application, or shall we consider that one's?
We do not discriminate between men and women, but we do have high professional standards and qualifications that the successful applicant must meet.

In addition to the three main types of conjunctions in the table on page 468, the English language has transitional adverbs and adverbial phrases called "conjunctive adverbs" that express relationships between two units of discourse (as two independent clauses, two complete sentences, or two or more paragraphs), and that function as conjunctions even though they are customarily classified as adverbs. The table on page 469 groups and illustrates conjunctive adverbs according to their functions.

Occurrence of a comma fault especially with conjunctive adverbs indicates that the writer has not realized that a comma alone will not suffice to join two sentences, and that a semicolon is required. The punctuation pattern with conjunctive adverbs is usually as follows:

clause + semicolon + conjunctive adverb + comma + clause

The following two sentences illustrate a typical comma fault and a rewrite that removes the error:

comma fault	*rewrite*
The clinic had flexible hours, however its employees were expected to abide by the hours they had selected for arrival and departure.	The clinic had flexible hours; however, its employees were expected to abide by the hours they had selected for arrival and departure.

Three Major Types of Conjunctions and their Functions

Type of Conjunction	Function	Example
coordinating conjunctions link words, phrases, dependent clauses, and complete sentences	*and* joins elements and sentences	[He ordered pencils, pens, *and* erasers.]
	but, yet exclude or contrast	[He is a brilliant *but* arrogant man.]
	or, nor offer alternatives	[You can wait here *or* go.]
	for offers reason or grounds	[The report is poor, *for* its data are inaccurate.]
	so offers a reason	[Her diction is good, *so* every word is clear.]
subordinating conjunctions introduce dependent clauses	*because, since* express cause	[*Because* she is smart, she is doing well in her job.]
	although, if, unless express condition	[Don't call *unless* you have the information.]
	as, as though, however express manner	[He looks *as though* he is ill.] [We'll do it *however* you tell us to.]
	in order that, so that express result	[She routes the mail early *so that* they can read it.]
	after, before, once, since, till, until, when, whenever, while express time	[He kept meetings to a minimum *when* he was administrator.]
	where, wherever express place or circumstance	[I don't know *where* he has gone.] [He tries to help out *wherever* it is possible.]
	whether expresses alternative conditions or possibilities	[It was hard to decide *whether* I should go or stay.]
	that introduces several kinds of subordinate clauses including those used as noun equivalents (as a subject or an object of a verb, or a predicate nominative)	[Yesterday I learned *that* he has been sick for over a week.]
correlative conjunctions work in pairs to link alternatives or equal elements	*either . . . or, neither . . . nor,* and *whether . . . or* link alternatives	[*Either* you go *or* you stay.] [He had *neither* looks *nor* wit.]
	both . . . and and *not only . . . but also* link equal elements	[*Both* typist *and* writer should understand style.] [*Not only* was there inflation, *but* there was *also* unemployment.]

Conjunctive Adverbs Grouped According to Meaning and Function

Conjunctive Adverbs	Functions	Examples
also, besides, further-more, in addition, in fact, moreover, too	express addition	[This employee deserves a sub-stantial raise; *furthermore,* she should be promoted.]
indeed, that is [to say], *to be sure*	add emphasis	[He is brilliant; *indeed,* he is a genius.]

anyway, however, nevertheless, on the contrary, on the one hand/on the other hand that is	express contrast or discrimination	[Practically speaking, *however,* the three most common causes of hypercalciuria are hyperpara-thyroidism, renal tubular acidosis, and the syndrome of idiopathic hypercalciuria.
		    —Hubbard E. Williams, MD
		        Medical Times]

e.g., for example, for instance, i.e., namely, that is	introduce illustrations or elaborations	[*For example,* patients on Cytoxan must drink at least two quarts of fluids a day . . . .
		    —*Am. J. of Nursing*]
		[Its mechanism of action appears to be competitive inhibition; *that is,* naloxone prevents narcotics from occupying their central nervous system receptors by binding to these sites itself.
		    —David J. Cullen, MD
		        Resident & Staff Physician]

accordingly, as a result, consequently, hence, therefore, thus, so	express or introduce conclusions or results	[*Consequently,* when things go wrong, the first cause identified by the layman is the physician. —*Bulletin of the ACP*]
first, second, further on, later, then, in conclusion, finally	orient elements of discourse as to time or space	[*First,* we can say that the account is long overdue; *second,* that we must consider consulting our attorneys.] [*Finally,* these patients are . . . overmedicated. —*Emergency Medicine*]

The following are general points of conjunction usage:

Conjunctions as meaning clarifiers   Properly used conjunctions ensure order and coherence in writing since they often serve to pinpoint shades of meaning, place special emphasis where required, and set general tone within sentences and para-graphs. Improperly used conjunctions may result in choppy, often cloudy writing, and in incoherent orientation of ideas. Therefore, the purpose of a conjunction is totally defeated if it creates ambiguities rather than makes things clear. The often misused conjunction-phrase *as well as* is an example:

ambiguous
Jean typed the report *as well as* Joan.
(Does the writer mean that both women
typed the report together, or that both
women typed the report equally well?)

clear
Jean typed the report just *as well as* Joan
did.
Jean and Joan typed the report equally well.
or
Both Jean and Joan typed the report.
Jean typed the report; so did Joan.
Jean typed the report, and so did Joan.

Coordinating conjunctions: proper use   These terms should link equal elements
of discourse—e.g., adjectives with other adjectives, nouns with other nouns, participles with other participles, clauses with other equal-ranking clauses, and so on.
Combining unequal elements may result in unbalanced sentences:

unbalanced
Having become disgusted *and* because he
was tired, he left the meeting.

balanced
Because he was tired *and* disgusted, he left
the meeting.
or
He left the meeting because he had become
tired *and* disgusted.
or
Having become tired *and* disgusted, he left
the meeting.

Coordinating conjunctions should not be used to string together excessively long
series of elements, regardless of their equality.

strung-out
Hypothermia is the prime cause of death
in the remote outdoors and hypothermia
occurs when there is a decrease in core
body temperature to a point that prevents normal muscular coordination and
cerebral function.

tightened
Hypothermia is the prime cause of death in
the remote outdoors. It occurs when core
body temperature is decreased to a point
that prevents normal muscular coordination and cerebral function.

Choice of just the right coordinating conjunction for a particular verbal situation
is important: the right word will pinpoint the writer's true meaning and intent, and
will highlight the most relevant idea or point of the sentence. The following three
sentences exhibit increasingly stronger degrees of contrast through the use of
different conjunctions:

neutral   He works hard *and* doesn't progress.

more contrast   He works hard *but* doesn't progress.

stronger contrast He words hard, yet he doesn't progress.

The coordinating conjunction *and/or* linking two elements of a compound subject often poses a problem as to the number (singular or plural) of the verb that
follows. A subject comprising singular nouns connected by *and/or* may be considered singular or plural, depending on the meaning of the sentence:

singular
All loss and/or damage *is* to be the responsibility of the sender. [one or the other and
possibly both]

plural
John R. Jones and/or Robert B. Flint *are*
hereby *appointed* as the executors of my
estate. [both executors are to act, or either
of them is to act if the other dies or is
incapacitated]

Subordinating conjunctions: proper use   Subordinating conjunctions introduce
dependent clauses, and also deemphasize less important ideas in favor of more

important ideas. Which clause is made independent and which clause is made subordinate has great influence in determining the effectiveness of a sentence. Notice how differently these two versions strike the reader:

When the emergency call came, we were just coming out of the door.

Just as we were coming out of the door, the emergency call came.

The writer must take care that the point he or she wishes to emphasize is in the independent clause and that the points of less importance are subordinated.

Faulty clause subordination can render a sentence impotent. Compare the following examples:

faulty subordination	*improved: two sentences*
Although cerebrovascular disease is predominantly a disease of later decades of life but since as many as 5% of all strokes occur in persons under 40 years of age, the occurrence of stroke in young adults cannot be construed as insignificant.	While cerebrovascular disease is predominantly a disease of the later decades in life, as many as 5% of all strokes nevertheless occur in persons under 40 years of age. Thus, the occurrence of stroke in young adults cannot be construed as insignificant.

Correlative conjunctions: proper use   These pairs of words also join equal elements of discourse. They should be placed as close as possible to the elements they join:

misplaced	*repositioned*
Either I must send a telex *or* make a long-distance call.	I must *either* send a telex *or* make a long-distance call.

The negative counterpart of *either . . . or* is *neither . . . nor*. The conjunction *or* should not be substituted for *nor* because its substitution will destroy the negative parallelism. However, *or* may occur in combination with *no*. Examples:

He received *neither* a promotion *nor* a raise.

He received *no* promotion *or* raise.

Interjection	**in·ter·jec·tion** . . . *n* . . . **3 a :** an ejaculatory word (as *Wonderful*) or form of speech (as *ah*) **b :** a cry or inarticulate utterance (as *ouch*) expressing an emotion

---

Interjections exhibit no characteristic features or forms. As independent elements not having close grammatical connections with the rest of a sentence, interjections may often stand alone.

Interjections may be stressed or ejaculatory words, phrases, or even short sentences, as

Stat!

Come on!

Listen to the patient!

or they may be so-called "sound" words (such as those representing shouts, hisses, etc.):

Ouch! That hurts.

Shh! The meeting has begun.

Psst! Come over here.

Ah, that's my idea of a terrific instrument.

Oh, you're really wrong there.

---

noun . . . *n* . . . **1** : a word that is the name of a subject of discourse (as a person, animal, plant, place, thing, substance, quality, idea, action, or state) and that in languages with grammatical number, case, and gender is inflected for number and case but has inherent gender **2** : a word except a pronoun used in a sentence as subject or object of a verb, as object of a preposition, as the predicate after a copula, or as a name in an absolute construction

Noun

Nouns exhibit these characteristic features: they are inflected for possession, they have number (singular, plural), they are often preceded by determiners (as *a, an, the; this, that, these, those; all, every,* and other such qualifiers; *one, two, three,* and other such numerical quantifiers; *his, her, their,* and other such pronominal adjectives), a few of them still have gender (as the masculine *host,* the feminine *hostess*), and many of them are formed by suffixation (as with the suffixes *-ance, -ist, -ness,* and *-tion*).

The only noun case indicated by inflection is the possessive which is normally formed by addition of *-'s* (singular) or *-s'* (plural) to the base word. (See Apostrophe, pages 447–448, for other examples.)

Number is usually indicated by addition of *-s* or *-es* to the base word, although some nouns (as those of foreign origin) have irregular plurals:

regular plurals

dog→dogs	grass→grasses
male→males	dish→dishes
X ray→X rays	buzz→buzzes
encephalograph→encephalographs	branch→branches

irregular, variant, and zero plurals
chemoreceptivity→chemoreceptivities
child→children
foot→feet
phenomenon→phenomena
fusarium→fusaria
matrix→matrices *or* matrixes
maximum→maxima *or* maximums
alga→algae
corpus delicti→corpora delicti
surgeon general→surgeons general
manus→manus
encephalitis→encephalitides
pediculosis→pediculoses

When in doubt of a plural spelling, the assistant should consult a dictionary. Nouns may be subgrouped according to type and function within a sentence as shown in the table on page 474.

Nouns may be used as follows in sentences:

1. as subjects
   The *office* was quiet.
2. as direct objects
   He locked the *office.*

3. as objects of prepositions
   The file is in the *office*.
4. as indirect objects
   He gave the *patient* the information.
5. as retained objects
   The patient was given the *information*.
6. as predicate nominatives
   Mr. Dow is the *administrator*.
7. as subjective complements
   Mr. Dow was named *administrator*.
8. as objective complements
   They made Mr. Dow *administrator*.
9. as appositives
   Mr. Dow, the *administrator,* wrote that memorandum.
10. in direct address
    Mr. Dow, may I present Mr. Lee?

Compound nouns Since English is not a static and unchanging entity, it experiences continuous style fluctuations because of preferences of its users. The styling (open, closed, or hyphened) variations of noun and other compounds reflect changing usage. No rigid rules can be set down to cover every possible variation or combination, nor can an all-inclusive list of compounds be given here. The assistant should consult a dictionary when in doubt of the styling of a compound.

Use of indefinite articles with nouns The use of *a* and *an* is not settled in all situations. In the examples below, some words or abbreviations beginning with a vowel letter nevertheless have a consonant as the first <u>sound</u> (as *one, union,* or *US*). Conversely, the names of some consonants begin with a vowel <u>sound</u> (as *F, H, L, M, N, R, S,* and *X*).

a

a. Before a word (or abbreviation) beginning with a consonant <u>sound</u>, *a* is usually spoken and written: *a BA degree, a CAT scanner, a door, a hat, a human, a one, a union, a US senator.*

b. Before *h-* in an unstressed (unaccented) or lightly stressed (lightly accented) first syllable, *a* is more frequently written, although *an* is more usual in speech whether or not the *h-* is actually pronounced. Either one certainly may be considered acceptable in speech or writing: *a historian—an historian, a heroic attempt—an heroic attempt, a hysterectomy—an hysterectomy.*

c. Before a word beginning with a vowel <u>sound</u>, *a* is occasionally used in speech: *a hour, a inquiry, a obligation.* (In some parts of the United States this may be more common than in others.)

an

a. Before a word beginning with a vowel <u>sound</u>, *an* is usually spoken and written: *an isoenzyme, an FDA ruling, an hour, an honor, an MIT professor, an nth degree polynomial, an orthopaedist, an Rh factor, an ultraviolet light source, an unknown.*

b. Before *h-* in an unstressed or lightly stressed syllable, *an* is more usually spoken whether or not the *h-* is pronounced, while *a* is more frequently written. Either may be considered acceptable in speech or writing. (See the examples above at point b.)

c. Sometimes *an* is spoken and written before a word beginning with a vowel in its spelling even though the first <u>sound</u> is a consonant: *an European city, an unique occurrence, such an one.* This is less frequent today than in the past and it is more common in Britain than in the United States.

d. Occasionally *an* is used in speech and writing before a stressed syllable beginning with *h-* in which the *h-* is pronounced: *an huntress, an heritage.* This is regularly the practice of the King James Version of the Old Testament.

Nouns Subgrouped According to Type and Function

Type of Noun	Function	Example
common nouns	identify general classes of things	[valley] [college] [company] [author]
proper nouns	identify particular members of classes of things, and are capitalized	[the Ohio Valley] [Amherst College] [The Macmillan Company] [Shakespeare]
abstract nouns	name qualities and ideas that do not have physical substance or configuration	[good] [evil] [honesty] [dishonesty] [science] [philosophy] [ruthlessness] [compassion]
concrete nouns	name animate and inanimate objects	[desk] [typewriter] [chair] [building] [floor] [ceiling] [finger] [abdomen]
mass nouns	identify things that are not ordinarily thought of in terms of numbered elements; they are usually singular in form, although in a few contexts the plural is appropriate especially when *types* of items within a class are being differentiated	[paper] [fruit] [water] [rice] [cotton] [Paper is costly today.] [Fruit is healthful.] [Water was scarce there.] [Rice grows in the Deep South.] [Cotton is raised in South Carolina.] *but* [Not all cottons have the same texture.]
count nouns	identify things considered as separate units that can be enumerated or counted NOTE: Many nouns have both count and non-count senses.	[paper clip] [peach] [desk] [chair] [five hundred paper clips] [many peaches] [two desks and various types of chairs] [Their firm manufactures the cloth for our book covers.] *but* [She used two cloths to cover the tray.]
collective nouns	identify things that can be construed either in terms of number or collectively; collective nouns are singular in form but are sometimes or always plural in construction	[The family was proud of her.] [The committee have been debating among themselves for an hour.] *but* [The group has decided.] [The mob was running wild.] [That audience was impolite.]

Preposition

prep·o·si·tion . . . *n* . . . : a linguistic form that combines with a noun, pronoun, or noun equivalent to form a phrase that typically has an adverbial, adjectival, or substantival relation to some other word

Prepositions are not characterized by inflection, number, case, gender, or identifying suffixes. Rather, they are identified chiefly by their positioning within sentences and by their grammatical functions.

Prepositions may occur in the following positions:

1. before nouns or pronouns
   below the desk
   beside them
2. after adjectives
   antagonistic *to*
   insufficient *in*
   symbolic *of*
3. after the verbal elements of idiomatically fixed verb + preposition combinations
   take *for*
   get *after*
   come *across*

Prepositions may be simple, i.e., composed of only one element (as *of, on, out, from, near, against,* or *without*); or they may be compound, i.e., composed of more than one element (as *according to, by means of,* or *in spite of*). Prepositions are chiefly used to link nouns, pronouns, or noun equivalents to the rest of a sentence:

He expected continued deterioration *in* the patient's condition.
I sat down *beside* her.

Prepositions may also be used to express the possessive:

one fourth *of* the employees
the top drawer *of* my desk

The following are general points of preposition usage:

Prepositions and conjunctions: confusion between the two   The words *after, before, but, for,* and *since* may function as either prepositions or conjunctions. Their positions within sentences clarify whether they are conjunctions or prepositions:

preposition	I have nothing left *but* hope.
	(*but* = "except for")
conjunction	I was a bit concerned *but* not panicky.
	(*but* links 2 adjectives)
preposition	The device conserves fuel *for* residual heating.
	(*for* + noun)
conjunction	The device conserves fuel, *for* it is battery-powered.
	(*for* links 2 clauses)

Implied or understood prepositions   If two words combine idiomatically with the same preposition, that preposition need not be repeated after both of them:

We were antagonistic [to] and opposed *to* the whole idea.
but
We are interested *in* and anxious *for* raises.

Prepositions terminating sentences   There is no reason why a preposition cannot end a sentence, especially when it is an essential element of an idiomatic, fixed verb phrase:

Their shyness must then be peculiar to the type of transcultural group they find themselves schooled *with*.
>   —*Adolescence*

What does all this add up *to?* Students used to believe when they entered medical school that if they worked . . . they would become professionals . . . deserving . . . respect.
>   —Irvine H. Page, MD

Use of *between* and *among*   The preposition *between* is ordinarily followed by words representing two persons or things:

between you and me

information exchange *between* the United States and the Soviet Union

and *among* is ordinarily followed by words representing more than two persons or things:

among the three of us
among various hospitals

However, *between* sometimes may be used to express an interrelationship between more than two things when those things are being considered individually rather than collectively:

. . . travels regularly *between* New York, Baltimore, and Washington.

Pronoun

> **pro·noun** . . . *n* . . . **:** a word belonging to one of the major form classes in any of a great many languages that is used as a substitute for a noun or noun equivalent, takes noun constructions, and refers to persons or things named or understood in the context

---

Pronouns exhibit all or some of the following characteristic features: case (nominative, possessive, objective), number (singular, plural), person (first, second, third person), and gender (masculine, feminine, neuter). Pronouns may be grouped according to major types and functions, as shown in the table on the next page.

Personal pronouns   A personal pronoun agrees in person, number, and gender with the word it refers to; however, the case of a pronoun is determined by its function within a sentence:

Everybody had *his* own office.
Everybody was given an office to *himself.*
Each employee was given an office to *himself.*
You and *I* thought the meeting was useful.
Just between *you* and *me*, the meeting was useful but far too lengthy.
My assistant and *I* attended the seminar.
The administrator told my assistant and *me* about the seminar.

The nominative case (as in the locutions "It is I" and "This is she") after the verb *to be* is considered standard English and is preferred by strict grammarians; however, the objective case (as in the locution "It's me") also may be used without criticism especially in spoken English.

   When a personal pronoun occurs in a construction introduced by *than* or *as*,

Types and Functions of Pronouns

Type of Pronoun	Function	Example
personal pronouns (such as *I, we, you, he, she, it, they*)	refer to beings and objects and reflect the person and gender of those antecedents	[Put the book on the table and close *it*.] [Put the baby in *his* crib and cover *him* up.]
reflexive pronouns (such as *myself, ourselves, yourself, yourselves, himself, herself, itself, themselves*)	express reflexive action on the subject of a sentence or add extra emphasis to the subject	[He hurt *himself*.] [They asked *themselves* if they were being honest.] [I *myself* am not afraid.]
indefinite pronouns (*all, another, any, anybody, anyone, anything, both, each, each one, either, everybody, everyone, everything, few, many, much, neither, nobody, none, no one, one, other, several, some, somebody, someone, something*)	are indistinguishable by gender, are chiefly used as third-person references, and do not distinguish gender	[*All* of the patients are here.] [*All* of them are here.] [Has *anyone* arrived?] [*Somebody* has called.] [Does *everyone* have his paper?] [*Nobody* has answered.] [A *few* have offered their suggestions.]
reciprocal pronouns	indicate interaction	[They do not quarrel with *one another*.] [Be nice to *each other*.]
demonstrative pronouns (*this, that, these, those*)	point things out	[*This* is your seat.] [*That* is mine.] [*These* belong to her.] [*Those* are strong words.]
relative pronouns (*who, whom, which, what, that, whose*) or combinations with *-ever* (as *whoever, whosever, whichever, whatever*)	introduce clauses acting as nouns or as modifiers	[The thrust of this memorandum is *that* there will be no cost overruns.] [I'll do *what* you want.] [I'll do *whatever* you want.]
interrogative pronouns (as *who, which, what, whoever, whichever, whatever*)	phrase direct questions	[*Who* is there?] [*What* is his title?] [His title is *what*?] [*Whom* did the article pan?] [*Whatever* is the matter?]

it should be in the nominative case:

I received a bigger bonus than *you* [did].
She has as much seniority as *I* [do].

The suffixes *-self* and *-selves* combine only with the possessive case of the first- and second-person pronouns (*myself, ourselves, yourself, yourselves*) and with the objective case of the third-person pronouns (*himself, herself, itself, themselves*). Other combinations (as "hisself" and "theirselves") are considered nonstandard and should not be used.

When one uses the pronoun *I* with other pronouns or with other peoples' names, *I* should be last in the series:

Mrs. Smith and *I* were trained together.

He and *I* were attending the meeting.

The memorandum was directed to Ms. Montgomery and *me*.

In composing letters for the doctor, the assistant should avoid using the pronoun *we* unless it has been dictated by the doctor or unless the practice is joint. The use of *we* could convey to the reader that the assistant is attempting to speak for the practice along with the doctor. The pronouns *I, he,* or *she* are more specific. Example:

Dr. Smith has asked *me* to thank you for sending *him* the reprint of your article that appeared in the January 1, 19— issue of the *Journal of the American Medical Association. He* has found the material to be most informative.

While the personal pronouns *it, you,* and *they* are often used as indefinite pronouns in spoken English, they can be vague or even redundant in some contexts and therefore should be avoided in precise writing:

vague	*explicit*
They said at the seminar that there would be a breakthrough in cancer research. (The question is: Who exactly is *they*?)	The doctors on the panel at the seminar predicted a breakthrough in cancer research.

redundant	*lean*
In the graph *it* says that hospital admissions fell off by 50%.	The graph indicates a 50% drop in hospital admissions.

Notwithstanding recent concern about sexism in language, the personal pronoun *he* and the indefinite pronoun *one* are still the standard substitutes for antecedents whose genders are mixed or irrelevant:

Each employee should check *his* W-2 form.

Present the letter to the physician for *his* approval.

If *one* really wants to succeed, *one* can.

Indefinite pronouns: agreement   Agreement in number between indefinite pronouns and verbs is sometimes a problem especially in contexts where the actual number of individuals represented by the pronoun is unclear. In some instances, there is also a conflict between written and spoken usage.

The following indefinite pronouns are clearly singular, and as such take singular verbs:

another	*much*	*other*
anything	*nobody*	*someone*
each one	*no one*	*something*
everything	*one*	

And these are clearly plural:

both
few
many
several

But depending on whether they are used with mass or count nouns, the following may be either singular or plural:

all	*none*
any	*some*
each	

with mass noun	*All* of the *equipment is* sterile.
with count noun	*All* of the *bandages are* sterile.

The following are singular in form, and as such logically take singular verbs; however, because of their plural connotations, informal speech has established the use of plural pronoun references to them:

anybody
anyone
everybody
everyone
somebody

The following citations illustrate usage variants involving indefinite pronouns:

. . . can hardly fail to occur to *anyone* who looks at the spectrum of the hydrogen atom . . . .
　　　　　　　—*Modern Astrophysics*

but

. . . it may be difficult for *anyone* to find *their* path through . . . a sort of maze.
　　　　　　　—Ford Madox Ford

. . . a small Mid-Western town were *everybody* knows you!
　　　　　　　—William A. Tyson, Jr.

Everybody drives just where *they* want to.
　　　　　　　—F. Scott Fitzgerald

Everybody has a right to describe *their* own party machine as *they* choose.
　　　　　　　—Winston Churchill

Everybody fights for *their* own team . . . .
　　　　　　　—Stuart Symington

I was calling *everybody* by *their* first names.
　　　　　　　—Marshall McLuhan

and

But *everyone* is aware that even the most lowly forms project on our consciousness an unmistakable flavor of identity.
　　　　　　　—*JAMA*

Somebody is always putting down a table of specifications for the good salesman.
　　　　　　　—*Printers' Ink*

but

Now that *everyone* goes to the Mediterranean for *their* holidays . . . .
　　　　　　　—*Times Literary Supplement*

. . . the minute *somebody* opens *their* mouth. . . . .
　　　　　　　—Robert A. Hall, Jr.

The question of number in pronoun phrases such as *each + of +* noun(s) or other pronoun(s), *none + of +* noun(s) or other pronoun(s), *either/neither + of +* noun(s) or other pronoun(s), and *some + of +* noun(s) or other pronoun(s), depends on the number of the headword. For example, when *either* means "one of two or more" or "any one of more than two," it is usually singular in construction and thus takes a singular verb. However, when *of* after *either* is followed by a plural, the verb that follows the whole phrase is often plural. This decision is really a matter of writer preference:

Either of the two measurements *is* standard.
Either of these measurements *is/are* standard.
or
Either of the two *is* satisfactory.
Either of them *are* satisfactory.

The word *none* involves similar variations:

. . . has two brothers and two sisters . . . *none* [i.e., *not any*] of them stutter.
        —*The Psychiatric Quarterly*

. . . *none* [i.e., *not any*] of us communicate this ideally or intellectually.
        —*Conjoint Family Therapy*

but

None [i.e., *not one*] of the larger viruses . . . has yielded . . . .
        —*Science*

Many systems . . . have been formulated but *none* [i.e., *not one*] of them is . . .
suitable.
        —*Biological Abstracts*

The indefinite pronoun *any* when used in comparisons   The indefinite pronoun
any is conventionally followed by *other(s)* or *else* when it forms part of a comparison of two individuals in the same class. Examples:

not   He is a better researcher than any in his field.
         (Is he a better researcher than all others including himself?)

but   He is a better researcher than any others in his field.
         He is a better researcher than anyone else in his field.

not   Boston is more interesting than any city in the U.S.
but   Boston is more interesting than any other city in the U.S.

Demonstrative pronouns   One problem involving demonstrative pronouns occurs
when a demonstrative introduces a sentence referring to an idea or ideas contained
in a previous sentence or sentences. One should be sure that the reference is definite and not cloudy:

a cloudy sentence
The heir's illness, the influence of a faith healer at court, massive military setbacks, general
strikes, mass outbreaks of typhus, and failed crops contributed to the revolution. *This* influenced the course of history.

*The question is: What exactly influenced the course of history? All of these factors, some
of them, or the last one mentioned?*

an explicit sentence
None of the participants in the incident kept records of what they said or did. *That* is quite
unfortunate, and it should be a lesson to us.

When demonstrative pronouns are used with the words *kind, sort,* and *type +* of
+ nouns, they should agree in number with both nouns:

not   We want these kind of pencils.
but   We want *this kind* of *pencil.*   *or*   We want *these kinds* of *pencils.*

Relative pronouns   While a relative pronoun itself does not exhibit number,
gender, or person, it does determine the number, gender, and person of the relative-clause elements that follow it because of its implicit agreement with its antecedent:

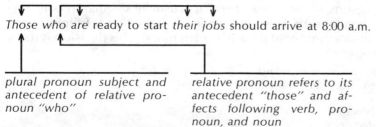

Those who are ready to start *their jobs* should arrive at 8:00 a.m.

plural pronoun subject and
antecedent of relative pronoun "who"

relative pronoun refers to its
antecedent "those" and affects following verb, pronoun, and noun

When the antecedent of a relative pronoun is doubtful (as when either of two nouns may be considered the antecedent), the number of the verb may vary according to the writer's preference. If a plural noun is closer to the verb, the writer may choose a plural verb. Examples:

He's one of those physicians who *worry* a lot.
or
He's a physician who *worries* a lot.

The relative pronoun *who* typically refers to persons and some animals; *which,* to things and animals; and *that,* to both beings and things:

a man *who* sought success

. . . a hummingbird *who* came to the bushes in front must have got very slim pickings.
    —Edmund Wilson

a drug *which* sold well
a dog *which* barked loudly

a drug *that* sold well
a dog *that* barked loudly
a man *that* we can trust

Relative pronouns can sometimes be omitted for the sake of brevity:

The man *whom* I was talking to is the chief resident.
or
The man I was talking to is the chief resident.

The relative pronoun *what* may be substituted for the longer and more awkward phrases "that which," "that of which," or "the thing which" in some sentences:

stiff   He was blamed for *that which* he could not have known.
easier   He was blamed for *what* he could not have known.

The problem of when to use *who* or *whom* has been blown out of proportion. The situation is very simple: standard written English makes a distinction between the nominative and objective cases of these pronouns when they are used as relatives or interrogatives, as

Who is she?
Who does she think she is, anyway?
She thinks she is the one *who* ought to be promoted.
She's the one individual *who* I think should be promoted.
Give me a list of the ones *who* you think should be promoted.
but
Whom are you referring to?
To *whom* are you referring?
He's a man *whom* everyone should know.
He's a man with *whom* everyone should be acquainted.

In speech, however, case distinctions and boundaries often become blurred, with the result that spoken English favors *who* as a general substitute for all uses of *whom* except in set phrases as "*To whom* it may concern." *Who,* then, may be used without criticism as the subject of the clause it introduces, as

I serve *who* I like.
    —*Irish Digest*

and *who* may be used as the object of a verb in a clause that it introduces, as

. . . old peasants . . . *who,* if isolated from their surroundings, one would expect to see in a village church. . . .
    —John Berger

Then I would have him select *who* he thought could make the best . . . candidate.
    —Joseph Napolitan

Who is used less frequently, however, as the object of a preceding or following preposition in the clause that it introduces:

. . . of *who* I know nothing.   *Who* are you going to listen to, anyway. . . .
                —Raymond Paton   —*National Review*

The relative pronoun *whoever* likewise lends itself without criticism to flexible grammatical relationships:

. . . performs a self-assigned role to win a . . . response from *whoever* may be witnesses.
                —*Saturday Review*

Whoever he picks has to have the stature of a collaborator, not a subordinate. . . .
                —*Time*

or

. . . permit the Mayor to name *whomever* he liked.
                —*Saturday Review*

. . . *whomever* this alleged autobiography . . . is about, it is a real life. . . .
                —*Springfield* (Mass.) *City Library Bulletin*

---

	verb . . . *n* . . . : a word that characteristically is the grammatical center of a predicate and expresses an act, occurrence, or mode of being, that in various languages is inflected for agreement with the subject, for tense, for voice, for mood, or for aspect, and that typically has rather full descriptive meaning and characterizing quality but is sometimes nearly devoid of these esp. when used as an
Verb	auxiliary or copula

Verbs exhibit the following characteristic features: inflection (*help, helps, helping, helped*), person (first, second, third person), number (singular, plural), tense (present, past, future), aspect (time relations other than the simple present, past, and future), voice (active, passive), mood (indicative, subjunctive, imperative), and suffixation (as by the typical suffixal markers -*ate*, -*en*, -*ify*, and -*ize*).

Regular verbs have four inflected forms signaled by the suffixes -*s* or -*es*, -*ed*, and -*ing*. The verb *help* as shown in the first sentence above is regular. Most irregular verbs have four or five forms, as

bring	*see*
brings	*sees*
bringing	*seeing*
brought	*saw*
	seen

but some, like *can, ought, put,* and *spread,* have fewer forms, as

can	*ought*	*put*	*spread*
could		*puts*	*spreads*
		putting	*spreading*

and one, the verb *be,* has eight:

be	*being*
is	*was*
am	*were*
are	*been*

When one is uncertain about a particular inflected form, one should consult a dictionary that indicates not only the inflections of irregular verbs but also those inflections resulting in changes in base-word spelling, as

blame; blamed; blaming
spy; spied; spying
picnic; picnicked; picnicking

in addition to variant inflected forms, as

bias; biased or *biassed; biasing* or *biassing*
counsel; counseled or *counselled; counseling* or *counselling*
diagram; diagramed or *diagrammed; diagraming* or *diagramming*
travel; traveled or *travelled; traveling* or *travelling*

all of which may be found at their applicable entries in *Webster's New Collegiate Dictionary.*

There are, however, a few rules that will aid one in ascertaining the proper spelling patterns of certain verb forms. These are as follows:

1. Verbs ending in a silent -*e* generally retain the -*e* before consonant suffixes (as -*s*) but drop the -*e* before vowel suffixes (as -*ed* and -*ing*):

   arrange; arranges; arranged; arranging
   hope; hopes; hoped; hoping
   require; requires; required; requiring
   shape; shapes; shaped; shaping

   Other such verbs are: *agree, arrive, conceive, grieve, imagine,* and *value.*

   NOTE: A few verbs ending in a silent -*e* retain the -*e* even before vowel suffixes in order to avoid confusion with other words:

   dye; dyes; dyed; dyeing (vs. *dying*)
   singe; singes; singed; singeing (vs. *singing*)

2. Monosyllabic verbs ending in a single consonant preceded by a single vowel double the final consonant before vowel suffixes (as -*ed* and -*ing*):

   gel; gelled; gelling
   grip; gripped; gripping
   pin; pinned; pinning

3. Polysyllabic verbs ending in a single consonant preceded by a single vowel and having an accented last syllable double the final consonant before vowel suffixes (as -*ed* and -*ing*):

   commit; committed; committing
   control; controlled; controlling
   occur; occurred; occurring
   omit; omitted; omitting

   NOTE: The final consonant of such verbs is not doubled when

   a. two vowels occur before the final consonant, as
      daub; daubed; daubing
      spoil; spoiled; spoiling

   b. two consonants form the ending, as
      help; helped; helping
      lurk; lurked; lurking
      peck; pecked; pecking

4. Verbs ending in -*y* preceded by a consonant regularly change the -*y* to -*i* before all suffixes except those beginning with -*i* (as -*ing*):

   carry; carried; carrying
   marry; married; marrying
   study; studied; studying

   NOTE: If the final -*y* is preceded by a vowel, it remains unchanged in suffixation, as

delay; delayed; delaying
enjoy; enjoyed; enjoying
obey; obeyed; obeying

5. Verbs ending in -c add a -k when a suffix beginning with -e or -i is appended, as

   mimic; mimics; mimicked; mimicking
   panic; panics; panicked; panicking
   traffic; traffics; trafficked; trafficking

   And words derived from this type of verb also add a k when such suffixes are added to them, as

   panicky
   trafficker

English verbs exhibit their two simple tenses by use of two single-word grammatical forms:

simple present = *do*
simple past   = *did*

The future is expressed by *shall/will* + verb infinitive:

I *shall do* it.
he *will do* it.

or by use of the present or progressive forms in a revealing context, as

I *leave* shortly for New York. (present)
I *am leaving* shortly for New York. (progressive)

Aspect is a property that allows verbs to indicate time relations other than the simple present, past, or future tenses. Aspect covers these relationships:

action occurring in the past and continuing to the present	has seen	*present perfect tense*
action completed at a past time or before the immediate past	had seen	*past perfect tense*
action that will have been completed by a future time	will have seen	*future perfect tense*
action occurring now	is seeing	*progressive*

In contexts that require it, the perfective and the progressive aspects can be combined to yield special verb forms, as

had been seeing

Voice enables a verb to indicate whether the subject of a sentence is acting (he *loves* = active voice) or whether the subject is being acted upon (he *is loved* = passive voice).

Mood indicates manner of expression. The indicative mood states a fact or asks a question (He *is* here. *Is* he here?). The subjunctive mood expresses condition contrary to fact (I wish that he *were* here). The imperative mood expresses a command or request (*Come* here. Please *come* here).

Verbs may be used transitively; that is, they may act upon direct objects, as

She *contributed* money.

or they may be used intransitively; that is, they may not have direct objects to act upon, as

She *contributed* generously.

There is another group of words derived from verbs and called *verbals* that deserve added discussion. The members of this group—the gerund, the participle, and the infinitive—exhibit some but not all of the characteristic features of their parent verbs.

A gerund is an -*ing* verb form, but it functions mainly as a noun. It has both the active (*seeing*) and the passive (*being seen*) voices. In addition to voice, a gerund's verbal characteristics are as follows: it conveys the notion of a verb—i.e., action of some sort; it can take an object; and it can be modified by an adverb. Examples:

Typing tabular *data daily* is a boring task.

gerund   noun object   adverb

He liked *driving cars fast.*

gerund   noun object   adverb

Nouns and pronouns occurring before gerunds are expressed by the possessive:

Her typing is good.
She is trying to improve *her typing.*
We objected to *their reproducing* our data.
We saw the *boy's whipping.* (i.e., the boy being whipped)
We expected the *physician's coming.* (i.e., his or her arrival)

Participles, on the other hand, function as adjectives and may occur alone (a *broken* typewriter) or in phrases that modify other words (*Having broken the typewriter,* she gave up for the day). Participles have active and passive forms like gerunds. Examples:

active-voice participial phrase modifying "he"
Having failed to pass the examination, he was forced to repeat the course.

passive-voice participial phrase modifying "he"
Having been failed by his instructor, he was forced to repeat the course.

Participles, unlike gerunds, are not preceded by possessive nouns or pronouns:

We saw the *boy whipping* his dog. (i.e., we saw the boy doing the whipping)
We saw the *physician coming.* (i.e., we saw him or her arrive)

Infinitives may exhibit active (*to do*) and passive (*to be done*) voices and they may indicate aspect (*to be doing, to have done, to have been doing, to have been done*).

Infinitives may take complements and may be modified by adverbs. In addition, they can function as nouns, adjectives, and adverbs in sentences. Examples:

noun use
To be known is *to be castigated.*
(subject)   (subjective complement)
He tried everything except *to bypass his superior.*
(object of preposition *except*)

adjectival use
They had found a way *to improve results* greatly.
(modifies the noun *way*)

adverbial use
He was too furious *to speak.*
(modifies *furious*)

Although *to* is the characteristic marker of an infinitive, it is not always stated but may be understood:

He helped [to] complete the pathology report.

The following are general points of verb and verbal usage:

Sequence of tenses If the main verb in a sentence is in the present tense, any other tense or compound verb form may follow it in subsequent clauses, as

I *realize* that you *are leaving.*
I *realize* that you *left.*
I *realize* that you *were leaving.*
I *realize* that you *have been leaving.*
I *realize* that you *had left.*
I *realize* that you *had been leaving.*
I *realize* that you *will be leaving.*
I *realize* that you *will leave.*
I *realize* that you *will have been leaving.*
I *realize* that you *can be leaving.*
I *realize* that you *may be leaving.*
I *realize* that you *must be leaving.*

If the main verb is in the past tense, that tense imposes time restrictions on any subsequent verbs in the sentence, thus excluding use of the present tense, as

I *realized* that you *were leaving.*
I *realized* that you *left.*
I *realized* that you *had left.*
I *realized* that you *had been leaving.*
I *realized* that you *would be leaving.*
I *realized* that you *could be leaving.*
I *realized* that you *might be leaving.*
I *realized* that you *would leave.*

If the main verb is in the future tense, it imposes time restrictions on subsequent verbs in the sentence, thus excluding the possibility of using the simple past tense, as

He *will see* you because he *is going* to the meeting too.
He *will see* you because he *will be going* to the meeting too.
He *will see* you because he *will go* to the meeting too.
He *will see* you because he *has been going* to the meetings too.
He *will see* you because he *will have been going* to the meetings too.

In general, most writers try to maintain an order of tenses throughout their sentences that is consistent with natural or real time, e.g., present tense = present-time matters, past tense = past matters, and future tense = matters that will take place in the future. However, there are two outstanding exceptions to these principles:

a. If one is discussing the contents of printed or published material, one conventionally uses the present tense, as

In *Medical Writing,* Morris Fishbein *discusses* style.

This report *gives* the laboratory test values needed.

In her latest paper on alcohol/drug abuse, Dr. Lee *writes* that . . . .

b. If one wishes to add the connotation of immediacy to a particular sentence, one may use the present tense instead of the future, as

I *leave* for the hospital tonight.

c. The sequence of tenses in sentences which express contrary-to-fact conditions is a special problem frequently encountered in writing. The examples below show the sequence correctly maintained:

If he *were* on time, we *would leave* now.

If he *had been* (not *would have been*) on time, we *would have left* an hour ago.

Subject-verb agreement   Verbs agree in number and in person with their grammatical subjects. At times, however, the grammatical subject may be singular in form, but the thought it carries—i.e., the logical subject—may have plural connotations. Here are some general guidelines:

a.   Plural and compound subjects take plural verbs even if the subject is inverted. Examples:
Neuropharmacology and psychopharmacology *are* grouped under the heading "pharmacology."
Both dogs and cats *were* tested for the virus.

b.   Compound subjects or plural subjects conveying a unitary idea take singular verbs in American English. Examples:
McKesson & Robbins *is* a pharmaceutical company.
Five hundred dollars *is* a stiff fee.
but:
Twenty-five milligrams of pentazocine *were* administered.

c.   Compound subjects expressing mathematical relationships may be either singular or plural. Examples:
One plus one *makes* (or *make*) two.
Six from eight *leaves* (or *leave*) two.

d.   Singular subjects joined by *or* or *nor* take singular verbs; plural subjects so joined take plural verbs. Examples:
A CMA-A or a CMA-AC *is* eligible for the position.
Neither CMA-A's nor CMA-C's *are* eligible for the position.
If one subject is singular and the other plural, the verb usually agrees with the number of the subject that is closer to it. Examples:
Either the staff nurses or the supervisor *has* to do the job.
Either the supervisor or the staff nurses *have* to do the job.

e.   Singular subjects introduced by *many a, such a, every, each,* or *no* take singular verbs, even when several such subjects are joined by *and:*
Many a physician *has* studied in Vienna.
No supervisor and no nurse *is* excused from the staff meeting.
Every needle, syringe, and narcotic *has* to be accounted for.

f.   The agreement of the verb with its grammatical subject ordinarily should not be skewed by an intervening phrase even if the phrase contains plural elements. Examples:
One of my reasons for resigning *involves* purely personal considerations.
The hospital administrator, as well as members of his staff, *has* arrived.
He, not any of the proxy voters, *has* to be present.

g.   The verb *to be* agrees with its grammatical subject, and not with its complement:
Her complaint *was* gastrointestinal distress and dizziness.
In addition, the verb *to be* introduced by the word *there* must agree in number with the subject following it. Examples:

There *are* many complications here.

There *is* no reason to worry about him.

NOTE: For discussion of verb agreement with indefinite-pronoun subjects, see pages 478–479. For discussion of verb number as affected by a compound subject whose elements are joined by *and/or,* see page 470.

Linking and *sense* verbs   Linking verbs (as the various forms of *to be*) and the so-called "sense" verbs (as *feel, look, taste, smell,* as well as particular senses of *appear, become, continue, grow, prove, remain, seem, stand,* and *turn*) connect subjects with predicate nouns or adjectives. The latter group often cause confusion, in that adverbs are mistakenly used in place of adjectives after these verbs. Examples:

He *is* an administrator.

He *became* administrator.

The temperature *continues* normal.

The patient's color *looks* bilious.

I *feel* awful.

This medication *tastes* good.

The ointment *smells* nice.

He *remains* healthy.

Split infinitives   The writer who consciously avoids splitting infinitives regardless of resultant awkwardness or changes in meaning is as immature in his or her position as the writer who consciously splits all infinitives as a sort of rebellion against convention. Actually, the use of split infinitives is no rebellion at all, because this construction has long been employed by a wide variety of distinguished English writers—Wycliffe, Byron, Coleridge, Browning (at least 23 times, according to one scholarly source), and Spenser—to name a few. Indeed, the split infinitive can be a useful device for the writer who wishes to delineate a shade of meaning or direct special emphasis to a word or group of words—emphasis that cannot be achieved with an undivided infinitive construction. For example, in the locution

to *thoroughly* complete the physical examination

the position of the adverb as close as possible to the verbal element of the whole infinitive phrase strengthens the effect of the adverb on the verbal element—a situation that is not necessarily true in the following reworded locutions:

to complete *thoroughly* the physical examination

thoroughly to complete the physical examination

to complete the physical examination *thoroughly*

In other instances, the position of the adverb may actually modify or change the entire meaning, as

original	*recast with new meanings*
. . . arrived in New York to *unexpectedly* find it in print.	. . . arrived in New York *unexpectedly* to find it in print.
—Harrison Smith	. . . arrived in New York to find it in print *unexpectedly.*

The main point is this: If the writer wishes to stress the verbal element of an infinitive or wishes to express a thought that is more clearly and easily shown with *to* + adverb + infinitive, such split infinitives are acceptable. However, very long adverbial modifiers such as

He wanted to *completely and carefully* examine the patient.

are clumsy and should be avoided or recast, as

He wanted to examine the patient *completely and carefully*.

Dangling participles and infinitives   Careful writers avoid danglers (as participles or infinitives occurring in a sentence without having a normally expected syntactic relation to the rest of the sentence) that may create confusion for the reader or seem ludicrous. Examples:

dangling	Falling out of bed, the patient's arm was broken.
recast	Having fallen out of bed, the patient broke her arm.
	The patient's arm was broken when she fell out of bed.
	The patient broke her arm when she fell out of bed.
dangling	Caught in the act, his excuses were unconvincing.
recast	Caught in the act, he could not make his excuses convincing.
dangling	Having been told that he was seriously ill, the physician admitted the patient to the hospital.
recast	Having told the patient that he was seriously ill, the physician had him admitted to the hospital.
	Having been told by his physician that he was seriously ill, the patient was admitted to the hospital.

Participial use should not be confused with prepositional use especially with words like *concerning, considering, providing, regarding, respecting, touching,* etc., as illustrated below:

prepositional usage
Concerning your complaint, we can tell you. . . .
Considering all the implications, you have made a dangerous decision.
Touching the matter at hand, we can say that. . . .

Having examined the eight parts of speech individually in order to pinpoint their respective characteristics and functions, we now view their performance in the broader environments of the phrase, the clause, and the sentence.

PHRASES
A phrase is a brief expression that consists of two or more grammatically related words and that may contain either a noun or a finite verb (i.e., a verb that shows grammatical person and number) but not both, and that often functions as a particular part of speech within a clause or a sentence. The table on page 490 lists and describes seven basic types of phrases.

CLAUSES
A clause is a group of words containing both a subject and a predicate and functioning as an element of a compound or a complex sentence (see pages 492–497 for discussion of sentences). The two general types of clauses are:

independent	It is hot, and I feel faint.
dependent	Because it is hot, I feel faint.

Like phrases, clauses can perform as particular parts of speech within a total sentence environment. The table on page 491 describes such performance.

Clauses that modify may also be described as restrictive or nonrestrictive. Whether a clause is restrictive or nonrestrictive has direct bearing on sentence punctuation.

Types of Phrases

Type of Phrase	Description	Example
noun phrase	consists of a noun and its modifiers	[*The concrete building* is huge.]
verb phrase	consists of a finite verb and any other terms that modify it or that complete its meaning	[She *will have arrived too late* for you to talk to her.]
gerund phrase	is a nonfinite verbal phrase that functions as a noun	[*Sitting on a patient's bed* is bad hospital etiquette.]
participial phrase	is a nonfinite verbal phrase that functions as an adjective	[*Listening all the time in great concentration,* he lined up his options.]
infinitive phrase	is a nonfinite verbal phrase that may function as a noun, an adjective, or an adverb	[*To do that* will be stupid.] [This was a performance *to remember.*] [It would be highly improper *to bypass your superior.*]
prepositional phrase	consists of a preposition and its object(s) and may function as a noun, an adjective, or an adverb	[Here is the desk *with the extra file drawer.*] [He now walked *without a limp.*] [*Out of here* is where I'd like to be!]
absolute phrase	is also called a nominative absolute, consists of a noun + a predicate form (as a participle), and acts independently within a sentence without modifying a particular element of the sentence	[He stalked out, *his eyes staring straight ahead.*]

Restrictive clauses are the so-called "bound" modifiers. They are absolutely essential to the meaning of the word or words they modify, they cannot be omitted without the meaning of the sentences being radically changed, and they are unpunctuated. Examples:

Women who aren't competitive should not aspire to high corporate office.

   ↑ | ↑
  no   *restrictive*   *no*
punctuation   *clause*   *punctuation*

In this example, the restrictive clause limits the classification of women, and as such is essential to the total meaning of the sentence. If, on the other hand, the restrictive clause is omitted as shown below, the classification of women is now not limited at all, and the sentence conveys an entirely different notion:

Women should not aspire to high corporate office.

Basic Types of Clauses with Part-of-speech Functions

Type of Clause	Description	Example
noun clause	fills a noun slot in a sentence and thus can be a subject, an object, or a complement	[*Whoever is qualified* should apply.] [I do not know *what his field is.*] [Route that journal to *whichever department you wish.*] [The trouble is *that she has no ambition.*]
adjective clause	modifies a noun or pronoun and typically follows the word it modifies	[His office assistant, *who was also a nurse,* was overworked.] [I can't see the reason *why you're uptight.*] [He is a man *who will succeed.*] [Anybody *who opts for a career like that* is crazy.]
adverb clause	modifies a verb, an adjective, or another adverb and typically follows the word it modifies	[They made a valiant effort, *although the risks were great.*] [I'm certain *that he is ill.*] [We accomplished less *than we did before.*]

Nonrestrictive clauses are the so-called "free" modifiers: They are not inextricably bound to the word or words they modify but instead convey additional information about them, they may be omitted altogether without the meaning of the sentence being radically changed, and they are set off by commas. Examples:

Our guide, who wore a green beret, was an experienced traveler.

    ↑ | ↑
  comma   *nonrestrictive*   *comma*
              clause

Obviously, the guide's attire is not essential to his experience as a traveler. Removal of the nonrestrictive clause does not affect the meaning of the sentence:

Our guide was an experienced traveler.

The following are basic points of clause usage:

Elliptical clauses   Some clause elements may be omitted if the context makes clear the understood elements:

I remember the first time [that] we met.
This typewriter is better than that [typewriter is].
When [she is] on the job, she is always competent and alert.

Clause placement   In order to achieve maximum clarity and to avoid the possibility that the reader will misinterpret what he reads, one should place a modifying clause as close as possible to the word or words it modifies. If intervening words cloud the overall meaning of the sentence, one must recast it. Examples:

cloudy   A memorandum is a piece of business writing, less formal than a letter, which serves as a means of interoffice communication.

The question is: Does the letter or the memorandum serve as a means of interoffice communication?

recast   A memorandum, less formal than a letter, is a means of interoffice communication.

Tagged-on *which* clauses Tagging on a "which" clause that refers to the total idea of a sentence is a usage fault that should be avoided by careful writers. Examples:

tagged-on	*recast*
The clinic is expanding, which I personally think is a wise move.	The expansion of the clinic is a wise move in my opinion.
	or
	I believe that the physicians' decision to expand the clinic is wise.

SENTENCES

A sentence is a grammatically self-contained unit that consists of a word or a group of syntactically related words and that expresses a statement (declarative sentence), asks a question (interrogative sentence), expresses a request or command (imperative sentence), or expresses an exclamation (exclamatory sentence). A sentence typically contains both a subject and a predicate, begins with a capital letter, and ends with a punctuation mark. The following table illustrates the three main types of sentences classified by their grammatical structure.

Sentences Classified by their Grammatical Structure

Description	Example
simple sentence is a complete grammatical unit having one subject and one predicate, either or both of which may be compound	[*Paper* is costly.] [*Bond* and *tissue* are costly.] [*Bond* and *tissue* are costly and *are* sometimes scarce.]
compound sentence comprises two or more independent clauses	[*I could arrange to arrive late, or I could simply send a proxy.*] [*This commute takes at least forty minutes by car, but we can make it in twenty by train.*] [*A few of the researchers had PhDs, even more of them had MDs, but the majority of them had both MSs and MDs.*]
complex sentence combines one independent clause with one or more dependent clauses (dependent clauses are italicized in examples)	[The committee meeting began *when the administrator and the chief of staff walked in.*] [*Although the new drug has been effective in reducing advanced bladder cancer,* it is not yet approved.]

How to construct sentences The following paragraphs outline general guidelines for the construction of grammatically sound sentences.

One should maintain sentence coordination by use of connectives linking phrases and clauses of equal rank. Examples:

faulty coordination with improper use of "and"
I was sitting in on a meeting, and he stood up and started a long rambling discourse on a new development in radiology.

recast with one clause subordinated
I sat in on a meeting during which he stood up and rambled on about a new development in radiology.

or—recast into two sentences
I sat in on that meeting. He stood up and rambled on about a new development in radiology.

faulty coordination with improper use of "and"
This company employs a full-time research staff and was founded in 1945.

recast with one clause subordinated
This company, which employs a full-time research staff, was founded in 1945.

or—recast with one clause reworded into a phrase
Established in 1945, this company employs a full-time research staff.

One should also maintain parallel, balanced sentence elements in order to achieve good sentence structure. Examples illustrating this particular point are as follows:

unparallel
The report gives statistics, but he does not list his sources for these figures.

parallel
The report gives statistics, but it does not list the sources for these figures.

unparallel
We are glad to have you as our patient, and please call us whenever you need help.

parallel
We are glad to have you as our patient, and we hope that you will call on us whenever you need help.

or recast into two sentences
We are glad to have you as our patient. Please do call on us whenever you need help.

Loose linkages of sentence elements such as those caused by excessive use of *and* should be avoided by careful writers. Some examples of this type of faulty coordination are shown below:

faulty coordination/excessive use of "and"
The XYZ Medical Center is a service-teaching facility, and its central laboratories serve four separate hospitals with a combined bed capacity of 2,000 and a 1,000-patient-per-day outpatient clinic.

recast into two shorter, more effective sentences
The XYZ Medical Center—a service-teaching facility—contains central laboratories serving four separate hospitals. These hospitals have a combined bed capacity of 2,000 as well as a 1,000-patient-per-day outpatient clinic.

In constructing one's sentences effectively, one should choose the conjunction that best expresses the intended meaning. Examples:

not
Overcrowding was a problem *and* we had to decentralize the labs.

but
We had to decentralize the labs *because* overcrowding was a problem.
Overcrowding was a problem, *so* we had to decentralize the labs.

or recast to
Overcrowding forced us to decentralize the labs.

Good writers avoid unnecessary grammatical shifts that interrupt the reader's train of thought and needlessly complicate the material. Some unnecessary grammatical shifts are shown below, and improvements are also illustrated:

unnecessary shifts in verb voice
Any information you *can give* us *will be* greatly *appreciated* and we *assure* you that discretion *will be exercised* in its use.

rephrased (note the italicized all-active verb voice)
We *will appreciate* any information that you *can give* us. We *assure* you that we *will use* it with discretion.

unnecessary shifts in person
One can use either erasers or correcting fluid to remove typographical errors; however, *you* should make certain that *your* corrections are clean.

rephrased (note that the italicized pronouns are consistent)
One can use either erasers or correcting fluid to eradicate errors; however, *one* should make certain that *one's* corrections are clean.
or
You can use either erasers or correcting fluid to eradicate errors; however, *you* should make certain that *your* corrections are clean.

unnecessary shift from phrase to clause
Because of the physician's vacation and *we are short-handed in the office,* we cannot book any appointments now.

rephrased
Because of the physician's vacation and a shortage of office personnel, we cannot book any appointments now.
or
Because the physician is on vacation and the office staff is short-handed, we cannot book any appointments now.

Always keeping in mind the reader's reaction, the writer should strive for a rational ordering of sentence elements. Closely related elements, for example, should be placed as close together as possible for the sake of maximum clarity. Examples:

not
We would appreciate your sending us the material on health insurance claims by mail or cable.
but
We would appreciate your sending us by mail or by cable the material on health insurance claims.
or
We would appreciate your mailing or cabling us the health insurance claims material.
or
We would appreciate it if you would mail or cable us the health insurance claims material.

One should ensure that one's sentences form complete, independent grammatical units containing both a subject and a predicate, unless the material is dialogue or specialized copy where fragmentation may be used for particular reasons (as to reflect speech or to attract the reader's attention). Examples:

poor
During the last three years, our anticoagulant sales soared. While our narcotic analgesic sales fell off.
better
During the last three years, our anticoagulant sales soared, but our narcotic analgesic sales fell off.

or, with different emphasis
While our narcotic analgesic sales fell off during the last three years, our anticoagulant sales soared.

sentences featuring the imperative for special effects
Come with me; I'm going to
visit the mother of a
Down's syndrome child. She
has much to tell us.
Listen while she speaks.
—Ralph Crawshaw, MD
Modern Medicine

sentences intended for advertising
A full line of quality generic products . . .
at the lowest possible price.

Sentence length   Sentence length is directly related to the writer's purpose: there is no magic number of words that guarantees a good sentence. For example, a writer covering broad and yet complex topics (as in a long memorandum) may choose concise, succinct sentences for the sake of clarity, impact, fast dictation, and reading. On the other hand, a writer wishing to elicit the reader's reflection upon what is being said may employ longer, more involved sentences. Still another writer may juxtapose long and short sentences to emphasize an important point. The longer sentences may build up to a climactic and forceful short sentence.

Sentence strategy   Stylistically, there are two basic types of sentences—the periodic and the cumulative or loose. The periodic sentence is structured so that its main idea or its thrust is suspended until the very end, thereby drawing the reader's eye and mind along to an emphatic conclusion:

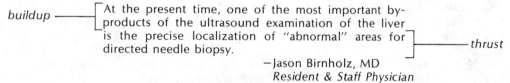

buildup ⎡At the present time, one of the most important by-
⎣products of the ultrasound examination of the liver
is the precise localization of "abnormal" areas for⎤
directed needle biopsy.   ⎦ —*thrust*
—Jason Birnholz, MD
Resident & Staff Physician

The cumulative sentence, on the other hand, is structured so that its main thought or its thrust appears first, followed by other phrases or clauses expanding on or supporting it:

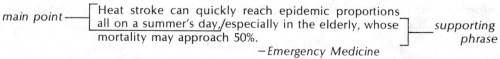

main point ⎡Heat stroke can quickly reach epidemic proportions
⎣all on a summer's day,/especially in the elderly, whose⎤ *supporting*
mortality may approach 50%.   ⎦ *phrase*
—*Emergency Medicine*

The final phrase in a cumulative sentence theoretically could be deleted without skewing or destroying the essential meaning of the total sentence. A cumulative sentence is therefore more loosely structured than a periodic sentence.

A writer may employ yet another strategy to focus the reader's attention on a problem or an issue. This device is the rhetorical question—a question that requires no specific response from the reader but often merely sets up the introduction of the writer's own views. In some instances, a rhetorical question works as a topic sentence in a paragraph; in other instances, a whole series of rhetorical questions may spotlight pertinent issues for the reader's consideration. The following excerpts illustrate rhetorical questions in action:

rhetorical question as ————— What should physicians do about the problem?
a topic sentence —————— Two important suggestions relate to protecting yourself
through how you practice: explain matters carefully to
author answers question ——— patients and write thorough notes on charts, explaining
posed earlier —————— your thinking at each step.
            —*Resident & Staff Physician*

series or rhetorical —————— Should one reassure that crocky patient over the phone,
questions focus on —————— or does this new complaint warrant an office visit?
specific issues —————— Is this chest pain something to be dismissed, or should
the patient go directly to the emergency room?
            —Michael J. Halberstam, MD

A writer uses either coordination or subordination or a mixture of both to create different stylistic effects. As shown in the subsection on clauses, coordination links independent sentences and sentence elements by means of coordinating conjunctions, while subordination transforms elements into dependent structures by means of subordinating conjunctions. While coordination tends to promote rather loose sentence structure which can become a fault, subordination tends to tighten the structure and to focus attention on a main clause. Examples:

coordination
During 1976, the 14 institutes sponsored 300 professional meetings *and* published 18 medical periodicals.
subordination
While the 14 institutes sponsored 300 professional meetings during 1976, they *also* published 18 medical journals.

A reversal of customary or expected sentence order is yet another effective stylistic strategy, when used sparingly, because it injects a dash of freshness, unexpectedness, and originality into the prose. Examples:

customary or expected order
I find that these realities are indisputable: the economy has taken a drastic downturn, health care costs have soared, and jobs are at a premium.
reversal
That the economy has taken a drastic downturn; that health care costs have soared; that jobs are at a premium—these are the realities that I find indisputable.

Interrupting the normal flow of discourse by inserting comments is a strategy that some writers employ to call attention to an aside, to emphasize a word or phrase, to render special effects (as forcefulness), or to make the prose a little more informal. Since too many interrupting elements may distract the reader and disrupt his train of thought, they should be used with discretion. Examples:

an aside   His evidence, if reliable, could constitute a major breakthrough.
emphasis   The vast majority—85% in fact—of renal stones are calcium phosphate, calcium oxalate, or mixtures of these minerals.
            —Philip H. Henneman, MD

While interruption breaks up the flow of discourse, parallelism and balance work together toward maintaining an even rhythmic flow of thoughts. Parallelism means a similarity in the grammatical construction of adjacent phrases and clauses that are equivalent, complementary, or antithetical in meaning. Examples:

These ecological problems are of crucial concern *to* scientists, *to* businessmen, *to* government officials, and *to* all citizens.

Our attorneys have argued *that* the trademark is ours, *that* our rights have been violated, and *that* appropriate compensation is required.

He was respected not only *for his intelligence* but also *for his integrity*.

Balance is the juxtaposition and equipoise of two or more syntactically parallel constructions (as phrases and clauses) that contain similar, contrasting, or opposing ideas, as shown in the following general quotations:

To err is human; to forgive, divine.
        —Alexander Pope

Ask not what your country can do for you—ask what you can do for your country.
        —John F. Kennedy

And finally, a series can be an effective way to emphasize a thought and to establish a definite rhythmic prose pattern:

The thing that interested me . . . about New York . . . was the . . . contrast it showed between the dull and the shrewd, the strong and the weak, the rich and the poor, the wise and the ignorant. . . .
        —Theodore Dreiser

PARAGRAPHS

The underlying structure of any written communication—be it a memorandum, a letter, or a report—must be controlled by the writer if the material is to be clear, coherent, logical in orientation, and effective. Since good paragraphing is a means to this end, it is essential that the writer be facile when using techniques of paragraph development and transition between paragraphs. While the writer is responsible for the paragraphing system, the assistant still should be able to recognize various kinds of paragraphs and their functions as well as the potential problems that often arise in structuring a logical paragraph system. In this way, the assistant can aid the writer, especially by pointing out possible discrepancies that might result in misinterpretation by the reader or that might detract from the total effect of the communication.

A paragraph is a subdivision in writing that consists of one or more sentences, that deals with one or more ideas, or that quotes a speaker or a source. The first line of a paragraph is indented in reports, studies, articles, theses, and books. However, the first line of a paragraph in business letters may or may not be indented, depending on the style being followed. See Chapter 15, section 15.7, for business-letter styling.

Uses of paragraphs   Paragraphs should not be considered as isolated entities that are self-contained and mechanically lined up without transitions or interrelationship of ideas. Rather, paragraphs should be viewed as components of larger groups or blocks that are tightly interlinked and that interact in the sequential development of a major idea or cluster of ideas. The overall coherence of a communication depends on this interaction.

Individual paragraphs and paragraph blocks are flexible: their length, internal structure, and purpose vary according to the writer's intention and his own style. For example, one writer may be able to express his point in a succinct, one-sentence paragraph, while another may require several sentences to make his point. Writers' concepts of paragraphing also differ. For instance, some writers think of paragraphs as a means of dividing their material into logical segments with each unit developing one particular point in depth and in detail. Others view paragraphs as a means of emphasizing particular points or adding variety to long passages.

Writers use paragraphs in the following ways:

1. To support a generalization with facts or examples
2. To give a reason or reasons
3. To define something
4. To classify—i.e., to present something as a member of a particular class and then to explain the characteristics of that class
5. To delineate (as facts) or to list (as details) usually in support of a proposition
6. To set forth points of comparison and contrast, or pros and cons
7. To describe (as a case, a situation, or a thing)
8. To limit, expand, elaborate, or restate (as an idea)
9. To narrate (as a history or a report)
10. To paraphrase or to quote (an individual or a source)
11. To analyze or summarize (as a situation)
12. To summarize (as findings)

There are two general types of paragraphs: the expository—a unit of facts, details, or ideas brought together to explain or describe; and the argumentative—a unit of facts, details, or ideas brought together to persuade or convince. A writer may use or modify one or both of these prototypes, depending on the major thrust.

Paragraph development and strategy   Depending on the writer's intentions, paragraph development may take any of these directions:

1. The paragraph may move from the general to the specific.
2. The paragraph may move from the specific to the general.
3. The paragraph may exhibit an alternating order of comparison and contrast.
4. The paragraph may chronicle events in a set temporal order—e.g., from the beginning to the end, or from the end to the beginning.
5. The paragraph may describe something (as a group of objects) in a set spatial order— e.g., the items being described may be looked at from near-to-far, or vice versa.
6. The paragraph may follow a climactic sequence with the least important facts or examples described first followed by a buildup of tension leading to the most important facts or examples then followed by a gradual easing of tension. Other material can be so ordered for effectiveness; for example, facts or issues that are easy to comprehend or accept may be set forth first and followed by those that are more difficult to comprehend or accept. In this way the easier material makes the reader receptive and prepares him or her to comprehend or accept the more difficult points.
7. Anticlimactic order is also useful when the writer's intent is to persuade the reader. With this strategy, the writer sets forth the most persuasive arguments first so that the reader, having then been influenced in a positive way by that persuasion, moves along with the rest of the argument with a growing feeling of assent.

Keys to effective paragraphing   The following material outlines some ways of building effective paragraphs within a text.

A topic sentence—a key sentence to which the other sentences in the paragraph are related—may be placed either at the beginning or at the end of a paragraph. A lead-in topic sentence should present the main idea in the paragraph, and should set the initial tone of the material that follows. A terminal topic sentence should be an analysis, a conclusion, or a summation of what has gone before it.

Single-sentence paragraphs can be used to achieve easy transition from a preceding to a subsequent paragraph (especially when those are long and complex), if it repeats an important word or phrase from the preceding paragraph, if it contains a pronoun reference to a key individual mentioned in a preceding paragraph, or if it is introduced by an appropriate conjunction or conjunctive adverb that tightly connects the paragraphs.

Since the very first paragraph sets initial tone, introduces the subject or topic under discussion, and leads into the main thrust of a communication, it should be worded so as to immediately attract the reader's attention and arouse interest. These openings can be effective:

a. a succinct statement of purpose or point of view
b. a concise definition (as of a problem)
c. a lucid statement of a key issue or fact

But these openings can blunt the rest of the material:

a. an apology for the material to be presented
b. a querulous complaint or a defensive posture
c. a rehash of ancient history (as a word-for-word recap of previous correspondence from the individual to whom one is writing)
d. a presentation of self-evident facts
e. a group of sentences rendered limp and meaningless because of clichés

The last paragraph ties together all of the ideas and points that have been set forth earlier and reemphasizes the main thrust of the communication. These can be effective endings:

a. a setting forth of the most important conclusion or conclusions drawn from the preceding discussion
b. a final analysis of the main problem or problems under discussion
c. a lucid summary of the individual points brought up earlier
d. a final, clear statement of opinion or position
e. concrete suggestions or solutions if applicable
f. specific questions asked of the reader if applicable

But the following endings can decrease the effectiveness of a communication:

a. apologies for a poor presentation
b. qualifying remarks that blunt or negate incisive points made earlier
c. insertion of minor details or afterthoughts
d. a meaningless closing couched in clichés

The following are tests of good paragraphs:

1. Does the paragraph have a clear purpose? Is its utility evident, or is it there just to fill up space?
2. Does the paragraph clarify rather than cloud the writer's ideas?
3. Is the paragraph adequately developed, or does it merely raise other questions that the writer does not attempt to answer? If a position is being taken, does the writer include supporting information and statistics that are essential to its defense?
4. Are the length and wording of all the paragraphs sufficiently varied, or does the writer employ the same types of locutions again and again?
5. Is the sentence structure coherent?
6. Is each paragraph unified? Do all the sentences really <u>belong</u> there; or does the writer digress into areas that would have been better covered in another paragraph or that could have been omitted altogether?
7. Are the paragraphs coherent so that one sentence leads clearly and logically to another? Is easy, clear transition among the paragraphs effected by a wise selection of transitional words and phrases which indicate idea relationships and signal the direction in which the author's prose is moving?
8. Does one paragraph simply restate in other terms what has been said before?

17.9

PROBLEMS IN MEDICAL WRITING

The introductory matter in section 17.2 states that mechanical style guidelines—especially those relating to abbreviations—vary according to the editorial policies of the journal or the publishing house to which a manuscript is being submitted. Differences in style also abound in the treatment of numerals, units of measure, and medical/scientific references. (See Chapter 16, "Special Typing Projects," section 16.2, for a full discussion of manuscript preparation and reference styling.) Obviously, it is not within the scope of this book to recognize and delineate all of the style variations that are current among medical journals and scientific publishers. However, the following paragraphs do highlight and expand on some of the more troublesome areas that will require the careful attention of both the writer and the typist during manuscript development.

ABBREVIATIONS: Special Problems

Clinical and technical designations In most instances, clinical and technical designations can be abbreviated in a text after they have first been written out in full. The written-out form is immediately followed by its proper abbreviation in parentheses. In subsequent references to the word or words, the abbreviation may then stand alone without glosses. If a writer wishes to coin an abbreviation, he or she ought to make sure first of all that a standard abbreviation for the term does not already exist. The writer should also avoid using or making up an abbreviation for a term involving a drug name (exception: *LSD*). And finally, the abbreviation should not contain within itself a unit of measure. If these three criteria have been satisfied, the writer can use the new abbreviation, provided that he or she first spells out the word or words and then includes the abbreviation in parentheses directly following the expansion.

Chemical element abbreviations and expressions One- or two-letter chemical element abbreviations (or combinations thereof) may be used in titles, texts, captions, and graphs. These abbreviations are <u>never</u> terminated by periods. The only exception to this rule lies with a chemical element abbreviation or formula that has been placed at the end of a declarative sentence in a running text. In this case, a single period may end the sentence. Examples:

correct
The elements studied in the experiment were As, Fe, Pb, and Hg.

incorrect
The elements studied in the experiment were As., Fe., Pb., and Hg.

correct
Phosphorus occurs in nature in the form of phosphates, chiefly of aluminum in the mineral *wavellite* $[4AlPO_4 \cdot 2Al(OH)_3 \cdot 9H_2O]$; of calcium in the minerals *apatite* $[Ca_3(PO_4)_2$ with some $CaCl_2$ or $CaF_2]$, and *phosphorite* $[Ca_3(PO_4)_2]$, and of iron in *vivianite* $[Fe_3(PO_4)_2 \cdot 8H_2O]$.

—Remington's Pharmaceutical Sciences

incorrect
Phosphorus occurs in nature in the form of phosphates, chiefly of aluminum in the mineral *wavellite* $[4Al.PO._4 \cdot 2Al.(OH.)_3 \cdot 9H_2O.]$; of calcium in the mineral *apatite* $[Ca._3(PO._4)_2 \ldots]$.

In the two correct examples in the pairs shown above, the chemical elements and formulas are run into the text, and some of them occur at the ends of the sentences. Therefore, final periods are in order to terminate the sentences. The other symbols within the sentences are unpunctuated.

Compare the above quotation from *Remington's Pharmaceutical Sciences* with the one below in which the chemical formula has been indented (or "displayed") for clarity and emphasis. In this situation, the typist does not insert a terminal period, even if the displayed formula or expression ends the entire sentence:

correct
Potassium laurate . . . has the structure:
$$CH_3(CH_2)_{10}COO^-K^+$$
Solutions of alkali soaps have a high pH; they start to . . . .
                                                    —Remington's Pharmaceutical Sciences

incorrect
Potassium laurate has the structure:
$$CH_3(CH_2)_{10}COO^-K.^+$$
Solutions of alkali soaps have a high pH; they start to . . . .

The typist should style chemical elements and formulas exactly as they have been set down by the writer. Even so-called "minor" changes that may seem totally unimportant to a nonspecialist can drastically alter the whole meaning of a formula or an expression. Thus, it is essential that the typist go over the material carefully in advance so that the writer can clear up any uncertain or confusing points before the material is typed. If the typist anticipates that long formulas or expressions may have to be divided at the ends of lines, the author should be asked to indicate where the line breaks should occur and how they should be indicated.

Journal title abbreviations in references   Most medical journals recommend that their writers adhere to the abbreviations of journal titles that are used in the *Index Medicus*. Such abbreviations are used by writers in parenthetic textual citations and in listed references. See Chapter 16, section 16.2 for examples and detailed discussion.

Mathematical abbreviations and expressions   Trigonometric terms and their abbreviations (as cos = cosine, sin = sine, and log = logarithm) should not be underscored or italicized. However, letters in mathematical expressions that designate unknown quantities or constants and letters that refer to geometric figures should be underscored or typed in italic typeface:

$$k = \frac{2.303}{t_{\frac{1}{2}}} \log \frac{c_o}{c_o/2} = \frac{0.693}{t_{\frac{1}{2}}}$$

$$\frac{d \log K_s}{dt} = \frac{\Delta H}{2.3 \, RT^2}$$

$$x + y = 12$$

$$\angle ABC = \angle ABD$$

Italicized material appearing in displayed formulas and equations also appears in italics when used in running texts, as
. . . in the equation where *x* equals *y*, and *n* represents the number of . . . .
      If an expression contains both superscript (i.e., ^{2}) and subscript (i.e., $_2$) numerals, the typist should type the subscript numeral first, followed by *no* space and the superscript numeral, as

$$12_2{}^2$$

Exponents are typewritten before all punctuation marks except the period of an abbreviation:

cm^2 *but* $in.^2$ *and* $a^2 + b^2 = c.^2$

As with chemical formulas, the typist should exercise great care with mathematical material. The material should be read through before it is typed, and the author should be queried regarding any unclear manuscript or any potential formatting/typing problems.

Units of measure In formal medical writing, some units of measure are typically written out rather than abbreviated. These are as follows: *acre, Bessey-Lowry units, calorie, day* (Note: usage is somewhat divided on whether or not to abbreviate *day*; consult the style guidelines of the publisher before using the abbreviation *da), dram, dyne, equivalent roentgen, farad, foot-lambert, gas volume, grain(s), joule, King-Armstrong unit, knot, liter, lumen, lux, megaunits, metric ton, microfarad, mile, millifarad, mole, newton, rad, radian, siemens, Somogyi unit, tonne,* and *unit*. If the writer has abbreviated any of the above terms in a manuscript, it would be helpful if the typist first consulted the style guide being followed and then tactfully queried the author about the appropriateness of the abbreviation(s).

THE HYPHEN: Special Problems
Chemical compounds Do not hyphen written-out chemical compounds occurring before and modifying nouns:

correct	incorrect
Sodium pentothal injections were	Sodium-pentothal injections were . . . .
Sulfuric acid burns were found	Sulfuric-acid burns were found . . . .

Dimensions, duration of time, and range of measurement The hyphen is used between numerical elements expressing dimensions, duration of time, and ranges of measurement when these elements function as adjectival compounds occurring before and modifying nouns. Examples:

a 9- to 12-month drug-free period
but
a drug-free period of 9 to 12 months

In the first example above, the expression *9- to 12-month* functions as a compound adjective modifying the noun *period.*
In the following example

a 3 × 5-inch card

3 × 5-inch functions adjectivally and modifies the noun *card.* Other examples are:

a 4- to 8-mg dose
a 4-, 8-, or 16-mg dose
but
a dose of 4 mg to 8 mg
a dose of 4 mg, 8 mg, or 16 mg

In the first two examples above, the expressions *4- to 8-mg* and *4-, 8-, or 16-mg* both function as compound adjectives and occur before the nouns they modify.
    In some expressions of range and direction used to modify nouns, the hyphen actually replaces a preposition (such as *to* or *through*). In these expressions the hyphen may be retained whether the modifier precedes or follows its noun. Examples:

errors in the 12%–15% range
a 200µg–400µg dose
and also
errors in the range of 12%–15% (or 12% to 15%)
a dose of 200µg–400µg (or 200µg to 400µg)

Disease names used as modifiers   Disease names that ordinarily are written as open compounds when standing alone are not hyphened when they are used attributively as modifiers of other nouns:

standing alone
grand mal
Rocky mountain spotted fever
equine encephalitis

modifying other nouns
grand mal seizures
Rocky mountain spotted fever epidemics
an equine encephalitis outbreak

However, if the disease name is itself a hyphened compound when standing alone, or if it contains a hyphened element, these hyphens are retained when the disease name is used as a unit modifier of another noun. Examples:

standing alone
Duchenne-Erb paralysis
diphtheria-pertussis-tetanus

modifying other nouns
Duchenne-Erb paralysis studies
diphtheria-pertussis-tetanus inoculations

GREEK LETTERS AND THEIR USE IN MANUSCRIPTS
The letters of the Greek alphabet—some of which are often used in medical writing—are as follows:

ALPHABET TABLE

GREEK

A α	alpha	a	H η	eta	ē	N ν	nu	n	T τ	tau	t
B β	beta	b	Θ θ	theta	th	Ξ ξ	xi	x	γ υ	upsilon	y, u
Γ γ	gamma	g, n	I ι	iota	i	O o	omicron	o	Φ φ	phi	ph
Δ δ	delta	d	K κ	kappa	k	Π π	pi	p	X χ	chi	ch
E ε	epsilon	e	Λ λ	lambda	l	P ρ	rho	r, rh	Ψ ψ	psi	ps
Z ζ	zeta	z	M μ	mu	m	Σ σ ς	sigma	s	Ω ω	omega	ō

Typical uses of Greek letters in medical writing include their appearance in units of measure (400μg), in clinical designations (γ-globulin; hemoglobin α chain deficiency), in statistical data ($\Sigma xB^2 = 2{,}393.82$), in mathematic expressions (πr^2), and in generic drug names and chemical terms (β-amylase; α-methylphenethylamine sulfate).

Greek letters in titles and subtitles of manuscripts and abstracts   Lowercase Greek letters are used at the beginning of and within the titles and subtitles of manuscripts and abstracts:

Hemoglobin α Chain Deficiency
α, β-Unsaturated Carbonyl Compounds: A Review

NOTE: The above examples are styled as they would appear on a manuscript title page. Notice in the second example that the first letter of the English word *Unsaturated* that directly follows the Greek letter for *beta* is capitalized, even though the whole expression forms a hyphened compound. This style applies to capitalized titles only.

Greek letters in sentences   In a sentence beginning with a Greek letter, it is not necessary to spell out the letter. Rather, the writer should retain the lowercase Greek letter but capitalize the first English word that follows that letter, as

α, β-Unsaturated carbonyl compounds are . . . .

Listing Greek letters in manuscripts   When submitting a manuscript to a publisher, it is helpful to include on a separate sheet a list of all Greek letters used in the manuscript. This practice will assist the editor and will later on help the typesetter.

ROMAN NUMERALS AND ARABIC NUMERALS: Special Usage Problems

Roman numerals should be avoided in formal medical writing unless they form a part of a personal name (as Walter M. Danvers, III, MD) or unless they are segments of established medical and technical terms (such as blood-clotting factors, ECG leads, or designations of cranial nerves):

Blood-clotting factor VII
lead II
The cranial nerves (II, IV, and IX) are . . . .

On the other hand, Arabic numerals are used regularly in medical writing and especially with terms designating blood platelet factors, virus and organism types, heart murmurs (indicating their intensity in grades 1 through 6), and with the terms *para, gravida,* and *abortus.* Typical examples of these uses are:

platelet factor 3
adenovirus type 2
B77 avian sarcoma virus RNA subunits
reovirus type 3
gr. i/6 systolic [heart] murmur
para 1
gravida 3
abortus 1

SYMBOLS AND SIGNS: General Guidelines

Every journal or publisher has its own specific rules regarding the symbols and signs that are acceptable or unacceptable in manuscripts. The most important general advice that can be given here is that both the writer and the typist should (1) become familiar with the particular publisher's Instructions to Authors, which are often printed in each issue in the case of a medical journal (2) be consistent in the use of symbols and signs, and (3) supply the publisher with a separate list of the symbols and signs used in the manuscript. The latter point is especially important because the publisher may have to ascertain whether or not the typesetter is capable of reproducing the needed symbols or signs.

Degree sign   Although usage is somewhat divided on this issue, it is generally recommended that the degree sign ° be omitted in expressions of temperature:

100F *not* 100°F
39C *not* 39°C

However, the word *degree* may be written out in expressions of latitude and longtitude, providing that the expressions do not also indicate *minutes* and *seconds*:

. . . . a difference in 10 degrees latitude.

It is acceptable to omit both *degree* and its symbol in expressions like

. . . latitude 39 North

but the symbol ° as well as the symbol ′ (minutes) and ″ (seconds) should appear in expressions like

. . . 6°40′10″ N

where degrees, minutes, and seconds are all elements of the total expression. Notice that the expression is unspaced, except for the compass point.

Diacritics   American writers now tend to omit diacritics and foreign accents whenever possible in English-language manuscripts. One reason for this trend is that excessive use of these marks unnecessarily complicates typesetting. For example, it is not necessary to include the bolle ° over the A in the word *Ångstrom*:

Ångstrom → *Angstrom.*

The umlaut ¨ can also be dropped from terms like *Schüller:*

Schüller-Christian disease → *Schuller-Christian disease*

and the acute accent marks ′′ can be dropped from terms like *Bárány chair:*

Bárány chair → *Barany chair.*

An exception to the rule is, however, a term whose meaning is determined by the presence or absence of diacritics. Example: *atu* which means a unit of atmospheric underpressure in the metric technical system, versus *atü* (note umlaut) which means a unit of atmospheric overpressure in the metric technical system. In cases such as this one, the marks should be retained.

Parentheses, brackets, and braces in formulas and equations   In chemical and mathematic formulas and equations, parentheses are often used in combination with brackets and/or braces to indicate aggregation. The standard order for such combinations is illustrated below, with the smallest unit of aggregation being in the center (i.e., the smaller parentheses):

$$\{\,[\,(\,\{\,[\,(\qquad)\,]\,\}\,)\,]\,\}$$

Since most typewriters feature only pica or elite parentheses and possibly brackets, the typist or the writer will have to insert braces and outsize symbols by hand. This should be done in black ink with a fine-point pen so that the manuscript will be readable and neat.

Percent sign: usage   If a specific amount is to be expressed, use figure(s) + the sign %. Do not space between the figure(s) and the symbol. Examples:

. . . observed the reaction in 0.6% of those tested.
. . . studied 5.2% of the patients. . . .
. . . found that in 91% of the slides . . . .
. . . observed the reaction in 80.5% of the subjects . . . .

Be sure to include the *percent* sign even if one of the numbers in a series or unit combination is *zero*:

. . . a variation of 0% to 10%.

However, with indefinite amounts not expressible in Arabic numerals, the words *percent* or *percentage* should be used instead of the symbol:

. . . only a small percent of the test animals . . . .
A greater percentage of the subjects experienced hallucinations . . . .

VIRGULE IN *PER* CONSTRUCTIONS: Points of Usage

In formal medical writing, it is generally recommended that the virgule when meaning *per* be used only when

1. the expression contains units of physical measurement or time measurement
2. at least one element of the expression is or has to do with a specific numerical quantity
3. each element of a pair is either a specific numerical quantity or a specific unit of measure.

If the construction satisfies these criteria, the virgule may be used in place of *per*. Examples:

Rats treated with $1W/cm^2$ for 10 min exhibited . . . .
. . . requires 2 mg/kg to produce a 5- to 10-min period of anesthesia.
Intravenous infusion, initially 4 mU/min for 10 min . . . .
. . . a hemoglobin level of 16 gm/100 cc.
. . . a leukocyte count of 5,000/cu mm indicated that . . . .
. . . a normal serum potassium value of 4.0–4.8 mEq/liter means that . . . .
Amylase test: 60–150 Somogyi units/100 ml
. . . indicated that ammonia in the urine measured 40 Eq/liter/36 hr . . . .

Note, however, that the virgule is <u>not</u> used in *per* constructions if a prepositional phrase occurs between two or more segments of the construction, as

40 units of insulin per day

where *of insulin* is the intervening prepositional phrase.
    The virgule is also omitted from the construction and *per* is written out if one segment of the construction contains a series, as

. . . 6, 8, and 10 mg per hour. . .

where *6, 8, and 10 mg* constitutes a series.
    Finally, the virgule is not used if the construction does not contain a specific quantity or amount expressed in numbers, as

half a dozen weeks per year
one or two hours per day
about seven times a week

where *half a dozen, one or two,* and *about seven times* are not exact numerical amounts or are not expressed in numbers. Notice that in the last example, *a* was used instead of *per*; in fact, *a* could have been used in the first two examples also.

VIRUS DESIGNATIONS: Problems of Styling

Usage is erratic as to the styling of virus designations. Thus, no set formula can be given regarding the capitalization or the wording of these terms. The following examples illustrate the situation:

human wart virus
vesicular stomatitis virus (serotype Indiana)
murine sarcoma-leukemia virus
mosquito iridescent virus
but
hemagglutinating virus of Japan
Sindbis virus
Junin virus
Rauscher leukemia virus
California encephalitis virus
Moloney leukemia virus
Epstein-Barr virus

The only general capitalization rule that is fixed is this: If the virus name contains a proper noun (as *California, Sindbis,* or *Epstein-Barr*),the proper noun is capitalized. Arabic numerals are used to designate types of viruses, as

B77 avian sarcoma virus
coxsackievirus B2
adenovirus type 2
reovirus type 3

Consult one of the major medical dictionaries (a list of titles is given in the Appendix) for the styling of virus names not shown here. Additional help may be obtained from the *Classification and Nomenclature of Viruses, First Report of the International Committee on Nomenclature of Viruses* (Basel, Switzerland: S. Karger AG, 1971).

18

CHAPTER EIGHTEEN

OFFICE COPYING EQUIPMENT: How to Make It Work for You

CONTENTS

18.1

REPROGRAPHICS EQUIPMENT AND PROCESSES

INTRODUCTION

Today's society depends on paper-based communications. An estimated 15 trillion pieces of paper are presently in circulation in U.S. business offices, and another million new pages are added each minute of each working day. Not only the influx of original material but also the constantly increasing use of multiple copies of documents have fundamentally altered the business scene. The production and handling of this paper barrage is dependent on the ever-increasing technological evolution of office machines which goes on at an almost unbelievable pace. Every issue of the business magazines and newspapers bombards its readers with "the newest" and "the best" in office copiers. The term designating this field is *reprographics:* this includes all the processes, techniques, and equipment employed in the multiple copying or reproduction of documents in a graphic form—hence *repro* plus *graphics.*

Not only have technological advancements created an impact on offices, but they have also altered the responsibilities and duties of assistants. The assistant's role has been expanded; now the assistant must understand the capabilities of each reprographic process, and must know how to operate commonly used copying equipment. Since the office function affects the profit-and-loss statement of a practice, the assistant also needs to be aware of the costs of each copying process. Often an assistant selects the reprographics equipment for the office; therefore, it is vital that the assistant understand which process will provide the office with the best copy quality in minimum time and at minimum cost.

No single office reproduction method can be described as the best for handling all situations, and requirements of each particular situation will suggest the appropriate reprographic process. However, the selection of a reprographic process should be based principally on quality/quantity/budget requirements with consideration given to one or more of the following factors:

1. **Appearance of copy desired**
   If the copy will be distributed within an office, generally a lower quality of reproduction is acceptable; however, if the copy is mailed to someone outside the office, a higher quality product is usually desired.

2. **Quantity needed**
   Most decisions involve the number of copies needed. If only a few copies are required, one process may be better than another. But if a large number of copies is needed, a process specifically applicable to large-volume reproduction requirements would probably be used.

3. **Cost**
   In general, the higher the quality of the copy, the higher the cost in materials and labor. Some of these costs can be substantially lowered where a large output is usual.

4. **Time demands**
   If a copy is needed instantly with no setup time, this limitation will determine the reprographic method to be used.

5. **Additional considerations**
   Any unusual requirements will affect the method of reproduction, since standard equipment cannot always accommodate unusual jobs. Such additional factors might include unusual sizes of copy, special copy design, and the need for color reproduction.

These factors are seldom considered separately, but rather in various combinations, depending on the requirements of each job. Though the priority of the factors may be determined by the office or the practice, it is the assistant who often must determine the most appropriate method in each situation.

Reprographics encompasses five basic processes of duplication:
1. Carbon Process (conventional and film)
2. Fluid Process
3. Stencil Process
4. Printing Process
5. Photocopy Process

Although medical assistants seldom need to know how all five of the processes work, they should, nevertheless, be *generally* familiar with each one. Hence, this chapter discusses all five processes for purposes of reference.

CARBON PROCESS

The carbon process can be effectively used to make from 2 to 15 copies of a document. Two types of carbon are available—conventional carbon paper and carbon film. Conventional carbon paper has long been a staple supply in offices. The selection of the grade and weight of conventional carbon paper depends on the number of copies that are required. The table below provides guidelines for the selection of conventional carbon paper.

Carbon Paper Recommendations for Typewriters

Electric Typewriters		Manual Typewriters	
Number of Copies	Weight Recommended	Number of Copies	Weight Recommended
1–5	Heavy (standard)	1–3	Heavy (standard)
6–8	Medium	4–5	Medium
8–10	Light	6–8	Light

The weight of carbon paper is often expressed as *heavy, medium,* or *light;* and the weight indicates the number of copies that can be successfully reproduced with one typing. A lighter-weight carbon paper should be used as the number of copies increases. Manufacturers usually suggest that conventional carbon paper can be used satisfactorily from five to eight times, but many typists stretch its reuse considerably.

Film carbon is a newer development that is gaining enthusiastic acceptance in the office. Film carbon is a tough polyester film coated with a plastic solvent. The increased durability of film carbon prevents tearing and eliminates wrinkling and curling. This strong but pliant carbon will produce up to 15 legible copies. Film carbon has the added advantage of not smearing or smudging hands or paper.

Additional factors affecting the suitability of carbon paper or carbon film include the weight of the original stationery and the second sheets, the sharpness of the typewriter typeface, the kind and condition of the typewriter platen, and the touch of the typist, particularly if a manual typewriter is being used.

An impression control device on electric typewriters regulates the pressure of the typeface striking the paper. This mechanism allows for a setting of one to ten, with the *one* setting being suitable for typing one or two copies and the *five* (or more) setting appropriate when the typist is making many copies. Electric typewriters also have a carbon copy lever which interacts with the impression control regulator to ensure that multiple copy impressions are properly made.

Carbon pack A carbon pack contains the original, the carbon paper, and the copy sheets. Two methods can be used when assembling a carbon pack:

1. **Desk Assembly Method**
   a. Assemble the materials by placing the copy (sometimes called the *second sheet*) on top of your desk; then place one sheet of carbon paper on top with the carbon side down.
   b. Add another copy sheet and the carbon paper to the stack. (A copy sheet topped with a carbon sheet should be added for every extra copy needed.)
   c. Place the original sheet of letterhead or bond paper on the top of the pack.
   d. Pick the carbon pack up carefully and straighten the edges by tapping the pack gently on the desk.
   e. Turn the pack until the glossy carbon side of the carbon paper is facing you.
   f. In order to keep the carbon pack from slipping, insert the pack into the fold of an envelope or into the crease of a folded piece of paper before inserting it into the typewriter.
   g. Insert the pack and the envelope or the folded paper into the typewriter with a quick turn of the cylinder, roll it around, and then remove the envelope or the folded paper from the pack.
   h. Use the paper-release lever on the typewriter after you have partially inserted the carbon pack to avoid wrinkling the carbon pack and to allow you to straighten it.

2. **Machine Assembly Method**
   a. Assemble one sheet of letterhead or bond stationery in front of the required number of copy sheets and begin inserting them into the typewriter.
   b. Turn the cylinder to a point where all of the sheets are gripped securely by the feed rolls. (Approximately seven-eighths of the paper will not have entered the typewriter.)
   c. Then, flip all of the sheets except the last sheet of copy paper toward you over the top of the typewriter.
   d. Place one sheet of carbon paper (with the glossy carbon side facing you) between each of the sheets of paper. Lay each sheet back as the carbon sheet is added.

e. After all carbon sheets have been inserted, continue rolling the pack into the regular typing position.

f. Use the paper-release lever on the typewriter to avoid wrinkling the carbon pack and to allow you to straighten it.

Note: Previously assembled carbon sets may be purchased. These sets consist of a lightweight sheet of carbon paper attached to the top of a sheet of copy paper. These carbon sets may be stacked to make several copies at one typing. Although the cost of the preassembled carbon sets is somewhat higher than the do-it-yourself packs, many users believe the savings in time more than compensate for the added cost.

After the typing is completed, the carbon pack can be removed from the typewriter by pulling the paper bail forward and using the paper-release lever. The carbon paper can be removed in one swift motion by giving the pack a quick downward shake. If the machine assembly method is used, the carbon extensions may be grasped and the carbon sheets pulled out all in one motion.

Correction of errors   Quality typing demands careful correction of errors. Although some typists follow the practice of correcting an error on all copies of a document, a growing trend today is to correct the errors only on the original and on those copies being sent outside the office. An exception to this practice occurs when an error is made on a number or date, or when the error might cause the message to be misunderstood. In those cases, corrections should be made on all copies. Errors should be corrected on all copies of statistical/technical typing.

A hard, abrasive typing eraser works best when one is correcting errors on an original, and a soft pencil eraser is most effective when one is correcting carbon copies. Erasures will be neat if the typist (1) makes sure that the hands are clean before making an erasure (2) checks to see that the eraser is clean (one can clean it by rubbing it on a rough surface such as sandpaper or an emery board) (3) erases with the grain of the paper, and (4) erases each letter separately with a light, short stroke (5) camouflages the erased area by applying a white charcoal film or by using a special white charcoal pencil. Also, a good quality white liquid correction fluid can be used to cover up difficult corrections, punctuation marks, and others. Tinted liquid correction fluid is available to match colored shades of stationery, but should be ordered at the time the stationery order is placed. If an erasing shield is used, it should be placed in front of the carbon paper. When correcting subsequent copies, the typist should transfer the shield, making sure that it is placed in front of the carbon each time.

When errors are discovered after the carbon pack has been removed from the typewriter, the typist inserts each sheet into the machine individually to make the correction. If it is important to keep the shading similar, a small piece of carbon can be placed over the erased spot before the correction is typed on the copy.

The typist ought to use the typewriter alignment scale and the variable line spacer to align the typing when reinserting typewritten work into the machine for correction. A good practice is to check the positioning of the typewriter typeface in relation to the alignment scale by first typing a few words on a sheet of scratch paper.

Use of colored carbon paper   Carbon paper is available in several colors. There may be occasions when one will want to highlight a word, a sentence, or a symbol in a second color. The typist inserts a small piece of colored carbon paper behind the typewriter ribbon (which affects the original) and additional pieces behind each sheet of carbon. The colored carbon pieces are removed as soon as the typist has completed typing the word(s) that are to be highlighted.

Disposal of carbon paper   Carbon paper should be discarded as soon as it no longer makes good, clean copies. The life of carbon paper varies, and this feature should be evaluated before the paper is purchased. The assistant should check carbon copies after typing numbers to be sure that the numbers can be easily read. Wrinkled carbon paper should not be used, since any characters striking the wrinkled section will be distorted.

Storage of carbon paper   Carbon paper should be stored in a flat folder with the carbon side down and away from heat. Used carbon paper should be put away as soon as possible to avoid the possibility of getting carbon marks on other papers, on clothing, or on the desk top.

Problem-solving tips for working with conventional (non-film) carbon paper   The following table describes some of the more common problems encountered with conventional (non-film) carbon paper and suggests some ways these problems may be solved (note that the characteristics of film carbon differ markedly from those of conventional carbon; therefore, the table that follows does not apply to film carbon):

Problem-solving Tips — Carbon Process

Condition	Probable Cause(s)	Guideline(s)/Solution(s)
Curling	usually the result of a change in temperature or humidity	Store carbon paper face down in a flat folder away from extreme temperature or excessive moisture; purchase curl-free carbon paper.
Limited durability	possibly due to poor-quality carbon paper or a soft finish on the carbon paper, or excessive wear caused by the use of the high impression settings on the typewriter	Select carbon paper having a hard finish; alternate the carbon sheets within the carbon pack for more even wear.
Illegibility	often due to excessive use of carbon paper beyond the manufacturer's recommendations	Typewriter may need cleaning; discard worn carbon paper and replace it with unused sheets; determine whether the finish and weight of the carbon paper are suitable for the number of copies being typed.
Cutting	results when the typewriter's typeface is excessively sharp	Use a heavier weight of carbon paper; if lightweight bond paper is used for the original, insert a second sheet of bond between the original and the first carbon.
Slippage	may be caused by using copy sheets with a slick finish	Slip the carbon pack into the fold of an envelope before inserting it into the typewriter; when typing near the bottom of a page, insert an extra sheet of bond paper between the last copy and the cylinder.

Smudging	may be caused by careless handling of carbon copies; may be aggravated by using glossy copy paper	Use carbon paper having a hard finish; select copy paper that will absorb carbon.
Treeing	results from wrinkled carbon paper	When inserting or removing a carbon pack, use the paper-release lever. This procedure tends to smooth out potential wrinkles.
Offsetting image	usually caused by excessive pressure on the carbon pack	Adjust the impression control mechanism on the typewriter; use lightweight carbon paper and copy paper; discourage roller marks by moving the rollers to the edge of the paper.

Advantages and disadvantages of the carbon process   Every reprographic process has superior features as well as limitations, and the carbon process is no exception. The following table describes some of the advantages and disadvantages most evident in this process:

Advantages
1. a relatively inexpensive method of producing copies
2. process can be used on a wide variety of papers relative to color, quality, and weight
3. all copies made at same time as original
4. entire process completed in one location; assistant does not have to leave work station
5. additional equipment not needed to make copies
6. file copies reproduced on lightweight paper, creating less bulk in files

Disadvantages
1. only a limited number of copies reproduced from one typing
2. time needed to make corrections on the original and all copies

Although reprographics is often associated with copier equipment, the assistant should recognize the suitability of the use of carbon paper or film in preparing a small number of copies. This process is often superior to any other for many office requirements.

FLUID PROCESS
Fluid duplicating is one of the older reprographic processes; and it is one that is seldom used in medical offices today. (The newer thermal spirit masters are discussed on page 528.) The fluid process involves the interaction of five elements: the carbon sheet, the master sheet, the moistening fluid, the duplicating paper, and a duplicator machine. The material is typed directly onto the spirit master. After the carbon sheet is removed, the master sheet is placed on the outside of the machine cylinder (sometimes called the *drum*) with the carbon copy side up. The paper is then fed through the moistening unit and between the cylinder and impression roller. As each sheet of moistened paper makes contact with the master on the cylinder, the moistening fluid on the paper dissolves a thin layer of the car-

bon deposit from the master. The copy that appears on the sheet of paper is the result of this layer of carbon deposit.

The master unit   The master unit consists of the original sheet of special glossy white paper (*master*) attached to a sheet of paper coated with a waxlike substance (*direct process/hectograph carbon*) which gives the appearance of carbon. Type-writing, handwriting, drawing, or printing on the face of the master causes this waxlike carbon to be transferred to the back of the master. A protective tissue slip-sheet separates the master from the carbon sheet and must be removed before any impressions are made on the master. After the master sheet has been com-pleted, the protective sheet should be replaced behind it to protect its content and to avoid unwanted carbon transfer that will stain other surfaces. Master units are available in the following range of sizes: 8½″ × 11″, 11″ × 8½″, 8½″ × 14″, 17″ × 11″, and 17″ × 14″. Special master units which provide printed guidelines to assist the typist in positioning the copy can be purchased for routine jobs.

Master units can be purchased in several colors, but purple is considered the standard color. Other available colors are red, green, blue, and black. These colors are often used to highlight words or pictures. Two or more colors can be used on the same master unit. Different colors can be obtained by inserting the color of carbon that has been selected behind the white glossy master, and then by typing, writing, or drawing the desired material. These colors will be reproduced on the final copy. Duplicating paper is available in white and also in a variety of colors; however, the most common colors are pink, green, blue, and yellow.

The fluid process is used for work to be distributed within a large organiza-tion. This process tends to produce adequately legible, but not high-quality copy. Each master is capable of making about 300 legible copies. The fluid duplicating process is the most economical process for duplicating up to 300 copies.

Preparation of a typed spirit master   The typeface on the typewriter must be clean. The ribbon should be left in the normal typing position. Then, the typist should experiment with several pressure settings to decide which one will result in the sharpest carbon image on the back of the master. Normally, the lowest pressure setting is the most effective; however, the highest pressure setting is better on some typewriters.

After removing the protective tissue sheet, the typist should insert the open end of the master unit into the typewriter to allow for easier correction of errors. The master unit is positioned in the same way that it is when one is typing on a regular sheet of bond paper. Allow a one-half-inch margin at the top of the master unit for clamping the master sheet onto the cylinder of the duplicator. Push the rollers on the paper bail to the side so they do not ride on the master. (If the platen is worn, a plastic backing sheet inserted under the master unit will produce a sharper copy.)

Preparation of artwork on a master   A ball-point pen, a stylus, or a pencil with hard lead should be used to draw on a master unit. Use firm, even pressure and work on a flat, smooth surface. It may be helpful to fold the carbon sheet back and sketch the proposed drawing in pencil on the master in order to position the sketch. Then replace the carbon sheet behind the master sheet and trace over the sketch. When making a sketch, one may prefer to fold the master unit carbon back and then insert a sheet of regular typing carbon between the master and the design one wishes to copy. After the design has been traced, the typing carbon is removed, the master unit carbon is slipped back into place, and the design is recopied on the master.

A shading plate may be used to provide the characteristics of halftone work on a drawing. Shading plates are made of thin pieces of plastic on which a pattern has been etched. The shading plate should be placed beneath the master unit. Then the master is rubbed with a stylus wherever the shading pattern design is desired. Lettering guides and tracing sheets can also be used to achieve the desired appearance.

Correction of errors   Errors can be corrected so that they are undetectable on final copies. For example, a scratcher or fiberglass brush eraser can be used to lightly scrape the carbon from the back of the master. However, care must be exercised to avoid damaging the surface of the master. Any remaining carbon crumbs should be removed by blowing or brushing them away.

Transparent tape, special correction tape, or strips of self-sticking labels can be used to block out a large area on the master. Press the tape over the material to be corrected, insert an unused strip of carbon over the tape and then redo the material. The master can be cut apart and taped back together—a feature that can be used to good advantage when the typist needs to add or delete any section of the master.

After an error in copy has been corrected on the master, place a new piece of carbon face-up under the spot where the error was removed. (Cut—do not tear—a small section from an unused corner of the master carbon since only a small piece of carbon is needed.) Type the correct letter and remove the extra piece of carbon. Check the back of the master to see that the correction is satisfactory. The correction on the front of the master will appear as a strikeover but will not affect the duplicated copies.

Reproduction of a master   The following procedure should be followed in running a spirit master.

1. Prepare the duplicator. Check to make sure an adequate supply of fluid is in the machine. Turn on the fluid feeding mechanism. Place paper (felt side up) neatly on the feed tray. Adjust the paper guides for the width of paper being used. Check the receiving tray to confirm that the position is suitable to receive the length of paper being used.
2. Set the pressure control knob or lever. Almost all runs use a medium setting. If larger quantities are to be·run, start with a light pressure setting and increase the pressure setting periodically. This procedure will allow a gradual wearing of the master so that all copies will be similar in shading.
3. Set the counter at zero before running the copies.
4. Open the master clamp lever; insert the master in the cylinder. Place the master with the carbon side up (reverse image). Close the master clamp. Avoid touching the carbon on the master.
5. Turn on the electric motor and activate the paper feeder mechanism. Run a few test copies to check copy quality; make any needed adjustments in the machine; complete the runoff of copies. (If a manual machine is used, turn the handle clockwise to run the copy.)
6. Remove the master by opening the clamp lever and lifting the master off the cylinder. Close the clamp lever. If the master will be used again, attach it to the protective tissue sheet; otherwise, fold the master with the carbon side inside and discard it.
7. It is very important to remember to turn the machine off. Set the pressure knob or lever on zero. Be sure to check to see that the clamp on the cylinder is also closed. Turn off the fluid feeding mechanism.
8. Clean up the work area. It is quite inconsiderate to leave the work area in a state of disarray for the next person who will use it.

Problem-solving tips for working with master units The table below shows the possible reasons for copying problems when one is using a fluid duplicator. Possible solutions to these problems are also provided.

Problem-solving Tips—Fluid Process

Condition	Probable Cause(s)	Guide(s)/Solution(s)
Wrinkled master	result of not loading the master squarely into the clamp of the duplicator	Remove the master from the drum and reinsert it into the clamp while making sure it is clamped squarely; press the master down where it fits into the clamp; gently pull the edges of the master in the area of the wrinkle and put a piece of transparent tape on the front of the master. This procedure may require a second person to help.
Wrinkled copy	impression paper possibly not feeding properly, due to moisture absorption in humid conditions	Use paper from a different ream.
	corner separators may be binding	Adjust the corner separators to cover the feed edges of the paper.
	feed table possibly overloaded	Check to determine if too much paper was loaded on the feed table.
Offsetting image	impression roller may contain excessive deposits from the direct-process carbon caused by the absence of paper during machine operation	Clean any carbon deposits from the impression roller periodically (use duplicating fluid as a cleaning agent).
	dark shadows or roller marks may appear down the sides of the copy	Discourage roller marks by moving the rollers to the ends of the paper bail.
Streaked copy	can be caused by a lint-covered wick	Wipe any accumulated lint from the moistening roller and wick. Change the wick if necessary.
	duplicator possibly not level, resulting in uneven distribution of fluid	Check to see that the duplicator is level. Revolve the drum several times without the master to ensure that the wick is uniformly coated with fluid.
Typing appearing on tissue	protective tissue not removed from master unit before typing	Place the protective tissue instead of master onto the drum. Usually a limited number of copies can be run from this protective tissue sheet.

Advantages and disadvantages of the fluid process   The following table shows some of the advantages and disadvantages of using the fluid process for duplicating materials.

Advantages

1. an inexpensive process, with each copy costing less than one cent
2. master usable on a variety of paper weights and colors
3. several colors usable simultaneously on a single copy
4. copies that can be made at a rate of over 100 a minute
5. equipment that is easy to use and that requires a minimum of training time

Disadvantages

1. a master must be prepared before any copies can be made
2. about 300 copies can be made from one master
3. copies not having a high-quality appearance when compared with more sophisticated copy work
4. copies not usually legible enough to be satisfactorily reproduced on a photo-copying machine
5. carbon is messy and requires careful handling
6. black masters tend to reproduce in a dull, gray shade rather than in black

STENCIL PROCESS

One of the better-known reprographic processes involves the use of a stencil and is technically referred to as the *stencil process*. Although the stencil process is rarely used in medical offices, it may be used in larger organizations such as hospitals, medical schools, and health-care corporations. This method of duplication is more versatile than the carbon paper process or the fluid process because electronic stencil-cutting equipment that allows one to reproduce photographs is available. The stencil process relies on four elements: the stencil, the ink, the paper, and the stencil duplicator machine. The stencil is prepared and placed on the cylinder of the stencil duplicator over an ink pad. Ink flows from the inside of the cylinder onto the ink pad and through the opening in the stencil. As paper is fed between the cylinder and the impression roller, the roller causes the paper to touch the stencil. Simultaneously, the ink flows from the ink pad through the openings in the stencil and produces a copy on the paper.

Stencil selection   Stencils are available to accommodate varying conditions relative to copies required, durability, guide markings, cushion coating, and preprinted designs. Because of the variety of stencils available, it is important that the intended use of a stencil be carefully considered. For instance, if 1,000 copies or less are required, an average-run stencil is suitable; however, if more than 1,000 copies are planned or if the stencil will be run at a later time, it is advisable to select a long-run stencil which can produce 5,000 or more satisfactory copies.

Special stencils   Manufacturers offer a variety of special stencils designed for specific kinds of jobs. Some of the more important special stencils available are:

1. **Addressing stencil**   This stencil provides 33 grid spaces in which names and addresses are to be typed. The stencil can be run off on regular paper or on sheets of gummed labels.
2. **Bulletin stencil**   This stencil is helpful in typing bulletins or double-page forms that would normally require a typewriter with a long carriage. Guidelines are provided for cutting the stencil apart, typing the copy, and cementing the stencil together before running.

3. **Continuous stencil**   This stencil has control holes punched along one or both sides and is used with automated data processing printout machines.
4. **Document stencil**   This stencil is intended for use when typing oversized documents.
5. **Electronic stencil**   This stencil is electronically produced and permits the reproduction of letterheads, office forms, and bulletin or memo headings with the use of an electronic scanner.
6. **Four-page folder stencil**   This stencil provides printed guidelines to help the typist avoid copy-positioning errors.
7. **Handwriting stencil**   This stencil is equipped with guides so that the assistant can keep the handwriting straight and well-spaced on it.
8. **Outline map stencil**   This stencil contains a precut geographical outline map. Outline map stencils are available for states and many countries. Locations and other data may then be typed or marked on the stencil.
9. **Thermal stencil**   This stencil is cut by running an original copy with a stencil through a special thermal photocopier, thereby eliminating the need to type the stencil.

Stencil pack   A stencil pack usually has four parts: (1) the stencil sheet, (2) the backing sheet, (3) the cushion sheet, and (4) the typing film (optional). The stencil sheet is made of a fine but tough fibrous tissue covered on both sides with a wax coating that will not allow ink to pass through the surface. This coating is pushed aside when the typewriter key or stylus strikes the stencil. The backing is the heavy, smooth sheet on which the stencil is mounted. The cushion sheet is placed between the stencil and the backing sheet. It supports the stencil, cushions the blow of the typeface, and makes the typed stencil easier to read. The typing film, considered an optional feature, is a thin sheet of plastic film lightly attached to the top of the stencil sheet. Use of the typing film sheet tends to make the copy more bold in appearance and minimizes the cutting out of letters on the stencil sheet.

Preparation of a stencil   The following steps are involved in the correct typing of a stencil:
1. Place the ribbon control lever on the typewriter in the "white" or "stencil" position.
2. Clean the typewriter keys with a stiff brush. Certain liquid type cleaners may be used only on conventional typebars, but never on elements or fonts.
3. Push the paper bail rollers to the sides of the paper bail.
4. Insert the cushion sheet between the stencil sheet and the backing sheet (glossy side up, if the cushion sheet is coated).
5. Insert the stencil pack into the typewriter and straighten it, using the paper-release lever on the typewriter.
6. On manual typewriters, use a firm, even, staccato touch; on electric typewriters, adjust the pressure regulator (starting with lowest pressure setting).
7. Proofread the material after typing has been completed.

Correction of errors   Errors can be corrected on a stencil by following these directions:
1. If you are using a coated (glossy) cushion sheet in the stencil pack, apply a thin coat of correction fluid to each character individually with a vertical, upward brushstroke.
2. If you are using a film-topped stencil, detach the film from the stencil and apply the correction fluid directly onto the stencil sheet.
3. If a tissue cushion sheet is being used, burnish (i.e., flatten out) the error first by rubbing it gently in a circular motion with the rounded end of a glass burnishing rod or a

paper clip. Then insert a pencil between the stencil sheet and the cushion sheet and apply the correction fluid; this creates an air pocket that will thoroughly seal off the error and will pave the way for a good correction.

4. Allow the correction fluid to dry and then type over the corrected error with a slightly lighter-than-normal touch.

Using stencil duplicating machines Though the kinds of stencil machines vary in minor details, their basic features are the same and the same procedures will ordinarily be followed with all machines. These procedures are given below:

1. Adjust the paper on the paper table. The left guide of the paper table should be set according to the scale indicated on the metal table, and the right guide should be moved in toward the paper stack until it lightly touches the right edge of the paper. Push the paper in until the corners are under the separators.
2. Raise the paper table to the correct height for the feed rollers.
3. Adjust the receiving tray to accommodate the size of paper being used.
4. To attach the stencil pack, move the right end clamps to release the right end of the protective cover on the ink pad. Then, open the left end clamp and remove the protective cover. Attach the stencil pack to the left end of the cylinder by hooking the stencil stub over the stencil hooks. Close the left clamp and remove the backing sheet by tearing it from the pack. Lay the stencil smoothly over the ink pad, ease out any wrinkles in the stencil, and attach the end of the stencil under the right cylinder clamps.
5. Release the brake, turn on the motor switch, raise the feed lever, and set the copy counter mechanism. Run the number of copies desired.
6. Turn off the copy counter mechanism and the motor switch.
7. When you have finished using the stencil duplicator, remove the stencil and cover the ink pad with a protective cover. Be sure that the ink cylinder is placed in the "Stop Here" position. This allows the ink to settle in the bottom of the cylinder and eliminates the possibility of the ink seeping through the ink pad.
8. Set the brake and clean up the work area.

If the position of the image on the paper is unacceptable, the stencil duplicator can be adjusted to correct the situation. When the copy image must be moved one-half inch or more horizontally from one side of the paper to the other, move the paper table guide rails and the paper supply in the same direction that the copy must be moved. The lateral adjustment knob can be used to make minor horizontal copy adjustments of less than one-half inch. Copy may be raised or lowered by using the vertical adjustment lever on the stencil duplicator. If the duplicated image is crooked, use the angular adjustment lever to correct this problem.

Color copies Multiple colors can be used with the stencil process. Either of the following two methods is acceptable when the addition of color is desired:

1. Use colored ink pads. It should be emphasized that this method is effective when used for short runs only, because the various colors of ink eventually overlap and blend. Cover the cylinder with a special wax-coated cover to prevent the black ink from flowing; attach a multicolor ink pad over the coated cover; outline the image area of the stencil with one or more colors of ink. Then, stretch the stencil over the ink pad to show where additional ink is needed. Pull the right edge of the stencil off the ink pad. Apply colored ink directly to the pad with a small brush. Paint on additional ink as needed. Fasten the loose end of the stencil and run off the copies.
2. Use colored ink cylinders for long runs. Some stencil duplicators allow the entire cylinder to be removed and replaced with another cylinder that is filled with a different color of ink. With this method, only the copy to be printed in any given color is cut in each stencil. Change the ink cylinder and the stencil after each run of copy until the desired result is obtained.

Problem-solving Tips—Stencil Process

Condition	Probable Cause(s)	Guideline(s)/Solution(s)
Visible corrections	excess keystroke pressure applied when correcting error	Type all corrections using normal keystroking pressure.
	error not completely covered with correction fluid	After correcting an error, see that all parts of the error have been covered with correction fluid.
	error typed over before correction fluid dried	Allow time for the correction fluid to dry properly.
Closed characters	dirty typewriter typeface	Clean the typewriter typeface.
Cut-out characters	excessively sharp typeface	Type on a typing film sheet placed on top of the stencil.
	keys struck too hard or machine impression lever set too high	Use a gentle stroke when typing; lower the impression setting.
Uneven quality	stroking possibly inconsistent or too light	Use a firm, even, staccato touch on a manual machine or adjust the pressure on an electric.
	strokes not printed clearly due to improper machine adjustments	Adjust the multiple copy control so that the stencil is held securely.
Setoff	newly-run sheets dropped into the receiving tray before the ink had dried on previous sheets— often caused by the use of a slow-drying ink	Check to see that the stencil duplicator is not overinked; use an ink that is quick-drying (oil-based inks are slower drying). Add a blank clean sheet or an inter-tray sheet as a separator between each printed sheet.
Poor signature(s)	signature(s) not cut deeply enough into the stencil	Write slowly with a uniform, heavy pressure on the stylus; use a rollpoint stylus; write the signature over a writing plate or on a hard surface.
Light spots	inadequate inking	Measure the ink supply in the cylinder for adequacy, adding ink if needed. Paint additional ink on the ink pad to ink especially dry areas on the pad, or change/agitate the ink pad.
	stencil duplicator not level	Place levelers under the stencil duplicator so that it is perfectly balanced.
	impression roller in poor condition	Replace the impression roller.
Copy in margins	typing extended beyond the guidelines on the stencil	Keep all the typing and drawings within the printed guidelines.

Drawing on a stencil   An illuminated drawing board designed for stencil preparation is available to hold the stencil. The drawing to be traced should be placed on
top of the drawing board. A flexible writing plate—a textured, translucent, plastic
sheet—goes on top of the drawing. The backing sheet of the stencil pack is inserted
through an opening at the top of the drawing board. The stencil is clipped to the
frame of the drawing board. By using the light under the drawing board, one can
easily trace a drawing onto the stencil. The proper drawing tools include an assortment of styli, plastic shading plates, and lettering guides.

Storage of stencils   Stencils that will be used again should be stored individually
in stencil folders (sometimes called *filing wrappers*) and ought to be kept in a cool,
dry area. The stencil should be placed in the folder with the ink side up. The stencil
must be carefully straightened to avoid wrinkling. Any excess ink on the stencil
will be absorbed by closing the folder and firmly rubbing the outside of the folder.
After five minutes, the folder should be opened and the stencil turned over to prevent it from sticking to the folder when it dries. Stencils may be cleaned with various
special preparations or they may be washed (depending on the kind of ink used)
so that handling and storage are facilitated (washed stencils may be hung on racks).
The contents of each stencil folder should be identified for filing purposes. Simple
techniques for doing so are these: (1) run the stencil folder through the stencil
duplicator before removing the stencil for storage (2) remove the stencil and blot
it on the stencil folder, thus reproducing a copy, or (3) tape one copy from the
stencil duplication on the outside of the folder.

Stencil maker   This piece of equipment will automatically transfer printed, typewritten, or pasted-up copy to an electronic stencil. The original and a blank electronic stencil are placed side-by-side on the cylinder of the stencil maker. When
the machine is activated, the image of the original is transferred to the blank
stencil.

Problem-solving tips for working with stencils   The table on page 520 offers some
solutions to the problems that are often encountered when one uses a stencil
duplicator.

Advantages and disadvantages of the stencil process   The following table lists
some of the advantages and disadvantages of the stencil process.

Advantages	Disadvantages
1. inexpensive process	1. stencil must be prepared before copies can be made
2. stencil duplicator generally uncompli- cated; operator can be easily trained	2. color can be produced, but the process is time-consuming and untidy
3. easy-to-type stencils; corrections easy to make	3. machine operation somewhat difficult if operator is improperly trained
4. legible copies with excellent contrast between black ink and paper	4. stencils may be cleaned for later runs, but doing so is a messy process
5. stencils repeatedly usable on paper of different weights and colors	
6. from 11 to 5,000 or more copies may be made from one stencil at a produc- tion rate of 7,500 to 12,000 copies an hour	

The stencil process is used primarily in small or medium-sized businesses. Considerable use of this process is also made by educational institutions, religious
organizations, and social groups.

PRINTING PROCESS
The five basic printing methods are: (1) letterpress (2) gravure (3) engraving (4) screen, and (5) offset. Since the offset process is the one most often used in business offices, it is described here, mainly for the benefit of medical secretaries employed in large organizations as opposed to private practices. Small, tabletop offset machines—very popular in offices today—are capable of producing quality copies, and they are relatively simple to operate. Some models are self-cleaning.

The fundamental parts of an offset duplicator are the master (or the *plate*) cylinder, the blanket cylinder, the impression cylinder, the ink fountain, and the water fountain. When the offset duplication process is begun, the master contacts the blanket cylinder leaving a mirror image. When paper passes between the blanket cylinder and the impression cylinder, the image is mirrored a second time and appears on the copy in correct, original form.

Classification of offset masters   The offset duplicating master may be paper, plastic, or metal. Paper masters are less durable and are normally used for short runs (from 50 to 1,000 copies) while plastic masters are designed for producing as many as 25,000 copies. Metal masters are the most durable, and the same metal master may be used repeatedly over a period of several years to produce 50,000 and more copies. Masters are available in a variety of sizes and weights, mountings (as straight-edge, slotted, or pin), and come in rolls, individual sheets, and fan-fold pockets. Each of these is designed for specific applications.

Imaging offset masters   Several methods can be used to transfer an image to a paper offset duplicating master:

1. **Direct image**   The image is made on an offset master by writing, drawing, or typing directly on the offset master. Special tools containing an oil-based substance that will attract ink must be used. Special pencils, crayons, ball-point pens, and rubber stamps can be purchased for this purpose. Typewriter ribbons suitable for use in the offset process are carbon ribbons (paper, polyethylene, and Mylar) or fabric ribbons (cotton, nylon, and silk).

2. **Electrostatic**   This method uses a copying feature available on many photocopying machines. The original copy is inserted into the machine and is projected onto a positive-charged photoconductive plate. This plate is passed through a toner solution and the emerging image is transferred, and then fused by the application of heat, onto a master. Many machines have the capability to produce paper and plastic masters, and several models of photocopying machines can also image metal masters. Masters can be made in seconds from any printed, typed, drawn, or bound original and will produce a minimum of 100 high-quality copies.

3. **Transfer**   This method uses a photographic camera process without the use of a separate negative. An image from an original is projected onto a light-sensitive sheet by way of gelatin transfer and photo-transfer methods. This process images a master. Self-contained photocopy units can deliver several masters a minute using this method.

4. **Pre-sensitized**   A photocopying machine is utilized in this process. An original and a special pre-coated master sheet are inserted into the machine. This master sheet has been pre-coated with a highly sensitive substance which is acted on by the photocopying machine and results in a master ready for use on an offset duplicator.

Two methods can be used to produce an image on a metal master:

1. **Pre-sensitized**   A graphic camera is used to make a film negative of an original. This film negative is exposed to a concentrated light source and onto a metal master. These film negatives can be stored and used many times to make additional metal masters when needed. Metal masters produce very high-quality copies. Photographs

can be effectively reproduced through the capability of this method to reproduce halftones.

2. **Transfer**   This method is basically the same as the one described for imaging paper and plastic masters. Photocopying machines can produce metal masters of the same size as the original, while a camera process can accommodate the enlargement or reduction of the original before imaging the metal master.

Typing paper offset masters   Medical secretaries employed in large organizations may be involved in writing or typing on paper offset masters. A discussion concerning the correct procedures to follow when typing paper offset masters is included in this section. Paper offset masters must be handled with care. The following steps can be followed in preparing typewritten offset masters:

1. Clean the typeface on your typewriter.
2. Check the typewriter fabric ribbon to make certain that it is suitable for typing on a paper offset master; certain kinds of film ribbon may be used in offset master preparation.
3. Push the paper bail rollers to the margin area of the master.
4. Type directly on the paper master with the same amount of pressure that is used in regular typing, but at a slightly slower pace. (A heavy touch tends to encourage the appearance of hollow characters on copies.)
5. The paper master should be handled with the utmost care. One's fingers should touch only the edges of the master to avoid smearing. Hand lotion containing lanolin or nail polish can produce smudge marks on copies. Also, paper offset masters should never be folded or creased.
6. If the paper master must be reinserted into the typewriter, slip a clean sheet of paper over the master to prevent it from being smudged by the feed rollers.
7. After typing the master, allow it to rest for a minimum of 30 minutes. This waiting period will provide time for the image to become fixed so that the master will produce a darker, sharper image when run on the offset duplicator.

Special offset pens, pencils, and crayons should be used when drawing, writing, or ruling on an offset master. When one is tracing a design on a paper master, offset carbon paper must be used. (The manufacturer of the offset duplicating equipment can provide the necessary information concerning the drawing tools needed for preparing various kinds of artwork on an offset master.)

Correction of errors on a paper offset master   For best results, errors should be corrected with a special eraser designed for use on paper offset masters. Offset erasers are very soft and do not contain abrasives that will mar the surface of the master. (If absolutely necessary, any soft nonabrasive eraser may be substituted; however, this practice is not recommended.) A light, quick stroke should be used in erasing an error. The eraser should be cleaned after each stroke by rubbing it on a clean sheet of paper or on a piece of sandpaper. One should not erase too heavily since the carbon deposit is removed rather easily. A slightly visible ghost image may remain on the master, but this image will not be reproduced on the copies. Only the surface ink should be removed. Deep erasures will remove the surface coating on the paper master, and these spots will reproduce in black. Offset deletion fluid can be used to make a correction which covers a large area of the master. The secretary can then type over the erased area with the same pressure used originally. Only a single erasure can be made in any one spot.

Storage of offset masters   Offset paper masters should be filed and stored in a plain paper folder and placed in a flat position. If more than one master is stored in a folder, each of the paper masters should be separated with a sheet of paper to prevent them from absorbing ink from each other. A cotton pad moistened with water can be used to remove any smudges left on the edges of a master before it is stored. If proper care is taken of paper offset masters, they can be rerun many times with excellent results. The same methods that have been suggested on page 521 for identifying the folders in which stencils are stored can be used in filing paper offset masters. Plastic and metal masters can be stored in paper folders in the same manner as paper masters; however, special cabinets are available in which these plates may be hung to that there is little danger of their touching each other.

Problem-solving tips for working with offset masters   Some of the more common problems encountered in working with offset masters are identified in the following table.

Problem-solving Tips—Offset Process

Condition	Probable Cause(s)	Guideline(s)/Solution(s)
Black correction smudges	errors erased too deeply on offset master, thereby removing surface coating	Typist must prepare a new offset master.
	dirty eraser	Use fountain solution on the eraser to try to clean the master error area.
Fingerprints	improper handling of offset master	Only the edges of the offset master should be touched; avoid using hand lotion with lanolin before touching the offset master.
Roll marks	excess pressure from typewriter rollers	Push the paper bail rollers to the margin area of the offset master; if reinserting the master, place a sheet of paper over the master.
Light image	offset master run immediately after preparation	Allow the offset master to rest from 30 minutes to two hours to allow the image to set.
	typing strokes too light	Type the master using a slightly heavier pressure or install a new offset fabric ribbon.
Uneven drawing	uneven pressure used when making outlines	Make all drawings on a flat, hard surface; use a firm, even pressure when making lines; use the artwork tool that is appropriate for the desired effect.

Advantages and disadvantages of the offset process   The following table lists the advantages and disadvantages of the offset process.

Advantages
1. high-quality printing closely resembling original
2. all copies of equal quality
3. copy reproducible on both sides of the paper

Disadvantages
1. equipment relatively expensive when compared with that used in fluid and stencil processes
2. more training required for operating personnel

4. printing can be in color
5. hourly production rate of 9,000 or more copies
6. only one metal master needed for more than 50,000 copies

3. equipment requires more maintenance than fluid and stencil process equipment
4. higher material costs than those used in fluid and stencil processes
5. more time needed both in preparing the machine for operation and in cleaning the machine after copies have been run off

Use of the offset printing process can result in excellent reproduction. If appearance is a primary requirement, offset duplication offers many advantages, particularly for business communications that will be distributed outside one's organization.

PHOTOCOPY PROCESS

The copying machine has rapidly become a necessity in the office. Copiers are now used in virtually all offices, large or small. These photocopying machines reproduce directly from original documents. No intermediate master is needed.

Copiers are usually classified in two ways. One classification is based on the chemical process by which the copier works; the second, which is used more frequently, concerns the type of paper used for making copies. The newest innovation in copying machines is the capability to produce copies in a variety of colors, including a range of seven colors. The major copier classifications are the *wet process* and the *dry process*. These are divided into a number of secondary processes. There are four basic wet processes and three dry processes. The wet processes are: (1) diazo (2) diffusion transfer (3) stabilization, and (4) dye transfer.

1. **Diazo process** uses a coated paper that is sensitive to light. After exposure to the original, the coated paper passes through a developing process which converts the coating into a duplicate of the original. Copies reproduced in this way are inexpensive. An added advantage is that oversize documents can be copied on diazo process equipment. This feature is often used for special applications such as copying engineering drawings. The equipment is rather complicated and generally requires considerable maintenance. Unfortunately, copies cannot be made from originals printed on both sides or from opaque paper.

2. **Diffusion transfer** is sometimes called a photo transfer. The original sheet and a negative sheet are rolled around a light source so that the light passes through the photo paper. The negative is then exposed by the reflection from the original. After exposure, the negative is placed with a sheet of positive sensitized paper and is developed. Both sheets emerge slightly dampened from the copier, and the negative sheet is peeled off and discarded. This process has the capacity to make very clear copies and can also reproduce colors. Although the equipment itself is relatively inexpensive, the per-copy cost tends to be expensive and the process is somewhat wasteful. Since the copies emerge from the machine in a damp condition, some drying time must elapse before the copies can be handled.

3. **Stabilization** exposes the original to a sheet coated with a silver-sensitive emulsion mixed with a developing agent. These sheets are then passed through a special solution which activates the developing agent and results in an emerging image. Next, the sheets are bathed in a stabilizing solution so as to set the image. This image is a reverse negative and produces a white-on-black copy. To obtain a more usable black-on-white copy, the reverse negative must be reinserted into the machine with a second coated sheet, and the entire process must be repeated a second time. The negatives can be filed and reused many times. The general complexity and increased costs associated with this photocopy process has diminished its use. The necessary repetition of steps as well as the time needed to dry the dampened copies is a disadvantage of the process.

4. **Dye transfer** uses an incandescent light source to expose a sensitized master (sometimes called a *matrix*) to the original. The master is developed in an activating solution and is then placed with a sheet of ordinary paper and passed through rollers. The rollers apply sufficient pressure to transfer the dye image from the master to the copy paper. This process requires that the two sheets be separated after they emerge from the machine. This process allows the copying of colors. Each master can reproduce about eight copies. Unfortunately, copies tend to be brownish in appearance. Copies are expensive unless several copies are made from each master: the more copies made from a master, the lower the cost per copy.

Dry photocopying processes are: (1) thermal (2) dual spectrum, and (3) electrostatic.

1. **Thermal** is a process by which an original and a heat-sensitive sheet are joined and exposed to an infrared light source. Because dark material absorbs more heat than light material does, this exposure images the dark outlines and produces a copy. Unfortunately, the copies made with this process have a tendency to become brittle as time passes.

2. **Dual spectrum** is a process in which a light-sensitive copy paper and a heat-sensitive copy paper are both needed to produce a copy. The original and the light-sensitive paper are exposed to a light source. Then, the original is removed and the light-sensitive copy paper and the heat-sensitive copy paper are placed together and are exposed to a source of heat. This step transfers the image to the heat-sensitive paper which becomes the final copy.

3. **Electrostatic** involves a *transfer* electrostatic process which is based on light reflecting an original through lenses and exposing a charged drum. The resulting particles of toner left on the drum become the image, which is then transferred and fused by heat onto the copy. A *direct* electrostatic process follows the same principles as the transfer electrostatic process except that the image appears directly on the copy paper and does not need to be transferred.

Photocopying machines are sometimes categorized as *coated-paper copiers* or *plain-paper copiers,* depending on the copy paper required for duplication. Earlier machines used coated papers, and although these photocopiers are still very prevalent, the present trend is definitely toward an increased use of plain-paper copying equipment. Some of the reasons given for the current popularity of plain-paper copiers include the following:

1. The appearance of the copies closely resembles the original, since the same grade and weight of paper is used in the duplication process

2. Plain-paper copies can be produced on letterhead stationery.

3. The slightly higher per-copy cost of plain-paper copies is often considered to be justified, because of the higher quality copies that can be made. The appearance of plain-paper copies is especially suitable and desirable for documents that will be sent outside the company.

4. Photocopying equipment manufacturers continue to develop special peripheral equipment used with plain-paper copiers that can easily and quickly produce offset masters, transparencies, and two-sided copies; that can automatically sort and collate copies; and that can provide for the cassette-loading of paper. Other available features include: slitters, perforators, folders, staplers, stitchers, and binding devices. Often, these mechanisms can be operated independently of the copier.

5. The ease of operating a plain-paper copier is appealing to office employees.

6. Special supply requirements are kept to a minimum.

Though coated-paper copiers are used in many offices, the copies made with these machines do have some limitations: (1) coated-paper copies do not resemble or feel like bond stationery, (2) writing is difficult on coated-paper copies, and (3) equipment tends to be complex and requires special materials for its use. Efforts are being made by manufacturers of coated-paper copiers to overcome some of these disadvantages. Even though the present costs of plain-paper copies are higher than the coated-paper copies, predictions are that by 1980, six out of every seven copies made will be reproduced on plain paper. Another apparent trend is towards the use of hybrid copier/duplicators. These machines can automatically develop masters and run copies in one step.

Control of photocopying machines The total volume of copies produced on an individual copying machine depends on the size of the office, the type of material copied, the availability of the copier, and whether or not use of the machine is supervised. The duplicating costs associated with a copier can be astonishingly high. An abnormally large part of an organization's reprographics budget is often spent on photocopiers. When copiers are very convenient and easy to operate, their use is often diverted to activities unrelated to the business or to the practice. One director of a large corporation has estimated that over ten percent of the copies made on unattended copiers was for the personal use of the employees. Several plans have been devised to discourage the personal use of copying machines as well as the indiscriminate copying of business communications. The following copy control systems are in use today:

1. **Key control plan** A key must be inserted into the photocopying machine in order to make copies.
2. **Card control method** A small card (plastic or computer) must be placed into the photocopier before it will function properly and produce copies.
3. **Coin control method** A pay-as-you-go practice is followed by which the insertion of a coin is required in order to activate the machine.
4. **Supervisory control plan** One person is placed in charge of the copying machine(s), and all work to be copied must be submitted to this person before copying is allowed.
5. **Audit system** A machine-recorded tally is kept of all work being processed on the copier. An audit system can be used independently or in conjunction with any of the previously mentioned plans.

Problem-solving tips for working with copiers Although most copiers work quite satisfactorily, an occasional problem may arise during their operation. The table on page 528 lists a few problems associated with some photocopiers, offers possible causes of the trouble, and suggests a few solutions.

Advantages and disadvantages of the photocopying process The following table provides an overall view of some of the strengths and weaknesses often associated with using a photocopying process.

Advantages	Disadvantages
1. copies easy to make	1. higher costs per copy than with other duplicating processes
2. copies reproducible very quickly	
3. machine that is easy to operate and requires little training	2. very attractive for copying material for personal use
4. no master needed—only a legible original	3. tendency toward making too many unnecessary copies of material
5. quality on all copies remains the same throughout a run	4. rather slow functioning of some copiers
6. pages from the firm's catalogs and from books (with copyright permission) can be copied on many machines	

Problem-solving Tips—Photocopying Machines

Condition	Probable Cause(s)	Guideline(s)/Solution(s)
Feeding difficulties	dimensional stability and tolerance of the paper affected feeding—perhaps paper was too stiff	Use 20-pound paper for best results; lighter paper is more difficult to handle.
	moisture content in the paper too high	Check your packaging and storing facility—humidity must be controlled.
Paper curls	inadequate weight of paper being used	Read the instruction manual to determine whether the proper kind of copy paper is being used. If so, call the sales office of the firm selling the equipment for further advice.
Poor duplication	attempting to copy show-through originals	Use only opaque originals.
Machine malfunction	any one of many mechanical difficulties	Call the authorized service representative.

A chart entitled "Summary of Methods of Copying and Duplicating" that shows some of the characteristics of the various reprographic processes is presented on pages 530 and 531 of this chapter.

18.2

NEW DEVELOPMENTS IN REPROGRAPHICS

Technological developments cause frequent changes in reprographic techniques; even the best copying method for a particular office application may become obsolete or too expensive overnight. A few of the technological developments that in time will probably change or alter office copying procedures are described here.

Thermal spirit masters   Photocopying machines that use the heat-transfer process can also be used to make thermal spirit masters. Of course, a special thermal spirit master pack is required, but these packs are not expensive. The original to be copied is inserted into the thermal carbon pack; then the pack is passed through the photocopying machine. This flexibility allows thermal spirit masters to be made of typewritten copy, letters, magazine articles, or handwritten copy. The master made by this process will produce from 40 to 50 legible copies.

Electronic stencil scanner   This office machine can create a stencil that produces up to 10,000 copies. The electronic scanner copies any original copy including typewritten copy, line drawings, hand lettering, and photographic halftones. Simple scanners recognize all colors as black, but more expensive models can be set to ignore specific colors in the original copy. Although these devices may require as much as 12 minutes to make one stencil, the machine can be left unattended.

Thermal stencils   The thermal photocopying process has also been incorporated into a special machine for making stencils. The machine requires a special, heat-sensitive stencil. This process can reproduce copy which is prepared in black ink. Photographic halftones cannot be reproduced. Care must be taken in order not to smudge the original copy, since this process reproduces all shades of any color as definite black impressions.

Facsimile copying   Images of telegram-size messages have been transmitted between offices over teletype telephone lines for years. The recent application of laser technology has broadened the size and volume capabilities as well as the speed with which messages can be transmitted. Facsimile copiers are designed for use anywhere that a telephone and an electric outlet are available. One master at the source office can cause single or multiple copies to be transmitted to many other offices which may be geographically separated. Documents, charts, pictures, electrocardiograms, and other recorded data can be transmitted or received within two to six minutes.

Micrographic copies   Many offices have used microfilm as a relatively inexpensive method of storing large files. This photoreduction process allows individual records to be retrieved, viewed, and copied. The term *micrographics* merely indicates a variety of microfilm record-storage processes. Photographs or architectural-engineering drawings are usually recorded on film that is larger than the kind used for standard letters. Each film exposure can be attached to a computer punch card for filing. An alternative is a plastic jacket that can contain one exposure or a strip of exposures. Modern computers can record their output on either microfilm or microfiche when a microform camera is attached directly to the computer. Computer Output Microfilm (COM) is gaining rapid acceptance because of its low storage cost coupled with its speed and the easy retrievability of the records it produces. Computer Output Microfilm stores pages of printed copy on rolls of film. Computer microfiche output stores pages of copy on sheets of film approximately 4″ x 6″ in size. While standard microfiche ratios store 100 or 220 exposures per film sheet, ultrafiche can store two to three times this number of exposures on the 4″ x 6″ film sheet. Each exposure on the fiche is a picture of an 8½″ x 11″ document. The stored information on fiche may be retrieved through the use of a microfiche reader. This reader is attached to some models of photocopying machines and printed copies may be made. This process is especially useful for storing large numbers of inactive patient files. (See also Chapter 9, section 9.9.)

NCR forms   NCR (no carbon required) forms are popular in many offices. The pressure-sensitive top sheets and duplicate sheets allow the reproduction of several copies without the use of carbon paper, which tends to become messy. Insurance and billing forms, telephone message pads, and other such preprinted material can be purchased with this feature. The materials are, however, more expensive than conventional carbon packs.

18.3

SUMMARY OF COPYING METHODS

The following chart summarizes the copying methods discussed earlier.

Summary of Methods of Copying and Duplicating

Factors to Consider	Carbon Paper	Fluid Duplicating
COPY APPEARANCE One of the first points to consider is what you want your copies to look like. Some methods are limited to one-color reproduction only. Others permit you to use multi-colors economically and/or reproduce pictures and illustrations.	single-color reproduction	multicolor reproduction
ECONOMICAL LENGTH OF RUN The copy ranges listed here do not represent the maximum length of run, but the most economical range for each method. There is usually a point where an economical length of run dictates the method used unless it is overruled by other considerations.	1 to 10 copies	11 to 300 copies
PAPER SIZE RANGE The size of the original to be copied or the size of the paper to be duplicated or printed will help determine the methods that you should use.	letter size legal size	11″ x 15″ maximum 3″ x 4″ minimum image: 11″ x 14″
COPY COST RANGE (8½″ x 11″) Cost per copy will vary with the method of master preparation, the types of supplies and paper used, and the length of the run. Because quantity purchasing can also affect costs, approximate copy cost ranges are shown.	1¢ and more	$\frac{3}{5}$¢ to 1¢ per copy
SPEED Speed is an important factor to consider because it is related to your investment in people and also to the urgency of the material to be duplicated. If it takes too long to get copies, costly minutes or hours can be lost.	copies made as original is typed	up to 120 copies/minute, or 7200 copies/hour
MASTERS The type of master will directly reflect on all of the above factors. Each process varies with the flexibility afforded by various methods of master generation.	none	*Direct Image* It is imaged by typing, writing, or drawing. Available in various colors: blue, black, red, and green; and in various length of run: long = 300+ copies, medium = 200+ copies, short = 100+ copies. *Thermal* With a faxable original copy, a short run spirit master can be created by a single pass through a thermal copier. Purple and black are available.

Stencil Duplicating	Offset Duplicating	Copier
multicolor reproduction	full-color reproduction	single-color reproduction or multicolor reproduction (up to 7 colors)
11 to 5000 or more copies	11 to 50,000 or more copies	1 to 10 copies

9" x 15" maximum
3" x 5" minimum
image: 7$\frac{5}{8}$" x 14"
	11" x 17" maximum
	 3" x 5" minimum
	maximum image:
	  tabletop 9$\frac{1}{2}$" x 13"
	  console 10$\frac{1}{2}$" x 16$\frac{1}{2}$"
		up to 10" x 15"

$\frac{1}{3}$¢ to 1$\frac{2}{5}$¢ per copy	$\frac{1}{3}$¢ to 1$\frac{1}{2}$¢ per copy	2¢ to 5¢ and more
fluid inks: up to 200 copies/minute, or 1200 copies/hour *paste inks:* up to 125 copies/minutes, or 7500 copies/hour	up to 9000 copies/hour	first copy in 3 to 10 seconds; various ranges of output up to 8,000+/ hour
Stencil It is imaged by any combination of typing, writing, or drawing. Various types are available for specific applications. It will produce thousands of copies. *Thermal Stencil* With a faxable original copy, a stencil can be created by a single pass through a thermal copier. It will produce thousands of copies. *Electronic Stencil* In a matter of minutes, a stencil can be produced from most originals including halftone photographs. It will produce thousands of copies.	*Direct image* It is imaged by any combination of typing, writing, or drawing. Lengths of run are from 50 to several thousand. *Electrostatic* It is imaged on an electrostatic copier. Copies are available in seconds. It will produce a minimum of 100 copies. *Metal Plate* With a photographic negative and concentrated light source, a metal plate is exposed and duplicated. Short run = 10,000 copies/side; long run = 25,000+ copies/side. *Camera/Processor* It is a photographic process using a separate negative. Self-contained units deliver several masters/minute. Length of run is in the thousands. All of the above masters will duplicate in any of hundreds of colors.	no master involved, as copying is not a transfer process unless teamed with offset duplicating; copy and masters are prepared from an original copy

APPENDIX
LATIN WORDS AND ABBREVIATIONS IN PRESCRIPTIONS

Abbreviation Used on Prescription	Complete Latin Word or Phrase	English Meaning
aa or $\overline{aa}$	ana	of each
a.c.	ante cibum or ante cibos	before meals
ad	ad	to (a specified amount)
add.	adde	add
	addatur	let it be added
	addantur	let them be added
ad lib.	ad libitum	at pleasure
ad sat.	ad saturandum	to saturation
ad us. exter.	ad usum externum	for external use
adv.	adversum	against
agit. a. us.	agita ante usum	shake before using
agit. bene	agita bene	shake well
aq.	aqua	water
aq. bull.	aqua bulliens	boiling water
aq. dest.	aqua destillata	distilled water
aq. ferv.	aqua fervens	warm water
bib.	bibe	drink
b.i.d.	bis in die	twice a day
c or $\overline{c}$	cum	with
cap.	capiat	let him take
cap. moll.	capsula mollis	soft capsule
cib.	cibus	food, meal
collut.	collutorium	mouthwash
comp.	compositus	compounded
cong.	congius	gallon
cons.	conserva	keep
consperg.	consperge	dust, sprinkle
conter.	contere	rub together
d.	da	give
	detur	let it be given
	dentur	let them be given
de d. in d.	de die in diem	from day to day
deglut.	deglutiatur	let it be swallowed
dil.	dilue	dilute
dim.	dimidius	one half
dir. prop.	directione propria	with proper direction
div.	divide	divide
d.t.d.	detur talis dosis	let such a dose be given
dur. dol.	durante dolore	while pain lasts

Abbreviation Used on Prescription	Complete Latin Word or Phrase	English Meaning
e	ex *or* e	out of, with
ead.	eadem	the same
ejusd.	ejusdem	of the same
e. m. p.	ex modo praescripto	in the manner prescribed
et	et	and
f.	fac	make
f. *or* ft.	fiat	let it be made
	fiant	let them be made
gr.	granum *pl* grana	grain, grains
grad.	gradatim	gradually
gtt.	gutta *pl* guttae	drop, drops
h.	hora	hour
h. d.	hora decubitus	at bedtime
h. s. *or* h. som.	hora somni	just before sleeping
in d.	in die	in a day
int. cib.	inter cibos	between meals
int. noct.	inter noctem	during the night
lat. dol.	lateri dolente	to the painful side
M.	misce	mix
mist.	mistura	mixture
m. dict. *or* mor. dict.	more dicto	as directed
noct.	nocte	at night
non rep. *or* non repet.	non repetatur	do not refill
O. D.	oculus dexter	right eye
	oculo dextro	in the right eye
omn. hor.	omni hora	every hour
omn. man.	omni mane	every morning
omn. noct.	omni nocte	every night
O. S.	oculus sinister	left eye
	oculo sinistro	in the left eye
p. ae. *or* part. aeq.	partes aequales	equal parts
part. vic.	partitis vicibus	in divided parts
p. c.	post cibum *or* post cibos	after meals
pond.	pondere	by weight
p. r. n.	pro re nata	as needed
pro dos.	pro dose	for a dose
pro rat. aet.	pro ratione aetatis	according to age
pro us. ext.	pro usu externo	for external use
q. d.	quaque die	every day
q. h. *or* qq. hor.	quaque hora	every hour
q. i. d.	quater in die	four times a day
q. o. d.		every other day

Abbreviation Used on Prescription	Complete Latin Word or Phrase	English Meaning
q. s.	quantum sufficiat	as much as needed
quot.	quoties	as often as needed
s. *or* s̄	sine	without
sem.	semi, semis	one half
semih.	semihora	half an hour
sesquihor.	sesquihora	an hour and one half
Sig. *or* S.	signa	write on label
sol.	solutio	solution
solv.	solve	dissolve
ss *or* s̄s̄	semissem	one half
stat.	statim	at once
stillat.	stillatim	by drops *or* in small amounts
sum. tal.	sumat talem	let him take one like this
syr.	syrupus	syrup
t.	ter	three times
ter.	tere	rub
t. i. d.	ter in die	three times a day
ut dict.	ut dictum	as directed
utend.	utendus	to be used
ut. supr.	ut supra	as above
vic.	vices	times

WEIGHTS AND MEASURES

Unit	Abbr or Symbol	Equivalents in Other Units of Same System	Equivalent in Indicated System
length			
English system			metric system
mile	mi	5280 feet 320 rods 1760 yards	1.609 kilometers
rod	rd	5.50 yards 16.5 feet	5.029 meters
yard	yd	3 feet 36 inches	0.914 meters
foot	ft or '	12 inches 0.333 yards	30.480 centimeters
inch	in or "	0.083 feet 0.027 yards	2.540 centimeters
metric system			English system
myriameter	myr	1×10^3 meters	6.2137 miles
kilometer	km	1000 meters	0.62137 miles
hectometer	hm	100 meters	109.36 yards
dekameter	dkm	10 meters	32.808 feet
meter	m	1 meter	39.370 inches
decimeter	dm	0.1 meters	3.9370 inches
centimeter	cm	0.01 meters	0.39370 inches
millimeter	mm	0.001 meters	0.039370 inches
micron	μ	1×10^{-6} meters	3.9370×10^{-5} inches
weight			
avoirdupois weight			metric system
ton	tn		
short ton		20 short hundredweight 2000 pounds	0.907 metric tons
long ton		20 long hundredweight 2240 pounds	1.016 metric tons
hundredweight	cwt		
short hundredweight		100 pounds 0.05 short tons	45.359 kilograms
long hundredweight		112 pounds 0.05 long tons	50.802 kilograms
pound	lb or lb av	16 ounces 7000 grains	0.453 kilograms
ounce	oz or oz av	16 drams 437.5 grains	28.349 grams
dram	dr or dr av	27.343 grains 0.0625 ounces	1.771 grams
grain	gr	0.036 drams 0.002285 ounces	0.0648 grams

Unit	Abbr or Symbol	Equivalents in Other Units of Same System	Equivalent in Indicated System
troy weight			metric system
pound	lb t	12 ounces 240 pennyweight 5760 grains	0.373 kilograms
ounce	oz t	20 pennyweight 480 grains	31.103 grams
pennyweight	dwt *also* pwt	24 grains 0.05 ounces	1.555 grams
grain	gr	0.042 pennyweight 0.002083 ounces	0.0648 grams
apothecaries' weight			metric system
pound	lb ap	12 ounces 5760 grains	0.373 kilograms
ounce	oz ap *or* ℥	8 drams 480 grains	31.103 grams
dram	dr ap *or* ℨ	3 scruples 60 grains	3.887 grams
scruple	s ap *or* ℈	20 grains 0.333 drams	1.295 grams
grain	gr	0.05 scruples 0.002083 ounces 0.0166 drams	0.0648 grams
metric system			apothecaries' weight
metric ton	MT *or* t	1×10^6 grams	2679.2 lbs
quintal	q	1×10^5 grams	267.92 lbs
kilogram	kg	1000 grams	2.6792 lbs
hectogram	hg	100 grams	3.2151 oz
dekagram	dag	10 grams	0.32151 oz
gram	g *or* gm	1 gram	0.032151 oz
decigram	dg	0.10 grams	1.5432 grains
centigram	cg	0.01 grams	0.15432 grains
milligram	mg	0.001 grams	0.015432 grains
microgram	μg	1×10^{-6} grams	1.5432×10^{-5} grains

capacity

Unit	Abbr or Symbol	Equivalents in Other Units of Same System	Equivalent in Indicated System
apothecaries' measure			metric system
gallon	gal	4 quarts (231 cubic inches)	3.785 liters
quart	qt	2 pints (57.75 cubic inches)	0.946 liters
pint	pt	4 gills (28.875 cubic inches)	0.473 liters
gill	gi	4 fluidounces (7.218 cubic inches)	118.291 milliliters

Unit	Abbr or Symbol	Equivalents in Other Units of Same System	Equivalent in Indicated System
fluidounce	fl oz *or* f ʒ	8 fluidrams (1.804 cubic inches)	29.573 milliliters
fluidram	fl dr *or* f ʒ	60 minims (0.225 cubic inches)	3.696 milliliters
minim	min *or* ♏	1/60 fluidram (0.003759 cubic inch)	0.061610 milliliters
metric system			apothecaries' measure
kiloliter	kl	1000 liters	264.18 gals
hectoliter	hl	100 liters	26.418 gals
dekaliter	dal	10 liters	2.6418 gals
liter	l	1 liter	1.0567 qts
deciliter	dl	0.10 liters	3.3815 fl oz
centiliter	cl	0.01 liters	2.7052 fl dr
milliliter	ml	0.001 liters	16.231 minims
microliter	μl	1×10^{-6} liters	0.016231 minims

METRIC AND TEMPERATURE CONVERSION FACTORS

Metric Conversion Factors

LENGTH

To convert from	to	multiply by
centimeters	inches	.394
meters	yards	1.094
meters	feet	3.281
kilometers	miles	.622
inches	centimeters	2.54
yards	meters	.914
feet	meters	.305
miles	kilometers	1.609

AREA

To convert from	to	multiply by
square centimeters	square inches	.155
square meters	square yards	1.196
square kilometers	square miles	.386
square kilometers	acres	247.16
square inches	square centimeters	6.452
square yards	square meters	.836
square miles	square kilometers	2.59
acres	square kilometers	.004

VOLUME

To convert from	to	multiply by
liters	fluidounces	33.81
liters	quarts	1.057
liters	gallons	.264
fluidounces	liters	.0296
quarts	liters	.946
gallons	liters	3.785

MASS

To convert from	to	multiply by
grams	ounces (avdp.)	.035
grams	pounds	.0022
kilograms	ounces	35.27
kilograms	pounds	2.205
ounces (avdp.)	grams	28.35
pounds	grams	453.6
ounces	kilograms	.0284
pounds	kilograms	.4536

Fahrenheit To Celsius Temperature Conversion

$C° = 5/9 (F° -32°)$

F°	C°	F°	C°	F°	C°	F°	C°
−27	−32.8	20	−6.7	67	19.4	114	45.6
−26	−32.2	21	−6.1	68	20.0	115	46.1
−25	−31.7	22	−5.6	69	20.6	116	46.7
−24	−31.1	23	−5.0	70	21.1	117	47.2
−23	−30.6	24	−4.4	71	21.7	118	47.8
−22	−30.0	25	−3.9	72	22.2	119	48.3
−21	−29.4	26	−3.3	73	22.8	120	48.9
−20	−28.9	27	−2.8	74	23.3	121	49.4
−19	−28.3	28	−2.2	75	23.9	122	50.0
−18	−27.8	29	−1.7	76	24.4	123	50.6
−17	−27.2	30	−1.1	77	25.0	124	51.1
−16	−26.7	31	−0.6	78	25.6	125	51.7
−15	−26.1	32	0.0	79	26.1	126	52.2
−14	−25.6	33	0.6	80	26.7	127	52.8
−13	−25.0	34	1.1	81	27.2	128	53.3
−12	−24.4	35	1.7	82	27.8	129	53.9
−11	−23.9	36	2.2	83	28.3	130	54.4
−10	−23.3	37	2.8	84	28.9	131	55.0
−9	−22.8	38	3.3	85	29.4	132	55.6
−8	−22.2	39	3.9	86	30.0	133	56.1
−7	−21.7	40	4.4	87	30.6	134	56.7
−6	−21.1	41	5.0	88	31.1	135	57.2
−5	−20.6	42	5.6	89	31.7	136	57.8
−4	−20.0	43	6.1	90	32.2	137	58.3
−3	−19.4	44	6.7	91	32.8	138	58.9
−2	−18.9	45	7.2	92	33.3	139	59.4
−1	−18.3	46	7.8	93	33.9	140	60.0
0	−17.8	47	8.3	94	34.4	141	60.6
1	−17.2	48	8.9	95	35.0	142	61.1
2	−16.7	49	9.4	96	35.6	143	61.7
3	−16.1	50	10.0	97	36.1	144	62.2
4	−15.6	51	10.6	98	36.7	145	62.8
5	−15.0	52	11.1	99	37.2	146	63.3
6	−14.4	53	11.7	100	37.8	147	63.9
7	−13.9	54	12.2	101	38.3	148	64.4
8	−13.3	55	12.8	102	38.9	149	65.0
9	−12.8	56	13.3	103	39.4	150	65.6
10	−12.2	57	13.9	104	40.0	151	66.1
11	−11.7	58	14.4	105	40.6	152	66.7
12	−11.1	59	15.0	106	41.1	153	67.2
13	−10.6	60	15.6	107	41.7	154	67.8
14	−10.0	61	16.1	108	42.2	155	68.3
15	−9.4	62	16.7	109	42.8	156	68.9
16	−8.9	63	17.2	110	43.3	157	69.4
17	−8.3	64	17.8	111	43.9	158	70.0
18	−7.8	65	18.3	112	44.4	159	70.6
19	−7.2	66	18.9	113	45.0	160	71.1

F°	C°	F°	C°	F°	C°	F°	C°
161	71.7	174	78.9	187	86.1	200	93.3
162	72.2	175	79.4	188	86.7	201	93.9
163	72.8	176	80.0	189	87.2	202	94.4
164	73.3	177	80.6	190	87.8	203	95.0
165	73.9	178	81.1	191	88.3	204	95.6
166	74.4	179	81.7	192	88.9	205	96.1
167	75.0	180	82.2	193	89.4	206	96.7
168	75.6	181	82.8	194	90.0	207	97.2
169	76.1	182	83.3	195	90.6	208	97.8
170	76.7	183	83.9	196	91.1	209	98.3
171	77.2	184	84.4	197	91.7	210	98.9
172	77.8	185	85.0	198	92.2	211	99.4
173	78.3	186	85.6	199	92.8	212	100.0

Celsius To Fahrenheit Temperature Conversion

$$F° = 9/5 \ C° + 32°$$

C°	F°	C°	F°	C°	F°	C°	F°
−31	−23.8	2	35.6	35	95.0	68	154.4
−30	−22.0	3	37.4	36	96.8	69	156.2
−29	−20.2	4	39.2	37	98.6	70	158.0
−28	−18.4	5	41.0	38	100.4	71	159.8
−27	−16.6	6	42.8	39	102.2	72	161.6
−26	−14.8	7	44.6	40	104.0	73	163.4
−25	−13.0	8	46.4	41	105.8	74	165.2
−24	−11.2	9	48.2	42	107.6	75	167.0
−23	−9.4	10	50.0	43	109.4	76	168.8
−22	−7.6	11	51.8	44	111.2	77	170.6
−21	−5.8	12	53.6	45	113.0	78	172.4
−20	−4.0	13	55.4	46	114.8	79	174.2
−19	−2.2	14	57.2	47	116.6	80	176.0
−18	−0.4	15	59.0	48	118.4	81	177.8
−17	1.4	16	60.8	49	120.2	82	179.6
−16	3.2	17	62.6	50	122.0	83	181.4
−15	5.0	18	64.4	51	123.8	84	183.2
−14	6.8	19	66.2	52	125.6	85	185.0
−13	8.6	20	68.0	53	127.4	86	186.8
−12	10.4	21	69.8	54	129.2	87	188.6
−11	12.2	22	71.6	55	131.0	88	190.4
−10	14.0	23	73.4	56	132.8	89	192.2
−9	15.8	24	75.2	57	134.6	90	194.0
−8	17.6	25	77.0	58	136.4	91	195.8
−7	19.4	26	78.8	59	138.2	92	197.6
−6	21.2	27	80.6	60	140.0	93	199.4
−5	23.0	28	82.4	61	141.8	94	201.2
−4	24.8	29	84.2	62	143.6	95	203.0
−3	26.6	30	86.0	63	145.4	96	204.8
−2	28.4	31	87.8	64	147.2	97	206.6
−1	30.2	32	89.6	65	149.0	98	208.4
0	32.0	33	91.4	66	150.8	99	210.2
1	33.8	34	93.2	67	152.6	100	212.0

STATISTICS SYMBOLS

||	absolute difference
χ^2	chi-square—used in comparisons of obtained deviations with expected deviations
r	correlation test
df	degrees of freedom
D	difference
$\overline{D}$	mean difference
type I	error designation—used in rejecting null hypothesis erroneously
type II	error designation—used in accepting null hypothesis erroneously
$n!$	(n) factorial
f	frequency
$\overline{X}, M$	mean of population
$\overline{x}, m$	mean of sample
N	number in population
n	number in sample
P	probability
X	raw score (population data)
x	raw score (sample data)
σ, SD	standard deviation
SE	standard error
SEM	standard error of the mean
z	standard score
t	student distribution
Σ	sum, summation
σ^2	variance (population)
s^2	variance (sample)
F	variance ratio
$\overline{\overline{X}}$	weighted mean

SELECTED REFERENCES

Abbreviations Dictionaries/General
Crowley ET (ed): *Acronyms, Initialisms, & Abbreviations Dictionary,*
ed 5. Detroit, Gale Research Co., 1976.
Paxton J (ed): *Dictionary of Abbreviations.* Totowa, NJ, Rowman &
Littlefield, 1973.
Spillner P: *World Guide to Abbreviations,* vol 1–3, ed 2. New York,
R. R. Bowker, 1973.

Abbreviations Dictionaries/Medical
Garb S, et al: *Abbreviations and Acronyms in Medicine and Nursing.*
New York, Springer Publishing Co., 1976.
Roody P, et al: *Medical Abbreviations and Acronyms.* New York,
McGraw-Hill, 1977.
Schertel A: *Abbreviations in Medicine.* Detroit, Gale Research Co., 1977.
Steen EB: *Abbreviations in Medicine,* ed 4. Philadelphia, Saunders, 1978.

Career Development
Blayney KD: Where in health are medical assistants and where in health
are they going? *The Professional Medical Assistant,* March–April 1977,
pp 37–40.
Parsons BJ: The medical assistant today: Profile of an emerging profession. *The Professional Medical Assistant,* March–April 1978,
pp 16–21.

Clinical Topics
Brunner LS, Suddarth D: *Textbook of Medical-Surgical Nursing,* ed 3.
New York, Lippincott, 1975.
French RM: *Guide to Diagnostic Procedures.* New York, McGraw-Hill,
1975.
Smith AL: *Microbiology and Pathology,* ed 10. St. Louis, C. V. Mosby,
1972.
Tilkian S, Conover M: *Clinical Implications of Laboratory Tests.*
St. Louis, C. V. Mosby, 1975.

English Handbooks
Irmscher WF: *The Holt Guide to English,* ed 2. New York, Holt, Rinehart
and Winston, 1976.
Perrin PG, Corder JW: *Handbook of Current English,* ed 4. Glenview, IL,
Scott Foresman, 1975.

Finance
American Medical Association: *The Business Side of Medical Practice.*
Chicago, AMA, 1973.
Blair V: Credit: Way of life. *The Professional Medical Assistant,* November–
December 1973 [reprint].
Blair V: How to shop for collection services. *The Professional Medical
Assistant,* January–February 1974 [reprint].
Blair V: Check list for checks. *The Professional Medical Assistant,* March–
April 1974 [reprint].
Cummings J, Euler L: Accuracy demanded in medical office accounting.
The Professional Medical Assistant, May–June 1975 [reprint].

Cummings J, Euler L: Medical office accounting: Accounts receivable. *PMA*, July–August 1975 [reprint].

Cummings J, Euler L: Medical office accounting: Accounts payable. *PMA*, September–October 1975 [reprint].

Cummings J, Euler L: The professional corporation and its effects on medical office bookkeeping. *PMA*, November–December 1975 [reprint].

Willis ME: Computer billing in medical practice. *PMA*, January–February 1976 [reprint].

Insurance

A Guide for Physicians and other Providers of Care under the Civilian Health and Medical Program of the Uniformed Services. Denver, OCHAMPUS, 1971.

Ehrlich A: Easier handling of insurance claims. *PMA*, March–April 1977, pp 13–14.

Eilers RD: *Regulation of Blue Cross and Blue Shield Plans.* Homewood, IL, Richard D. Irwin, 1963.

Euler L: The ins and outs of insurance: I. Insurance terminology. *PMA*, September–October 1976, pp 16–18.

Euler L: The ins and outs of insurance: II. Historical perspective. *PMA*, November–December 1976, pp 30–32.

Euler L: The ins and outs of insurance: III. Types of plans. *PMA*, January–February 1977, pp 14–19.

Euler L: The ins and outs of insurance: IV. Completing insurance forms. *PMA*, March–April 1977, pp 10–12.

Follmann JF Jr.:   *Medical Care and Health Insurance: A Study in Social Progress.* Homewood, IL, Richard D. Irwin, 1963.

Fordney MT: *Insurance Handbook for the Medical Office.* Philadelphia, W. B. Saunders, 1977.

Law and Ethics

American Medical Association: *Opinions and Reports of the Judicial Council.* Chicago, AMA, 1977.

Bliss BP, Johnson AG: *Aims and Motives in Clinical Medicine: A Practical Approach to Medical Ethics.* Brooklyn Heights, NY, Beekman, 1975.

Brody H: *Ethical Decisions in Medicine.* Boston, Little, Brown, 1976.

Dedek JF: *Contemporary Medical Ethics.* Mission, KS, Sheed Andrews & McMeel, 1975.

Ehrlich A: *Ethics and Jurisprudence.* Champaign, IL, The Colwell Company, 1975.

Gorovitz S: *Moral Problems in Medicine.* Englewood Cliffs, NJ, Prentice-Hall, 1976.

Hunt R, Arras J (eds):   *Ethical Issues in Modern Medicine.* Palo Alto, CA, Mayfield Publishing Co., 1977.

Institute of Medicine: *Ethics of Health Care,* Tancredi L (ed). National Academy of Science, 1974.

Masters NC, Shapiro HA: *Medical Secrecy and the Doctor-Patient Relationship.* New York, International Publications Service, 1966.

Ramsey P: *The Patient as Person: Exploration in Medical Ethics.* New Haven, Yale University Press, 1974.

Vaux K: *Biomedical Ethics.* New York, Harper & Row, 1976.

Veatch RM: *Case Studies in Medical Ethics.* Cambridge, Harvard University Press, 1977.

Medical Dictionaries
Critchley M (ed): *Butterworth's Medical Dictionary,* ed 2. Woburn, MA, Butterworths, 1977.
Dorland's Illustrated Medical Dictionary, ed 25. Philadelphia, W. B. Saunders, 1974.
Osol A, et al: *Blakiston's Gould Medical Dictionary,* ed 3. New York, McGraw-Hill, 1972.
Stedman's Medical Dictionary, ed 22. New York, Robert E. Krieger Publishing Co., 1972.

Medical Librarianship
Annan GL, Felter JW (eds): *Handbook of Medical Library Practice,* ed 3. Chicago, Medical Library Association, 1970.

Medical Record Administration
American Hospital Association: *Medical Record Departments in Hospitals: Guide to Organization.* Chicago, AHA, 1972.
American Hospital Association: *Hospital Medical Records: Guidelines for Their Use and Release of Medical Information.* Chicago, AHA, 1972.
Cash MS: The medical record practitioner. *Med Rec News,* August 1976, pp 58–60.
Cross H, Bjorn J: *The Problem-Oriented Private Practice of Medicine— A System for Comprehensive Health Care.* Chicago, Modern Hospital Press, 1970.
Finnegan R: Outpatient medical records—the future. *Med Rec News* 41:142–149, 1970.
Gordon BL: *Simplified Medical Records System.* Acton, MA, Publishing Sciences Group, 1975.
Mosier A, Pace FJ: *Medical Records Technology.* Allied Health Series. Indianapolis, Bobbs-Merrill, 1975.
Patrikas EO, et al: *Medical Records Administration Continuing Education Review.* Flushing, NY, Medical Examination Publishing Co., 1975.
Weed LL, et al (eds): *Implementing the Problem-Oriented Medical Record,* vol 2. Seattle, Medical Computer Services Association, 1976.

Medical Spelling Books
Byers EE: *Ten Thousand Medical Words.* New York, McGraw-Hill, 1972.
Carlin HL: *Medical Secretary Medi-Speller.* Springfield, IL, Charles C Thomas, 1973.
Johnson CE: *Medical Spelling Guide.* Springfield, IL, Charles C Thomas, 1966.
Lee RV, Hofer DJ: *How to Divide Medical Words.* Carbondale, IL, Southern Illinois University Press, 1972.
Pease RW Jr. (ed): *Webster's Medical Speller.* Springfield, MA, Merriam-Webster Inc., 1975.
Prichard RW, Robinson RE: *Twenty Thousand Medical Words.* New York, McGraw-Hill, 1972.

Medical Terminology Guides
American Medical Association: *Current Procedural Terminology,* ed 4.
Chicago, AMA Scientific Publications Division, 1977.
Bennet A, et al (eds):   *Selected Medical Terminology.* New York, Preston
Publishing Co., 1968.
Rimer EH: *Harbech's Glossary of Medical Terms.* Menlo Park, CA, Pacific
Coast Publishers, n.d.
Sloane SB: *The Medical Word Book: A Spelling and Vocabulary Guide to
Medical Transcription.* Philadelphia, W. B. Saunders, 1973.
Stegeman W: *Medical Terms Simplified.* St. Paul, MN, West Publishing
Co., 1975.
Strand HR: *An Illustrated Guide to Medical Terminology.* Baltimore, MD,
Williams & Wilkins, 1968.
U.S. Department of Health, Education and Welfare: *International
Classification of Diseases, Adapted for Use in the United States.*

Medical Writing
DeBakey L: *The Scientific Journal: Editorial Policies and Practices.*
St. Louis, C. V. Mosby, 1976.
Fishbein M: *Medical Writing: The Technic and the Art,* ed 4. Springfield,
IL, Charles C Thomas, 1972.
Marti-Ibanez F (ed):   *Medical Writing.* New York, MD Publications, 1956.
Thorne C: *Better Medical Writing.* New York, Grune & Stratton, 1971.

Speeches
Dudley H: *The Presentation of Original Work in Medicine and Biology.*
New York, Churchill Livingstone, 1977.

Style Manuals/Medical and General
A Manual of Style, ed 12, Chicago, University of Chicago Press, 1974.
American Medical Association: *Stylebook/Editorial Manual of the AMA.*
Chicago, AMA Scientific Publications Division, 1976.
American Psychological Association: *Publication Manual,* ed 2. Washington, DC,
APA, 1974.
Council of Biology Editors Committee on Form and Style: *CBE Style
Manual,* ed 3. Washington, DC, American Institute of Biological
Sciences, 1974.

Style/Nomenclature
International Committee for Nomenclature and Nosology of Renal Disease:
A Handbook of Kidney Nomenclature. Boston, Little, Brown, 1975.
International Committee on Nomenclature of Viruses: *Classification and
Nomenclature of Viruses: First Report.* Basel, Switzerland, S. Karger,
AG, 1971.
International Congress of Zoology (XV):   *International Code of Zoological
Nomenclature.* London, The International Trust for Zoological
Nomenclature, 1964.

Transcription
Alcazar CC: *Medical Typist's Guide for Histories and Physicals,* ed 2.
Flushing, NY, Medical Examination Publishing Co., 1974.
Bradbury PF (ed):   *Transcriber's Guide to Medical Terminology.* Flushing,
NY, Medical Examination Publishing Co., 1973.

Davis PE: *Medical Shorthand.* New York, Wiley-Medical (John Wiley), 1967.

Eshom M: *Medical Secretary's Manual.* New York, Appleton-Century-Crofts, 1966.

Medical Records Input Systems Workbook.   Lanier Business Products, Executive Communication Systems, n.p.

Smither EB: *Gregg Medical Shorthand Manual and Dictionary.* New York, McGraw-Hill, 1953.

Writing, Scientific/Technical

Barnett MY: *Elements of Technical Writing.* Albany, NY, Delmar Publishers, 1974.

Dagher JB: *Technical Communication: A Practical Guide.* Englewood Cliffs, NJ, Prentice-Hall, 1978.

Ehrlich EH, Murphy D: *Art of Technical Writing: A Manual for Scientists, Engineers, and Students.* Scranton, PA, Apollo Editions, 1969.

King LS: *Why Not Say It Clearly: A Guide to Scientific Writing.* Boston, Little, Brown, 1978.

Mitchell JH: *Writing for Technical and Professional Journals.* New York, Wiley-Interscience (John Wiley).

Trelease SF: *How to Write Scientific and Technical Papers.* Cambridge, MA, MIT Press, 1969.

TABLE OF AIR AND ROAD DISTANCES

A complete list of air mileage from cities in the United States to foreign cities is shown in the *Official Airline Guide*. This guide, commonly called the *OAG*, also lists complete airline schedules and is updated frequently. It is an essential reference for the executive who travels regularly.

TABLES OF AIRLINE DISTANCES

All Distances in Statute Miles

Between Principal Cities in the United States

FROM/TO	Albuquerque, N. Mex.	Atlanta, Ga.	Baltimore, Md.	Boise, Idaho	Boston, Mass.	Brownsville, Tex.	Buffalo, N. Y.	Chicago, Ill.	Cincinnati, Ohio	Cleveland, Ohio	Denver, Colo.	Des Moines, Iowa	Detroit, Mich.	El Paso, Tex.	Fargo, N. Dak.	Fort Worth, Tex.	Galveston, Tex.	Hastings, Nebr.	Hot Springs, Ark.	Houghton, Mich.	Jacksonville, Fla.	Kansas City, Mo.	Los Angeles, Calif.
Albuquerque, N. Mex.	....	1273	1670	774	1967	838	1577	1126	1248	1417	332	833	1360	228	968	561	803	588	773	1252	1492	717	663
Atlanta, Ga.	1273	...	575	1830	933	960	695	583	368	550	1208	738	595	1293	1112	750	688	901	498	947	286	675	1935
Baltimore, Md.	1670	575	...	2055	358	1525	273	603	423	305	1505	913	398	1750	1143	1239	1245	1154	964	808	682	962	2313
Boise, Idaho	774	1830	2055	...	2266	1610	1872	1453	1663	1754	637	1155	1671	969	975	1263	1538	934	1384	1367	2008	1158	663
Boston, Mass.	1967	933	358	2266	....	1881	398	849	737	550	1766	1159	613	2067	1304	1574	1598	1415	1302	922	1015	1250	2590
Brownsville, Tex.	838	960	1525	1610	1881	....	1575	1234	1184	1402	1047	1102	1358	682	1445	471	287	1013	650	1543	1025	923	1370
Buffalo, N. Y.	1577	695	273	1872	398	1575	....	454	392	175	1368	762	218	1690	923	1221	1289	1019	956	560	880	862	2195
Chicago, Ill.	1126	583	603	1453	849	1234	454	....	249	307	918	310	236	1249	571	820	954	566	585	367	861	413	1741
Cincinnati, Ohio	1248	368	423	1663	737	1184	392	249	....	218	1090	509	234	1333	818	839	897	742	569	589	628	541	1892
Cleveland, Ohio	1417	550	305	1754	550	1402	175	307	218	....	1223	617	94	1521	838	1046	1116	871	787	518	768	700	2044
Denver, Colo	332	1208	1505	637	1766	1047	1368	918	1090	1223	....	607	1153	554	642	643	925	353	749	970	1468	555	828
Des Moines, Iowa	833	738	913	1155	1159	1102	762	310	509	617	607	....	545	980	397	640	851	256	488	458	1024	180	1433
Detroit, Mich.	1360	595	398	1671	613	1398	218	236	234	94	1153	545	....	1475	745	1018	1111	800	761	427	832	643	1976
El Paso, Tex.	228	1293	1750	969	2067	682	1690	1249	1333	1521	554	980	1475	....	1161	543	723	757	802	1422	1481	836	702
Fargo, N. Dak.	968	1112	1143	975	1304	1445	923	571	818	838	642	397	745	1161	....	973	1218	440	875	393	1400	548	1426
Fort Worth, Tex.	561	750	1239	1263	1574	471	1221	820	839	1046	643	640	1018	543	973	....	283	544	273	1093	943	460	1212
Galveston, Tex.	803	688	1245	1538	1598	287	1289	954	897	1116	925	851	1111	723	1218	283	....	808	375	1277	799	677	1423
Hastings, Nebr.	588	901	1154	934	1415	1013	1019	566	742	871	353	256	800	757	440	544	808	....	513	666	1178	226	1177
Hot Springs, Ark.	773	498	964	1384	1302	650	956	585	569	787	749	488	761	802	875	273	375	513	....	901	728	326	1437
Houghton, Mich.	1252	947	808	1367	922	1543	560	367	589	518	970	458	427	1422	393	1093	1277	666	901	....	1216	633	1787
Jacksonville, Fla.	1492	286	682	2098	1015	1025	880	861	628	768	1468	1024	832	1481	1400	943	799	1178	728	1216	....	952	2153
Kansas City, Mo.	717	675	962	1158	1250	923	862	413	541	700	555	180	643	836	548	460	677	226	326	633	952	....	1352
Los Angeles, Calif.	663	1935	2313	663	2590	1370	2195	1741	1892	2044	828	1433	1976	702	1426	1212	1423	1177	1437	1787	2153	1352	....
Louisville, Ky.	1174	317	498	1823	823	1093	483	268	92	309	1035	477	315	1253	818	751	807	693	480	636	595	480	1825
Memphis, Tenn.	938	335	792	1506	1133	777	802	481	410	627	878	485	621	978	882	448	492	591	176	830	591	370	1602
Miami, Fla.	1710	610	958	2368	1258	1100	1184	1190	957	1088	1732	1338	1156	1662	1721	1150	941	1468	983	1545	328	1247	2355
Minneapolis, Minn.	980	905	918	1140	1125	1335	733	356	603	632	609	235	542	1156	219	870	1087	399	722	272	1192	413	1522
Missoula, Mont.	805	1790	1947	252	2124	1706	1740	1348	1578	1640	670	1074	1552	1115	819	1312	1505	891	1385	1208	2070	1117	910
Nashville, Tenn.	1117	218	597	1631	941	952	626	394	239	456	1018	523	468	1169	900	643	666	697	370	760	502	472	1777
New Orleans, La.	1030	427	1001	1713	1359	536	1087	831	708	922	1079	825	938	986	1221	470	288	870	358	1187	511	678	1675
New York, N. Y.	1810	747	170	2153	188	1695	291	711	568	404	1628	1023	483	1902	1213	1398	1415	1275	1125	849	838	1097	2446
Norfolk, Va.	1696	507	167	2137	467	1465	435	696	474	429	1562	983	522	1755	1258	1226	1195	1216	955	946	548	1009	2352
Oklahoma, Okla.	518	753	1173	1138	1490	659	1117	888	755	946	503	469	905	573	786	188	456	357	260	926	988	293	1182
Omaha, Nebr.	718	815	1026	1044	1280	1061	883	432	620	738	485	122	666	875	390	590	828	135	490	547	1098	165	1312
Philadelphia, Pa.	1748	663	90	2113	268	1614	278	664	501	343	575	972	444	1834	1186	1324	1335	1222	1051	827	758	1037	2388
Phoenix, Ariz.	330	1592	2002	733	2295	1023	1904	1451	1578	1745	585	1154	1685	347	1225	858	1065	901	1094	1550	1800	1045	357
Pittsburgh, Pa.	1498	520	194	1863	478	1424	178	411	258	115	1320	718	208	1592	952	1097	1140	967	825	530	703	784	2135
Portland, Me.	2015	1022	446	2282	100	1961	438	892	802	603	1803	1197	657	2126	1313	1642	1678	1454	1371	924	1113	1300	2631
Portland, Oreg.	1107	2172	2367	349	2553	1944	2167	1765	1987	2063	985	1479	1975	1286	1248	1612	1885	1271	1733	1638	2442	1397	825
Richmond, Va.	1628	470	128	2060	471	1428	375	618	399	353	1488	905	445	1695	1180	1170	1154	1142	897	870	953	937	2283
St. Louis, Mo.	938	467	731	1389	1036	975	662	259	305	490	793	270	452	1033	658	568	697	455	325	591	755	238	1585
Salt Lake City, Utah	483	1580	1858	292	2099	1317	1701	1260	1450	1567	372	952	1490	689	865	977	1249	708	1116	1242	1840	922	577
San Francisco, Calif.	893	2133	2451	516	2696	1675	2298	1855	2037	2163	946	1547	2087	993	1447	1454	1693	1297	1648	1833	2375	1500	345
Schenectady, N. Y.	1823	840	278	2120	150	1770	249	702	605	408	1618	1012	467	1930	1157	1445	1487	1267	1175	776	960	1107	2445
Seattle, Wash.	1178	2180	2341	405	2508	2015	2130	1743	1974	2035	1020	1470	1945	1373	1206	1658	1938	1288	1759	1588	2450	1505	956
Shreveport, La.	764	548	1064	1433	1410	510	1080	725	688	904	799	624	891	752	1002	209	233	615	142	1043	733	326	1420
Spokane, Wash.	1028	1960	2110	290	2279	1852	1900	1514	1746	1804	827	1243	1715	1238	976	1470	1753	1061	1552	1360	2239	1286	939
Springfield, Mass.	1889	863	282	2196	79	1805	325	774	639	473	1692	1085	540	1990	1240	1495	1524	1340	1224	860	957	1173	2515
Vermillion, S. Dak.	742	917	1083	973	1314	1161	916	479	694	785	468	187	705	920	284	689	938	167	605	510	1203	280	1291
Washington, D. C.	1648	542	33	2045	392	1493	290	594	403	303	1490	895	397	1726	1141	1210	1214	1139	936	813	647	943	2295

These tables showing airline distances between principal cities of the United States, between representative cities of the United States and Latin America, between principal cities of Europe, and between principal cities of the world are reprinted from pages 346 and 347 of *Webster's Atlas and Zip Code Directory* (Springfield: G. & C. Merriam Company, 1973), a book prepared by the staff of Hammond, Inc.

Louisville, Ky.	Memphis, Tenn.	Miami, Fla.	Minneapolis, Minn.	Missoula, Mont.	Nashville, Tenn.	New Orleans, La.	New York, N.Y.	Norfolk, Va.	Oklahoma, Okla.	Omaha, Nebr.	Philadelphia, Pa.	Phoenix, Ariz.	Pittsburgh, Pa.	Portland, Me.	Portland, Oreg.	Richmond, Va.	St. Louis, Mo.	Salt Lake City, Utah	San Francisco, Calif.	Schenectady, N.Y.	Seattle, Wash.	Shreveport, La.	Spokane, Wash.	Springfield, Mass.	Vermillion, S. Dak.	Washington, D.
1174	938	1710	980	895	1117	1030	1810	1696	518	718	1748	330	1498	2015	1107	1628	938	483	893	1823	1178	764	1028	1889	742	1648
317	335	610	905	1790	218	427	747	507	753	815	663	1592	520	1022	2172	470	467	1580	2133	840	2180	548	1960	863	917	542
498	792	958	948	1947	597	1001	170	167	1173	1026	90	2002	194	416	2367	128	731	1858	2451	278	2341	1064	2110	282	1083	33
1623	1506	2368	1140	252	1631	1713	2153	2137	1138	1044	2113	733	1863	2282	349	2060	1389	292	516	2120	405	1433	290	2196	973	2045
823	1133	1258	1125	2124	941	1359	188	467	1490	1280	268	2295	478	100	2553	471	1036	2099	2696	150	2508	1410	2279	79	1314	392
1093	777	1100	1335	1706	952	536	1695	1465	659	1061	1614	1023	1424	1961	1944	1428	975	1317	1675	1770	2015	510	1852	1805	1161	1493
483	802	1184	733	1740	626	1087	291	435	1117	883	278	1904	178	438	2167	375	662	1701	2298	249	2130	1080	1900	325	916	290
268	481	1190	356	1348	394	831	711	696	689	432	664	1451	411	892	1765	618	259	1260	1855	702	1743	725	1514	774	479	594
92	410	957	603	1578	239	708	568	474	755	620	501	1578	258	802	1987	399	308	1450	2037	605	1974	688	1746	659	694	403
309	627	1088	632	1640	456	922	404	429	946	738	343	1745	115	603	2063	353	490	1567	2163	408	2035	904	1804	478	785	303
1035	878	1732	699	670	1018	1079	1628	1562	503	485	1575	585	1320	1803	985	1488	793	372	946	1618	1020	799	827	1692	468	1490
477	485	1338	235	1074	523	825	1023	983	469	122	972	1154	718	1197	1479	905	270	952	1547	1012	1470	624	1243	1085	187	895
315	621	1156	542	1552	468	938	483	522	905	666	444	1685	208	657	1975	445	452	1490	2087	467	1945	891	1715	540	705	397
1253	978	1662	1156	1115	1169	986	1902	1755	578	875	1834	347	1592	2126	1286	1695	1033	689	903	1930	1373	752	1238	1990	920	1726
818	882	1721	219	819	900	1221	1213	1258	786	390	1186	1225	952	1313	1248	1180	658	865	1447	1157	1206	1002	976	1240	284	1141
751	448	1150	870	1312	643	470	1398	1226	188	590	1324	858	1097	1642	1612	1170	568	977	1454	1445	1658	209	1470	1495	689	1210
807	492	941	1087	1595	666	288	1415	1195	456	828	1336	1065	1140	1078	1885	1154	697	1249	1693	1487	1938	233	1753	1524	938	1214
693	591	1468	399	891	697	870	1275	1216	357	135	1222	901	967	1454	1271	1142	455	708	1297	1267	1288	615	1061	1340	167	1139
480	176	983	722	1385	370	358	1125	955	260	490	1051	1094	825	1371	1733	897	325	1116	1648	1175	1759	142	1552	1224	605	936
636	830	1545	272	1208	760	1187	849	946	926	547	827	1550	630	924	1638	870	591	1242	1833	776	1588	1043	1360	860	510	813
595	591	328	1192	2070	502	511	838	548	988	1098	758	1800	703	1113	2442	953	755	1840	2375	960	2450	733	2239	957	1203	647
480	370	1247	413	1117	472	678	1097	1009	203	165	1037	1045	784	1300	1397	937	238	922	1500	1107	1505	326	1286	1173	280	943
1825	1602	2355	1522	910	1777	1675	2446	2352	1182	1312	2388	357	2135	2631	825	2283	1585	577	345	2445	956	1420	939	2515	1291	2295
....	319	923	605	1550	153	623	650	528	675	579	980	1512	345	892	1953	457	242	1400	1983	695	1945	598	1720	745	663	473
319	....	878	700	1483	195	358	953	778	422	529	873	1264	660	1205	1852	722	242	1250	1800	1010	1867	279	1652	1055	642	763
923	878	....	1516	2359	821	681	1095	802	1233	1402	1023	1998	1014	1357	2716	831	1067	2098	2603	1229	2740	950	2528	1210	1510	927
605	700	1516	....	1010	695	1050	1019	1047	692	291	985	1279	745	1145	1435	964	464	988	1585	975	1403	859	1173	1056	238	936
1550	1483	2359	1010	....	1582	1733	2030	2045	1162	978	1997	932	1754	2133	430	1967	1331	435	762	1978	395	1457	170	2060	887	1940
153	195	821	695	1582	....	470	758	586	602	604	683	1445	472	1015	1970	526	253	1399	1958	820	1973	470	1752	863	704	567
623	358	681	1050	1733	470	....	1173	932	575	845	1090	1318	923	1445	2063	899	599	1433	1923	1259	2098	280	1898	1287	960	968
650	953	1095	1019	2030	758	1173	....	293	1324	1144	83	2142	313	277	2455	287	873	1972	2568	142	2419	1230	2190	120	1189	204
528	778	802	1047	2045	586	932	293	....	1186	1095	220	2027	316	565	2458	79	771	1925	2510	426	2440	1037	2211	411	1166	145
675	422	1233	692	1162	602	575	1324	1186	....	405	1256	843	1013	1550	1488	1122	456	862	1386	1354	1523	297	1324	1412	502	1150
579	529	1402	291	978	604	845	1144	1095	405	....	1094	1032	837	1318	1373	1020	352	833	1425	1133	1372	617	1149	1205	115	1012
580	878	1023	985	1997	683	1090	83	220	1256	1094	....	2079	254	360	2419	205	808	1923	2518	205	2388	1153	2159	201	1143	122
1512	1264	1998	1279	932	1445	1318	2142	2027	843	1032	2079	....	1829	2339	1007	1960	1270	504	652	2152	1112	1067	1020	2220	1043	1980
345	660	1014	745	1754	472	923	313	316	1013	837	254	1829	....	545	2174	242	561	1670	2264	350	2145	939	1918	400	891	188
892	1205	1357	1145	2133	1015	1445	277	565	1550	1318	360	2339	545	....	2563	565	1094	2127	2725	197	2513	1484	2285	159	1345	480
1953	1852	2716	1435	430	1970	2063	2455	2458	1488	1373	2419	1007	2174	2563	....	2381	1723	636	536	2405	143	1783	295	2488	1293	2360
457	722	831	964	1967	526	899	287	79	1122	1020	205	1960	242	565	2381	....	699	1850	2436	406	2362	985	2133	407	1089	96
242	242	1067	464	1331	253	599	873	771	456	352	808	1270	561	1094	1723	699	....	1158	1738	898	1722	466	1500	958	450	710
1400	1250	2098	988	435	1390	1433	1972	1925	862	833	1923	504	1670	2127	636	1850	1158	....	592	1950	697	1155	548	2027	785	1845
1983	1800	2603	1585	762	1958	1923	2568	2510	1386	1425	2518	652	2264	2725	536	2436	1738	592	....	2548	680	1655	730	2625	1383	2437
695	1010	1229	975	1978	820	1259	142	426	1354	1133	205	2152	350	197	2405	406	898	1950	2548	....	2363	1290	2139	86	1165	313
1945	1867	2740	1403	395	1973	2098	2419	2440	1523	1372	2388	1112	2145	2513	143	2362	1722	697	680	2363	....	1820	229	2445	1282	2335
598	279	950	859	1457	470	280	1230	1037	297	617	1153	1067	939	1484	1783	985	466	1155	1655	1290	1820	....	1621	1333	726	1035
1720	1652	2528	1173	170	1752	1898	2190	2211	1324	1149	2159	1020	1918	2285	295	2133	1500	548	730	2139	229	1621	....	2216	1055	2105
745	1055	1210	1056	2060	863	1287	120	411	1412	1205	201	2220	400	159	2488	407	958	2027	2625	86	2445	1333	2216	....	1242	321
663	642	1510	238	887	704	960	1189	1166	502	115	1143	1043	891	1345	1293	1089	450	785	1383	1165	1282	726	1055	1242	....	1073
473	763	927	936	1940	567	968	204	145	1150	1012	122	1980	188	480	2360	96	710	1845	2437	313	2335	1035	2105	321	1073	....

Between Principal Cities of the World

FROM/TO	Azores	Bagdad	Berlin	Bombay	Buenos Aires	Callao	Cairo	Cape Town	Chicago	Istanbul	Guam	Honolulu	Juneau	London	Los Angeles	Melbourne	Mexico City	Montreal	New Orleans	New York	Panama	Paris	Rio de Janeiro	San Francisco	Santiago	Seattle	Shanghai	Singapore	Tokyo	Wellington
Azores	···	3906	2148	5930	5385	4825	3325	5670	3305	2880	8985	7421	4715	1562	5034	12190	4584	2548	3718	2604	3918	1617	4312	5114	5718	4720	7324	8338	7370	11475
Bagdad	3906	···	2040	2022	8215	8618	785	4923	6490	1085	6380	8445	6210	2568	7695	8150	8155	5814	7212	6066	7807	2385	7012	7521	8876	6848	4468	4443	5242	9782
Berlin	2148	2040	···	3947	7411	6937	1823	5949	4405	1068	7158	7384	4638	575	5849	9992	6119	3776	5182	4026	5902	540	6246	5744	8523	5121	5218	6226	5623	11384
Bombay	5930	2022	3947	···	9380	10530	2698	5133	8144	3043	4831	8172	6638	4526	8810	6140	9818	7582	8952	7875	9832	4391	8438	8523	10127	7830	3219	2425	4247	7752
Buenos Aires	5385	8215	7411	9380	···	1982	7428	4332	5598	7638	10516	7653	7964	6919	6148	7336	4609	5619	4902	5295	3319	6891	1230	6487	731	6956	12295	9940	11601	6341
Callao	4825	8618	6937	10530	1982	···	7870	6195	3765	7666	9760	5993	5806	6376	4155	8196	2619	3954	2990	3633	1450	6455	2400	4500	1548	4964	10760	11700	9740	6696
Cairo	3325	785	1823	2698	7428	7870	···	4476	6231	780	7175	8925	6352	2218	7554	8720	7807	5502	6862	5701	7230	2020	6242	7554	8100	6915	5290	5152	6005	10360
Cape Town	5670	4923	5949	5133	4332	6195	4476	···	8551	5210	8918	11655	10382	5975	10165	6510	8620	7975	8390	7845	7090	5732	3850	10340	4553	10305	8179	6025	9234	7149
Chicago	3305	6490	4405	8144	5598	3765	6231	8551	···	5530	7510	4315	2310	3975	1741	9837	1690	750	827	727	2320	4219	5320	1875	5325	1753	7155	9475	6410	8465
Istanbul	2880	1085	1068	3043	7638	7666	780	5210	5530	···	7015	8200	5665	1540	6895	9189	7160	4825	6220	5060	6797	1390	6420	6770	8230	6124	5084	5440	5649	10790
Guam	8985	6380	7158	4831	10516	9760	7175	8918	7510	7015	···	3896	5225	7605	6255	3497	7690	7842	7895	8115	9220	7675	11710	5952	9946	5785	1945	2990	1596	4206
Honolulu	7421	8445	7384	8172	7653	5993	8925	11655	4315	8200	3896	···	2825	7320	2620	5581	3846	4902	4305	5051	5211	7525	8400	2407	6935	2707	4963	6722	3850	4676
Juneau	4715	6210	4638	6638	7964	5806	6352	10382	2310	5665	5225	2825	···	4496	1835	8162	2647	2860	2860	2874	4456	4700	7611	1530	7320	870	5009	6874	4117	7501
London	1562	2568	575	4526	6919	6376	2218	5975	3975	1540	7605	7320	4496	···	5496	10590	5605	3370	4656	3500	5310	210	5747	5440	7275	4850	5841	6818	5940	11790
Los Angeles	5034	7695	5849	8810	6148	4155	7554	10165	1741	6895	6255	2620	1835	5496	···	8098	1545	2468	1695	2466	3025	5711	6330	345	5134	961	6598	8955	5600	6806
Melbourne	12190	8150	9992	6140	7336	8196	8720	6510	9837	9189	3497	5581	8162	10590	8098	···	8599	10553	9455	10541	9211	10500	8340	7970	7130	8330	4967	3768	5172	1655
Mexico City	4584	8155	6119	9818	4609	2619	7807	8620	1690	7160	7690	3846	2647	5605	1545	8599	···	2247	940	2110	1532	5800	4810	1870	4122	2339	8120	10495	7035	7003
Montreal	2548	5814	3776	7582	5619	3954	5502	7975	750	4825	7842	4902	2860	3370	2468	10553	2247	···	1390	340	2545	3490	5110	2557	5461	2309	7141	9280	6546	9206
New Orleans	3718	7212	5182	8952	4902	2990	6862	8390	827	6220	7895	4305	2860	4656	1695	9455	940	1390	···	1171	1600	4846	4798	1960	4553	2137	7830	10255	6993	7950
New York	2604	6066	4026	7875	5295	3633	5701	7845	727	5060	8115	5051	2874	3500	2466	10541	2110	340	1171	···	2211	3600	4810	2606	5134	2440	7460	9617	6846	9067
Panama	3918	7807	5902	9832	3319	1450	7230	7090	2320	6797	9220	5211	4456	5310	3025	9211	1532	2545	1600	2211	···	5440	3311	3349	3000	3680	9430	11800	8560	7580
Paris	1617	2385	540	4391	6891	6455	2020	5732	4219	1390	7675	7525	4700	210	5711	10500	5800	3490	4846	3600	5440	···	5680	5710	7325	5080	5855	6730	6132	11865
Rio de Janeiro	4312	7012	6246	8438	1230	2400	6242	3850	5320	6420	11710	8400	7611	5747	6330	8340	4810	5110	4798	4810	3311	5680	···	6655	1852	6945	11510	9875	11600	7510
San Francisco	5114	7521	5744	8523	6487	4500	7554	10340	1875	6770	5952	2407	1530	5440	345	7970	1870	2557	1960	2606	3349	5710	6655	···	5960	692	6245	8440	5250	6800
Santiago	5718	8876	8523	10127	731	1548	8100	4553	5325	8230	9946	6935	7320	7275	5134	7130	4122	5461	4553	5134	3000	7325	1852	5960	···	6466	10850	10270	10850	5925
Seattle	4720	6848	5121	7830	6956	4964	6915	10305	1753	6124	5785	2707	870	4850	961	8330	2339	2309	2137	2440	3680	5080	6945	692	6466	···	5780	8200	4863	7310
Shanghai	7324	4468	5218	3219	12295	10760	5290	8179	7155	5084	1945	4963	5009	5841	6598	4967	8120	7141	7830	7460	9430	5855	11510	6245	10850	5780	···	2395	1095	6080
Singapore	8338	4443	6226	2425	9940	11700	5152	6025	9475	5440	2990	6722	6874	6818	8955	3768	10495	9280	10255	9617	11800	6730	9875	8440	10270	8200	2395	···	3350	5360
Tokyo	7370	5242	5623	4247	11601	9740	6005	9234	6410	5649	1596	3850	4117	5940	5600	5172	7035	6546	6993	6846	8560	6132	11600	5250	10850	4863	1095	3350	···	5730
Wellington	11475	9782	11384	7752	6341	6696	10360	7149	8465	10790	4206	4676	7501	11790	6806	1655	7003	9206	7950	9067	7580	11865	7510	6800	5925	7310	6080	5360	5730	···

Reprinted from **Webster's Atlas and Zip Code Directory** courtesy of Hammond, Incorporated.

Between Principal Cities of Europe

	Amsterdam	Athens	Baku	Barcelona	Belgrade	Berlin	Brussels	Bucharest	Budapest	Cologne	Copenhagen	Istanbul	Dresden	Dublin	Frankfort	Hamburg	Leningrad	Lisbon	London	Lyon	Madrid	Marseilles	Milan	Moscow	Munich	Oslo	Paris	Riga	Rome	Sofia	Stockholm	Toulouse	Vienna	Warsaw	Zurich
Amsterdam	....	1340	2218	770	875	365	105	1100	710	128	381	1360	385	468	228	232	1090	1140	220	458	912	627	517	1325	415	568	257	820	808	1073	695	625	580	673	375
Athens	1340	....	1395	1160	500	1112	1292	460	698	1200	1320	350	1022	1765	1113	1250	1535	1770	1476	1100	1463	1025	900	1388	925	1610	1300	1310	650	335	1495	1215	795	990	1000
Baku	2218	1395	....	2427	1487	1867	2240	1220	1562	2127	1980	1070	1837	2490	2055	2020	1570	3050	2435	2238	2742	2238	2028	1852	1912	2118	2335	1590	1360	1175	1862	2425	1700	1555	2050
Barcelona	770	1160	2427	....	998	925	658	1210	924	692	1085	1380	860	919	652	910	1740	610	707	327	316	211	450	2490	648	1112	518	1440	530	1072	1410	156	830	1150	513
Belgrade	875	500	1487	998	....	618	850	295	205	750	840	502	530	1327	652	760	1165	1555	1068	752	1235	750	540	1160	475	1005	1000	1050	530	193	1220	930	345	510	590
Berlin	365	1112	1867	925	618	....	401	798	425	300	225	1068	95	815	268	165	815	1410	575	691	1149	725	570	995	310	520	540	520	730	810	503	815	322	320	410
Brussels	105	1292	2240	658	850	401	....	1110	700	110	475	1345	407	521	198	301	1175	998	202	521	807	521	435	1175	372	672	170	900	705	883	793	515	568	720	312
Bucharest	1100	460	1220	1210	295	798	1110	....	295	1010	970	272	725	1560	808	950	1080	1842	1285	1080	1518	1020	819	965	476	1245	770	685	500	345	820	875	342	580	855
Budapest	710	698	1562	924	205	425	700	295	....	590	629	650	272	1515	345	572	1292	2005	1540	965	1690	1030	435	1080	227	1245	634	523	585	315	1340	762	135	342	460
Cologne	128	1200	2127	692	750	300	110	1010	590	....	400	1240	292	475	93	180	1222	1126	390	370	875	521	390	1090	250	635	250	805	675	945	750	700	460	460	259
Copenhagen	381	1320	1980	1085	840	225	475	970	629	400	....	1240	315	768	412	180	708	1520	540	760	906	720	500	720	520	303	634	453	948	1010	330	1340	598	415	595
Istanbul	1360	350	1070	1380	502	1068	1345	272	650	1240	1240	....	852	1830	671	995	1292	2005	1540	995	1690	1205	1030	1180	592	1505	1390	1115	630	315	1340	1400	852	852	1090
Dresden	385	1022	1837	860	530	95	407	725	272	292	315	852	....	1152	236	238	885	1380	1015	592	1380	435	476	965	345	523	480	585	630	768	350	1130	233	235	342
Dublin	468	1765	2490	919	1327	815	521	1560	1515	475	768	1830	1152	....	671	480	1440	975	300	720	880	1015	880	1728	1200	786	900	1175	1040	852	948	1040	768	480	193
Frankfort	228	1113	2055	652	652	268	198	808	345	93	412	671	236	671	....	250	1301	1160	392	323	888	492	323	1240	193	448	392	697	698	860	504	640	370	370	193
Hamburg	232	1250	2020	910	760	165	301	950	572	180	180	995	238	480	250	....	880	1301	575	580	1098	730	570	1100	378	502	459	810	810	954	780	965	460	432	432
Leningrad	1090	1535	1570	1740	1165	815	1175	1080	1292	1222	708	1292	885	1440	1301	880	....	2235	975	1420	1980	1540	1315	391	1208	1980	1335	300	1540	1440	1635	640	975	1218	1225
Lisbon	1140	1770	3050	610	1555	1410	998	1842	2005	1126	1520	2005	1380	975	1160	1301	2235	....	975	850	313	810	1350	1940	1208	1690	890	1940	1150	1685	1848	640	1700	1415	1058
London	220	1476	2435	707	308	575	202	1285	900	390	540	1540	1015	300	392	575	975	975	....	455	777	620	595	1540	526	531	210	890	985	1235	550	550	710	762	480
Lyon	458	1100	2238	327	752	691	557	1080	965	370	760	995	592	720	323	580	1420	850	455	....	557	170	210	1560	352	1005	248	1122	462	928	1080	228	850	850	206
Madrid	912	1463	2742	316	1235	1149	807	1518	1690	875	906	1690	1380	880	888	1098	1980	313	777	557	....	394	728	2120	910	1474	645	1670	840	1385	1598	344	1410	1110	765
Marseilles	627	1025	2238	211	750	725	521	1020	1030	521	720	1205	435	1015	492	730	1540	810	620	170	394	....	238	1612	215	1165	410	1238	372	895	1225	196	620	620	318
Milan	517	900	2028	450	540	570	435	819	435	390	500	1030	476	880	323	570	1315	1350	595	210	728	238	....	1408	215	1000	400	1010	295	715	1020	400	385	385	137
Moscow	1325	1388	1852	2490	1160	995	1175	965	1080	1090	720	1180	965	1728	1240	1100	391	1940	1540	1560	2120	1612	1408	....	1220	1030	1538	520	1462	1100	770	1770	1028	705	158
Munich	415	925	1912	648	475	310	372	476	227	250	520	592	345	1200	193	378	1208	1208	526	352	910	215	215	1220	....	810	425	800	430	672	811	570	222	222	158
Oslo	568	1610	2118	1112	1005	520	672	1245	1245	635	303	1505	523	786	448	502	1980	1690	531	1005	1474	1165	1000	1030	810	....	830	531	1242	1295	267	1140	835	653	869
Paris	257	1300	2335	518	1000	540	170	770	634	250	634	1390	480	900	392	459	1335	890	210	248	645	410	400	1538	425	830	....	1050	690	1080	950	431	845	276	295
Riga	820	1310	1590	1440	1050	520	900	685	523	805	453	1115	585	1175	697	810	300	1940	890	1122	1670	1238	1010	520	800	531	1050	....	1155	985	276	1335	685	350	930
Rome	808	650	1360	530	530	730	705	500	585	675	948	630	630	1040	698	810	1540	1150	985	462	840	372	295	1462	430	1242	690	1155	....	545	1220	1281	470	810	421
Sofia	1073	335	1175	1072	193	810	883	345	315	945	1010	315	768	852	860	954	1440	1685	1235	928	1385	895	715	1100	672	1295	1080	985	545	....	1170	1062	500	345	780
Stockholm	695	1495	1862	1410	1220	503	793	820	1340	750	330	1340	350	948	504	780	1635	1848	550	1080	1598	1225	1020	770	811	267	950	276	1220	1170	....	1281	770	500	908
Toulouse	625	1215	2425	156	930	815	515	875	762	700	1340	1400	1130	1040	640	965	640	640	550	228	344	196	400	1770	570	1140	431	1335	1281	1062	1281	....	725	345	425
Vienna	580	795	1700	830	345	322	568	342	135	460	598	852	233	768	370	460	975	1700	710	850	1110	620	385	1028	222	835	845	685	470	500	770	725	....	345	640
Warsaw	673	990	1555	1150	510	320	720	580	342	460	415	852	235	480	370	432	1218	1415	762	850	1110	620	385	705	222	653	276	350	810	345	500	345	345	....	365
Zurich	375	1000	2050	513	590	410	312	855	498	259	595	1090	342	193	193	206	1225	1058	480	206	765	318	137	158	158	869	295	930	421	780	908	365	640	365	....

Reprinted from **Webster's Atlas and Zip Code Directory** courtesy of Hammond, Incorporated.

New York to	Miles	San Francisco to	Miles	Seattle to	Miles	Washington to	Miles
Buenos Aires.........	5,295	Buenos Aires.......	6,487	Buenos Aires.......	6,956	Buenos Aires.......	5,205
Bogota............	2,474	Bogota...........	3,863	Bogota...........	4,166	Bogota..........	2,344
Caracas............	2,100	Caracas...........	3,900	Caracas...........	4,100	Caracas..........	2,040
Guatemala City.....	2,060	Guatemala City...	2,525	Guatemala City..	2,930	Guatemala City....	1,835
Havana............	1,302	Havana..........	2,600	Havana..........	2,805	Havana..........	1,110
La Paz............	3,905	La Paz..........	5,080	La Paz..........	5,110	La Paz.....	3,780
Panama...........	2,211	Panama..........	3,349	Panama..........	3,680	Panama..........	2,020
Para.............	3,281	Para...........	5,430	Para...........	5,550	Para.....	3,270
Managua...........	2,100	Managua.........	2,860	Managua.........	3,240	Managua........	1,920
Rio de Janeiro......	4,810	Rio de Janeiro...	6,655	Rio de Janeiro....	6,945	Rio de Janeiro....	4,710
San Jose...........	2,200	San Jose.........	3,070	San Jose........	3,430	San Jose.....	2,030
Santiago...........	5,134	Santiago.........	5,960	Santiago.........	6,466	Santiago.....	4,965
Tampico...........	1,880	Tampico.........	1,790	Tampico........	2,200	Tampico....	1,665

Between Representative Cities of the United States and Latin America

Chicago to	Miles	Denver to	Miles	Los Angeles to	Miles	New Orleans to	Miles
Buenos Aires.........	5,598	Buenos Aires.......	5,935	Buenos Aires.......	6,148	Buenos Aires......	4,902
Bogota............	2,691	Bogota...........	3,100	Bogota...........	3,515	Bogota........	1,996
Caracas............	2,480	Caracas...........	3,105	Caracas...........	3,610	Caracas.......	1,990
Guatemala City......	1,870	Guatemala City...	1,935	Guatemala City...	2,190	Guatemala City ..	1,050
Havana............	1,315	Havana..........	1,760	Havana..........	2,320	Havana..........	672
La Paz............	4,130	La Paz..........	4,445	La Paz..........	4,805	La Paz..........	3,480
Panama...........	2,320	Panama..........	2,620	Panama..........	3,025	Panama..........	1,600
Para.............	3,820	Para...........	4,580	Para...........	5,110	Para..........	3,470
Managua...........	2,060	Managua.........	2,230	Managua.........	2,540	Managua.......	1,250
Rio de Janeiro......	5,320	Rio de Janeiro....	5,900	Rio de Janeiro....	6,330	Rio de Janeiro....	4,798
San Jose...........	2,100	San Jose.........	2,420	San Jose........	2,725	San Jose........	1,425
Santiago...........	5,320	Santiago....	5,495	Santiago.........	5,595	Santiago....	4,553
Tampico.....,....	1,460	Tampico.........	1,240	Tampico.........	1,470	Tampico....	720

Reprinted from **Webster's Atlas and Zip Code Directory** courtesy of Hammond, Incorporated.

FOREIGN CURRENCY TABLE

The following money table, reprinted from pages 742 and 743 of *Webster's New Collegiate Dictionary*, lists countries, the names of their currencies, currency symbols and currency subdivisions. Because rates of exchange change so rapidly, they must be checked almost daily if current quotations are required. These rates, not shown here, can be obtained from most banks and some newspapers.

MONEY

NAME	SYMBOL	SUBDIVISIONS	COUNTRY
afghani	Af	100 puls	Afghanistan
baht or tical	Bht or B	100 satang	Thailand
balboa	B/	100 centesimos	Panama
bolivar	B	100 centimos	Venezuela
cedi	¢	100 pesewas	Ghana
colon	₡ or ¢	100 centimos	Costa Rica
colon	₡ or ¢	100 centavos	El Salvador
cordoba	C$	100 centavos	Nicaragua
cruzeiro	$ or Cr$	100 centavos	Brazil
dalasi	D	100 bututs	Gambia
deutsche mark	DM	100 pfennigs	West Germany
dinar	DA	100 centimes	Algeria
dinar	BD	1000 fils	Bahrain
dinar	ID	5 riyals 20 dirhams 1000 fils	Iraq
dinar	JD	1000 fils	Jordan
dinar	KD	1000 fils	Kuwait
dinar	LD	1000 dirhams	Libya
dinar	£SY	1000 fils	Southern Yemen
dinar	D	1000 millimes	Tunisia
dinar	Din	100 paras	Yugoslavia
dirham	DH	100 francs	Morocco
dollar	$	100 cents	Australia
dollar	B$	100 cents	Bahamas
dollar	$	100 cents	Barbados
dollar	$	100 cents	Bermuda
dollar		100 sen	Brunei
dollar	$	100 cents	Canada
dollar	Eth$ or E$	100 cents	Ethiopia
dollar	$F	100 cents	Fiji
dollar	G$	100 cents	Guyana
dollar	HK$	100 cents	Hong Kong
dollar	$	100 cents	Jamaica
dollar	$	100 cents	Liberia
dollar	M$	100 cents	Malaysia
dollar	NZ$	100 cents	New Zealand
dollar	S$	100 cents	Singapore
dollar	TT$	100 cents	Trinidad and Tobago
dollar	$	100 cents	United States
dollar — see YUAN, below			

NAME	SYMBOL	SUBDIVISIONS	COUNTRY
dong	D	100 xu	North Vietnam
drachma	Dr	100 lepta	Greece
escudo	E or F°	100 centesimos / 1000 milesimos	Chile
escudo	$ or Esc	100 centavos	Portugal
florin — see GULDEN, below			
forint	F or Ft	100 filler	Hungary
franc	Fr or F	100 centimes	Belgium
franc	FBu	100 centimes	Burundi
franc	Fr or F	100 centimes	Cameroon
franc	Fr or F	100 centimes	Central African Republic
franc	Fr or F	100 centimes	Chad
franc	Fr or F	100 centimes	Congo (Brazzaville)
franc	Fr or F	100 centimes	Dahomey
franc	Fr or F	100 centimes	France
franc	Fr or F	100 centimes	Gabon
franc	Fr or F	100 centimes	Guinea
franc	Fr or F	100 centimes	Ivory Coast
franc	Fr or F	100 centimes	Luxembourg
franc	Fr or F or FMG	100 centimes	Malagasy Republic
franc	Fr or F	100 centimes	Mali
franc	Fr or F	100 centimes	Mauritania
franc	Fr or F	100 centimes	Niger
franc	Fr or F	100 centimes	Rwanda
franc	Fr or F	100 centimes	Senegal
franc	Fr or F	100 centimes or rappen	Switzerland
franc	Fr or F	100 centimes	Togo
franc	Fr or F	100 centimes	Upper Volta
gourde	G or G or Gde	100 centimes	Haiti
guarani	G or G	100 centimos	Paraguay
gulden or guilder or florin	F or Fl or G	100 cents	Netherlands
kip	K	100 at	Laos
koruna	Kčs	100 halers	Czechoslovakia
krona	Kr	100 aurar	Iceland
krona	Kr	100 öre	Sweden
krone	Kr	100 öre	Denmark
krone	Kr	100 öre	Norway
kwacha	K	100 tambala	Malawi
kwacha	K	100 ngwee	Zambia
kyat	K	100 pyas	Burma
lek	L	100 qintar	Albania
lempira	L	100 centavos	Honduras
leone	Le	100 cents	Sierra Leone
leu	L	100 bani	Rumania
lev	Lv	100 stotinki	Bulgaria
lira	L or Lit	100 centesimi	Italy
lira or pound	£T or LT or TL	100 kurus or piasters	Turkey
mark or ostmark	M or OM	100 pfennigs	East Germany
mark — see DEUTSCHE MARK, above			
markka	M or Mk	100 pennia	Finland
naira	₦	100 kobo	Nigeria
ostmark — see MARK, above			
pa'anga	T$	100 seniti	Tonga
pataca	P or $	100 avos	Macao
peseta	Pta or P (pl Pts)	100 centimos	Equatorial Guinea
peseta	Pta or P (pl Pts)	100 centimos	Spain
peso	$	100 centavos	Argentina
peso	$B	100 centavos	Bolivia
peso	$ or P	100 centavos	Colombia
peso	$	100 centavos	Cuba
peso	RD$	100 centavos	Dominican Republic
peso	$	100 centavos	Mexico
peso	₱ or P	100 sentimos or centavos	Philippines
peso	$	100 centesimos	Uruguay
piaster	Vn$ or Pr	100 cents	South Vietnam
pound	£	1000 mils	Cyprus
pound	£E	100 piasters / 1000 milliemes	Egypt
pound	£	100 pence	Ireland
pound or lira	I£ or IL	100 agorot	Israel
pound	L£ or LL	100 piasters	Lebanon
pound	£	100 pence	Malta
pound	£	20 shillings / 240 pence	Rhodesia
pound	£S or LSd	100 piasters / 1000 milliemes	Sudan
pound or lira	£S or LS	100 piasters	Syria
pound	£	100 pence	United Kingdom
pound — see LIRA, above			
quetzal	Q or Q	100 centavos	Guatemala
rand	R	100 cents	Botswana
rand	R	100 cents	Lesotho
rand	R	100 cents	South Africa
rand	R	100 cents	Swaziland
rial	R or Rl	100 dinars	Iran
rial	R	1000 baizas	Oman
rial	YR	40 buqshas	Yemen
riel	₵ or CR	100 sen	Cambodia
riyal	R or SR	20 qursh / 100 halala	Saudi Arabia
ruble	R or Rub	100 kopecks	U.S.S.R.
rupee	Re (pl Rs)	100 paise	Bhutan
rupee	Re (pl Rs)	100 cents	Sri Lanka
rupee	Re (pl Rs)	100 paise	India
rupee	Re (pl Rs)	100 cents	Mauritius
rupee	Re (pl Rs)	100 paise	Nepal
rupee	Re (pl Rs)	100 paisa	Pakistan
rupee	Re (pl Rs)	100 cents	Seychelles
rupiah	Rp	100 sen	Indonesia
schilling	S or Sch	100 groschen	Austria
shilling or shilling	Sh	100 senti	Tanzania
shilling	Sh	100 cents	Kenya
shilling	Sh or So Sh	100 cents	Somalia
shilling	Sh	100 cents	Uganda
sol	S/ or $	100 centavos	Peru
sucre	S/	100 centavos	Ecuador
taka		100 paisa	Bangladesh
tala	WS$	100 senes	Western Samoa
tical — see BAHT, above			
tugrik		100 mongo	Outer Mongolia
won	W	100 jun	North Korea
won	W	100 chon	South Korea
yen	¥ or Y	100 sen	Japan
yuan	$	10 chiao / 100 fen	China (mainland)
yuan or dollar	NT$	10 chiao	China (Taiwan)
zaire	Z	100 makuta (sing: likuta) / 10,000 sengi	Zaire
zloty	Zl or Z	100 groszy	Poland

INDEX